# BIOCHEMISTRY

Solved Question Papers

# BIOCHEMISTRY
## Solved Question Papers

**Eighth Edition**

**Singi Yatiraj**
Kalaburagi, Karnataka
India

*Foreword*
***Late* Jagadish B Ingin**

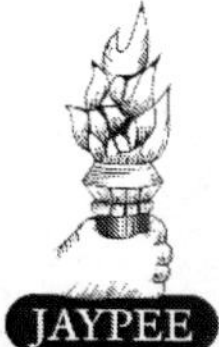

JAYPEE
JAYPEE BROTHERS MEDICAL PUBLISHERS
*The Health Sciences Publisher*
New Delhi | London

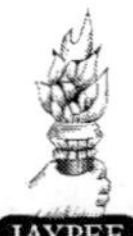

**Jaypee Brothers Medical Publishers (P) Ltd**

**Headquarters**
EMCA House
23/23-B, Ansari Road, Daryaganj
New Delhi 110 002, India
Landline: +91-11-23272143, +91-11-23272703
+91-11-23282021, +91-11-23245672
E-mail: jaypee@jaypeebrothers.com

**Corporate Office**
4838/24, Ansari Road, Daryaganj
New Delhi 110 002, India
Phone: +91-11-43574357
Fax: +91-11-43574314
E-mail: jaypee@jaypeebrothers.com

**Overseas Office**
J.P. Medical Ltd
83 Victoria Street, London
SW1H 0HW (UK)
Phone: +44 20 3170 8910
E-mail: info@jpmedpub.com

**EU GPSR** Authorised Representative
Logos Europe, 9 rue Nicolas Poussin
17000, La Rochelle, France
Phone: +33 (0) 6 67 93 73 78
E-mail: contact@logoseurope.eu

Website: www.jaypeebrothers.com
Website: www.jaypeedigital.com



***Biochemistry Solved Question Papers***

*First Edition* : *2004*
*Second Edition* : *2006*
*Third Edition* : *2007*
*Fourth Edition* : *2008*
*Fifth Edition* : *2011*
*Sixth Edition* : *2012*
*Seventh Edition* : *2014*
*Eight Edition* : 2017
*Reprint* : **2026**

ISBN 978-93-5270-147-6

*Printed at: Samrat Offset Pvt. Ltd.*

॥ ॐ श्री फलौदी ब्रम्हाणी देवी नमः ॥

*Om Shri Falaudi Brahmani Devi Namah*

## Dedicated to

*That person*
*Who has brought happiness in my life;*
*Who has given me a reason to smile;*
*Who has trusted me all the time; and*
*Showed me that I can do it.*

*This book is a tribute to my respectable*
**Late Sister Anupama**
***and***
**Grandmother Rajubai**

# Foreword

It gives me immense pleasure to write the foreword to this book written by my student, Singi Yatiraj because it is always heartening to see one's student excel.

I feel he has made a sincere attempt to answer the question papers of the Rajiv Gandhi University of Health Sciences (RGUHS), Karnataka, India, in best possible way referring numerous books, both undergraduate and postgraduate.

He has included flow charts of pathways wherever necessary, which is the best way of answering any biochemistry question as it consumes least possible time but describes everything like the precursors, product, enzymes, co-enzymes, etc.

An undergraduate student is sure to benefit from this book as it contains information from numerous books with a clear presentation idea. Moreover, it is well-known fact that in examinations, questions tend to repeat. Thus, this book will serve as question bank and an easy referral guide just before examinations.

I feel this book will help students to perform better and score well not only in the university examination but also in the other tests and internals conducted during the academic year.

Wishing him the best, the life has in offering.

***Late* Jagadish B Ingin**
*Formerly*, Professor and Head
Department of Biochemistry
MR Medical College
Kalaburagi, Karnataka, India

# Preface

Dear students,

Examinations are very crucial event in a student's life. They decide whether one would pass and go to the next phase or not. Every student tries his best to clear their examinations but call it bad fate; few fail. Not because they did not study, but because they could not revise at the eleventh hour or could not impress the examiners with their presentation.

With increasing competition, it is becoming imperative to score well in the university examinations. After strenuous night out and hard work, it is the right of the student to farewell in examinations, but he may be denied this just for lack of experience in presenting the answer in an excellent manner. Though he may know every nook and corner of a textbook, but it may happen that he may waste his time writing some answers more than needed and find it difficult to meet both ends of rope on the last bell during an examination.

During my examinations time, I could not have access to such book and wasted a lot of time procuring the syllabus, pattern of question papers, previous years question papers and searching answers for the questions in them; so this thought struck to me to prepare such a book, which combines all these into one and help the students. As they say *Necessity is the Mother of Invention.*

Therefore, book which will solve all the worries of the students during preparation of any examination, is in your hands right now. It includes the question papers of Rajiv Gandhi University of Health Sciences (RGUHS) in solved format as to reduce the workload on a student to refer numerous books for a single question. Also needed for perfect preparation are the Course Contents and the University Examination Pattern. Students should not waste time procuring these materials, as it is also included in this book. In short, I can say that this is a comprehensive manual for preparation of any examinations.

The most common suggestion received by me was to make this book chapterwise, so that it could be used even during college internals which have limited syllabus. But from updating point of view, this suggestion is impracticable. For every university examinations, three question papers are generated (including Revised Scheme 3). So in a year, 6 question papers have to be added to the book which will benefit the students only. Therefore, I always refuted this suggestion. Moreover, as the title of the book suggests, these are the solved question papers; so it looks ridiculous to make it chapterwise with the same title. However, considering infinite requests and suggestions, a new system of *Chapterwise Page References* were devised after considerable thinking, permutations and combinations, which has following advantages:

- The questions are arranged in chapterwise format
- Under each chapter, they are further subclassed in *Long Essays, Short Essays* and *Short Answers*
- The next column has page number from this book only on which the answer for the question is located
- Final column has the list of examination in which this question is appeared
- The originality of the questions is maintained, thus it also serves as an index
- Overall, a chapterwise question bank with solved answers.

This book is presented in a handy form for easy handling during examinations. The books referred to write the answers are the ones that are commonly read by the students; so as not to cause confusion and avoid perpetuation of the tension at eleventh hour. The questions that are repeated have been referred. The emphasis is on the revised scheme 3, as it is applicable to the present batches.

My loyal readers would have found that by purchasing my books, they made no mistake during these examinations. Such is importance of such books because they let you revise in nick of time. They also help you understand the various modes of presenting answers to score well. But by far and large and also in the opinion of the students, the significance of this book lies in 3 marks questions which they are answered schematically and precisely.

Another important aspect of this book is that it contains a combination of different authors in a particular answer. A student cannot afford to read numerous books on a single subject in the prescribed time of one year for the first phase. So, this book will help the students prepare answers to the bouncer questions or answer the questions which are not there in the textbook opted by the students.

I have tried to provide all the necessary and latest information as possible. But let me make it clear that the book can never be a substitute to a textbook.

I sincerely solicit your valuable comments to improve this book and make it more useful. So please do write your comments to my mail *singi_yatiraj@yahoo.com* or contact me in Facebook on my page *Singi Yatiraj*.

I hope, even this edition, would receive same warm response as the previous ones and my other books.

In conclusion, I would like to thank my readers for their overwhelming support and wish my new readers *Best Wishes* for upcoming examinations.

**Singi Yatiraj**
www.drsingiyatiraj.5u.com

# Acknowledgments

I would like to thank:

- Dr B Mallikarjun, Former Dean, MR Medical College, Kalaburagi, Karnataka, India, for his encouragement and support.
- *Late* Dr Jagadish B Ingin, Professor and Head, Department of Biochemistry, MR Medical College, Kalaburagi, for his active interest and time for going through the entire script and correcting it and giving a foreword.
- Dr SS Ronad, Dr BC Bandi and rest of the staff members of Department of Biochemistry, MR Medical College, Kalaburagi, for their selfless excellent teaching.
- Dr Hanumanth Rao, Dr MS Dharpurkar, Dr MN Patil, Mr Shivaraj Shankar and Mr Shivashankar AR, former staff members of Department of Biochemistry, MR Medical College, Kalaburagi, for their selfless excellent teaching.
- Mr Kalburgi and *Late* Sri Puranik of Computer Section, MR Medical College, Kalaburagi, for providing me the question papers of the respective examinations.
- My teachers, for they are the ones who made me this capable.
- My friends Kiran, Nagaraj and Wali, for their help, support, suggestions and encouragement throughout the project.
- Mr Md Bari, Mr Yousuf Patel and Mr Rashid, Star Computers, for all the assistance in timely and neat computer printing of the manuscript.
- My all friends and well-wishers, for their best wishes.
- Shri Jitendar P Vij (Group Chairman), Mr Ankit Vij (Group President), Ms Ritu Sharma (Director–Content Strategy) and Mr KK Raman (Production Manager) of M/s Jaypee Brothers Medical Publishers (P) Ltd, New Delhi, India, for publishing the book in the same format as wanted well in time.
- Mr Venugopal (Associate Director–South) and their staff members of Jaypee Brothers, Bengaluru Branch, for taking this book to every corner of Karnataka.
- Ms Sunita Katla (PA to Group Chairman and Publishing Manager), Ms Samina Khan (Executive Assistant to Director–Content Strategy), Ms Seema Dogra, Ms Uma Adhikari, Mr Laxmidhar Padhiary, and others at M/s Jaypee Brothers Medical Publishers (P) Ltd, New Delhi, for their painstaking effort to make this book attractive and lucid.
- Mr Tarun, Mr Gopal and Mr Balaji, for introducing me to Jaypee Brothers and being a close associate.
- All the students, for their overwhelming response and support to my prior endeavors.
- All those who have helped me directly or indirectly.
- Most important of all, my parents, sister, uncles and cousins aunties, for their eternal love, care and support.

Thank you all of you,

Without you, this book would not have been a reality.

# Contents

1. MBBS Phase I Examination – June 2005 (Revised Scheme 2) ..... 1
2. MBBS Phase I Examination – December 2005 (Revised Scheme 2) ..... 22
3. MBBS Phase I Examination – June 2006 (Revised Scheme 2) ..... 36
4. MBBS Phase I Examination – December 2006 (Revised Scheme 2) ..... 50
5. MBBS Phase I Examination – June 2007 (Revised Scheme 2) ..... 58
6. MBBS Phase I Examination – December 2007 (Revised Scheme 2) ..... 82
7. MBBS Phase I Examination – June 2008 (Revised Scheme 2) ..... 90
8. MBBS Phase I Examination – December 2008 (Revised Scheme 2) ..... 102
9. MBBS Phase I Examination – June 2009 (Revised Scheme 2) ..... 117
10. MBBS Phase I Examination – December 2009 (Revised Scheme 2) ..... 131
11. MBBS Phase I Examination – June 2010 (Revised Scheme 2) ..... 144
12. MBBS Phase I Examination – December 2010 (Revised Scheme 2) ..... 158
13. MBBS Phase I Examination – June 2011 (Revised Scheme 2 & 3) ..... 170
14. MBBS Phase I Examination – December 2011 (Revised Scheme 2 & 3) ..... 178
15. MBBS Phase I Examination – June 2012 (Revised Scheme 2 & 3) ..... 190
16. MBBS Phase I Examination – December 2012 (Revised Scheme 2 & 3) ..... 201
17. MBBS Phase I Examination – June 2013 (Revised Scheme 2 & 3) ..... 212
18. MBBS Phase I Examination – December 2013 (Revised Scheme 2 & 3) ..... 229
19. MBBS Phase I Examination – June 2014 (Revised Scheme 2 & 3) ..... 247
20. MBBS Phase I Examination – December 2014 (Revised Scheme 2 & 3) ..... 259
21. MBBS Phase I Examination – June 2015 (Revised Scheme 2 & 3) ..... 270
22. MBBS Phase I Examination – December 2015 (Revised Scheme 2 & 3) ..... 283
23. MBBS Phase I Examination – June 2016 (Revised Scheme 2 & 3) ..... 297
24. MBBS Phase I Examination – December 2016 (Revised Scheme 2 & 3) ..... 305
25. MBBS Phase I Examination – June 2017 (Revised Scheme 2 & 3) ..... 315
26. MBBS Phase I Examination – December 2017 (Revised Scheme 2 & 3) ..... 322
27. MBBS Phase I Examination – Sample Paper-1 ..... 327
28. MBBS Phase I Examination – Sample Paper-2 ..... 350

*Annexure* ..... *371*

*Index* ..... *375*

---

* October 2017 question paper is renamed as December 2017 to maintain uniformity in the book.

# Course Contents

## THEORY

I. Introduction and scope of biochemistry
II. Cell and subcellular structures
  a. Cell membrane—composition
  b. Functions of subcellular structures.
  c. Transport across the cell membrane
    i. Active transport
    ii. Facilitated diffusion
    iii. Receptor-mediated transport
    iv. Endocytosis.
III. Acid-base imbalance
  a. Hydrogen ion concentration, acids, bases, buffers, Henderson-Hasselbach equation.
IV. Isotopes, radioactive isotopes and their application in medicine
V. Chemistry of carbohydrates
  a. Definition, classification and biological importance.
  b. Monosaccharides: Structure, classification and properties—isomerism.
  c. Stereoisomerism
  d. Oligosaccharides: Disaccharides—structure and their importance.
  e. Polysaccharides: Homo- and heteropolysaccharides—structure and their functions.
VI. Chemistry of proteins, amino acids and peptides
  a. Proteins: Definition, classification and functions.
  b. Amino acids: Classification, properties, side chains of amino acids, charge properties.
  c. Peptides: Biologically important peptides—GSH, insulin and structure.
  d. Structural organization, conformation and denaturation.
VII. Chemistry of lipids
  a. Definition, classification and biological importance.
  b. Simple lipids: Triacylglycerol and waxes—structure and composition.
  c. Compound lipids: Phospholipids, sphingolipids, glycolipids and their composition and function.
  d. Derived lipids: Fatty acids—saturated and unsaturated and their properties, eicosanoids, terpenes.
VIII. Chemistry of nucleic acids
  a. Definition, biological importance.
  b. Classification and composition.
  c. Purine and pyrimidine bases, nucleosides, nucleotides and biologically important nucleotides.
  d. DNA: Structure and functions.
  e. RNA: Types of RNA—structure and functions.
IX. Enzymes and clinical enzymology
  a. Definition, classification, specificity, coenzymes, cofactors activators.
  b. Mechanism of enzymes action.
  c. Factors affecting enzymes activity—Km value and its importance.
  d. Enzyme inhibition: Reversible and irreversible, competitive and other types, in clinical application.
  e. Regulatory enzymes: Proenzymes or zymogen, isoenzymes, allosteric enzymes and feedback control.
  f. Diagnostic and therapeutic importance of enzymes including enzyme immunoassay.
  g. ELISA and RIA.
X. Vitamins
  a. Definition and classification.

  b. A brief account of chemistry, source, deficiency diseases and biochemical role, recommended dietary allowances (RDA).
  c. Vitamin antagonists.
  d. Hypervitaminosis.
  e. A brief account of role of antioxidants and free radicals.

XI. Biological oxidation
  a. Mitochondria electron transport chain, oxidative phosphorylation, mechanism, uncouplers and inhibitors.

XII. Digestion and absorption from gastrointestinal tract
  a. Digestion and absorption of carbohydrates, lipids, proteins and nucleic acids.
  b. Malabsorption syndromes.

XIII. Carbohydrates metabolism
  a. Glycogenesis, glycogenolysis and glycogen storage disease.
  b. Glucose transporters, glycolysis, Rapoport-Luebering cycle, pyruvate oxidation, citric acid cycle.
  c. Pentose phosphate pathway.
  d. Uronic acid pathway.
  e. Gluconeogenesis and Cori's cycle.
  f. Metabolism of fructose and galactose.
  g. Regulation of metabolic pathways.
  h. Disorders of carbohydrates metabolism.
  i. Regulation of blood sugar, glucose tolerance test, diagnostic and prognostic importance of glycated hemoglobin and diabetes mellitus.

XIV. Lipid metabolism
  a. Oxidation of fatty acids, propionate metabolism, formation and utilization of ketone bodies, ketosis, outline the synthesis of cholesterol (reactions up to mevalonate in detail), breakdown of cholesterol and metabolic disorders of lipids.
  b. Lipogenesis, de novo synthesis of fatty acids, chain elongation, desaturation, phospholipid biosynthesis (lecithin and cephalin only) and their breakdown.
  c. Fatty liver and lipotropic factors.
  d. Prostaglandins and their biological functions.
  e. Plasma lipoproteins—classification, functions and disorders.

XV. Protein and amino acid metabolism
  a. Breakdown of tissue proteins and amino acid pool, general reactions of amino acids.
  b. Disposal of ammonia: Urea cycle, glutamate and glutamine formation.
  c. Metabolism of individual amino acids (glycine, serine, sulfur-containing amino acids, aromatic amino acids, histidine and arginine).
  d. Metabolic disorders of amino acids, aminoacidurias.
  e. Synthesis of creatine, phosphocreatine, formation of creatinine and clinical significance of creatinine clearance.

XVI. Purine and pyrimidine metabolism
  a. Source of various atoms of purine and pyrimidine, biosynthesis of purine and pyramidine nucleotides and their breakdown.
  b. Salvage pathways.
  c. Disorders of purine and pyrimidine metabolism.

XVII. Intermediary metabolism
  a. Introduction, methods of study of intermediary metabolism.

XVIII. Minerals
  a. Calcium, phosphorous, sodium, potassium, chlorides, iron, copper, iodine, zinc, fluoride, magnesium, manganese and selenium.

XIX. Molecular genetics and protein biosynthesis
  a. DNA, RNA metabolism.
  b. Replication, transcription, reverse transcription and post-transcriptional modifications.
  c. Translation—amino acid activation, initiation, elongation and termination, post-translation modifications.
  d. Regulation of gene expression.

e. Mutations.
f. Recombinant DNA technology, PCR and gene therapy.

XX. Tissue biochemistry
a. Heme metabolism: Outline of heme biosynthesis, degradation of heme and functions of normal hemoglobin.
b. Abnormal hemoglobin.
c. Jaundice.
d. Porphyria.
e. Plasma proteins: Separation, functions and importance.
f. Immunoglobins: Structure and functions.
g. pH of blood, its regulation, acidosis, alkalosis, principles of estimation of body fluids, role of kidneys and lungs in blood pH maintenance.

XXI. Liver functions and kidney functions
a. Liver function tests, kidney function tests.
b. Detoxification, mechanisms and metabolism of xenobiotics.

XXII. Nutrition and energy metabolism
a. BMR and its importance.
b. Calorific values of food, RQ, SDA, balanced diet.
c. Protein energy malnutrition, biological value of proteins, nitrogen equilibrium.
d. Dietary fibers.
e. Biochemistry of starvation.

XXIII. Biochemisty of cancer
a. Oncogenes.
b. Growth factors.
c. Tumor markers
i. Definition
ii. Clinically important tumor markers—CEA, alpha fetoprotein (AFP).
iii. Human chorionic gonadotropins (hCG), calcitonin, prostate-specific antigen (PSA).

XXIV. Endocrine function
a. Hormone actions: Mechanism of action of insulin, glucagon, epinephrine, steroids.
b. Thyroid function tests.

XXV. Biochemical tests for atherosclerosis and myocardial infarction
a. Lipid profile, apoprotein, homocysteine and C-reactive protein.
b. CKMB, troponins.

XXVI. SI units, quality control and standardization
a. Clinical chemistry: Interpretation and reference values of blood glucose, urea, creatinine, uric acid, cholesterol, calcium, proteins, albumin and A/G ratio.
b. Instrumentation including autoanalyzer.

XXVII. Biomedical waste management
a. Types, potential risks and their safe management.

## PRACTICALS

### To be Done by the Students

*Qualitative Analysis*

a. Reactions of monosaccharides—glucose and fructose.
b. Reactions of disaccharides—lacotse, maltose and sucrose.
c. Reactions of polysaccharides—starch.
d. Identification of unknown carbohydrates.
e. Precipitation and coagulation reactions of protein.
f. Color reactions of protein—albumin and casein.
g. Identification of unknown proteins.

h. Identification of substances of physiological importance.
i. Normal constituents of urine.
j. Organic: Urea, uric acid and creatinine.
k. Inorganic: Ca, P, Cl, $SO_4$ and $NH_3$, specific gravity.
l. Analysis of abnormal urine.
m. Spectroscopic examination of hemoglobin derivatives and preparations of hemin crystals.
n. Spot test for PKU, alkaptonuria and homocystinuria.
o. Spotters.

*Quantitative Estimation*

a. Estimation of blood glucose and interpretation.
b. Estimation of blood urea and interpretation.
c. Estimation of serum inorganic phosphorus and interpretation.
d. Estimation of total serum proteins, serum albumin and A:G ratio.
e. Estimation of urinary creatinine and interpretation of creatinine clearance.
f. Interpretation of charts and case reports.

### Demonstration Only

a. Colorimetry.
b. Paper chromatography.
c. Paper electrophoresis.
d. Glucose tolerance tests.
e. Determination of AST (SGOT) and ALT (SGPT).
f. Estimation of serum cholesterol (Kit method).
g. Determination of ascorbic acid.
h. Principle of flame photometry.
i. Determination of glucose and proteins in CSF.
j. Estimation of albumin in urine and tests for Bence Jones proteins in urine.

## UNIVERSITY EXAMINATION PATTERN

*Eligibility for Writing the University Examination*

The candidate should have at least 35% aggregate in the two of the three internals conducted by the college and should also have minimum 75% attendance in Theory and Practical classes conducted.

*Criteria for Passing the University Examination*

The candidate should secure minimum 50% in the university theory examination (University theory + Viva voce) and the university practical examinations separately. Internal assessment marks would not be considered for passing criteria, however, they would be added to final marks to determine class of passing.

### Distribution of Marks

| | *Internal assessment* | | *University examination* | |
|---|---|---|---|---|
| | *Maximum marks* | *Minimum marks to qualify* | *Maximum marks* | *Minimum marks to pass* |
| Theory examination | 20 marks | 7 marks | 100 marks | 60 marks |
| Viva voce | — | — | 20 marks | |
| Practical examination | 20 marks | 7 marks | 40 marks | 20 marks |

## Theory Examination

There shall be two papers of 50 marks each in a common question paper carrying 100 marks. The pattern of questions in each paper would be of three types.

| | | |
|---|---|---|
| 1 Long Essay Questions | 1 × 10 marks | 10 marks |
| 5 Short Essay Questions | 5 × 5 marks | 25 marks |
| 5 Short Answer Questions | 5 × 3 marks | 15 marks |
| | **Total** | **50 marks** |

*Distribution of Chapters in Paper I and II for University Examination with Weightage of Marks*

| ***Paper I*** | | ***Paper II*** | |
|---|---|---|---|
| *Topics* | *Marks* | *Topics* | *Marks* |
| Cell structures and functions, subcellular organelles, cell membranes, transport across the membranes | 5 | Nucleotides and nucleic acid chemistry | 5 |
| Chemistry, digestion, absorption and metabolism of carbohydrates | 10 | Purine and pyramidine nucleotide metabolism, DNA metabolism, RNA metabolism, protein biosynthesis | 10 |
| Chemistry, digestion, absorption and metabolism of lipids | 10 | Vitamins | 10 |
| Amino acids and protein chemistry, general reactions of amino acids, digestion and absorption, urea cycle and metabolism of amino acids | 10 | Minerals | 10 |
| Endocrine functions and biochemical tests | 5 | Molecular genetics, regulation of gene expression, recombinant DNA technology, PCR and gene therapy | 5 |
| Detoxification and xenobiotics | 5 | Electrolyte and water balance, acid-base balance | 10 |
| Enzymes | 10 | Nutrition and energy metabolism | 10 |
| Biological oxidation, integration of metabolism, TCA cycle and regulation of metabolism | 10 | Heme metabolism, normal and abnormal hemoglobin, plasma proteins and immunoglobulins | 10 |
| Free radicals and antioxidants | 5 | Liver function tests | 5 |
| Biochemistry of cancer, oncogenes and tumor markers | 5 | Kidney function tests | 5 |
| | | Clinical chemistry, quality control, interpretation and reference values and analysis | 5 |

***Note:***

a. Marks allotted to each topic under each paper add up to more than 50 marks and they have been allotted marks only to signify the importance of the chapter.
b. Long essays may be asked from topics carrying 10 marks but short essays and short answers can be asked from any of the topic.
c. Topics assigned to the different papers are generally evaluated under those sections. However, a strict division of the subject may not be possible and some overlapping of topics is inevitable and students are advised to be prepared to answer overlapping topics.

## Practical Examination

Practical examination consists of two exercises of one-hour duration and 20 marks each.

*Distribution of Practicals in Session I and II for University Examination with Marks*

| | *Marks* |
|---|---|
| *Exercise I* | |
| Quantitative estimation (every candidate shall perform one given procedure) | |
| a. Principle and procedure for the estimation asked in the question should be written by the candidate in first 5 minutes | 5 marks |
| b. After collecting papers, correct procedure for the estimation is given and practical examination is done. Marks can be awarded for<br>i. Results (values)<br>ii. Calculations and reporting<br>iii. Interpretation of results and application of estimate | 10 marks |
| Discussion of case studies, graphs and charts (5 in number 1 mark each) | 5 marks |
| *Exercise II* | |
| a. Qualitative analysis (every candidate shall perform one given procedure such as identification of carbohydrates, proteins, substance of physiological importance, analysis of normal urine, analysis of abnormal urine) | |
| i. For selection of appropriate reactions | 5 marks |
| ii. For reasoning of analysis and correct reporting | 5 marks |
| iii. For interpretation of results and application of estimation | 5 marks |
| b. Five spotters, biochemical techniques—chromatography, electrophoresis, osazone preparation, biochemical tests and reagents | 5 marks |

## Viva Voce

The viva voce examination shall carry 20 marks and all the examiners will conduct the viva examination separately for each candidate.

# Chapterwise Page References

| Questions | Page No. | Examinations |
|---|---|---|
| **SECTION ONE: CHEMICAL CONSTITUENT OF LIFE** | | |
| **BIOMOLECULES AND THE CELL** | | |
| **Short Essays** | | |
| 1. Draw a neat diagram of a cell and its organelles. Explain the functions of each. | 205 | D12(RS3) |
| 2. Mitochondrial structure and important functions. | 195 | D05 |
| 3. Lysosomes. | 166 | J07 |
| **Short Answers** | | |
| 1. Name subcellular organelles. Which are metabolic functions of cytosols? | 206 | J05(RS2) |
| 2. Endoplasmic reticulum. | 155 | J10(RS2) |
| 3. Give metabolic function of endoplasmic reticulum and mitochondria. | 206 | J07(RS2) |
| 4. Mitochondria. | 195 | J12(RS3) |
| 5. Lysosomes (metabolic functions and clinical significance). | 166 | D10(RS2), D16 |
| 6. Golgi complex. | 345 | D08(OS) |
| 7. Peroxisomes. | 366 | J11(OS) |
| **CARBOHYDRATES** | | |
| **Short Essays** | | |
| 1. Function of carbohydrates. | 105 | D08(RS2) |
| 2. Epimerization. | 256 | J11 |
| 3. Invert sugar. | 344 | J98 |
| 4. What are mucopolysaccharides (glycosaminoglycans)? Give their biomedical importance with examples (name the functions and composition of four mucopolysaccharides). | 284 | D15(RS3), J16(RS3), J04, J12 |
| 5. Chondroitin sulfate. | 285 | J99, D04 |
| **Short Answers** | | |
| 1. Epimerism and anomerism. | 256 | J14(RS3) |
| 2. What are epimers? Give examples (name two epimers of alpha D-glucose). | 256 | D07 |
| 3. Mutarotation. | 56 | D06(RS2), J06 |
| 4. Glycosidic linkage. | 366 | J09 |
| 5. What is the clinical importance of glycosides? | 347 | D06 |
| 6. Invert sugar. | 344 | D14, D15 |
| 7. Compare and contrast starch and glycogen. | 289 | D15(RS3), J00 |
| 8. Glycosaminoglycans. | 284 | J06(RS2), J08, J14 |
| 9. Name mucopolysaccharides. Mention their functions. | 284 | J05(RS2) |
| 10. Give the composition of hyaluronic acid. | 285 | J13 |
| **LIPIDS** | | |
| **Long Essay** | | |
| 1. Define lipids. Classify lipids with an example for each. Mention the functions of the lipids. | 201 | D12(RS3) |
| **Short Essays** | | |
| 1. Classify of lipid with examples. What are essential fatty acids? Mention one function of each. | 201, 308 | D11 |
| 2. Compound lipids. | 201 | D98 |
| 3. What are essential fatty acids? What are the functions of essential fatty acids? | 308 | D16(RS3) |

Contd...

| QUESTIONS | PAGE No. | EXAMINATIONS |
|---|---|---|
| 4. Phospholipids—define, classify with examples, significance (functions), composition and functions of any two. | 136 | D09(RS2), D01, D03, J04, J08, D10, J12 |
| **Short Answers** | | |
| 1. Unsaturated fatty acid. | 308 | J09 |
| 2. Give two examples of polyunsaturated fatty acids. | 308 | D05 |
| 3. Essential fatty acids and their importance. | 308 | D05(RS2), D15(RS3), J99, J00, D07, D08, D12, J14, J15 |
| 4. Rancidity. | 98 | J08(RS2), J06 |
| 5. Lipid peroxidation—clinical importance. | 86 | D07(RS2) |
| 6. Phospholipids (name any two with their composition and functions). | 136 | D13(RS3), D06, J10, D12 |
| 7. Lecithin. | 136 | J99 |
| 8. Name the components of sphingomyelin. | 136 | D13 |
| 9. Surfactant—composition and function. | 347 | J02, J15 |
| **PROTEINS AND AMINO ACIDS** | | |
| **Long Essays** | | |
| 1. Classify amino acid based on their structure giving examples. | 247 | J14(RS3) |
| 2. How will you differentiate a native protein from a denatured protein? Explain the bonds at different levels of three dimensional structure of a native protein. | 352 | J11(OS) |
| **Short Essays** | | |
| 1. Essential amino acids. | 138 | D09(RS2) |
| 2. Describe the decarboxylation reactions of amino acids with four examples. Give its significance. | 41 | J11(RS2), J17(RS3) |
| 3. Structural organization of proteins. | 181 | J09, D12 |
| 4. Define primary, secondary, tertiary and quaternary structure of protein. What are the noncovalent forces which preserve the secondary structure? | 181 | D11(RS3) |
| 5. Secondary structure of proteins. | 182 | J08(RS2), J07 |
| 6. Give the salient features of α-helical structure and quaternary structure of proteins. | 182 | D13 |
| 7. Describe the bonds that contribute to (stabilize) protein structure. | 352 | J98, D03 |
| 8. Classify proteins based on their function giving an example for each class. | 217 | J13(RS3) |
| 9. Biologically active peptides (biological importance of peptides). | 46 | J08, D16 |
| 10. Glutathione. | 208 | D99 |
| **Short Answers** | | |
| 1. Name two hydroxy amino acids. | 247 | J07 |
| 2. Nutritional classification of amino acids. | 154 | J10(RS2) |
| 3. Essential amino acids and their importance (functions). | 138 | J11(RS2), D98, J09, J03, J06, D09, D10, J11 |
| 4. Peptide bond. | 353 | J10 |
| 5. Secondary structure of proteins. | 182 | D13(RS3), D10 |
| 6. Tertiary and quaternary structure of proteins. | 183 | D14(RS3) |
| 7. Bonds stabilizing protein structure. | 181 | J15(RS3) |
| 8. Give brief account on quaternary structure of proteins. | 183 | J05(RS2) |
| 9. What is isoelectric pH? What is the application of isoelectric pH? State properties of a protein at its isoelectric pH. | 344 | J07, D07, J13 |


Contd...

| Questions | Page No. | Examinations |
|---|---|---|
| 10. Denaturation of proteins and factors causing denaturation. | 156 | J10(RS2), J15(RS3), D16(RS3), J99, J08, J11, D12 |
| 11. Functional classification of proteins. | 217 | D07(RS2) |
| 12. What is complete protein? | 142 | D09(RS2) |
| 13. Biologically active peptides and their functions. | 46 | J06(RS2), D06 |
| 14. Glutathione and its significance (role in erythrocytes). | 208 | D12(RS3), D16(RS3), D12 |
| **NUCLEIC ACIDS AND NUCLEOTIDES** | | |
| **Long Essay** | | |
| 1. Draw neat diagram of Watson Crick model of DNA, explain its characteristics and the bonds that play a role in the stability of DNA structure. | 146 | J15(RS3) |
| **Short Essays** | | |
| 1. Structure and function of DNA. | 146 | D01, J08 |
| 2. RNA—types, salient features and functions. | 218 | J13(RS3) |
| 3. Structure and functions of mRNA. | 218 | J11(RS2) |
| 4. Structure and functions of tRNA. Mention the unusual bases present in it. | 219 | D13(RS3), J01, D06, D12 |
| **Short Answers** | | |
| 1. Distinguish between RNA and DNA. | 34 | D05(RS2), J06, J12 |
| 2. Cyclic nucleotides. | 49 | J06(RS2), J11 |
| 3. Which are biologically important nucleotides? Mention their functions. | 20 | J05(RS2), D05 |
| 4. Mention the functions of DNA. | 147 | J02 |
| 5. Salient features of Chargaff's rule. | 226 | D10, D15 |
| 6. Salient features of Watson-Crick model of DNA. | 146 | D11 |
| 7. Base-pairing rule and Wobble hypothesis. | 226 | J13(RS3) |
| 8. Base-pairing rule and its importance. | 226 | D07(RS2), J14 |
| 9. Types of RNA and their function. | 218 | J07(RS2), D00, J09 |
| 10. Ribosomal RNA. | 220 | J15(RS3) |
| 11. Messenger RNA (mRNA)—structure and functions. | 218 | J98, J05, J08 |
| 12. What is the role of tRNA? | 220 | D09 |
| 13. Draw a neat labeled diagram of tRNA. | 219 | D14(RS3) |
| **ENZYMES** | | |
| **Long Essays** | | |
| 1. Define enzymes. Explain the mechanism of enzyme action. Add a note on inhibition of enzymes. | 350, 64, 329 | D10(OS) |
| 2. What are enzymes? Classify enzymes with one example each. Explain any four factors that affect enzyme activity. Add a note on enzyme specificity. | 212 | J13(RS3), J14 |
| 3. Classify enzymes giving an example with the reaction catalyzed. | 212 | D15(RS3) |
| 4. Explain the influence of various factors on enzyme activity. | 213 | D06(RS2), D16(RS3) |
| 5. Define the enzyme inhibition. Explain the features of competitive and noncompetitive inhibition. Mention the therapeutic importance of competitive inhibition. | 64 | D16 |
| 6. Define isoenzymes. Mention the principles used for separation of isoenzymes. Write about the clinical importance of isoenzymes. | 82 | D07(RS2) |



Contd...

| Questions | Page No. | Examinations |
|---|---|---|
| **Short Essays** | | |
| 1. Define and classify enzymes (IUB classification) with one example for each class indicating the reaction catalyzed. | 212 | J02, D09, J11, J12 |
| 2. Factors affecting enzyme action (reaction). | 213 | D06, D10 |
| 3. Km value (Michaelis-Menten constant) of an enzyme and its significance with a suitable example. | 164 | D10(RS2), J12(RS3), J08 |
| 4. Effect of pH and temperature on enzyme catalyzed reaction. | 214 | J10 |
| 5. Explain competitive and noncompetitive inhibition. Mention significance of competitive inhibition. | 64 | J07(RS2) |
| 6. Competitive inhibition—features, examples, importance in medicine (clinical use). | 64 | D08(RS2), J99, D02, D04, D07, D14 |
| 7. Noncompetitive enzyme inhibition. | 64 | J10(RS2) |
| 8. Explain enzyme specificities with examples. | 194 | J12(RS3), J15 |
| 9. Coenzyme and their role in metabolism with four examples. | 242 | J07, J09 |
| 10. Allosteric enzymes. | 184 | J14(RS3), D99 |
| 11. Explain the mechanism of action of allosteric enzymes? Name the allosteric inhibitor and allosteric activator for phosphofructokinase and acetyl CoA—carboxylase. | 184 | D11(RS3) |
| 12. Describe the regulation of enzyme activity. | 329 | J04, J05 |
| 13. Proenzymes. | 141 | D98 |
| 14. Therapeutic uses of enzymes. | 12 | J05(RS2) |
| 15. Diagnostic importance of enzymes (Enzymes in clinical diagnosis)—diagnostic enzymology. | 173 | J11(RS2), J08, D08, D12, D13 |
| 16. How does estimation of enzymes in serum help in clinical diagnosis (Clinical significance of serum enzyme estimation)? Illustrate with five examples. | 173 | J01 |
| 17. Name five enzymes of diagnostic significance. Give the normal serum level and one clinical condition associated with their increase. | 173 | D01 |
| 18. Isoenzymes and their clinical importance citing three examples. | 82 | D05(RS2), J16(RS3), J17(RS3), D17(RS3), D16 |
| 19. What are isoenzymes? Discuss the isoenzyme forms of LDH | 82 | D15 |
| 20. What are isoenzymes? Name the isoenzymes forms of LDH and CK. What is their clinical significance? | 82 | J03 |
| 21. What are isoenzymes? Explain the enzyme profile in myocardial infarction. | 260 | D11 |
| 22. Clinical importance of enzymes in assessment of cardiac disease and liver function. | 236 | D13(RS3) |
| 23. Name three enzymes commonly estimated in myocardial infarction. Give its importance and limitations. | 260 | D14(RS3) |
| 24. Diagnostic enzymes used in the assessment of different liver functions. | 237 | D15(RS3) |
| **Short Answers** | | |
| 1. Classify enzymes with suitable examples. | 212 | J01, D04, J06 |
| 2. Lyases. | 212 | J98 |
| 3. $K_m$ value of enzymes and its significance. | 164 | D05(RS2), J01, D04, D08, J11, J13 |
| 4. Explain the relationship between $K_m$ and affinity. | 311 | D16(RS3) |
| 5. Explain how change in temperature alters the enzyme activity. | 213 | J00 |
| 6. Explain how change in ph alters the enzyme activity. | 214 | D00 |
| 7. Competitive inhibition of enzyme activity (give two examples). | 64 | J16(RS3), D05 |
| 8. Methanol poisoning can be alleviated by ethanol, justify. | 48 | J06(RS2) |

Contd...

| Questions | Page No. | Examinations |
|---|---|---|
| 9. Mention the actions and uses of two competitive enzyme inhibitors. | 65 | J03, D03 |
| 10. Define absolute specificity of enzyme. Give two examples. | 194 | D02 |
| 11. Coenzymes. | 242 | D13(RS3) |
| 12. What is meant by lock and key mechanism of enzymes? | 350 | D09 |
| 13. Define allosteric enzyme with an example and name modulators for the enzyme. | 184 | D06, D12 |
| 14. Define zymogens (proenzymes). Give two examples. | 141 | D09(RS2), J00, D02, J03, J04, D08, D10 |
| 15. What are ribozymes? Mention one use of ribozymes. | 367 | D09 |
| 16. Give three/two examples of enzymes having therapeutic use and indicate their specific applications. | 12 | D12(RS3), D02 |
| 17. Enzymes of diagnostic importance. | 173 | J13(RS3), J09, D14 |
| 18. Serum amylase and its diagnostic significance. | 155 | J10(RS2), J99 |
| 19. Mention the significance of serum amylase and alkaline phosphatase estimation. | 155, 83 | J05 |
| 20. Define isoenzymes. Give one example. | 82 | D05, J06, J08 |
| 21. Name the isoenzymes of LDH. Mention their significance. | 83 | D03 |
| 22. CPK isoenzymes and its clinical significance. | 83 | J99, J07, J15 |
| 23. Diagnostic significance of serum alkaline phosphatase. | 83 | D15 |
| 24. Explain troponin as a marker for myocardial infarction. | 261 | D05(RS2) |
| 25. Explain enzyme profile in myocardial infarction. | 260 | J07(RS2) |
| **VITAMINS** | | |
| **Long Essays** | | |
| 1. Give an account on chemistry, sources, absorption, daily requirement, biochemical functions. Manifestations of deficiency and toxic effects of vitamin A. | 133 | D09(RS2), D98, D03, J06 |
| 2. How provitamin D is converted to its active form? Give an account of chemistry, sources, daily requirement, biochemical functions and deficiency manifestations of vitamin D. | 73 | J03 |
| 3. Discuss the chemistry, source, requirement, metabolic functions and deficiency manifestations of vitamin C (ascorbic acid) in the human body. | 25 | D05(RS2), D99 |
| 4. What are the sources, functions, deficiency manifestations and daily recommended allowance of thiamine? | 13 | D17(RS3), D09 |
| 5. Name the coenzyme forms of vitamin involved in amino acid metabolism. Discuss the biochemical functions and deficiency manifestations of this vitamin. | 40 | J06(RS2) |
| 6. Discuss RDA. Functions and deficiency manifestations of folic acid. How is it interlinked to vitamin $B_{12}$? | 305 | D16(RS3) |
| **Short Essays** | | |
| 1. Name a provitamin form of vitamin A. Add a note on sources, functions, daily requirement, causes and features of deficiency of vitamin A. | 134 | J09(RS2), J10(RS2), D11(RS3), J12(RS3), D02, J05, J09 |
| 2. Wald's visual cycle. | 134 | J08 |
| 3. Active form of vitamin D and its biochemical role. | 73 | D08 |
| 4. Vitamin D metabolism. Add a brief note hepatic osteodystrophy. | 73 | D05 |
| 5. Synthesis of calcitriol in the body and its uses. | 73 | J00 |
| 6. Biochemical functions and causes and features of deficiency of vitamin D. | 73 | J07(RS2), J11(RS2), J04 |
| 7. Vitamin E. | 46 | J99, D04 |
| 8. Sources, daily requirements, functions and deficiency manifestation of vitamin C. | 25 | D07(RS2), J08(RS2), D07, D11 |

Contd...

| Questions | Page No. | Examinations |
|---|---|---|
| 9. Explain the following aspects of thiamine: (a) Coenzyme form, (b) Biochemical function and (c) Deficiency. | 13 | J05(RS2), D01, D14 |
| 10. Mention the functions of thiamine pyrophosphate (TPP) citing the reactions in which it is involved. | 13 | J14 |
| 11. Explain the following aspects of riboflavin (a) Coenzyme forms, (b) Biochemical functions. | 361 | D02 |
| 12. Give the biochemical functions of niacin with examples and manifestation of its deficiency. | 220 | J13(RS3) |
| 13. Name the coenzyme form of vitamin $B_6$ (pyridoxine). Describe the biochemical reactions involving it/biochemical functions of pyridoxine (pyridoxal phosphate co-decarboxylase). | 40 | D10(RS2), D98, J02, D14 |
| 14. Give the coenzyme role of pantothenic acid and its importance. | 275 | J15(RS3) |
| 15. Chemistry, sources, daily requirement, coenzyme forms and functions of folic acid. | 305 | D06(RS2), J04 |
| 16. Hyperhomocysteinemia. | 344 | J07 |
| 17. Coenzyme form of vitamin $B_{12}$ and its biochemical functions. | 285 | D15(RS3) |
| **Short Answers** | | |
| 1. Vitamin A—functions (antioxidant role), RDA, deficiency manifestations. | 133 | D08(RS2), J01, D04, D10, J11, D16 |
| 2. Visual cycle. | 134 | J00 |
| 3. Mention causes and clinical features of hypervitaminosis A. | 135 | J14 |
| 4. Vitamin D—biochemical functions, deficiency symptoms. | 73 | D00 |
| 5. Vitamin E—functions/antioxidant role. | 46 | J06(RS2), J15, D15 |
| 6. Vitamin K—biochemical role and requirement. | 200 | J12(RS3), D15(RS3), J02, J05, J10, J14 |
| 7. Vitamin C—functions (role in iron absorption), deficiency manifestations (scurvy). | 25 | D10(RS2), J09, J12 |
| 8. Cause of Scurvy and beriberi. | 228 | J13(RS3) |
| 9. Thiamine—sources, daily requirements, role, deficiency manifestations. | 13 | D99, D05, J06, D10, J11 |
| 10. TPP as a coenzyme in two metabolic reaction of the body. | 13 | J00 |
| 11. Types and causes of beriberi. | 14 | J12(RS3), J11(RS2), D11 |
| 12. What is the coenzymic form of niacin and give one reaction where it is utilized? | 220 | D06 |
| 13. Niacine—coenzymic forms and deficiency manifestations (pellagra). | 220 | J17(RS3), J00, D14, D15 |
| 14. Functions of pyridoxal phosphate. | 41 | J07(RS2) |
| 15. How is histamine formed? What is the role of histamine? | 367 | J10 |
| 16. Biotin. | 341 | D00 |
| 17. Name the anti-egg white injury factor, its source and coenzyme function. | 341 | J01, D04 |
| 18. Describe two carboxylation reactions. | 342 | J05, J08 |
| 19. Functions of folic acid. | 305 | J00 |
| 20. Explain the role of folic acid in DNA synthesis. | 307 | D16 |
| 21. Formiminoglutamic acid (FIGLU). | 255 | J14(RS3), D98, D00 |
| 22. FIGLU excretion test. | 224 | J13(RS3), D15 |
| 23. Coenzymic form of vitamin $B_{12}$ and folic acid. | 285, 305 | D11 |
| 24. What are the coenzymic forms of cobalamin? | 285 | D05 |
| 25. Name the biochemical functions of vitamin $B_{12}$. | 285 | D01 |
| 26. Methyl folate trap. | 363 | J12(OS) |
| 27. Provitamins. | 318 | J17(RS3), D00 |
| 28. Mention the functions of vitamin E and K. | 46, 200 | J04 |


Contd...

| Questions | Page No. | Examinations |
|---|---|---|
| 29. What is the daily requirement of thiamine, niacin and pyridoxine? | 129 | J09(RS2) |
| 30. Write coenzyme forms of niacin and riboflavin. | 372 | D00 |
| 31. Coenzyme form of niacin and folic acid. | 372 | D08 |
| **SECTION TWO: PHYSIOLOGICAL BIOCHEMISTRY** | | |
| **DIGESTION AND ABSORPTION** | | |
| **Long Essay** | | |
| 1. Write in detail about the digestion and absorption of lipids? Write about causes of fatty stools. | 283 | J98 |
| **Short Essays** | | |
| 1. Give an account of digestion of carbohydrates from GIT. | 271 | D13 |
| 2. Explain the mechanism involved in the absorption of glucose. Describe the causes and features of lactose intolerance. | 273, 346 | J99, J02, D04 |
| 3. Lactose intolerance. | 346 | D05 |
| 4. Write in brief about the digestion and absorption of proteins. | 261 | D14(RS3), J06, J13 |
| 5. Digestion and absorption of lipids. | 283 | D15(RS3), J12 |
| 6. Enzymes involved in the digestion of lipids (lipases). | 283 | D05 |
| **Short Answers** | | |
| 1. Give an example of proteolytic enzyme and its specificity. | 261 | D06, D14 |
| 2. Name the enzymes involved in carbohydrate digestion. | 272 | D09 |
| 3. Digestion and absorption of disaccharides. | 210 | D12(RS3) |
| 4. Describe the absorption of glucose. | 273 | J04 |
| 5. Lactose intolerance—causes and features. | 346 | D98, D99, J04, D08, J12 |
| 6. Role of hydrochloric acid in protein digestion. | 261 | J01, D04 |
| 7. How is pepsinogen activated? What is the function of pepsin? | 261 | J10 |
| 8. Pepsinogen activation and action of trypsin. | 261 | D11 |
| 9. Name the two endopeptidases with their specifications. | 127 | J09(RS2) |
| 10. What is steatorrhea? Mention the causes. | 196 | J12(RS3), J02, J03, D16 |
| **PLASMA PROTEINS** | | |
| **Long Essay** | | |
| 1. What are plasma proteins? Write a note on their separation and functions. | 266, 295 | D08 |
| **Short Essays** | | |
| 1. How plasma proteins are separated? Explain the significance of M band. What is A/G ratio? What is its clinical significance? | 295, 207 | J04 |
| 2. What is electrophoresis? Name five plasma proteins and their functions. | 295, 266 | D11 |
| 3. Name and explain the functions of plasma proteins with clinical significance. | 266 | D14(RS3) |
| 4. What is normal serum protein level? Mention three important functions of albumin. | 206 | D12(RS3) |
| 5. Enumerate the functions of albumin. Mention the causes of hypoalbuminemia and consequences of hypoalbuminemia. | 206 | J11(RS2), J03 |
| 6. List conditions when albumin/globulin (A/G) ratio is altered. | 207 | D12(RS3) |
| 7. Transport proteins of blood. | 126 | J09(RS2) |
| 8. Acute phase proteins. | 154 | J10(RS2) |
| 9. Immunoglobulins—enumerate, structure and functions. | 167 | J03, D12, D16 |

Contd...

| Questions | Page No. | Examinations |
|---|---|---|
| **Short Answers** | | |
| 1. What is the normal level of plasma proteins? Name a disease which features hypoalbuminemia. | 206 | D05 |
| 2. Hypoalbuminemia. | 207 | D17(RS3) |
| 3. Describe how plasma protein are separated in the clinical laboratory. | 295 | D17(RS3) |
| 4. What is electrophoresis? Enumerate major classes of proteins separated on electrophoresis. | 295 | J01, D04 |
| 5. Normal values of serum proteins and its fractions. | 266 | J99 |
| 6. Plasma proteins—enumerate and functions of plasma proteins. | 266 | J16(RS3), J06, D10, D12 |
| 7. Serum albumin—functions. | 207 | D06(RS2), J10 |
| 8. Negative acute phase reactants. | 154 | D15 |
| 9. Immunoglobulins—enumerate, structure and functions. Outline the structure of immunoglobulins. | 167 | D10(RS2), D12(RS3), D07, J08, D10 |
| 10. Immunoglobulin G (IgG). | 168 | J98 |
| 11. Structure of immunoglobulin M. | 168 | J14 |
| 12. Immunoglobulin A (IgA) and immunoglobulin M (IgM). | 168 | J11(RS2) |
| 13. Bence Jones proteins—significance and detection. | 33 | D05(RS2), J06(RS2), D11(RS3), D01, D08 |
| 14. Anticoagulants. | 100 | J08(RS2) |
| **HEMOGLOBIN AND PORPHYRIA** | | |
| **Long Essays** | | |
| 1. Outline heme synthesis. Write a note on its function and abnormal hemoglobin. | 109, 231 | J09 |
| 2. Describe the synthesis and breakdown of hemoglobin. Write a note on hemoglobinopathies. | 229 | D13(RS3) |
| **Short Essays** | | |
| 1. Name five heme proteins and their functions. | 109 | D08(RS2) |
| 2. What is methemoglobin? How it is formed? Mention the causes for methemoglobinemia. How it is detected? | 302 | J16(RS3), D99 |
| 3. Hemoglobinopathies (abnormal hemoglobins). | 231 | D05(RS2) |
| 4. Sickle cell hemoglobin. | 87 | J98 |
| 5. Discuss the manifestations, molecular basis and laboratory diagnosis of sickle cell disease. What is the biological advantage of sickle cell trait? | 87 | J01 |
| 6. Heme synthesis (regulation). | 109 | J17(RS3), D00, D11 |
| 7. Porphyrias—causes and general features. | 276 | D16(RS3), J13 |
| 8. What are porphyries? How are they classified? Name the enzymatic defect and biochemical findings in any one/four of the porphyries. | 276 | J15(RS3), J00, J03 |
| 9. What is porphyria? Mention the defect and signs and symptoms of acute intermittent porphyria. | 276 | D09(RS2), D11(RS3) |
| 10. Congenital erythropoietic porphyria. | 278 | J99, D04 |
| 11. Catabolism (degradation) of heme (hemoglobin) in the body adding a note on clinical significance. | 71 | D07(RS2), D14(RS3), D98, J00, D01, D08 |
| 12. Bile pigments (bilirubin)—describe the metabolism (formation, transport and detoxification). Write the normal values of serum bilirubin. Name the abnormalities associated with bilirubin metabolism. | 71 | J07(RS2), J09(RS2), J14(RS3), J16(RS3), J99, D04, J14, D14 |
| 13. How are bile acid synthesized? Mention two functions of bile acids. | 273 | J15(RS3), D10 |

Contd...

| QUESTIONS | PAGE No. | EXAMINATIONS |
|---|---|---|
| 14. Jaundice. | 334 | D12 |
| 15. Hemolytic jaundice. | 334 | D99 |
| 16. Unconjugated hyperbilirubinemia. | 110 | D08(RS2) |
| 17. Hepatocellular jaundice. | 334 | D09 |
| **Short Answers** | | |
| 1. What is Dubin-Johnson disease? | 361 | J01, D04 |
| 2. Mention the normal types of hemoglobin. | 366 | D11(OS) |
| 3. Hemoglobin as buffering agent. | 296 | D15(RS3) |
| 4. 2,3 BPG. | 48 | J06(RS2) |
| 5. Carboxyhemoglobin . | 99 | J08(RS2), J99 |
| 6. Methemoglobin. | 302 | J10(RS2) |
| 7. Name the hemoglobinopathies (abnormal hemoglobins). | 231 | D07, D09 |
| 8. Sickle cell hemoglobin—biochemical defects, alteration in function. | 87 | J06, J07, D13 |
| 9. Sickle cell anemia—causes, molecular defect and consequences. | 87 | D07(RS2), J11(RS2), D08, D12 |
| 10. Biochemical defect in thalassemia. | 227 | J13(RS3) |
| 11. Name the levels at which heme synthesis is regulated. | 109 | D02, D07 |
| 12. What porphyrias? Name one disorder indicating the underlying cause. | 276 | J04 |
| 13. Name two porphyrias and the enzyme defect in them. | 277 | J08 |
| 14. Explain any two types of porphyrias. | 277 | D10 |
| 15. Acute intermittent porphyria. | 277 | J14(RS3), D99, D13 |
| 16. Degradation of heme. | 71 | J05(RS2), D06(RS2), J04 |
| 17. Fate of bilirubin. | 71 | D15 |
| 18. How is bilirubin conjugated (made water soluble)? | 71 | J06(RS2) |
| 19. Define jaundice. Mention one cause for different types of jaundice. | 334 | D03 |
| 20. Obstructive jaundice and its diagnosis (biochemical findings). | 244 | D13(RS3), J02, D08 |
| 21. Physiological jaundice. | 365 | J11 |
| 22. Name two congenital hyperbilirubinemias and defect in each of them. | 360 | D01 |
| 23. What is Crigler-Najjar syndrome? Name the enzymatic defect. | 361 | D02, D05 |
| 24. Give enzyme defect in the following conditions:<br>a. Drug-induced hemolytic anemia.<br>b. Criggler-Najjar syndrome. | 129 | J09(RS2) |
| 25. Gilberts syndrome. | 258 | J14(RS3) |
| **BIOLOGICAL OXIDATION** | | |
| **Long Essays** | | |
| 1. Describe the components of electron transport chain. Write a note on uncouplers and inhibitors. | 66 | D08 |
| 2. Discuss in detail oxidative phosphorylation and enumerate its inhibitors. | 144 | J10(RS2) |
| **Short Essays** | | |
| 1. Write the different components of electron transport chain. Mention four inhibitors of ETC. | 66 | J14(RS3), D16 |
| 2. Describe the single electron carrier components of respiratory chain. Indicate the sites of ATP formation during electron transport. Name two inhibitors of electron transport. | 66 | J07(RS2), D07(RS2), D02, J03, D03, J08, J10, J13 |

Contd...

| Questions | Page No. | Examinations |
|---|---|---|
| 3. What are cytochromes? Indicate their location and functions. | 188 | D99 |
| 4. What is oxidative phosphorylation? Explain its mechanism (chemiosmotic theory). Mention inhibitors and uncouplers of oxidative phosphorylation. | 144 | J05(RS2), J06(RS2), D98, J01, J04, J06, D06, J14, D14, D15 |
| 5. What is P:O ratio? Which are inhibitors of electron transport chain? | 68 | D05(RS2) |
| 6. What are uncouplers? Mention the uncouplers of oxidative phosphorylation. | 145 | J16(RS3), J15 |
| 7. Shuttle systems to transport extra mitochondrial reducing equivalents. | 224 | D05 |
| **Short Answers** | | |
| 1. Name the inhibitors of cytochrome oxidase. | 69 | D06 |
| 2. Expand ATP. What is its free energy of hydrolysis? | 365 | D11 |
| 3. High energy (phosphate) compounds. | 223 | J13(RS3), J02, D16 |
| 4. Components of electron transport chain. | 66 | J17(RS3), D11 |
| 5. Diagrammatic representation of mitochondrial electron transport chain and location of ATP formation sites. | 68 | D09(RS2) |
| 6. Cytochromes. | 188 | D11(RS3) |
| 7. P:O ratio. | 69 | J09, D09, J11 |
| 8. Oxidative phosphorylation—mechanism (chemiosmotic theory), inhibitors, uncouplers (with two examples). | 144 | D06(RS2), J08(RS2), J11(RS2), J15(RS3), D17(RS3), J98, J03, J05, D12, D13, D16 |
| 9. List the site inhibitors of electron transport chain. | 68 | D16(RS3) |
| 10. Ionophores. | 209 | D12(RS3) |
| 11. Mitochondrial shuttle systems. | 224 | J13(RS3) |
| 12. Describe malate—aspartate shuttle. What is its significance? | 225 | J01, D04 |
| **SECTION THREE: METABOLISMS** | | |
| **INTRODUCTION TO METABOLISM** | | |
| None | | |
| **METABOLISM OF CARBOHYDRATES** | | |
| **Long Essays** | | |
| 1. Describe the reactions of glycolysis indicating the enzymes. Add a note on net yield of ATP under aerobic and anaerobic conditions. | 248 | D17(RS3) |
| 2. Give a detailed account on glycolysis. Explain the energetics and regulation of this pathway. What is the significance of Rapoport Luebering cycle? | 248, 151 | J98, J08, D12 |
| 3. Describe the process of aerobic glycolysis. What is substrate level phosphorylation? What is the effect of insulin and cortisol on blood glucose level? | 248, 132 | D11 |
| 4. Why TCA cycle is called as common metabolic pathway? Describe in detail the tricarboxylic acid cycle (Krebs citric acid cycle), energy production and its significance. How is it regulated? What is its amphibolic role? Explain how carbohydrates, lipids and amino acids enter this cycle. | 90 | J08(RS2), D13(RS2), J04, J10, D14 |
| 5. Describe in detail the major catabolic pathway for acetyl CoA in aerobic organisms. How does it play a pivotal role in metabolism? | 90 | D05 |
| 6. What is gluconeogenesis? Write in detail about gluconeogenesis in humans from its predominant precursor (conversion of lactate to glucose) and mention its significance. Write about glucose alanine cycle. | 117 | D11(RS3), D98, D00, J03 |
| 7. Discuss the formation of glucose from noncarbohydrate substances. | 117 | J15 |
| 8. Trace the pathway of gluconeogenesis starting from alanine. Mention the key enzymes and how they are regulated | 117 | J09(RS2) |


Contd...

| Questions | Page No. | Examinations |
|---|---|---|
| 9. Discuss about the metabolism of glycogen. | 58 | J99 |
| 10. What is the biomedical importance of muscle and liver glycogen? Describe the process of glycogen synthesis with its regulation. Name two glycogen storage diseases. | 58, 50 | D06, J11 |
| 11. Define glycogenesis and glycogenolysis. Write the reactions of glycogenesis and glycogenolysis in liver. How are these two pathways reciprocally regulated? | 58 | J07(RS2) |
| 12. Describe the reactions of pentose phosphate pathway (hexose monophosphate shunt). Why is it called multifunctional? Mention the significance of this pathway. | 234 | J02, J09, D10, D15 |
| **Short Essays** | | |
| 1. How is glycogen digested and absorbed? Describe glycogenolysis in the liver. | 271, 59 | J15(RS3) |
| 2. Glucose transporters. | 340 | D06 |
| 3. What is the difference between oxidative and substrate level phosphorylation? Give two examples of substrate level phosphorylation with complete reaction. | 259 | D10(RS2), J13(RS3), D14(RS3), J99, D04 |
| 4. Regulation of glycolysis. | 250 | J07 |
| 5. Discuss the Embden-Meyerhof pathway that occurs in RBC. Add a note on its energetics. | 248 | J14(RS3) |
| 6. 2,3 biphosphoglycerate pathway in erythrocytes (Rapoport-Luebering cycle). | 151 | J10(RS2), D10(RS2), D06 |
| 7. Fate of pyruvate. | 355 | D06 |
| 8. Pyruvate oxidation. | 355 | J99, D04 |
| 9. Pyruvate dehydrogenase complex—enzymes and coenzymes components, mechanism of action and biomedical importance. | 36 | D07(RS2), J12 |
| 10. Citric acid (TCA) cycle—reactions, energy releasing steps, amphibolic role. | 90 | J09(RS2), D11(RS3), J12(RS3), J06, J13 |
| 11. Gluconeogenesis—(key) reactions (from lactate/alanine), key enzymes, significance, | 117 | D05(RS2), J06(RS2), J13(RS3), D16(RS3), D02, D05, D08, D09, D16 |
| 12. Cori's cycle. | 120 | J12(RS3), J14 |
| 13. Glucose alanine cycle. | 120 | J08 |
| 14. Synthesis of glycogen (glycogenesis)—reactions and its significance. | 58 | J08(RS2), D07, J12, D13 |
| 15. Glycogenolysis—reactions, regulation. | 59 | J10(RS2), J11(RS2), J16(RS3), J02, D02, J05 |
| 16. Glycogen storage disease. | 50 | D06(RS2), J17(RS3), J00, J03, J06, J14 |
| 17. Hexose monophosphate shunt—reactions (oxidative phase), significance. | 234 | D13(RS3), J17(RS3), D06 |
| 18. Uronic acid pathway. | 127 | J13 |
| 19. Metabolism of galactose. | 353 | D00, D07 |
| 20. Metabolism of fructose. | 331 | J00 |
| 21. Fructose intolerance. | 332 | D98 |
| **Short Answers** | | |
| 1. What are the major differences between hexokinase and glucokinase? | 346 | J05 |
| 2. Glucokinase. | 346 | D99 |
| 3. Explain substrate level phosphorylation with two examples. | 259 | D01, D02, D07, J11, J12 |
| 4. Energetics in aerobic and anaerobic pathway of EM pathway (glucose oxidation). | 249 | D99, J09 |
| 5. Write short note on Rapoport-Luebering cycle. | 151 | J16(RS3), D17(RS3), D12 |
| 6. Conversion of pyruvate to acetyl CoA. | 355 | J06 |
| 7. Pyruvate dehydrogenase complex. | 36 | J14(RS3) |

Contd...

| QUESTIONS | PAGE No. | EXAMINATIONS |
|---|---|---|
| 8. Amphibolic role of citric acid cycle. | 91 | D10 |
| 9. Anaplerosis and its significance. | 92 | J00, D00, J03 |
| 10. Any three enzymes unique to gluconeogenesis. | 120 | J11(RS2) |
| 11. Name the key gluconeogenic enzymes. | 120 | J13 |
| 12. Cori's cycle. | 120 | J11 |
| 13. Describe glucose alanine cycle. Mention its significance. | 120 | J01, D01, D04 |
| 14. Glycogen storage disorders. | 50 | J13(RS3) |
| 15. Von Gierke's disease. | 51 | D17(RS3), D99 |
| 16. Muscle phosphorylase deficiency. | 51 | D98 |
| 17. Mention significance of HMP shunt pathway. | 235 | D05(RS2), J08(RS2), J08, J12 |
| 18. Glucose 6 phosphate dehydrogenase deficiency. | 86 | D07(RS2) |
| 19. UDP-Glucuronic acid. | 280 | J15(RS3) |
| 20. Give the significance of uronic acid pathway. | 127 | J09(RS2) |
| 21. Galactosemia–enzyme defect, clinical features and biochemical findings. | 311 | D16(RS3), D99, D02, J05, D12, D16 |
| 22. Name the enzyme defective in galactosemia and hereditary fructose intolerance. | 373 | J02, D06 |
| 23. Aldolase B deficiency. | 332 | J98 |
| **METABOLISM OF LIPIDS** | | |
| **Long Essays** | | |
| 1. What is carnitine and its role in oxidation of fatty acids? Enumerate the steps of beta oxidation of saturated fatty acids (palmitic acid). Write a note on energetic of palmitic acid. Explain the regulation of acetyl CoA in our body. | 102, 270 | D08(RS2), J15(RS3), J01, D02, D04, J05, J06, D07, D10, D13, J15 |
| 2. Describe the process of ketogenesis and ketolysis. Write a note on ketosis. | 170 | J11(RS2), J11 |
| 3. What is ketosis? What are the causes? What are ketone bodies? Enumerate the steps of formation and utilization of ketone bodies. | 170 | J00 |
| 4. Name the ketone bodies. Give two conditions characterized by excessive production of ketone bodies. Explain the metabolic derangements and consequences of ketosis. | 170 | J05(RS2) |
| 5. Describe in detail the de novo synthesis of fatty acids. Add a note on short- and long-term mechanisms that regulate lipogenesis. | 237, 361 | J07 |
| 6. Give an account of cholesterol biosynthesis with its regulation. Add a note on atherosclerosis. | 297 | J16(RS3) |
| 7. What are lipoproteins? How are they classified? How are chylomicrons metabolized? | 10 | D09 |
| **Short Essays** | | |
| 1. List various types of fatty acid oxidation. Write about activation of fatty acids for oxidation. | 102 | D07(RS2), J07 |
| 2. Describe the beta oxidation of fatty acids. Add a note on energetics of palmitic acid oxidation. | 102 | D05(RS2), D14(RS3), D16(RS3), D05, J09 |
| 3. Ketone bodies—enumerate, formation (ketogenesis), utilization (ketolysis), clinical significance (ketosis). | 170 | J06(RS2), D09(RS2), D00, D06, J09, D12, D14 |
| 4. Ketosis. | 171 | J08 |
| 5. Outline the de novo synthesis of fatty acid. What are the advantages of having a multifunctional enzyme complex? | 237, 38 | D13(RS3) |
| 6. Fatty acid synthase complex | 38 | J11(RS2), D06, J09 |
| 7. Synthesis of triacylglycerol in adipose tissue | 332 | D98(OS) |
| 8. Microsomal chain elongation of fatty acids. | 354 | D98(OS) |

Contd...

| Questions | Page No. | Examinations |
|---|---|---|
| 9. Mention the defect and clinical features of four lipid storage disorder. | 358 | D16 |
| 10. Name the ring structure present in cholesterol. Write the key regulatory step in the synthesis of cholesterol. Name four compounds derived from cholesterol. | 297, 124 | D17(RS3) |
| 11. Outline the steps for synthesis of cholesterol. Discuss the rate limiting step and regulation of synthesis of cholesterol. | 297 | D11(RS3) |
| 12. How is HMG CoA formed? What is its importance? | 297 | D13 |
| 13. Catabolic products of cholesterol. Describe the biomedical importance of three derivatives of cholesterol. | 124 | J09(RS2), D10(RS2), J98, J03 |
| 14. Lipoproteins—enumerate, composition and functions. | 10 | J05(RS2), J13(RS3), J14(RS3), J02, D02, D03, J06, J10 |
| 15. Chylomicrons (metabolism). | 10 | J10(RS2) |
| 16. Give an account of metabolism of LDL. | 10 | D13 |
| 17. Fatty liver (causes) and lipotropic factors. | 52 | D06(RS2), J07(RS2), D08(RS2), D14(RS3), D07, D08, J13, D15 |
| **Short Answers** | | |
| 1. Role of carnitine in β-oxidation (carnitine cycle). | 102 | J06(RS2), J12, D13 |
| 2. Give enzyme defect in the methylmalonyl aciduria and homocystinuria. | 373 | D16 |
| 3. Refsum's disease | 98 | J08(RS2) |
| 4. Ketone bodies. | 170 | D08 |
| 5. Name the ketone bodies. Mention two causes of ketosis. | 170 | D02, J03, J04 |
| 6. Ketosis. | 171 | J17(RS3) |
| 7. Name the ketone bodies and the tests to detect them. | 368 | D99(OS), J08(OS) |
| 8. Name two lipid storage disorders and indicate the corresponding enzyme defect. | 358 | D07 |
| 9. Niemann-Pick disease. | 155 | J10(RS2) |
| 10. Name four substances synthesized from cholesterol. | 300 | D06 |
| 11. Name bile acids. How are they formed? | 273 | J10 |
| 12. Bile salts—enumerate, functions (role in digestion). | 274 | J99, J05, D08, D09, D11, J12 |
| 13. Describe the role of bile salts in lipid metabolism. | 274 | J13 |
| 14. Reverse cholesterol transport. | 280 | J15(RS3), D05 |
| 15. What is normal serum level of cholesterol? Name its four biological functions. | 299 | J07(RS2) |
| 16. What is the normal level of serum cholesterol? Name one bile acid formed from cholesterol. | 299, 273 | J07 |
| 17. Plasma lipoproteins—enumerate, functions. | 10 | J17(RS3), D98, J08, D12 |
| 18. HDL cholesterol. | 10 | D99, J12 |
| 19. Name the cholesterol rich lipoproteins. | 10 | D06 |
| 20. What are functions of apolipoproteins? | 127 | J09(RS2) |
| 21. Fatty liver—causes. | 52 | J00, D03, J06, J12, J14 |
| 22. Lipotropic factors. | 53 | J98, J13, D14 |
| 23. Enumerate the consequences of obesity. | 364 | J11 |
| 24. What is the significance of brown adipose tissue? | 346 | J04 |
| 25. Mention two inborn errors of lipid metabolism and indicate the enzyme defect. | 373 | D03 |

Contd...

| Questions | Page No. | Examinations |
|---|---|---|
| 26. Name the biochemical defect in:<br>a. Niemann-Pick disease<br>b. Gauchers disease. | 373 | J03 |
| **METABOLISM OF AMINO ACIDS** | | |
| **Long Essays** | | |
| 1. What are the sources of ammonia in the body? Add a note on its transportation. Describe how ammonia is detoxified in the body and name two inborn errors associated with this process. | 178 | D01, J05, D06, J12, D16 |
| 2. Describe in detail the steps of urea cycle. How is it linked to TCA cycle? What is the reference range for serum urea? Write the causes of uremia. | 178 | D11(RS3) |
| 3. Describe the urea cycle. What is the normal blood urea level? Name two conditions in which blood urea level increases. | 178 | D02 |
| 4. Describe the metabolism, metabolic defects and special products formed from glycine giving their biomedical importance. Why is glycine nutritionally nonessential? | 22 | D05(RS2), J02, J04, D07 |
| 5. How is creatinine synthesized? Discuss about creatinine clearance and its clinical significance. | 23, 30 | J99 |
| 6. What are biologically important compounds derived from tyrosine? Describe the metabolism of phenylalanine and tyrosine. Outline the synthesis of different products obtained from Phenylalanine. Discuss the inborn errors associated with metabolism (tyrosinemia). | 158 | D10(RS2), J12(RS3), J17(RS3), D99, J01, D04, J07, J08, J10 |
| 7. Name the sulfur-containing amino acids. Describe in detail the metabolism of essential sulfur containing amino acid and add a note on the special products synthesized from it. Add a note on inborn errors associated with its pathway. | 232, 108 | D05, D12 |
| 8. What is the active form of methionine? How it is formed? What are its function? Enumerate the steps of methionine metabolism. Write the disorders associated with its metabolism. | 233, 108 | J00 |
| **Short Essays** | | |
| 1. What are nitrogen producing substances in the body? Explain how they are excreted from the body. | 322 | D17(RS3) |
| 2. Write about aminoaciduria. | 358 | J07 |
| 3. What are transamination reactions? Giving two examples discuss the importance of these reactions. | 41 | J13(RS3), D16(RS3), J06, J11, D15 |
| 4. Describe transamination. Mention the clinical significance of serum transaminases. | 41, 236 | J05 |
| 5. Name the coenzyme forms of vitamin $B_6$. Write the mechanism of transamination. | 41 | J01 |
| 6. Transamination and deamination. | 41, 339 | J09(OS) |
| 7. How ammonia is detoxified in the body? | 178 | J06(RS2), J09 |
| 8. Urea cycle (urea formation in liver)—steps, regulations, disorders. | 178 | D06(RS2), J07(RS2), D00, D03, D10, D12, D14 |
| 9. How is urea synthesized in the body? Give the reactions. What is the significance of urea cycle? | 178 | D13(RS3) |
| 10. Disorders associated with urea cycle. | 180 | D15 |
| 11. How is glycine synthesized in the body? Name the products synthesized from glycine (biomedical importance/metabolic role/fate of glycine). | 22 | D06(RS2), D17(RS3), J98, D09, D15 |
| 12. Compounds synthesized from glycine and enumerate the steps of synthesis of creatine. | 22 | J12 |
| 13. How creatine phosphate is synthesized? Mention the significance of estimation of urinary creatinine. | 23, 30 | D01 |
| 14. How is creatine synthesized? Add a note on creatinine clearance test with respect to its reference range and significance. | 23, 30 | D11 |

Contd...

| QUESTIONS | PAGE No. | EXAMINATIONS |
|---|---|---|
| 15. Biochemical importance of phenylalanine. | 158 | J15 |
| 16. Is tyrosine an essential amino acid? Justify. Write the reactions of three important biological products formed from tyrosine. | 158 | D12(RS3) |
| 17. List the important products formed from tyrosine and write the metabolic pathways leading to the formation of any two of them. | 158 | D07(RS2) |
| 18. Name and explain the steps of formation of three important compounds formed from tyrosine. | 158 | J14 |
| 19. Mention the catecholamines. How are they formed? | 309 | D16(RS3), D03 |
| 20. Outline the synthesis of epinephrine and give its functions. | 309 | J15(RS3) |
| 21. What is PKU (phenylketonuria)? What are the alternate metabolic pathways for the accumulated phenylalanine? How is it diagnosed biochemically? | 160 | D09(RS2), D10 |
| 22. Discuss phenylketonuria under: (i) enzyme defect, (ii) Manifestation, (iii) Diagnostic test. | 160 | D15(RS3) |
| 23. Describe tryptophan metabolism. | 300 | J16(RS3) |
| 24. Serotonin. | 197 | J08(RS2), D98, D99 |
| 25. Describe the fate and functions of methionine. | 231 | D13(RS3) |
| 26. Explain how S-adenosyl methionine is formed. Give examples of five transmethylation reactions. | 233 | J15 |
| 27. S-Adenosyl methionine—formation, functions. | 233 | D00, D09 |
| 28. Metabolic functions of methionine. | 232 | D05, D13 |
| 29. Transmethylation reactions with examples. | 150 | J09(RS2), J10(RS2), J12(RS3), J12 |
| 30. Describe the conversion of methionine to cysteine. Add a note on homocystinuria. | 8, 275 | J15(RS3) |
| 31. Metabolic functions of cysteine. | 7 | J05(RS2) |
| 32. Disorders of sulfur-containing amino acids. | 108 | D08(RS2) |
| 33. Cystinuria and homocystinurias. | 108 | J11 |
| 34. Describe one carbon metabolism. What is its significance? | 286 | D15(RS3), D07 |
| 35. Maple syrup urine disease | 126 | J09(RS2) |
| 36. Name the biochemical defect in the following disorders of amino acid metabolism.<br>a. Phenylketonuria.<br>b. Alkaptonuria.<br>c. Maple syrup urine disease.<br>d. Albinism.<br>e. Homocystinuria. | 373 | D01 |
| 37. Name the enzyme defective in:<br>a. Alkaptonuria.<br>b. Niemann-Pick disease.<br>c. Albinism.<br>d. Gaucher's disease. | 373 | D05 |
| **Short Answers** | | |
| 1. Carbamoyl phosphate synthetases. | 368 | D08(OS) |
| 2. Transamination reaction and clinical importance. | 41 | J09(RS2), D13(RS3) |
| 3. Formation of ammonia and its toxicity in brain. | 140 | D09(RS2) |
| 4. Formation of glutamine and its importance. | 362 | D12 |
| 5. Carbamoyl phosphate synthetase deficiency. | 180 | J98 |
| 6. What is the normal level of npn substances in the blood? | 81 | J08 |
| 7. Significance of non-protein nitrogenous substances. | 81 | J07(RS2) |

Contd...

| Questions | Page No. | Examinations |
|---|---|---|
| 8. Mention the compounds formed from glycine. | 22 | D03, J13, D14 |
| 9. How is creatinine synthesized? | 23 | J15, D16 |
| 10. Name the amino acid used for the synthesis of creatinine. | 23 | J07 |
| 11. Biologically important compounds derived from tyrosine. | 158 | D08(RS2), J11, D11 |
| 12. Melanin synthesis. | 159 | D15 |
| 13. Name two metabolic disorders of amino acids metabolism and indicate the enzyme defect. | 373 | D07 |
| 14. Phenylketonuria (PKU). | 160 | D00 |
| 15. Indicate the biochemical defect in phenylketonuria. | 160 | J14 |
| 16. Mention the enzyme defects in phenylketonuria and homocystinuria. | 373 | J05 |
| 17. Name the enzyme defect in: (a) Phenylketonuria, (b) Alkaptonuria. | 373 | D14 |
| 18. Alkaptonuria. | 161 | D14(RS3), J12, D15 |
| 19. Albinism. | 162 | J13 |
| 20. Derivatives of tryptophan. | 197 | J12(RS3), D05, D16 |
| 21. Serotonin—formation, functions of serotonin. | 197 | D12(RS3), J00, D00 |
| 22. Melatonin. | 198 | D15(RS3) |
| 23. Name the sulfur-containing amino acids. List two disorders of their metabolism. | 108 | D02 |
| 24. Hartnup's disease. | 197 | J12(RS3), J17(RS3), D14 |
| 25. S-adenosyl methionine (active methionine)—formation. | 233 | D98, D11 |
| 26. Homocysteine. | 367 | J09 |
| 27. Functions of cysteine. | 7 | D15 |
| 28. Enumerate the metabolic disorders associated with cysteine metabolism indicating the defect. | 108 | J02 |
| 29. What is meant by inborn error of metabolism? What is homocystinuria? | 108 | D11 |
| 30. Maple syrup urine disease. | 126 | J00 |
| 31. Name the deficient enzyme in: (a) Hyperargininemia, (b) Phenylketonuria. | 373 | J13 |
| 32. What is carnitine? Mention its biochemical role (in β oxidation). | 102 | J02, J13, D14 |
| 33. Polyamines. | 293 | D15(RS3) |
| 34. Name the biochemical defect in: a. Phenylketonuria. b. Maple syrup urine disease. | 373 | J03 |
| **INTEGRATION OF METABOLISM** | | |
| **Short Essay** | | |
| 1. Discuss the biochemical/metabolic changes during starvation. | 253 | J14(RS3), J03, J13, D14 |
| **Short Answers** | | |
| 1. Sources and fate of acetyl CoA. | 270 | D01, J12 |
| 2. Biochemical changes in starvation. | 253 | J16(RS3) |
| **METABOLISM OF NUCLEOTIDES** | | |
| **Long Essays** | | |
| 1. What are nucleotides? Explain the catabolism of purine nucleotides. Write briefly on the metabolic disorders associated with purine metabolism. | 62 | J07(RS2) |
| 2. What are sources of C and N atoms of purine? Describe the biosynthesis of purine and add a note on its regulation. | 214 | J13(RS3) |

Contd...

| Questions | Page No. | Examinations |
|---|---|---|
| 3. Enumerate the reactions of purine degradation and add a note on Gout. | 62 | J13 |
| 4. Describe the synthesis of pyrimidine and its regulation. | 203 | D12(RS3) |
| **Short Essays** | | |
| 1. What are nucleotides? What are the sources of C and N atoms of purine nucleotide? Mention the metabolic disorders associated with purine metabolism. | 214, 62 | J14(RS3) |
| 2. Briefly outline the steps of de novo synthesis of purine. | 214 | D11(RS3), J12(RS3) |
| 3. Purine salvage pathways. | 31 | D06(RS2), J15(RS3), D08, J11, D13, D14 |
| 4. Salvage pathway. | 31 | J12(RS3), D05(RS2) |
| 5. Catabolism (degradation) of purines and related disorders. | 62 | D06(RS2), D09(RS2), D10(RS2), D13(RS3), D09, J11 |
| 6. Synthesis of uric acid. | 62 | J98 |
| 7. How is uric acid formed in the body? What is gout? What is the treatment? Explain the basis for the treatment. | 62 | D15(RS3) |
| 8. Hyperuricemia—causes, features and drugs to lower plasma uric acid levels. | 63 | J04, J10 |
| 9. What is gout? Give its biochemical basis, clinical manifestations and line of treatment. | 63 | D12(RS3), D16(RS3), D99, D00, D07, D11 |
| 10. Lesch-Nyhan syndrome and orotic aciduria. | 15 | J05(RS2), D08(RS2) |
| 11. Degradation of pyrimidines. | 97 | J08(RS2) |
| **Short Answers** | | |
| 1. Indicate sources of various (carbon and nitrogen) atoms of purine ring by a diagrammatic representation. | 214 | D09(RS2), D03, D07 |
| 2. Describe two reactions of salvage pathway of purine nucleotide synthesis. | 31 | J05 |
| 3. Mention any two causes of hyperuricemia. | 63 | J06 |
| 4. Gout—causes. | 63 | J05(RS2), D01 |
| 5. What is the normal serum uric acid level? Name two pathological conditions associated with hyperuricemia. | 63 | D02 |
| 6. Lesch-Nyhan syndrome—causes, features. | 15 | J10(RS2), D14(RS3), D03, J08, J15 |
| 7. Identify the sources of carbon and nitrogen atoms of pyrimidine ring. | 203 | D13 |
| 8. Deficiency features of orotic aciduria. Explain the biochemical basis of manifestations. | 16 | J11(RS2), J07, J10, D16 |
| **MINERAL METABOLISM** | | |
| **Long Essays** | | |
| 1. Describe in detail the sources, daily requirement, absorption, distribution, functions, normal level and factors regulating blood calcium level. Discuss about any clinical condition with abnormal blood calcium level (tetany). | 121 | D06(RS2), J09(RS2), D00, D01, J12, D14 |
| 2. Explain the metabolism of iron under the following headings. (a) Absorption and transport, (b) Biochemical functions, (c) Hemosiderosis. | 76, 338 | D13 |
| **Short Essays** | | |
| 1. List any three trace elements with their biological function. | 316 | J17(RS3) |
| 2. Calcium—sources, daily requirements, factors affecting absorption, biochemical role (functions) and deficiency signs of calcium. | 121 | J12(RS3), J98, D99, D03, J09, D11 |
| 3. Intestinal absorption of calcium. | 121 | J15 |
| 4. Calcium homeostasis (regulation of blood calcium level)—by vitamin D, PTH and calcitonin. | 122 | D09(RS2), J00, J02, D07, D13 |

Contd...

| Questions | Page No. | Examinations |
|---|---|---|
| 5. Write briefly about the role of parathyroid hormone in the regulations of serum calcium level. | 123 | J06 |
| 6. Give an account of phosphorus metabolism. | 221 | J13(RS3) |
| 7. What are the major biochemical functions of sodium and potassium? Mention their normal serum levels. | 207 | D12(RS3), D03 |
| 8. What is the normal range of serum potassium and write about hypokalemia. | 165 | D10(RS2) |
| 9. Iron—source, daily requirement, absorption, factors affecting iron absorption, transports, storage and physiological role iron. | 76 | J07(RS2), D12(RS3), D16(RS3), D98, D99, D02, J04, J07, J10, J13, D15 |
| 10. What are the causes and consequences of iron toxicity? | 338 | D16 |
| 11. What is Wilson's disease? State the cause and treatment policy. | 323 | D17(RS3) |
| 12. Functions of iodine. | 174 | J11(RS2) |
| 13. Biological role of zinc in the body. | 43 | J06(RS2) |
| 14. Functions of selenium. | 153 | J10(RS2) |
| **Short Answers** | | |
| 1. Trace elements. | 316 | D06(RS2), D08(RS2) |
| 2. Functions of calcium. | 122 | J11, D16 |
| 3. Calcitriol. | 123 | J98 |
| 4. What is the normal serum calcium level? Explain its regulation. | 121 | D05(RS2), J05 |
| 5. List the hormones in plasma calcium regulation. | 123 | D06 |
| 6. Write short note on rickets. | 74 | J13 |
| 7. Functions of magnesium. | 317 | J09 |
| 8. Hyponatremia (causes). | 363 | J98 |
| 9. Describe the functions of potassium. | 207 | J05 |
| 10. Iron—absorption, transport and storage. | 76 | D10(RS2), D00, D10 |
| 11. Ferritin. | 79 | D08 |
| 12. Causes of hemochromatosis. | 338 | J01, D04 |
| 13. What is hemosiderosis? How it is caused? | 338 | D02 |
| 14. Functions of copper. | 317 | J12(RS3), D09 |
| 15. Copper containing protein and its clinical significance. | 317 | J98 |
| 16. Four enzymes with copper as integral component. | 317 | D12(RS3), J02, D08 |
| 17. Wilson's disease. | 323 | J00 |
| 18. Menkes disease. | 199 | J12(RS3) |
| 19. Iodine metabolism. | 87 | D07(RS2) |
| 20. Importance of iodine. | 174 | J14(RS3) |
| 21. Describe the functions of iodine and fluorine. | 174, 317 | J05 |
| 22. Mention the functions of:<br>a. Iodine<br>b. Zinc. | 174<br>43 | D01 |
| 23. Functions (metabolic roles) of zinc and selenium. | 43, 153 | J05(RS2), J01, D04 |
| 24. Biological role of zinc in the body. | 43 | D98, J99, J08, J10, J12, J14 |
| 25. Name a zinc containing enzyme and its catalytic role. | 43 | D05 |

Contd...

| Questions | Page No. | Examinations |
|---|---|---|
| 26. Fluorosis. | 99 | J08(RS2) |
| 27. Metabolic role of selenium. | 153 | D99, D08, J15 |
| 28. Functions of fluoride in dental health. | 317 | J07 |
| **SECTION FOUR: CLINICAL BIOCHEMISTRY AND NUTRITION** | | |
| **HORMONES** | | |
| **Short Essays** | | |
| 1. General mechanism of action of steroid hormones. | 95 | J08(RS2) |
| 2. Give a diagrammatic representation of mechanism of steroid hormone action. | 95 | D12(RS3) |
| **Short Answers** | | |
| 1. What is second messenger? Give an example. | 365 | D11 |
| 2. Mechanism of action of steroid hormones. | 95 | D14(RS3) |
| 3. Give a diagrammatic representation of action of a steroid hormone. | 95 | J05 |
| 4. Cyclic AMP—functions. | 369 | D03 |
| 5. Laboratory diagnosis for hypothyroidism. | 304 | J16(RS3) |
| 6. Thyroid function test—routine and anti-TPO. | 186 | D11(RS3) |
| 7. Reference range of TSH and its significance. | 143 | D11 |
| Clinical interpretation of estimation of thyroid stimulating hormone (TSH) in blood. | 143 | D09(RS2) |
| **ORGAN FUNCTION TEST** | | |
| **Short Essays** | | |
| 1. Liver function tests (based on secretary/metabolic and excretory functions). | 110 | D08(RS2), J14(RS3), J98, J01, D03, J06, J10, D10, J11 |
| 2. Vander Bergh's reaction (principle) and its clinical significance. | 111 | D00, J13, J15 |
| 3. Serum enzymes estimated to access the liver function. | 114 | D98 |
| 4. Hippuric acid test. | 113 | D15 |
| 5. Describe renal function tests. | 175 | J02, J05 |
| 6. Clearance tests. | 29 | J06(RS2), J15 |
| 7. Define renal clearance. Name clearance tests used to asses kidney function. Explain any one of the clearance tests and mention its significance. | 29 | D05(RS2) |
| 8. Creatinine clearance test. | 30 | D08 |
| 9. Standard urea clearance test. | 194 | J12(RS3) |
| 10. Concentration dilution test. | 176 | D15 |
| **Short Answers** | | |
| 1. Test for urobilinogen. | 349 | J99 |
| 2. Enumerate three/four functions of the liver and tests with reference ranges to assess them. | 110 | D11(RS3), D07 |
| 3. Describe Vander Bergh's reaction. Mention its significance. | 111 | J99, J04, D14 |
| 4. Write short note on enzyme assays for liver function/Marker enzymes of liver function test. | 114 | D16(RS3), D13 |
| 5. Enumerate renal function tests. | 175 | J11(RS2), D03 |
| 6. Tests to assess renal tubular function. | 319 | J17(RS3) |
| 7. Tests of renal distal tubular function. | 320 | J16(RS3) |
| 8. What is meant by renal clearance? How is creatinine clearance calculated? | 29 | D14(RS3) |

Contd...

| Questions | Page No. | Examinations |
|---|---|---|
| 9. Clearance tests. | 29 | D06(RS2) |
| 10. Creatinine clearance test. | 30 | J09(RS2), J13(RS3), D14 |
| 11. Name any two tests of assessment of gastric function and define the basal acid out. | 343 | J10(OS) |
| **WATER, ELECTROLYTE AND ACID-BASE BALANCE** | | |
| **Long Essays** | | |
| 1. What is the normal pH of blood? Explain the mechanism of how it is regulated. | 190 | J12(RS3) |
| 2. What is the importance of maintaining acid-base balance in the body? Write in detail how kidney helps in maintaining acid-base balance. | 190 | D07(RS2) |
| **Short Essays** | | |
| 1. Regulation of water balance. | 338 | J08(OS) |
| 2. Hormonal regulation of fluid and electrolyte. | 185 | D11(RS3), D16 |
| 3. Discuss the regulation of water by rennin-angiotensin system. | 185 | D17(RS3) |
| 4. Define pH and buffer. Mention the buffer systems present in plasma, erythrocytes and urine. | 190 | J02 |
| 5. What is Henderson-Hasselbalch equation? Describe the buffer systems in blood and urine. | 252, 190 | J05 |
| 6. What are buffers? Discuss any two buffer system of the body. | 190 | J13(RS3) |
| 7. What are Buffers? Explain the plasma buffers in maintaining acid-base balance. | 190 | J16(RS3) |
| 8. Name the buffer system of body fluids. Explain any one of them. | 190 | D05(RS2) |
| 9. Blood buffers and their role in acid-base balance. | 190 | J06(RS2), D99, J06 |
| 10. Write the Henderson-Hasselbalch equation and its significance in bicarbonate buffer system. | 252 | J14(RS3) |
| 11. Bicarbonate buffer system of blood. | 191 | J09(RS2) |
| 12. Extracellular buffers. | 191 | J10(RS2) |
| 13. What are buffers? Explain the role of the kidneys in homeostasis of pH of blood. | 190 | D11 |
| 14. Use of phosphate buffer in maintaining acid base balance. | 191 | D10 |
| 15. Renal regulation and respiratory regulation of body pH. | 191 | D00, D01, D03 |
| 16. Role of lungs in pH maintenance (respiratory regulation of pH). | 193 | D08 |
| 17. Renal regulation of acid-base balance (give the key reactions of renal mechanism in acid base balance). | 191 | D06(RS2), D09(RS2), D11(RS3), D12(RS3), J15(RS3), J09, J12, J14, D14 |
| 18. Chloride shift. | 95 | J08(RS2) |
| 19. What is anion gap? Explain normal anion gap acidosis and high anion gap acidosis with examples. | 15 | J05(RS2), D10(RS2), D09 |
| 20. How does metabolic alkalosis differ from respiratory alkalosis? Explain the cause and compensatory mechanism involved? | 312 | J00 |
| 21. Metabolic acidosis—causes, biochemical findings. | 96 | J08(RS2), J98, J11 |
| 22. Explain metabolic and respiratory acidosis. | 79 | J07(RS2) |
| 23. What are the causes of respiratory acidosis? List the primary abnormalities of respiratory acidosis. | 265 | D14(RS3), J01 |
| 24. Respiratory alkalosis. | 289 | D15(RS3) |
| **Short Answers** | | |
| 1. Hormones that regulate water balance. | 281 | J15(RS3) |
| 2. Define buffers. Name the blood buffer system. | 190 | J00, J01, D04, J08, D14 |


Contd...

| QUESTIONS | PAGE No. | EXAMINATIONS |
|---|---|---|
| 3. What are buffers? Write the importance of bicarbonate buffer system? | 190 | D13 |
| 4. Bicarbonate buffer. | 191 | J15 |
| 5. How does a buffer maintain the pH? Give an example of blood buffer. | 190 | D06 |
| 6. List the major kidney mechanism for regulation of pH of extracellular fluid. | 191 | D09 |
| 7. Carbonic anhydrase. | 346 | D99, D15 |
| 8. Discuss the role of carbonic anhydrase in the acid-base regulation. | 325 | D17(RS3) |
| 9. Reclamation of bicarbonate by kidneys. | 192 | J01, D04 |
| 10. Chloride bicarbonate shift. | 95 | D98 |
| 11. Give an account of anion gap. | 15 | J14 |
| 12. What is anion gap? Mention two causes for increased anion gap. | 15 | J03 |
| 13. Define anion gap. What happens to anion gap in acidosis resulting from renal failure? | 15 | J07 |
| 14. Metabolic acidosis—causes and features. | 96 | J04 |
| 15. Define respiratory acidosis. How is it compensated? | 265 | D13 |
| 16. Respiratory acidosis—causes. | 265 | J10 |
| 17. Alkalosis. | 312 | D16(RS3) |
| **TISSUE PROTEINS AND BODY FLUIDS** | | |
| **Short Answer** | | |
| 1. Discuss the nutritional role of milk and dairy products. | 325 | D17(RS3) |
| **NUTRITION** | | |
| **Short Essays** | | |
| 1. Basal metabolic rate (BMR)—definition, determination, normal value, factors affecting. | 45 | J06(RS2), D07(RS2), J09(RS2), D13(RS3), J08, J09, J12 |
| 2. What is meant by dietary fiber? What are the sources of dietary fibers? Discuss the importance of it in nutrition. Outline the functions of proteins. | 264, 279 | D14(RS3), J15(RS3) |
| 3. Nitrogen balance—factors affecting. | 17 | J05(RS2), J11(RS2) |
| 4. Define biological value of protein. What do you mean by complementary proteins? Give examples. What is the requirement of protein in diet? | 315 | J17(RS3), J14 |
| 5. What is a balanced diet? Discuss the components of a balanced diet. | 279 | J15(RS3), D13 |
| 6. Protein energy malnutrition. | 152 | J10(RS2), D11(RS3), D08 |
| 7. Describe the causes and features of kwashiorkar and marasmus. | 152 | J05 |
| **Short Answers** | | |
| 1. Respiratory quotient (RQ)—definition, RQ values of carbohydrate, lipids and proteins, factor affecting, conditions associated with lowering RQ. | 157 | J10(RS2), D01, J04, J05, D05, D10, D14, D15 |
| 2. Basal metabolic rate (BMR)—definition, factors affecting, causes of increased BMR. | 45 | J02, J04, D09, J10 |
| 3. Specific dynamic action (SDA) and basal metabolic rate (BMR). | 199, 45 | D12(RS3) |
| 4. Specific dynamic action (SDA) of food stuff. | 199 | J12(RS3), J15(RS3), J16(RS3), D07, D12, J15 |
| 5. Dietary fiber—sources, examples, beneficial effects (role in health and disease). | 264 | D07(RS2), D08(RS2), J10(RS2), D10(RS2), J00, J01, J02, D04, D10, J13 |
| 6. Nitrogen balance. | 17 | D11 |
| 7. Positive nitrogen balance. | 18 | D10 |
| 8. Biological value of protein. | 315 | J15 |

Contd...

| Questions | Page No. | Examinations |
|---|---|---|
| 9. Limiting amino acid. | 100 | J08(RS2) |
| 10. Balanced diet. | 279 | J16(RS3), J98, D99, D13 |
| 11. Protein energy malnutrition (biochemical changes). | 152 | J07(RS2), D10(RS2), D16(RS3), J13 |
| 12. Kwashiorkor—biochemical findings. | 153 | D02, D15 |
| 13. Marasmus | 152 | D98, J06 |
| 14. List two differences between marasmus and kwashiorkor. | 152 | D01 |
| 15. Nutritional deficiency anemias. | 35 | D05(RS2) |
| **SECTION FIVE: MOLECULAR BIOLOGY AND BIOTECHNOLOGY** | | |
| **DEOXYRIBONUCLEIC ACID (DNA)—REPLICATION, RECOMBINATION AND REPAIR** | | |
| **Long Essays** | | |
| 1. Discuss the structure and replication of DNA. | 146 | J10(RS2) |
| 2. Describe the synthesis of DNA. Write a note on replication of DNA. | 147 | D15(RS3) |
| 3. Define replication. Describe in detail the process of replication in eukaryotes. Mention its inhibitors. | 147 | D14(RS3), J16(RS3) |
| 4. Write about DNA replication and repair. | 147, 327 | J13 |
| **Short Essays** | | |
| 1. What is replication? Describe the steps of replication. | 147 | D00, D02, D07 |
| 2. Describe the replication of DNA. | 147 | J05 |
| 3. Replication of lagging strand. | 149 | D07(RS2) |
| 4. Mutations (point mutation). | 16 | J05(RS2) |
| 5. Point mutation—define and effects. | 17 | D17(RS3) |
| 6. Base excision DNA repair mechanism. | 327 | J10 |
| **Short Answers** | | |
| 1. Name bacterial DNA polymerases. Mention its significance. | 34 | D05(RS2) |
| 2. What is nucleotide excision repair? | 328 | J07 |
| 3. Causes for xeroderma pigmentosum. | 211 | D12(RS3) |
| 4. Replication of DNA. | 147 | D98, J09 |
| 5. What is meant by semiconservative mechanism of replication? | 147 | J10 |
| 6. Okazaki fragments. | 318 | J17(RS3), J15, D16 |
| 7. What is mutation? List two examples. | 16 | J02, D14 |
| 8. Mutagens. | 317 | J17(RS3) |
| 9. Point mutation with two examples. | 17 | J15(RS3), D15(RS3), J12 |
| 10. Missense mutation—list the effects. | 17 | J10, D15 |
| 11. Silent mutation. | 17 | J15 |
| **TRANSCRIPTION AND TRANSLATION** | | |
| **Long Essays** | | |
| 1. Give a detailed account of the eukaryotic transcription process. How is it regulated? Name the inhibitors of transcription. | 53 | J14 |
| 2. Define translation (protein biosynthesis). Describe the steps of translation. Name four inhibitors and their action. | 1 | J14(RS3), J17(RS3) |
| 3. What is genetic code? Describe the process of eukaryotic translation. | 173, 1 | J11(RS2) |


Contd...

| QUESTIONS | PAGE No. | EXAMINATIONS |
|---|---|---|
| 4. What is Lac operon? Explain the steps of activation, initiation, elongation and termination of protein biosynthesis and its regulation. | 240, 1 | J05(RS2), D08(RS2), D10(RS2), D11 |
| **Short Essays** | | |
| 1. Transcription (factors required). | 53 | D06(RS2), D01, J06 |
| 2. Post-transcriptional modifications of mRNA. | 139 | D09(RS2), D16(RS3), J10, D12 |
| 3. Genetic code—definition (Codon), salient features, initiating and terminating codon. | 173 | D06(RS2), J08(RS2), J17(RS3), D17(RS3), D03, J15 |
| 4. Write part played by ribosomes in proteins biosynthesis. | 347 | J00 |
| 5. Post-translational modification. | 225 | D15 |
| **Short Answers** | | |
| 1. RNA polymerase. | 313 | D16(RS3), D15 |
| 2. Name the post-transcriptional modifications of m-RNA. | 139 | D06 |
| 3. Name two inhibitors of RNA synthesis. | 56 | D05 |
| 4. Reverse transcriptase and its significance. | 343 | J01, J03, D04, J06 |
| 5. Codon and its characteristics. Name the chain initiating codon and chain terminating codons. | 173 | J99, D99, J05, D07 |
| 6. Genetic code—characteristic features. | 173 | D09(RS2), D10(RS2) |
| 7. Degeneracy of codon. | 173 | J01, D04, D09 |
| 8. Write short note on codon and 'Wobble hypothesis.' | 173, 226 | D13 |
| 9. Wobble phenomenon. | 226 | J15 |
| 10. Which are inhibitors of protein biosynthesis? | 5 | J07(RS2) |
| 11. Post-translational modifications with examples. | 225 | J13(RS3), D07 |
| **REGULATION OF GENE EXPRESSION** | | |
| **Short Essays** | | |
| 1. Describe with an example regulation of gene expression. | 240 | D13(RS3) |
| 2. Lac operon concept of gene regulation. | 240 | D17(RS3), J11 |
| **Short Answer** | | |
| 1. Operon concept. | 240 | D11(RS3) |
| **RECOMBINANT DNA TECHNOLOGY** | | |
| **Long Essay** | | |
| 1. Discuss in detail recombinant DNA technology and its clinical application. | 93 | J08(RS2) |
| **Short Essays** | | |
| 1. Recombinant DNA technology and its applications. | 93 | D08(RS2), J16(RS3), D16(RS3), J17(RS3), J03, J04, D08, D10, D15 |
| 2. What is the difference between endonuclease and restriction endonuclease? Give two examples for endonuclease. | 287 | D15(RS3) |
| 3. What is a restriction endonuclease? Give any two examples with their biomedical importance. Explain their role in recombinant DNA technology. | 287 | J13(RS3), J16(RS3) |
| 4. What is plasmid? What is its application in recombinant DNA technology? | 75 | J07(RS2), J10 |
| 5. Explain the principle, requirements, steps of polymerase chain reaction and its application. | 43 | D14(RS3), J15, D16 |

Contd...

| Questions | Page No. | Examinations |
|---|---|---|
| **Short Answers** | | |
| 1. What is the difference between endonuclease and restriction endonuclease? Give two examples of restriction endonuclease. | 287 | D08(RS2) |
| 2. What are restriction enzymes? List three features of restriction enzymes. | 287 | D14(RS3) |
| 3. What are restriction endonucleases? Give two examples. | 287 | D03 |
| 4. What is a chimeric (recombinant) DNA molecule? Give the applications of recombinant technology. | 189, 94 | D09(RS2), D11(RS3), D05, D11, D12 |
| 5. Southern blot techniques. | 258 | J14(RS3) |
| 6. What is polymerase chain reaction (PCR)? Mention application of PCR. | 43 | J05(RS2), J06(RS2), J09(RS2), J14(RS3), J04 |
| 7. What are DNA probes? Mention the types DNA probes. | 324 | D17(RS3) |
| 8. What is restriction fragment length polymorphism? Give one clinical application for the same. | 345 | J07 |
| **SECTION SIX: CURRENT TOPICS** | | |
| **HUMAN GENOME PROJECT** | | |
| None | | |
| **GENE THERAPY** | | |
| **Short Essay** | | |
| 1. Gene therapy—its application in medicine. | 85 | D07(RS2), D13(RS3), D09, D12 |
| **Short Answer** | | |
| 1. What is gene therapy? Name vectors used for gene therapy. | 85 | D05(RS2) |
| **BIOINFORMATICS** | | |
| None | | |
| **METABOLISM OF XENOBIOTICS (DETOXIFICATION)** | | |
| **Short Essays** | | |
| 1. What is biotransformation? Discuss the different phases of biotransformation with an example. | 27 | J14(RS3) |
| 2. Detoxification with examples of reactions involved. | 27 | D05(RS2), J05, J13 |
| 3. Define detoxification. Give any four reactions of phase II detoxification. | 27 | J17(RS3) |
| 4. What is detoxification? Explain the role of oxidation and conjugation reactions in the liver for detoxification. | 27 | D11 |
| 5. Detoxification by oxidation. | 27 | J11(RS2) |
| 6. Detoxification by conjugation with examples | 28 | D10 |
| **Short Answers** | | |
| 1. What are xenobiotics? What is the role of Glutathione in detoxification. | 166 | D10(RS2) |
| 2. What is biotransformation? Give two examples. | 27 | D02 |
| 3. Detoxification. | 27 | D17(RS3), J11 |
| 4. Explain any one detoxification mechanism with an example. | 27 | D12 |
| 5. Detoxification reaction—phase I. | 27 | D14(RS3) |
| 6. Give two examples of detoxification by oxidation and reduction. | 27 | D09(RS2) |
| 7. Detoxification of alcohol. | 129 | J09(RS2) |
| 8. Role of cytochrome $P_{450}$ in detoxification reaction | 114 | D08(RS2), D14 |
| 9. Conjugation as detoxification mechanism with two examples. | 28 | J06(RS2), J07(RS2), D98 |

Contd...

| Questions | Page No. | Examinations |
|---|---|---|
| **PROSTAGLANDINS AND RELATED COMPOUNDS** | | |
| **Short Essays** | | |
| 1. What are eicosanoids? Mention their biomedical importance. | 267 | J02 |
| 2. Prostaglandins—classification and biological action. | 268 | J09(RS2), D98, J07 |
| **Short Answers** | | |
| 1. Eicosanoids—names/functions. | 267 | D14(RS3), J08, D16 |
| 2. What are prostaglandins? Mention their biological functions. | 268 | D06(RS2), D13(RS3), D01, D10 |
| 3. What is arachidonic acid? Mention two uses of arachidonic acid. | 267 | J10 |
| **BIOLOGICAL MEMBRANES AND TRANSPORT** | | |
| **Short Essays** | | |
| 1. Cell membrane—fluid mosaic model. | 137 | D09(RS2), D17(RS3), J14 |
| 2. Transport across cell-membrane. | 290 | D09, J11 |
| 3. Facilitated diffusion. | 292 | D10 |
| 4. Active transport. | 290 | J15 |
| 5. Sodium-potassium pump. | 360 | J10 |
| 6. Classify transport mechanisms across cell membranes. Define uniport, symport and antiport. Give an example of each. | 180 | D11(RS3) |
| **Short Answers** | | |
| 1. Write four structural features of cell membrane. | 138 | J13 |
| 2. Cell membrane—functions. | 138 | D07(RS2), J09 |
| 3. Transport across cell membrane. | 290 | D15(RS3) |
| 4. Define the term active and passive transport. | 290 | J13 |
| 5. Describe secondary active transport. Mention one disorder of secondary active transport. | 290 | J05 |
| 6. Active transport. | 290 | J11(RS2), D06 |
| 7. What is uniport and symport transport system? Give an example. | 181 | D11 |
| 8. Endocytosis. | 290 | D08, J11 |
| **FREE RADICALS AND ANTIOXIDANTS** | | |
| **Short Essays** | | |
| 1. Antioxidants. | 94 | J08(RS2), J99, D04 |
| 2. Antioxidant vitamins. | 94 | D06 |
| **Short Answers** | | |
| 1. Free radicals—definition, generation, functions. | 18 | J05(RS2), J12(RS3), D10 |
| 2. Reactive oxygen species (ROS)—enumerate, formation, characteristics. | 115 | D08(RS2), D10(RS2) |
| 3. Free radicals and disease. | 18 | J11(RS2) |
| 4. Antioxidants with examples. | 94 | D06(RS2), D11(RS3), D12(RS3), J15(RS3), D98, D03 |
| 5. What are antioxidants? Name chain breaking and preventive antioxidants. | 94 | J07(RS2) |
| 6. Nonenzymatic antioxidants. | 94 | J16(RS3) |
| 7. Mention the dietary antioxidants. | 94 | J14 |
| **ENVIRONMENTAL BIOCHEMISTRY** | | |
| None | | |

Contd...

| Questions | Page No. | Examinations |
|---|---|---|
| **INSULIN, GLUCOSE HOMEOSTASIS AND DIABETES MELLITUS** | | |
| **Long Essay** | | |
| 1. What is the normal blood glucose level? Why does it need to be regulated? Describe the regulation of blood glucose. What are the causes of hyperglycemia and hypoglycemia? | 131 | D09(RS2), D14(RS3), D03 |
| **Short Essays** | | |
| 1. Regulation of blood sugar. | 131 | D12 |
| 2. Mechanisms of action of glucagon. | 83 | D07(RS2) |
| 3. Explain the role of hypoglycemic hormones (insulin) in regulation of blood glucose. | 6 | J05(RS2) |
| 4. Glucose tolerance test (GTT). | 335 | D02, J07, D09 |
| 5. Diabetes mellitus (metabolic changes). | 106 | D08(RS2), D12(RS3) |
| **Short Answers** | | |
| 1. How does insulin regulate blood glucose? | 132 | D13 |
| 2. Name two physiological actions of insulin. | 6 | D05 |
| 3. Intracellular insulin receptor. | 49 | J06(RS2) |
| 4. What are metabolic effects of glucagon? | 84 | J04 |
| 5. Name the insulin antagonists. | 132 | D01 |
| 6. Glucose tolerance test. | 335 | J11 |
| 7. What are the features of a normal glucose tolerance curve? | 336 | J10 |
| 8. GTT graph for renal glycosuria. | 188 | D11(RS3) |
| 9. Renal threshold for glucose and its significance. | 167 | D10(RS2) |
| 10. Renal glycosuria. | 157 | J10(RS2), J99, J12, J14, J15 |
| 11. What is renal glycosuria? How do you differentiate it from diabetic glycosuria? | 157 | J03 |
| 12. What is glycosuria? Mention the causes of different types of glycosuria. | 345 | J04 |
| **CANCER** | | |
| **Short Essays** | | |
| 1. Proto-oncogenes and oncogenes (mechanisms involved in activation of proto-oncogenes to oncogenes) | 163 | D10(RS2), D16 |
| 2. What are oncogenes? Discuss two tumor markers and their clinical application. | 163, 69 | D15(RS3) |
| 3. Tumor markers. | 69 | J07(RS2) |
| 4. Clinical importance of alpha-fetoprotein (AFP) and prostate specific antigen (PSA). Give their normal values. | 208 | D12(RS3) |
| **Short Answers** | | |
| 1. Cell cycle. | 318 | J17(RS3) |
| 2. Mechanism of carcinogenesis. | 142 | D09(RS2) |
| 3. Oncogenes—definition, examples, role in carcinogenesis. | 163 | J05(RS2), D06(RS2), D11(RS3), J04, J06, J09 |
| 4. Plasmids and oncogenes. | 244 | D13(RS3) |
| 5. Growth factors—enumerate, functions, role in carcinogenesis. | 32 | D05(RS2), D07(RS2) |
| 6. Tumor markers—definition, examples, diagnostic significance. | 69 | D08(RS2), D14(RS3), D15(RS3), D02 |
| 7. Prostate-specific antigen (PSA). | 208 | J08(RS2) |
| 8. Anticancer agents. | 244 | D13(RS3) |


Contd...

| Questions | Page No. | Examinations |
|---|---|---|
| **ACQUIRED IMMUNODEFICIENCY SYNDROME (AIDS)** | | |
| None | | |
| **SECTION SEVEN: BASICS TO LEARN BIOCHEMISTRY** | | |
| **INTRODUCTION TO BIOORGANIC CHEMISTRY** | | |
| None | | |
| **OVERVIEW OF BIOPHYSICAL CHEMISTRY** | | |
| **Short Essay** | | |
| 1. Radioactive isotopes of iodine and their clinical application. | 165 | D10(RS2) |
| **Short Answers** | | |
| 1. Define radioactivity. Name the uses of:<br>a. $I^{131}$<br>b. $Co^{60}$ | 246 | D01 |
| 2. Radioisotopes. | 245 | D13(RS3) |
| 3. Mention two isotopes and mention their application in medicine. | 246 | D08(RS2), D03, J07 |
| **TOOLS OF BIOCHEMISTRY** | | |
| **Short Essays** | | |
| 1. Chromatography. | 356 | J00 |
| 2. Electrophoresis. | 295 | D00 |
| 3. Write the components and principle of colorimeter. | 339 | J09(OS) |
| **Short Answers** | | |
| 1. Principle of chromatography. | 356 | J15 |
| 2. Electrophoresis—principle, normal pattern of serum proteins, diagnosis importance. | 295 | D15(RS3), D16(RS3), D03, J10, J12 |
| 3. Immunoelectrophoresis. | 99 | J08(RS2) |
| **IMMUNOLOGY** | | |
| **Short Answer** | | |
| 1. Monoclonal antibodies. | 256 | J14(RS3) |
| **MISCELLANEOUS** | | |
| **Long Essay** | | |
| 1. Discuss the significance of multienzyme complexes with respect to carbohydrate and lipid metabolism. | 36 | J06(RS2) |
| **Short Essay** | | |
| 1. Multienzyme complexes. | 36 | D07 |
| **Short Answers** | | |
| 1. Multienzyme complex. | 36 | D17(RS3) |
| 2. Abnormal components of urine. | 245 | D13(RS3) |
| 3. Indicate the biochemical defect in lactose intolerance and Gilbert's disease. | 373 | D13 |
| 4. Name the enzyme defects in the following cases: (1) Refsum's disease, (2) Alkaptonuria. | 373 | D13 |
| 5. Gamma-aminobutyric acid (GABA), polyunsaturated fatty acids (PUFA) and severe acute malnutrition (SAM) and their importance. | 255 | J14(RS3) |
| 6. What is reference range/values? How is it calculated? | 89 | D07(RS2), J16(RS3) |
| 7. Name two inborn errors of metabolism and the associated enzyme. | 373 | J09 |
| 8. Reference range of potassium and albumin in the serum. | 374 | D09 |

Contd...

| Questions | Page No. | Examinations |
|---|---|---|
| 9. Normal values of:<br>a. Serum creatinine (0.7–1.5 mg/dL).<br>b. Serum amylase (50–120 IU/L). | 374 | D99 |
| 10. Mention the normal serum values for:<br>a. AST (8–20 IU/L)<br>b. ALT (10–35 IU/L)<br>c. Urea (15–40 mg/dL)<br>d. Creatinine (0.7–1.5 mg/dL). | 374 | J02 |
| 11. Normal serum levels of:<br>a. Serum calcium (9–11 mg/dL)<br>b. Serum phosphorus (3–4.5 mg/dL). | 374 | J06, D08 |
| 12. Mention the normal levels of:<br>a. Serum protein (6–8 g/dL)<br>b. Urea (15–40 mg/dL)<br>c. Creatinine (0.5–1.5 mg/dL). | 57 | D06(RS2) |
| 13. Give the normal blood level of the following:<br>a. Fasting blood glucose (70–100 mg/dL)<br>b. Total protein (6–8 g/dL)<br>c. Urea (15–40 mg/dL)<br>d. Bicarbonate (24–30 mEq/L)<br>e. Sodium (135–145 mEq/L)<br>f. Potassium (3.5–5 mEq/L). | 130 | J09(RS2) |
| 14. Give the normal values of:<br>a. Fasting blood glucose (70–100 mg/dL)<br>b. Cholesterol (150–200 mg/dL). | 374 | D13 |
| 15. Name the normal serum levels of:<br>a. Sodium (135-145 mEq/L)<br>b. Potassium (3.5-5 mEq/L). | 374 | J14 |
| 16. Give the normal values of:<br>a. Fasting blood glucose (70–100 mg/dL)<br>b. Blood urea (15–40 mg/dL). | 374 | D14 |

# MBBS PHASE I EXAMINATION
## JUNE 2005
## (Revised Scheme 2)

### LONG ESSAYS

**1. Name the ketone bodies. Give two conditions characterized by excessive production of ketone bodies. Explain the metabolic derangements and consequences of ketosis.**

Refer Question No. 1 June 2011 (RS2).

**2. Explain the steps of activation, initiation, elongation and termination of protein biosynthesis.**

- Protein biosynthesis is an important process of genetic expression
- Also called translation
- Process by which genetic information present in form of a sequence of bases in mRNA is expressed to produce a sequence of amino acids in a protein.

#### Intracellular site

- Cytoplasm.

#### Reactions

| *Requirement* | *Steps* | |
|---|---|---|
| a. Activation of amino acids to form aminoacyl-tRNA<br>First and essential step | | |
| • 20 amino acids<br>• tRNAs corresponding to amino acids<br>• Amino acid activating enzyme (amino acyl-tRNA synthetases)<br>• Adenosine triphosphate (ATP) | • In first step, amino acid reacts with ATP to form aminoacyl AMP releasing pyrophosphate<br>• In second step, aminoacyl group of aminoacyl AMP is transferred to 3′ end of adenine nucleotide of CCA sequence in tRNA<br>• Each aminoacyl-tRNA synthetase is specific for amino acid and corresponding tRNA and specificity is responsible for correct incorporation of amino acid in protein<br>• Also provides energy for peptide chain elongation | 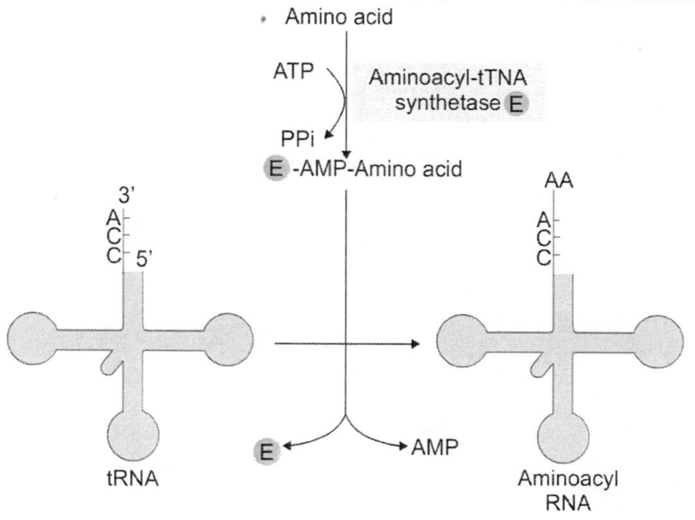 <br>**Fig. 1:** Activation of amino acids |

*Contd...*

Contd...

| *Requirement* | *Steps* | |
|---|---|---|
| b. Initiation of protein synthesis | | |
| • mRNA template<br>• 40s and 60s ribosomal units (which assemble to form complete 80s ribosome on which protein synthesis occurs)<br>• Initiation factors (proteins) 1, 2 and 3<br>• Methionyl-tRNA<br>• GTP | • Ternary complex formation<br>– By binding of methionyl-tRNA with GTP and IF2<br>• Preinitiation complex formation<br>– By binding of ternary complex with 40s ribosome subunit in presence of initiation factors eIF-3 and eIF-1<br>• Initiation complex formation<br>– Binding of mRNA to preinitiation complex in presence of initiation factor eIF-4E, eIF-4A and eIF-4F<br>• Attachment of aminoacyl-tRNA<br>– Attachment of anticodon (3'-UAC-5') of methionyl-tRNA to initiation codon (AUG) due to recognition of this codon by anticodon of methionly-tRNA and aminoacyl-tRNA is attached to ribosome by its TΨC arm<br>• Formation of 80s ribosome<br>– By attachment of 60s ribosome subunit to initiation complex to form 80s initiation complex with energy provided by hydrolysis of GTP to GDP and Pi<br>– Thus at end of initiation, complete initiation complex with 80s ribosome and attached mRNA is formed<br>– This ribosome has two sites called P (peptidyl) site and A (amino acyl) site<br>– P site contains methionyl-tRNA and A site is vacant | 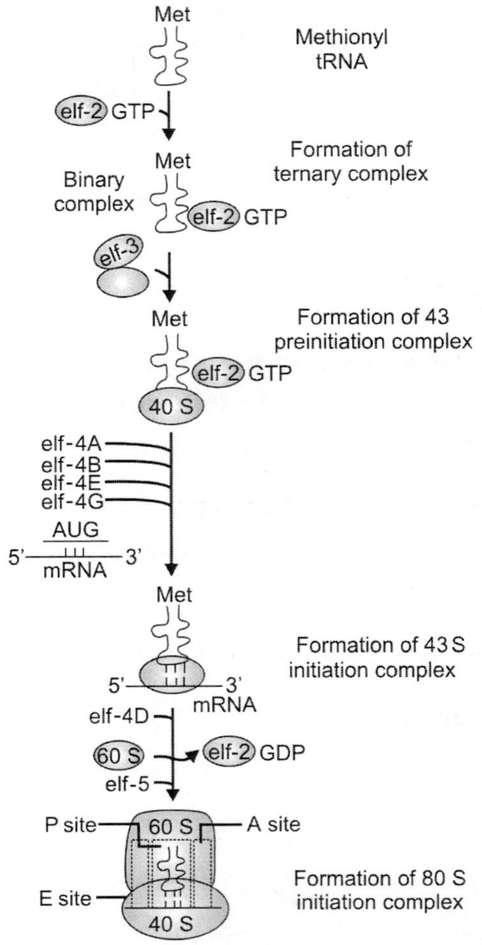 Met<br>Methionyl tRNA<br>elf-2 GTP<br>Met<br>Binary complex<br>elf-2 GTP<br>Formation of ternary complex<br>elf-3<br>Met<br>elf-2 GTP<br>40 S<br>Formation of 43 preinitiation complex<br>elf-4A<br>elf-4B<br>elf-4E<br>elf-4G<br>AUG<br>5' mRNA 3'<br>Met<br>5' 3'<br>mRNA<br>Formation of 43 S initiation complex<br>elf-4D<br>60 S<br>elf-2 GDP<br>elf-5<br>P site<br>60 S<br>A site<br>E site<br>40 S<br>Formation of 80 S initiation complex<br>**Fig. 2:** Initiation of protein systhesis |

Contd...

Revised Scheme 2

Contd...

| Requirement | Steps | |
|---|---|---|
| c. Elongation step | | |
| • Elongation factors (EF1 and EF2)<br>• GTP<br>• Amino acyl-tRNAs<br>• Peptidyl transferase<br>• mRNA template<br>• 40S and 60S ribosomal units | • Each aminoacyl-tRNA complexes with EF1 and GTP<br>• Depending on second codon, anticodon of appropriate aminoacyl-tRNA EF1-GTP complex binds to A site with release of EF1, GDP and Pi<br>• Peptidyl transferase forms peptide bond between carboxyl group of previous amino acid and $NH_2$ group of next amino acid resulting in attachment of peptide to tRNA in A site<br>• Protein synthesis starts from $NH_2$ terminal with $NH_2$ group of methionine as free amino end<br>• P site now has only tRNA (no amino acid) which is discharged to vacate P site<br>• Peptidyl-tRNA is translocated from A site to P site by energy provided by splitting of GTP into GDP and Pi<br>• At same time, ribosome moves along mRNA in 5'→'3 direction by one codon along with release of EF2<br>• Above cycle repeats a number of times till a 'chain termination' codon is approached and at this stage P site contains tRNA with its attached polypeptide | **Fig. 3:** Elongation of protein chain |

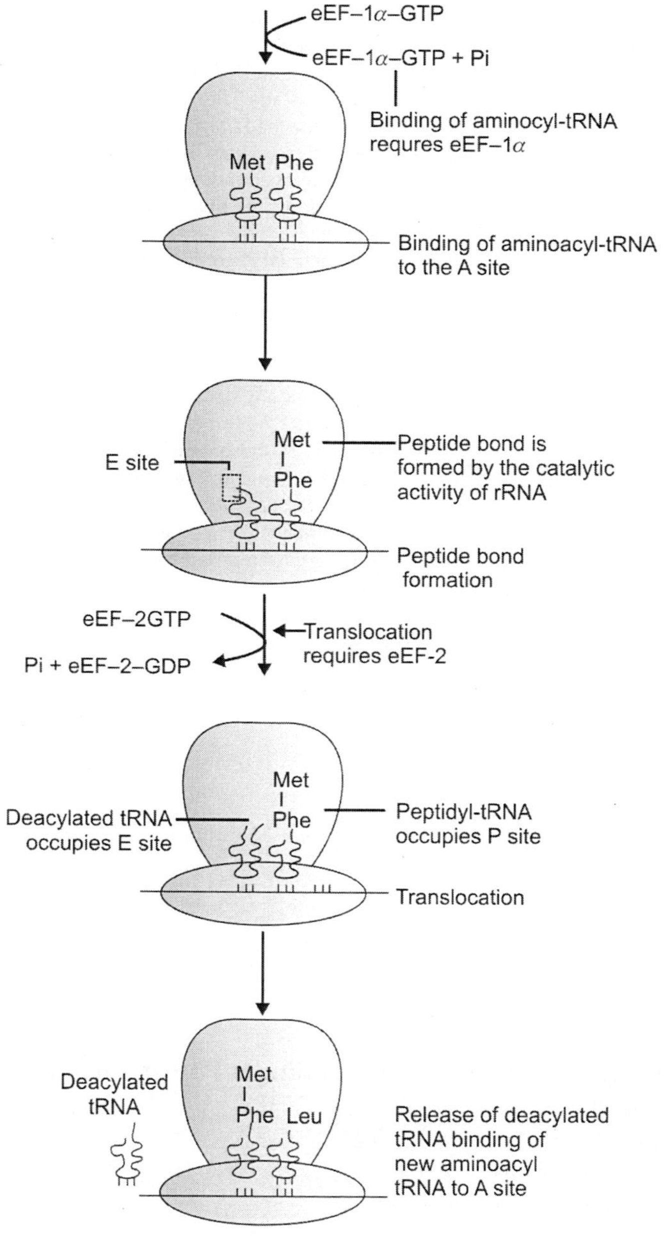

Contd...

*Contd...*

| ***Requirement*** | ***Steps*** | |
|---|---|---|
| d. Termination step | | |
| • Releasing factor<br>• GTP<br>• Peptidyl transferase | • Chain elongation continues till a 'chain termination' or stop codon (UAA, UAG and UCA) is approached and at this stage P site contains tRNA with its attached polypeptide<br>• Releasing factor with GTP and peptidyl transferase brings about hydrolysis of bond between polypeptide and tRNA<br>• Upon hydrolysis, entire protein synthesizing machinery dissociates to polypeptide, tRNA, 40s and 60s ribosome units, mRNA, releasing factor, GDP and Pi<br>• At a time, many ribosomes may be attached to a single mRNA at intervals and as each ribosome moves along the mRNA strand in 5'→ 3' direction, it weaves a copy of same protein<br>• An assembly of many ribosomes on a single mRNA is called 'Polysome' | 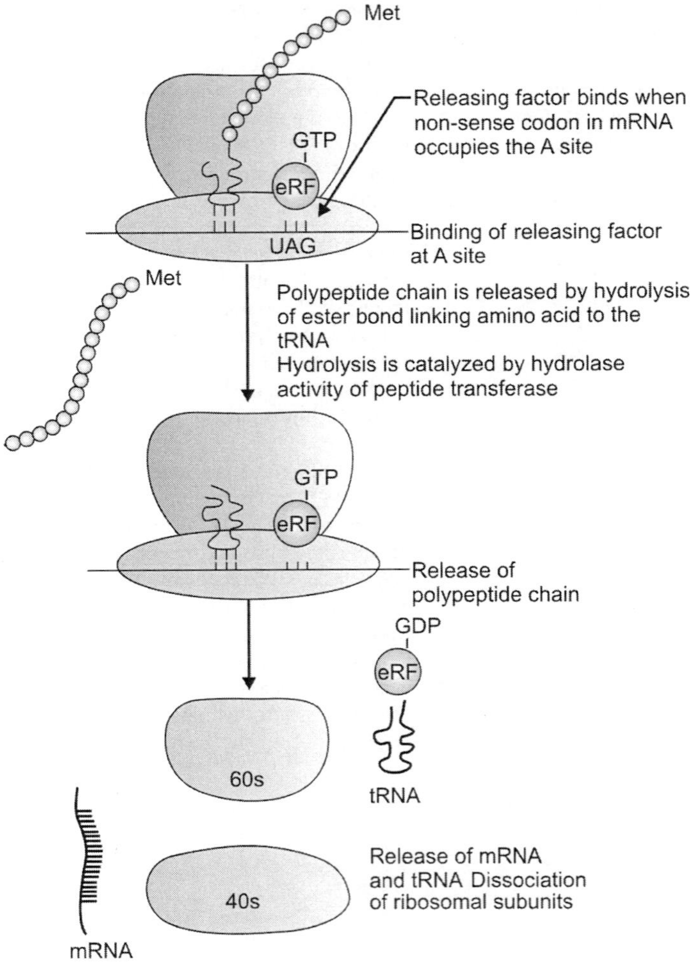 **Fig. 4:** Termination steps of protein synthesis |

## Energetics (for Formation of Single Peptide Bond)

| ***Steps*** | ***ATP used*** |
|---|---|
| • Formation of aminoacyl-tRNA | 2 ATP |
| • Entry of aminoacyl-tRNA into A site | 1 GTP = 1 ATP |
| • Translocation of peptidyl-tRNA from A site to P site | 1 GTP = 1 ATP |
| **Total** | **4 ATPs** |

Revised Scheme 2

## Regulation

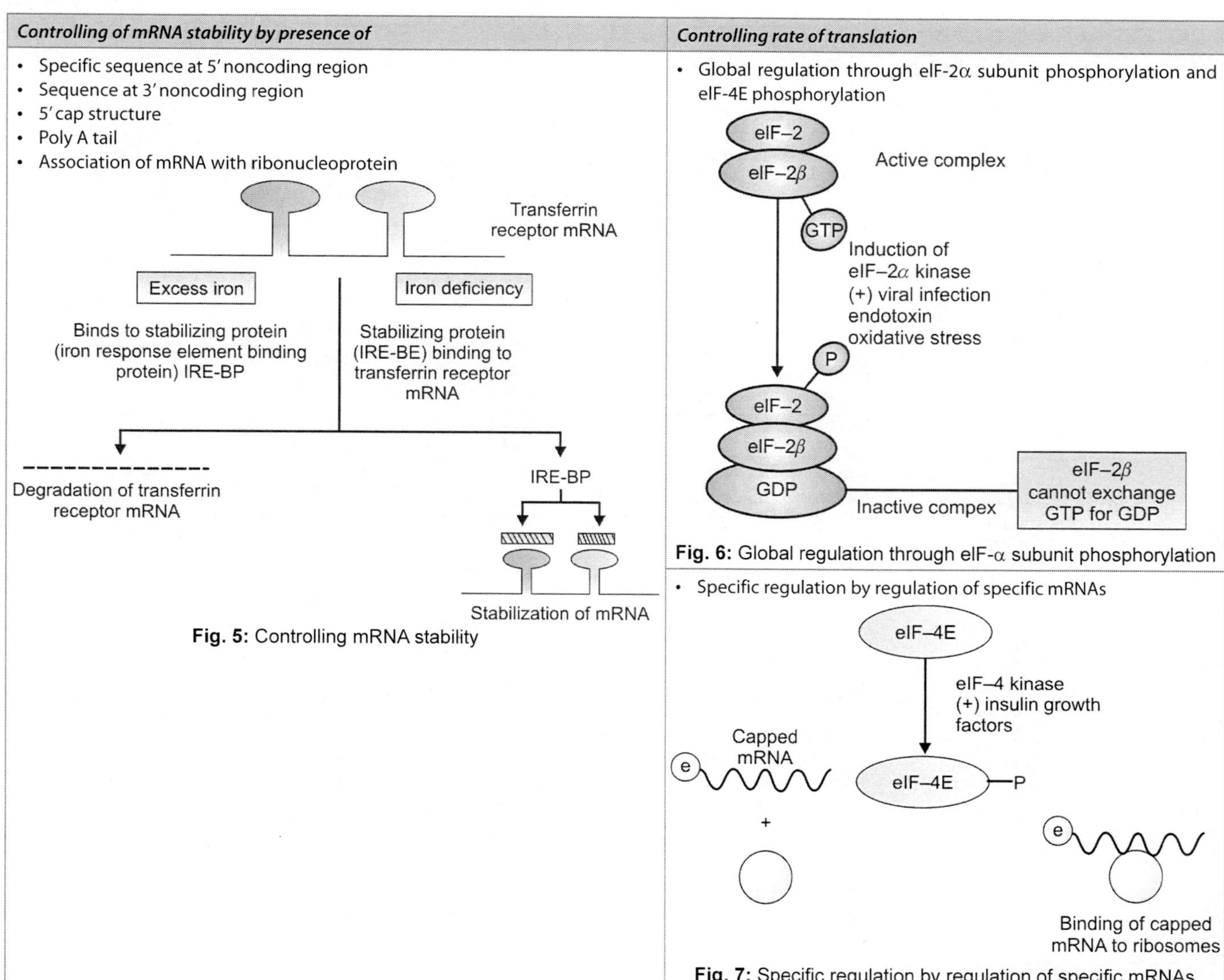

| *Controlling of mRNA stability by presence of* | *Controlling rate of translation* |
|---|---|
| • Specific sequence at 5′ noncoding region<br>• Sequence at 3′ noncoding region<br>• 5′ cap structure<br>• Poly A tail<br>• Association of mRNA with ribonucleoprotein | • Global regulation through eIF-2α subunit phosphorylation and eIF-4E phosphorylation |
| | • Specific regulation by regulation of specific mRNAs |



**Fig. 5:** Controlling mRNA stability

**Fig. 6:** Global regulation through eIF-α subunit phosphorylation

**Fig. 7:** Specific regulation by regulation of specific mRNAs

## Inhibitors

- Many substances inhibit protein synthesis at some specific steps but their actions differ in prokaryotes and eukaryotes.

| *In eukaryotes* | *In prokaryotes (used as antibiotics)* |
|---|---|
| • Diphtheria toxin: Prevents translocation by inactivating elongation factor $eEF_2$ by catalyzing its ADP ribosylation<br>• Ricin: Binds to 60s subunit and removes 1 adenine residue from 28s rRNA<br>• Cycloheximide: Inhibits peptidyl transferase thus blocking peptide chain elongation<br>• Puromycin: Structurally similar to aminoacyl-tRNA, thus gets incorporated into growing peptide chain causing its release | • Aminoglycosides: Interferes with binding of methionly tRNA to ribosomes and thereby inhibits initiation process and it also leads to misreading of mRNA<br>• Tetracycline: Binds to 30s subunit of ribosome and inhibits binding of aminoacyl-tRNA to A site thus inhibiting initiation process<br>• Chloramphenicol: Competitive inhibition of peptidyl transferase thus interfering with chain elongation<br>• Erythromycin: Inhibits translocation of peptidyl-tRNA to P site by binding with 50s subunit ribosome<br>• Puromycin: Structurally similar to aminoacyl-tRNA, thus gets incorporated into growing peptide chain causing its release |

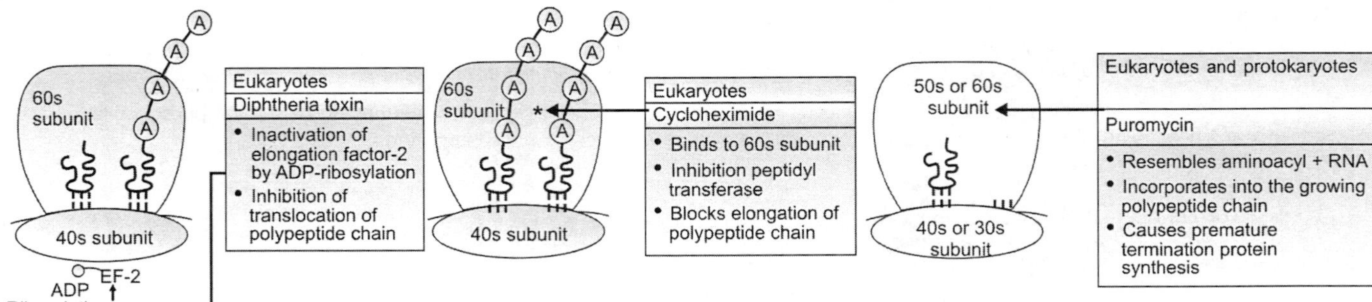


**Fig. 8A:** Inhibition of protein biosynthesis in eukaryotes

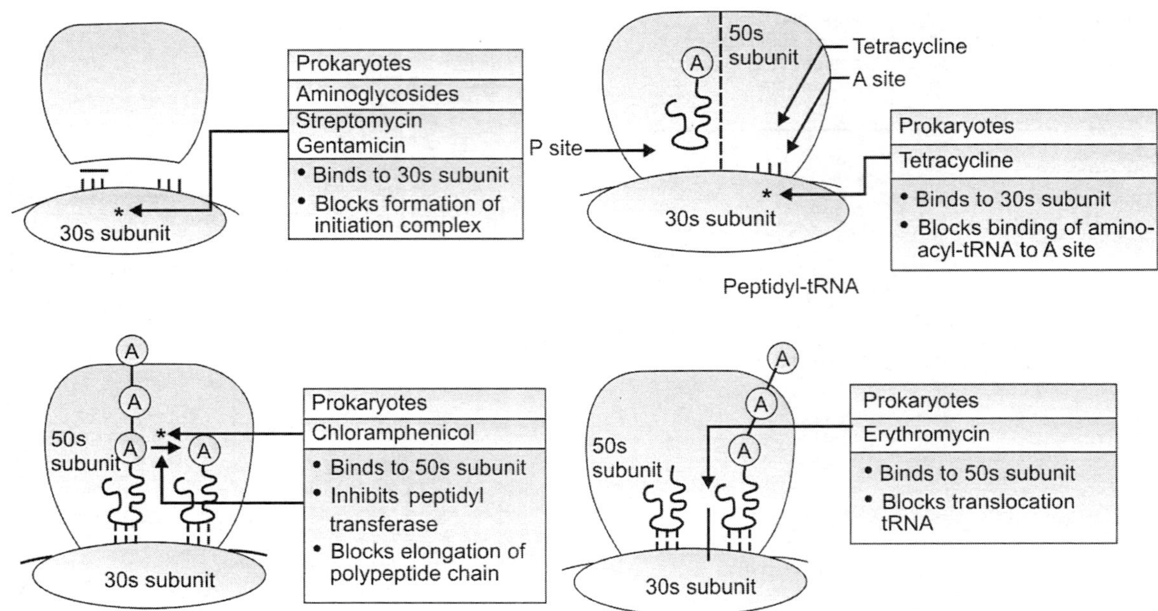


**Fig. 8B:** Inhibition of protein biosynthesis in prokaryotes



## SHORT ESSAYS

### 3. Explain the role of hypoglycemic hormones.

- Insulin is the only hormone reducing blood sugar level (hypoglycemic hormone).

| *Chemistry* | *Source* | *Regulation of secretion* |
|---|---|---|
| • 51 amino acid containing polypeptide hormone consisting of 2 chains, A and B chains (21 and 30 amino acids respectively) | • β-cells of islets of Langerhans of pancreas<br>• Synthesized as a single polypeptide preproinsulin (108 amino acids) which undergoes proteolytic processing to give proinsulin (86 amino acids) and finally insulin and C-peptide (used as indicator for endogenous insulin production)<br>• Gene for insulin is located on chromosome 11 | Stimulants<br>• Glucose (most important)<br>• Amino acids<br>• GIT hormones (secretin, gastrin, pancreozymin)<br>Inhibitors<br>• Epinephrine (most potent inhibitor) |

#### Actions of Insulin

- Insulin plays a vital role in regulating blood sugar level
- An important hormone regulating metabolism of carbohydrates, proteins and fats

| | |
|---|---|
| a. Carbohydrate metabolism<br>Only antidiabetic hormone in body | • Increases transport and uptake of glucose (muscles, adipose tissue, leukocytes and mammary glands require insulin for glucose uptake)<br>• Increases peripheral utilization of glucose or glycolysis (by stimulating glycolytic enzymes like glucokinase, phosphofructokinase, pyruvate kinase)<br>• Prevents rise in blood glucose level by inhibiting gluconeogenesis (by suppressing pyruvate carboxylase, phosphoenol carboxykinase, and G-6-phosphatase) and glycogenolysis (by inactivating glycogen phosphorylase)<br>• Promotes glycogenesis by stimulating glycogen synthase thus stores excess glucose in form glycogen<br>• Promotes HMP shunt |
| b. Protein metabolism<br>Prevents cellular utilization of proteins and causes synthesis and storage of proteins | • Facilitates entry of amino acids in cell<br>• Accelerates protein synthesis by influencing DNA transcription and translation of mRNA<br>• Inhibits protein catabolism, by inhibiting proteolytic enzymes |
| c. Lipid metabolism<br>Causes synthesis and storage of fat | • Promotes lipogenesis (synthesis of fatty acids and triglycerides)<br>• Inhibits lipolysis by inhibiting lipase and inhibits ketogenesis by decreasing activity of HMG CoA synthase<br>• Incorporates free fatty acids into neutral fats<br>• Facilitates entry of free fatty acid into adipocytes |
| d. Nucleic acid metabolism | • Promotes synthesis of DNA and RNA and thus help in tissue growth |
| e. Mineral metabolism | • Influences $K^+$, $Na^+$ and $Ca^{2+}$ metabolism |
| f. Growth | • Insulin promotes growth, by virtue of its anabolic action on protein metabolism |

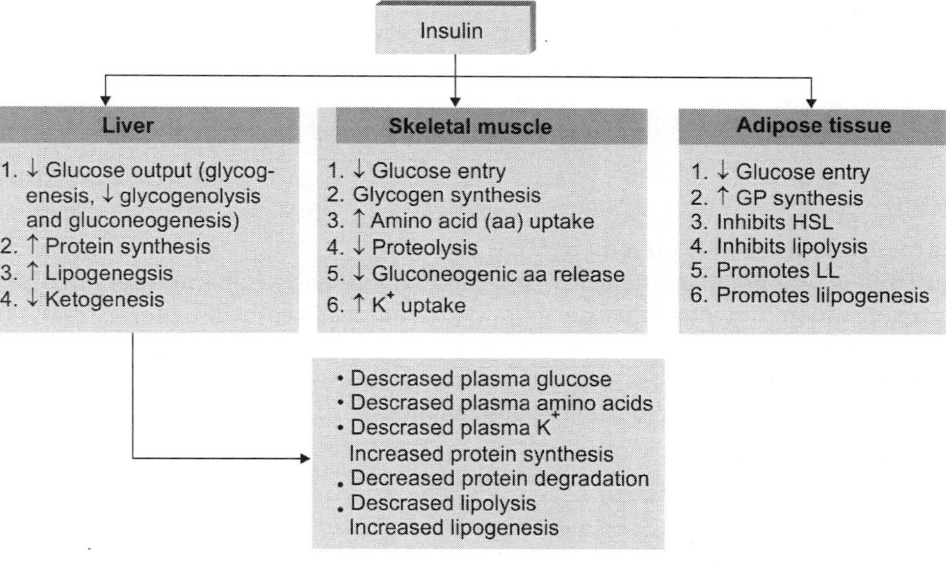


**Fig. 9:** Actions of insulin

## Significance

- Insulin is the only hypoglycemic or antidiabetic hormone in human body making it most essential for regulation of blood sugar level
- Deficiency of insulin hampers blood sugar regulation resulting in diabetes mellitus whereas any excess can lead to hypoglycemia which can be life threatening
- Commercial insulin preparations are manufactured similar to human insulin for treatment of diabetes mellitus.

## 4. Metabolic functions of cysteine.

- Cysteine is a sulfur containing, aliphatic, non-essential amino acid.

## Biosynthesis

- Cysteine is formed from methionine as follows

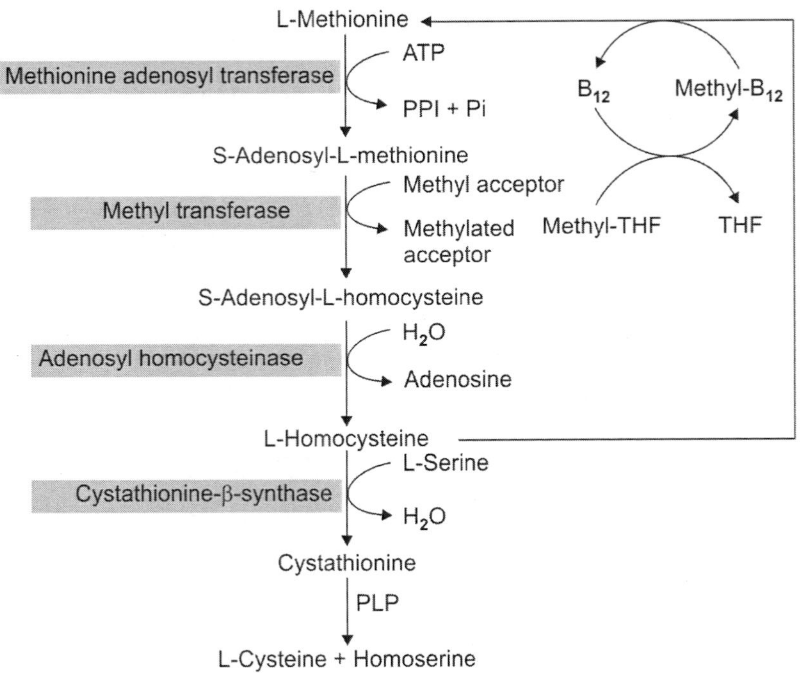


**Fig. 10:** Biosynthesis of cysteine



## Metabolic Functions

- Cysteine is used for synthesis of body proteins
- Cysteine is a particularly prominent amino acid in proteins of nails, hairs, hoofs and keratin of skin (scleroproteins)
- Cysteine is also a constituent of many other polypeptide hormones like insulin and vasopressin, etc. where it is of great importance in maintaining secondary and tertiary structures
- Gluconeogenesis
  - Cysteine is catabolised to pyruvic acid which is glucogenic

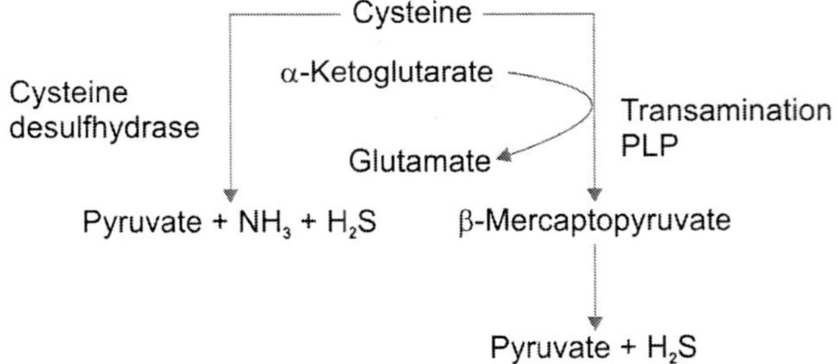


**Fig. 11:** Gluconeogenesis from cysteine

- Glutathione synthesis
  - Glutathione is a tripeptide containing glycine, cysteine and glutamic acid.

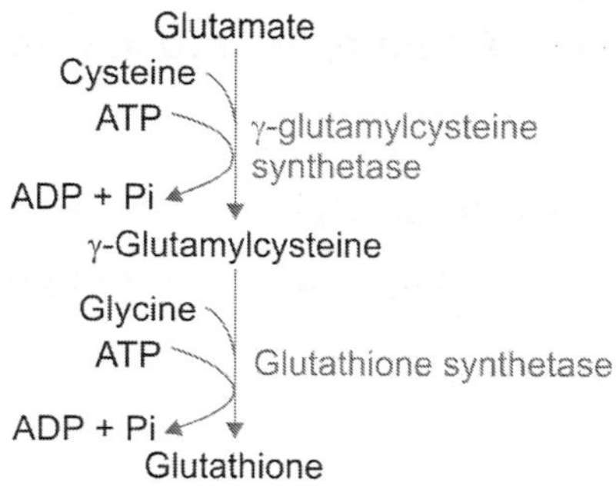


**Fig. 12:** Glutathione synthesis

*Functions*

- Keep enzymes in reduced state (active state)
- Suppress oxidative stress in the cell (antioxidant function)
- Maintain RBC membrane stability
- Prevent oxidation of hemoglobin to methemoglobin
- Amino acid transport (γ-glutamyl cycle).

- Taurine synthesis

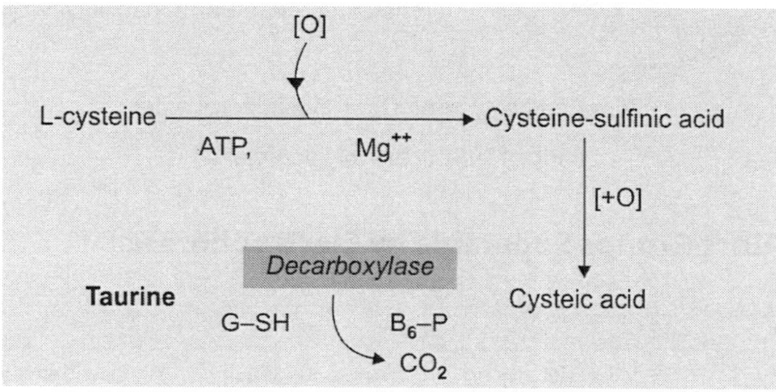


**Fig. 13:** Synthesis of taurine

*Functions*

- Required for formation of bile acids, taurocholate and taurochenodexycholate
- Acts as inhibitory neurotransmitter in brain
- Regulates ion flux across membranes in tissue such as heart
- Has membrane stabilizing effect.

- Mercaptoethanolamine synthesis
  - Mercaptoethanolamine is an important constituent of coenzyme A.

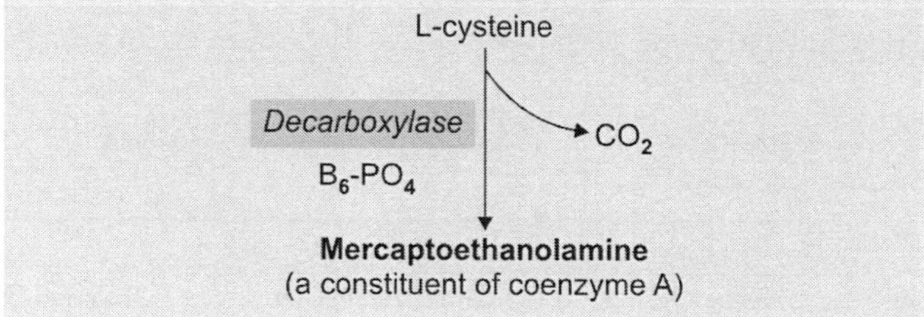


**Fig. 14:** Synthesis of mercaptoethanolamine

- Detoxification
  - Cysteine couples with certain aromatic compounds which then undergo acetylation to form mercapturic acid which are excreted in urine
    - Bromobenzene + cysteine + acetic acid → bromophenyl mercapturic acid
    - Naphthalene + cysteine + acetic acid → naphthyl mercapturic acid.

## 5. What is oxidative phosphorylation? Explain chemiosmotic theory.

Refer Question No. 1 June 2010 (RS2).

## 6. Classify lipoproteins. Mention their functions.

- Plasma lipoproteins are conjugated proteins or complex lipids consisting of lipid as prosthetic part and apolipoprotein as protein part
- Apolipoprotein makes lipids soluble and thus helps in their transport.

### Structure

- Triglyceride and cholesterol ester core surrounded by apolipoprotein shell, phospholipids and free cholesterol.

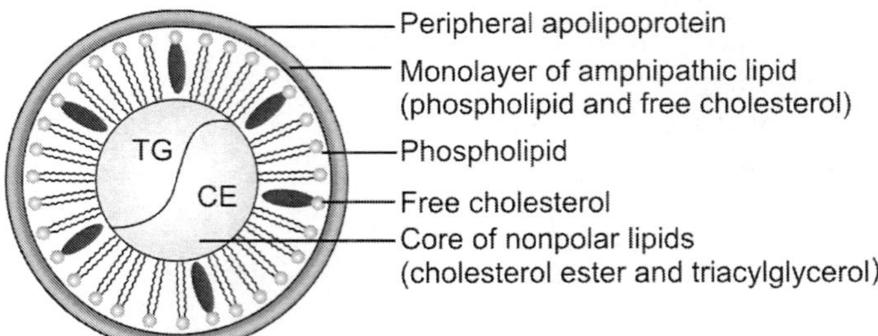


TG =Triacylglycerol, CE = Cholesterol ester

**Fig. 15:** Structure of lipoprotein

### Classification (Into Five Distinct Groups Separable by Electrophoresis)

| | *Chylomicrons* | *VLDL* | *IDL* | *LDL* | *HDL* |
|---|---|---|---|---|---|
| a. Electrophoretic mobility | Lowest density lipoprotein, remaining at origin on electrophoresis | Very low density on ultracentrifugation and migrate to prebeta position on electrophoresis | Intermediate density on ultracentrifugation and migrate to broad beta position on electrophoresis | Low density of ultracentrifugation and migrate to beta position on electrophoresis | High density of ultracentrifugation and migrate to alpha position on electrophoresis |
| b. Size | 90–1000 nm | 30–90 nm | 25–35 nm | 20–25 nm | 10–20 nm |
| c. Density | <0.95 | <1.006 | 1.006–1.019 | 1.019–1.063 | >1.063 |
| d. Composition | | | | | |
| i. Proteins | 2% Apoliprotein B-48 Apoliprotein C | 10% Apolipoprotein B-100 Apolipoprotein C | 15% Apolipoprotein B-100 Apolipoprotein E | 25% Apolipoprotein B-100 Apolipoprotein E | 40% Apolipoprotein AI Apolipoprotein AII |
| ii. Lipids | 98% | 90% | 85% | 75% | 60% |
| - Tricacylglycerol | 85% | 57% | 35% | 10% | 8% |
| - Cholesterol | 5% | 15% | 35% | 45% | 22% |
| - Phospholipids | 8% | 18% | 15% | 20% | 30% |
| e. Metabolism | | | | | |
| i. Synthesis | Initially nascent chylomicrons are assembled in intestine from triglycerides, phospholipids cholesterol and apo A, apo B48 and transported to blood via lymphatics | Liver synthesizes nascent VLDL of triglycerides, phospholipids, cholesterol esters, cholesterol, apo B100, apo C and apo E | Synthesized in liver from VLDL consisting of triglycerides, phospholipids, cholesterol esters, cholesterol, apo B100 and apo E | Obtained from VLDL, consisting of triglycerides, phospholipids, cholesterol and its esters and apo B100 | Synthesized in liver and intestine consisting of triglycerides, phospholipids, cholesterol and its esters, apo A, apo C and apo E |

Contd...

Contd...

| | *Chylomicrons* | *VLDL* | *IDL* | *LDL* | *HDL* |
|---|---|---|---|---|---|
| | In blood apo C and apo E are added to chylomicrons from HDL to form complete chylomicron | It becomes complete VLDL after addition of extra apo C and apo E from HDL | | | Serves as reservoir of apo C and apo E for formation of chylomicrons and VLDL |
| ii. Catabolism | In extrahepatic tissues, capillaries, lipoprotein lipase hydrolyses triglycerides to glycerol and free fatty acids<br>Free fatty acids are esterified back to triglycerides and stored by adipose tissue<br>Glycerol is circulated to liver<br>Chylomicrons depleted of triglycerides lose apo A and apo C to form chylomicron remnant which is degraded in liver<br>Apo A and apo C return to HDL | VLDL is hydrolyzed to release its triglycerides<br>Then it loses its apo C and becomes intermittent density lipoprotein called VLDL remnant | IDL is hydrolyzed to release its triglycerides<br>Then it loses apo E to become LDL | About half of circulating LDL is taken up by extrahepatic tissues and rest is degraded in liver | Degraded in liver |
| f. Functions | Transport of dietary triglycerides and cholesterol esters from intestine to peripheral tissues | Transport of endogenous triglycerides from liver to extrahepatic tissues | Transport of endogenous triglycerides and cholesterol from liver to extrahepatic tissues | Transport of cholesterol from liver to extrahepatic tissues (cholesterol influx) | Transport of cholesterol from extrahepatic tissues to liver in esterified form (cholesterol efflux) |

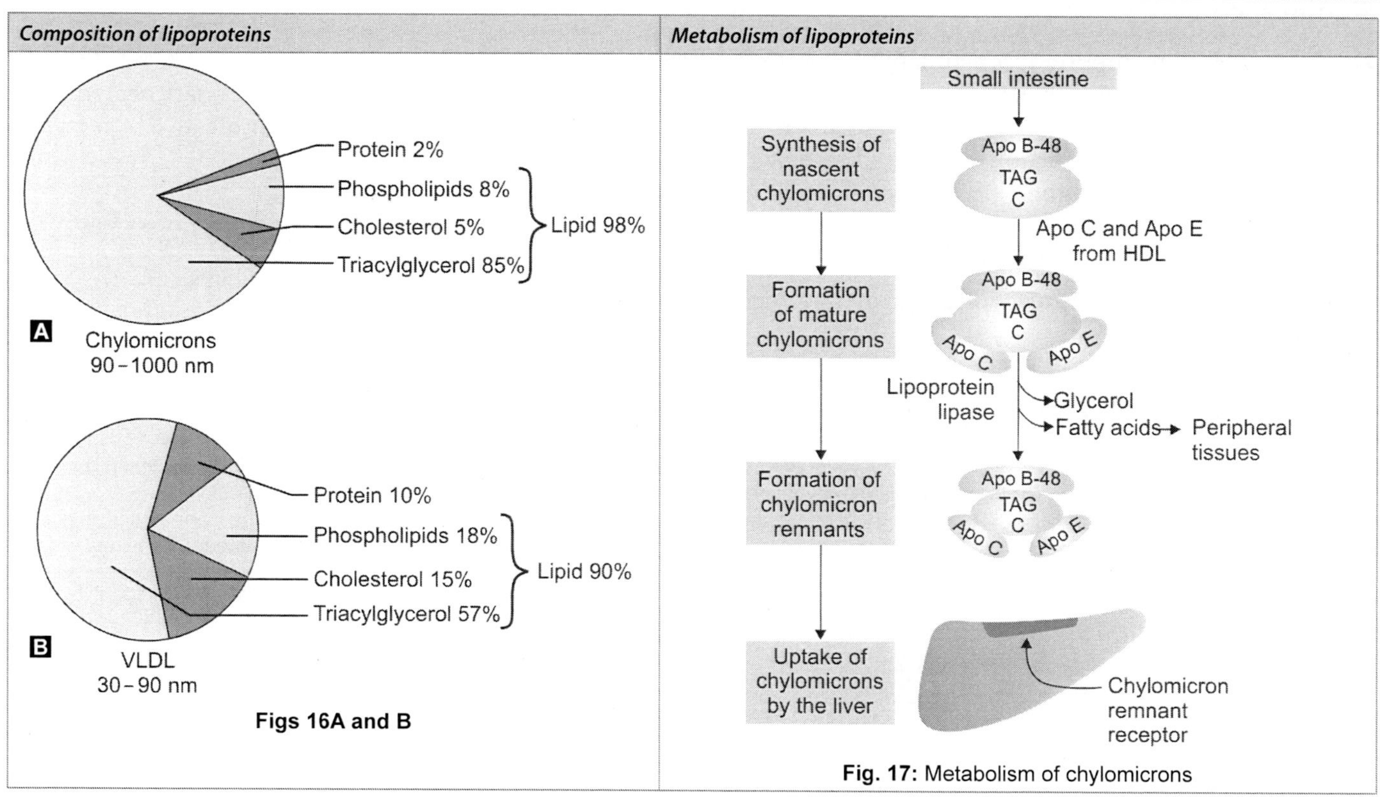


**Figs 16A and B**

**Fig. 17:** Metabolism of chylomicrons

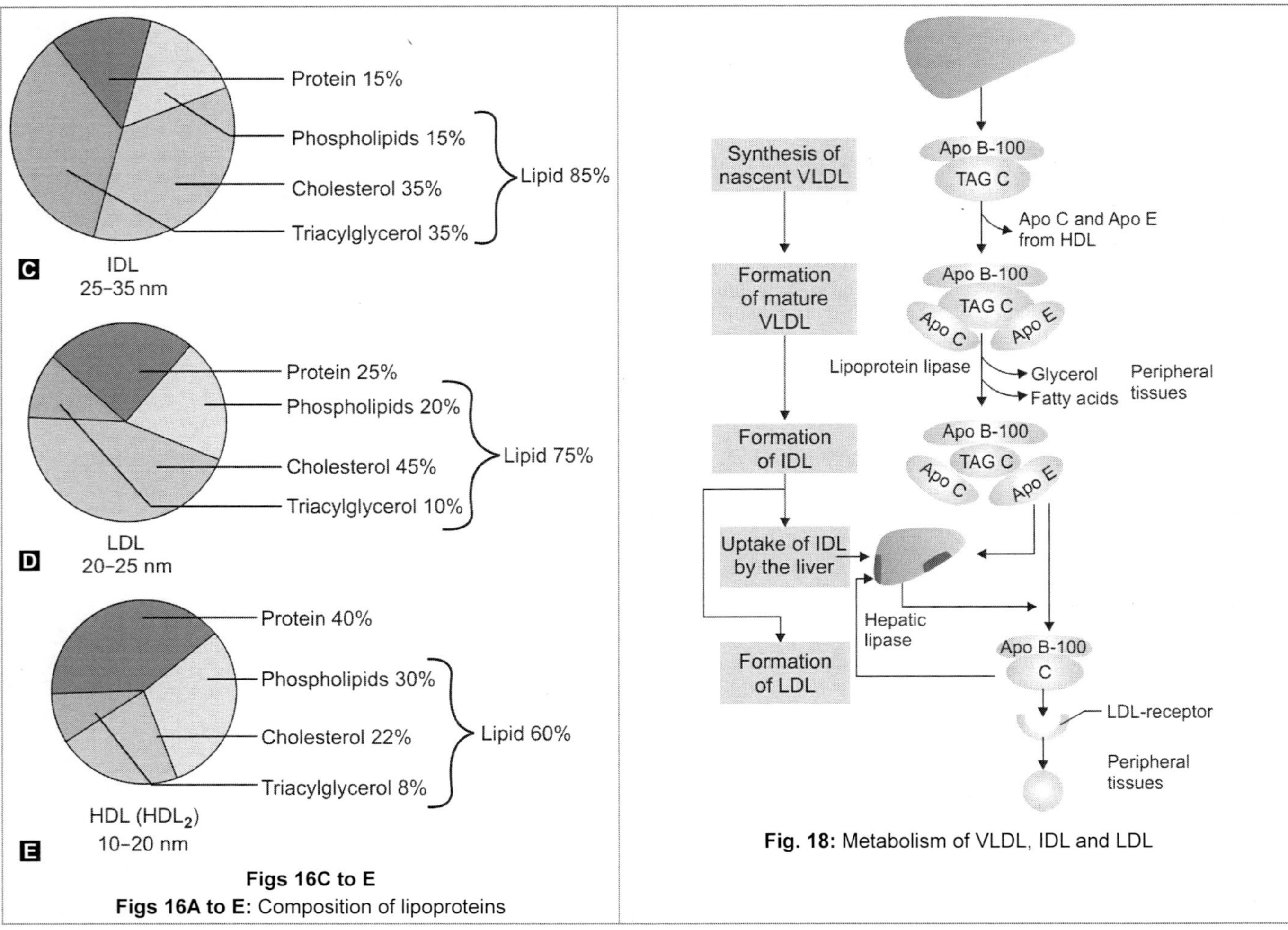


Figs 16C to E

**Figs 16A to E:** Composition of lipoproteins

**Fig. 18:** Metabolism of VLDL, IDL and LDL



## Significance

- Lipoproteins are important constituent of body lipid stores and are store house of cholesterol
- Increased lipoproteins (hyperlipoproteinemias) is an important risk factors for development of coronary heart disease
- VLDL and LDL are mostly incriminated in atherosclerosis whereas HDL is considered cardioprotective by it reverse cholesterol transport function
- Ratio of LDL to HDL is good indicator of risk of atherosclerosis.

## 7. Therapeutic uses of enzymes.

- Besides catalyzing body reactions, enzymes are also used clinically to treat numerous conditions.

## Therapeutic Uses

| *Enzymes* | *Therapeutic uses* |
|---|---|
| • Streptokinase<br>• Urokinase<br>• Alteplase<br>• Arvin<br>• Tissue plasminogen activator | As a thrombolytic agent in myocardial infarction, unstable angina, ischemic stroke, pulmonary embolism, deep vein thrombosis and acute peripheral arterial occlusion<br>• Activates plasminogen (a plasma protein) to plasmin which then digests fibrin (in clot) to form soluble degradation products and dissolves the clot; thus helps in tissue reperfusion in event of clot-induced ischemia |

*Contd...*

Contd...

| *Enzymes* | *Therapeutic uses* |
|---|---|
| • L-asparaginase | As a anticancer drug in some cases of lymphoblastic leukemia and reticulum cell sarcoma<br>• Some tumor cells require non-essential amino acid asparagine for their growth because they do not contain sufficient asparagine synthase activity to meet their metabolic demands and enzyme asparaginase hydrolyses asparagine to aspartate resulting in suppression of tumor growth |
| • Pancreatin | As a replacement therapy in chronic pancreatitis, obstruction caused by cancer of head of pancreas, cystic fibrosis and after total gastrectomy and pancreatectomy |
| • Diastase | As a digestant |
| • Pepsin and papain | As a digestant in gastric achalysia |
| • Papain | Anti-inflammatory |
| • Pancreatic dornase | As a mucolytic agent in cough |
| • Hyaluronidase | To promote rapid absorption of drugs and fluids given subcutenously or intramuscularly |
| • Streptodornase<br>• Trypsin | For debridement of chronic ulcers along with streptokinase |
| • Chymotrypsin | For traumatically induced inflammation and edema of soft tissues |
| • Alpha chymotrypsin | For dissolving suspensory ligament of lens to facilitate dissection of lens during intracapsular extraction of cataract |
| • Alpha-1 antitrypsin | To treat emphysema |
| • Collagenase | Debridement of dermal ulcers and severe burns |
| • Adenosine deaminase | Treatment of adenosine deaminase deficiency (gene therapy) |

## 8. Explain metabolic role of thiamine and its deficiency manifestations.

- Thiamin (vitamin $B_1$) is a water-soluble vitamin belonging to B complex group of vitamins.

| *Chemistry* | *Dietary sources* | *RDA* |
|---|---|---|
| • Thiamine contains thiazole and pyridine rings held together by methylene bridge<br>• Contains sulfur | Vegetable<br>• Cereals, pulses, oil seeds, nuts and yeast<br>Animal<br>• Pork, liver, heart, kidney, milk | Children<br>• 0.7–1.2 mg/day<br>Adults<br>• 1–1.5 mg/day<br>Pregnancy and lactation, old age and alcoholics<br>• 2 mg/day |

### Coenzyme Form

- Thiamine pyrophosphate (TPP) (formed by estimation of OH group with phosphate donated by ATP).

### Metabolic (Biochemical) Functions

a. TPP acts as a coenzyme for:
   i. Pyruvate dehydrogenase complex

$$\text{Pyruvate} \xrightarrow[\text{TPP, lipoamide and FAD}]{\text{Pyruvate dehydrogenase complex}} \alpha \text{ Acetyl CoA}$$

   ii. Ketoglutarate dehydrogenase complex of TCA cycle

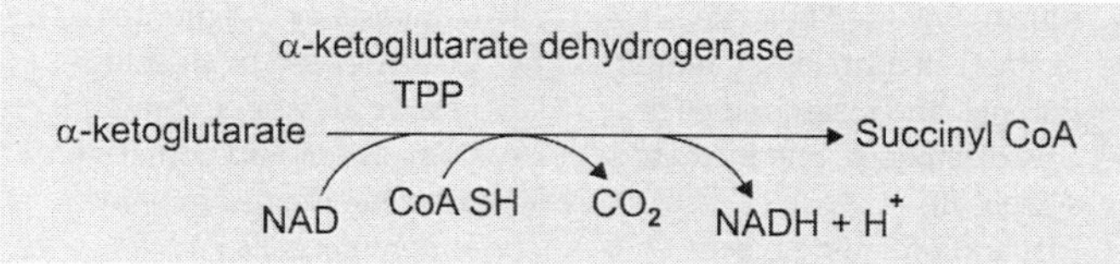

iii. α-keto acid (branched chain) dehydrogenase complex.

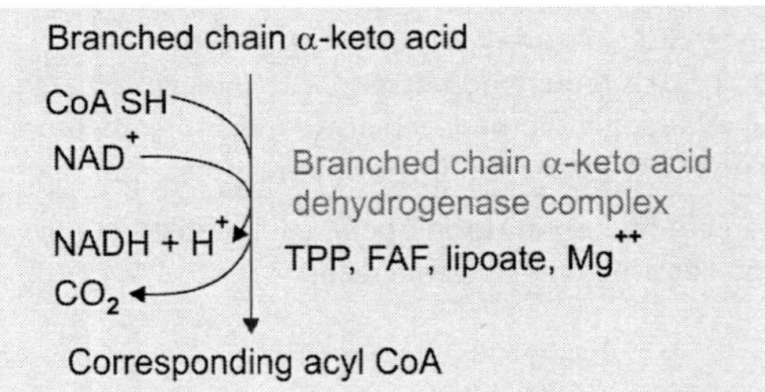


iv. Transketolase of HMP pathway.

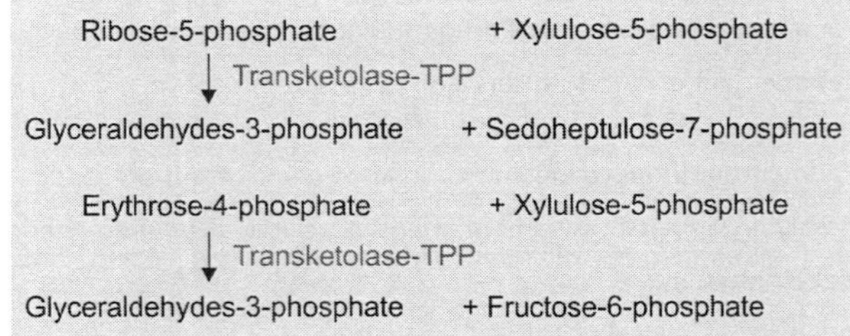


v. Decarboxylation step of degradation of α keto derivatives of branched chain amino acids, i.e. valine, leucine and isoleucine.

b. TPP plays an important role in transmission of nerve impulse (by acetylcholine synthesis and ion translocation in neural tissue).



## Deficiency Disorders

Beriberi (Sinhalese = I cannot)

| *Causes* | *Clinical features (common to all)* | *Diagnosis* | *Treatment* |
|---|---|---|---|
| • Inadequate intake (consumption of excessively polished rice)<br>• Ingestion of raw fish (contains microbial thiaminase)<br>• Impaired absorption (small intestinal disorders)<br>• Increased requirement (pregnancy, alcoholics) | • Anorexia, nausea, vomiting<br>• Weight loss, lassitude<br>• Rise in blood pyruvate level | • Elevated pyruvate and lactate concentration in serum and urinary excretion (due to ↓ activity of pyruvate dehydrogenase complex)<br>• Accumulation of pentose sugars<br>• Decreased RBC transketolase activity in erythrocytes (most common test for diagnosing thiamine deficency)<br>• Decreased thiamine excretion in urine | • Dietary supplementation |

## Types (Features)

| *Dry or neurotic beriberi (predominant CNS manifestations)* | *Wet or edematous beriberi (predominant CVS manifestations)* | *Infantile beriberi* | *Wernicke-Korsakoff syndrome or cerebral beriberi* |
|---|---|---|---|
| • Hyperaesthesia, paralysis and blindness (due to inflammation of peripheral nerves)<br>• Lesion in ventral horn of spinal cord, inflammation of dorsal root ganglia<br>• Loss of deep reflexes<br>• Mental confusion and anxiety | • Edema of legs, face, trunk and serous cavities<br>• Palpitation and breathlessness (due to enlarged heart)<br>• Tender calf muscles are tender<br>• Pulsatile and distended neck<br>• Low diastolic BP and increased systolic BP<br>• Fast and pounding pulse<br>• Weak heart resulting in heart failure | • Seen in infants born to/ breastfed by mothers suffering from thiamine deficiency<br>• Manifests by 2–4 months<br>• Characterized by sleeplessness, restlessness, vomiting<br>• Convulsions and bouts of screaming resembling abdominal colic<br>• Death due to cardiac failure | • Seen in chronic alcoholics<br>• Characterized by lesion and hemorrhage near third ventricle<br>• In-coordination and paralysis of eye movements<br>• Insomnia<br>• Abnormal gait and stance<br>• Mental confusion, depression, deranged mental function, disorientation, extreme anxiety and severe loss of memory |

## 9. What is anion gap? Explain normal anion gap acidosis and high anion gap acidosis with example.

- Anion gap is a mathematical approximation of difference between anions (chloride and bicarbonate—86%) and cations (sodium and potassium—95%) routinely measured in serum
- Refers to unmeasured anions in serum.

### Reason

- Due to presence of unmeasured cations like calcium, magnesium and unmeasured anions like protein, sulphate, phosphate and organic acids.

| *Calculations* | *Normal range* |
|---|---|
| Anion gap $= (Na^+ + K^+) - (Cl^- + HCO^-)$<br>$= (136 + 4) - (98 + 25)$<br>$= 140 - 123$<br>$= 17$ | • 12 to 20 mmol/L |

| | *Normal anion gap acidosis (Inorganic acidosis)* | *High anion gap acidosis (Organic acidosis)* | *Decreased anion gap* |
|---|---|---|---|
| Definition | • When there is loss of both anions and cations<br>• Thus though anion gap is normal but acidosis prevails | • Anion gap increases due to accumulation of other buffer anions but there is no change in chloride level | |
| Causes/ Examples | • Loss of intestinal secretions as in diarrhea, intestinal fistula<br>• Renal tubular acidosis<br>• Carbonic anhydrase inhibitors<br>• Drugs (antacids, lithium) | • Renal failure<br>• Diabetic ketosis<br>• Hypoxic states (accumulation of lactic acids—lactic acidosis)<br>• Salicylates<br>• Methanol<br>• Amino aciduria, organic aciduria<br>• Drugs (steroids, nitrates) | • Hypoalbuminemia<br>• Multiple myeloma<br>• Bromide intoxication<br>• Hypercalcemia |
| Treatment/ Compensation | • Restoration of ECF volume | • Through elimination of $CO_2$ rate and depth of respiration is increased<br>• Renal compensation is not very effective unless GFR increases<br>• In lactic acidosis and ketoacidosis, $HCO_3^-$ is used up but new bicarbonate is generated by activation of carbonic anhydrase<br>• $H^+$ excretion is increased | |

### Significance

- Anion gap helps for better understanding of pathophysiology of acid-base imbalance
- For quality control of laboratory results for $Na^+$, $K^+$, $Cl^-$ and $CO_2$
- For differential diagnosis of metabolic acidosis.

## 10. Lesch Nyhan syndrome and orotic aciduria.

### Lesch-Nyhan Syndrome

- Inherited disorder of salvage pathway of purine nucleotide synthesis

| *Inheritance* | *Deficient enzyme* | *Clinical feature* | *Treatment* |
|---|---|---|---|
| X-linked recessive | Hypoxanthine guanine phosphoribosyltransferase (HGPRT) | Excessive uric acid production causing gouty arthritis and neurological abnormalities such as mental retardation, aggressive behavior and learning disabilities<br>Patients have an urge for self mutilation by biting their own fingers and lips | Allopurinol to reduces uric acid formation<br>(Does not improve neurologic symptoms) |

## Orotic Aciduria

- Rare genetic metabolic disorder of pyramidine synthesis.

*Deficient Enzymes*

- Orotate phosphoribosyl transferase and OMP decarboxylase.

*Types*

- Type 1: Severe deficiency of orotate phosphoribosyl transferase and OMP decarboxylase
- Type 2: Inherited deficiency of OMP decarboxylase only.

*Causes*

- Inherited deficiency of enzymes
- Ornithine transcarbamoylase deficiency (less severe form)
  - Accumulation of carbamoyl phosphate in liver mitochondria → leakage → accumulation in cytosol
- Drug induced
  - Allopurinol or 6-azauridine inhibit OMP decarboxylase.

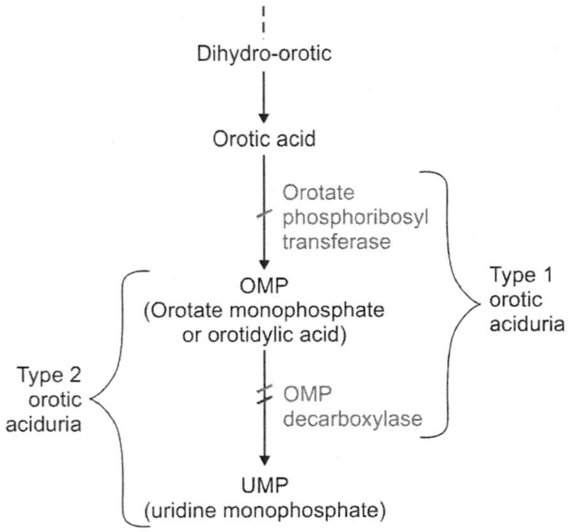

**Fig. 19:** Orotic aciduria—types

## Clinical Features

- Orotic aciduria (due to accumulation of orotic acid)
- Megaloblastic anemia and retarded growth (due to non-availability of pyrimidine bases).

## Treatment

- Diet rich in uridine and/or cytidine because these compounds through phosphorylation provide pyramidine nucleotides required for DNA and RNA synthesis and UTP inhibits carbomoyl phosphate synthetase II and blocks synthesis of orotic acid.

### 11. What is mutation? Give an account on point mutation.

- Mutation is a random undetected heritable variation caused by an alteration in nucleotide sequence at some point of DNA of cell, which may be in form of addition, deletion or substitution of one or more bases
- Mutation is a natural event, taking place all the time at a particular frequency of $10^{-2}$ to $10^{-10}$ per bacterium per division.

| *Causes* | *Features* | *Mechanism* |
|---|---|---|
| • Spontaneous<br>• Chemical mutagens (substances increasing frequency of mutation)<br>– Alkylating agents, acridine dyes, 5-bromouracil and 2-aminopurine<br>• Irradiation<br>– UV rays, ionizing radiations<br>• Error in DNA proofreading<br>• Error in DNA repair<br>• Error in DNA recombination | • May affect any gene and hence may modify any character<br>• Mostly goes unrecognized as it may be lethal or it may affect some minor function<br>• Best appreciated when it involves a readily observable function like nutritional requirements, biochemical reaction, antigenic structure, morphological features, colony form, drug susceptibility, virulence and host range, etc. | • During DNA replication, some error creeps in while progeny strands are copied<br>Example<br>• While replication guanine may bind with thymine instead of adenine due to tautomerism |

## Types

a. Point mutations

| *Base substitution mutation* | | *Frameshift mutation* |
|---|---|---|
| • Mutation where one base pair is replaced by another | | • Insertion or deletion of base in gene resulting in altered reading frame of mRNA<br>• Example: Thalassemia characterized by abnormal Hb chain synthesis |
| ↓ | ↓ | |
| *Transition* | *Transversion* | |
| • A base, either purine or pyramidine replaced by another base of same type<br>• Example: Hb C where adenine is substituted by guanine | • A purine base replaced by a pyramidine base or vice versa<br>• Example: HbS where adenine is substituted by uracil | |
| Transition mutation → Purine base replaced by purine base<br>Lysine: A A A ← HbA<br>↓<br>G A A ← HbC: Glutamic acid (codon in mRNA)<br>**Fig. 20A:** Transition mutation | Transversion mutation → Purine base replaced by pyrimidine base<br>Glutamic acid: G A A ← HbA<br>G U A ← HbS: Valine (codon in mRNA)<br>**Fig. 20B:** Transversion mutation | |

b. Large mutations

| *Deletions* | *Insertions* | *Recombination (Deletions and duplications)* |
|---|---|---|
| • Larger deletions may affect a portion of a gene or an entire gene<br>• Example: Duchenne's muscular dystrophy | • Insertions of gene may occur by retro-transposition<br>• Example: Appearance of a repeat sequence in blood clotting factor VIII gene as a cause of hemophilia A | • Results from non-aligned recombination<br>• A mismatch during recombination of two separate genes of similar sequence leading to deletion of some genes on one strand and duplication of some genes in other strand<br>• Example: Hemoglobin lepore with mismatch in combination of a and d chains |



## Effects of Mutation

| *Silent mutation* | *Missense mutation* | *Nonsense mutation* |
|---|---|---|
| • May go unnoticed because of degeneracy of the codon<br>• Example: Codon UCA codes for serine and any point mutation causing change in third base, i.e. UCO may not cause biochemical abnormality because codon UCO also codes for amino acid serine | • Mutated codon codes for different amino acid which may be acceptable, partially acceptable or unacceptable with regard to function of protein molecule<br>• Example: Hemoglobinopathies | • Makes a codon a terminating codon which acts as a stop signal for protein synthesis<br>• Example: Substitution of A for U in middle codon of leucine (UUG) results in generation of non-sense codons (UAG) |

## 12. What is nitrogen balance? Explain factors affecting nitrogen balance.

- Nitrogen balance is defined as quantitative difference between nitrogen intake and nitrogen output
- An adult healthy individual maintaining constant weight is said to be in nitrogen balance or nitrogenous equilibrium if his amount of intake of N in food as dietary proteins is equal to excretion of N in urine and sweat as urea, uric acid, creatine, creatinine, amino acids and in feces as unabsorbed N [Nitrogen Balance – Dietary Intake = Loss of protein through Urine + Feces + Skin]

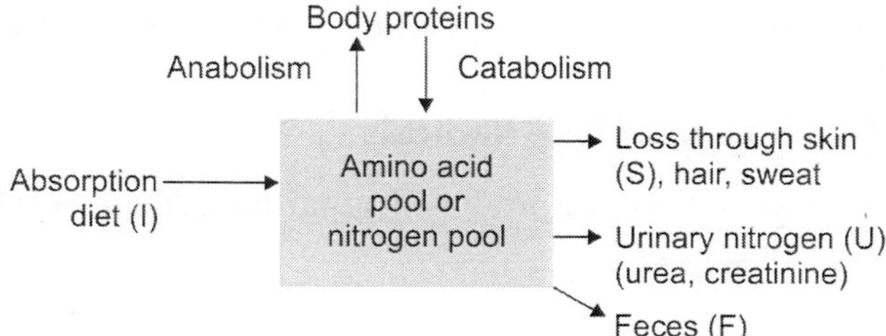


**Fig. 21:** Nitrogen balance

- Similarly a person can be in positive nitrogen balance or negative nitrogen balance:

| | *Positive Nitrogen Balance* | *Negative Nitrogen Balance* |
|---|---|---|
| Definition | • Nitrogen intake is higher than output | • Nitrogen output is higher than input |
| Causes | • Growing children, adolescents, pregnant women<br>• During recovery after serious illness<br>• Administration of growth hormone, Insulin and anabolic steroids | • Increased tissue catabolism: Fever, infections, muscle wasting, hyperthyroidism and conditions associated with cortisol excess<br>• Increased loss of proteins in urine: Nephrotic syndrome<br>• Increased loss of protein in stool: Protein loosing enteropathy<br>• Decreased intake of protein: Malnutrition |
| Factors influencing | • Growth, pregnancy (due to growth of fetus)<br>• Growth hormones, insulin and androgen<br>• Convalescence (due to active regeneration of tissues) | • Protein deficiency (starvation), acute illness<br>• Corticosteroids, thyroid hormones<br>• Chronic illness (cancer, uncontrolled diabetes) |

## SHORT ANSWERS

### 13. Define oncogene. Give examples of oncogene.

Refer Question No. 3 Dec. 2010 (RS2).

### 14. Name mucopolysaccharides. Mention their function.

Refer Question No. 5 Dec. 2015 (RS2).



### 15. Give brief account on quarternary structure of proteins.

Refer Question No. 4 Dec. 2011 (RS2).

### 16. Define free radicals. How free radicals are generated in the body?

- Free radicals are atoms or molecules containing 1 or more unpaired electrons in an outer orbit and is capable of independent existence
- They are usually generated by partial reduction of $O_2$ and they are highly reactive and create havoc in living systems. Hence, also called reactive oxygen species or ROS
- They are highly reactive species and have a tendency either to lose an electron thereby acting as reducing agent or gain an electron acting as oxidizing agent
- Thus they can initiate chain reaction by extracting an electron from a neighboring molecule to complete its own orbit.

| *Biologically important free radicals* | *Important characteristics* |
|---|---|
| • Superoxide radical ($O_2^-$)<br>• Hydrogen peroxide ($H_2O_2$)<br>• Hydroxyl peroxide ($OH^-$)<br>• Lipid peroxide radical ($ROO^{\cdot}$)<br>• Nitric oxide ($NO^-$)<br>• Peroxy nitrite ($ONOO^-$)<br>• Hypochlorous acid (HOCl)<br>**Note:** Hydrogen peroxide and singlet oxygen are not free radicals; however, because of their extreme reactivity, they are included in group of reactive oxygen species | • Extreme reactivity<br>• Short life span<br>• Generation of new ROS by chain reaction<br>• Damage to various tissues |

### Generation of Free Radicals

- Free radicals are produced by partial reduction of $O_2$ within mitochondrial inner membrane catalyzed by cytochrome oxidase

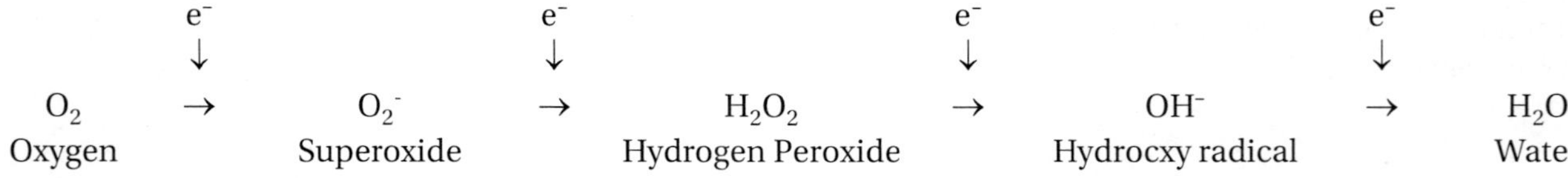

**Functions (Beneficial Effect)**

- Free radicals are implicated in causation and progression of several diseases like atherosclerosis, cancer, aging, etc.
- But their beneficial function in human body include bactericidal action during phagocytosis
- HClO and $H_2O_2$ produced by NADPH oxidase, superoxide dismutase and myeloperoxiadse mediate bactericidal action by oxidative degradation of bacterial lipids, proteins and DNA.

**Role in Diseases**

a. Chronic inflammation
   - Chronic inflammatory diseases like rheumatoid arthritis are self perpetuated by free radicals released by neutrophils
   - Free radical induced tissue damage is responsible for chronic ulcerative colitis, chronic glomerulonephritis.

b. Acute inflammation
   - Free radicals are produced by macrophages and neutrophils at inflammatory site.

c. Respiratory diseases
   - Reactive oxygen species are incriminated in adult respiratory distress syndrome (ARDS)
   - Free radicals from cigarette smoke causes lung damage.

d. Cardiovascular diseases
   - Oxidized low density lipoproteins formed by action of free radicals promote atherosclerosis.

e. Diabetes
   - Accumulation of free radicals leads to destruction of islets of pancreas causing pathogenesis of insulin dependent diabetes mellitus.

f. Diseases of eye
   - Cataract is result of photochemical generation of free radicals
   - Retrolental fibroplasia (retinopathy of prematurity) is caused by free radicals, causing thromboxane release, sustained vascular contracture and cellular injury.

g. Reperfusion injury
   - Reperfusion injury after myocardial ischemia is caused by free radicals.

h. Shock related injury
   - Free radicals released from phagocytes cause release of leukotrienes from platelets and proteases from macrophages which bring about increased vascular permeability resulting in tissue edema.

i. Carcinogenesis
   - Free radicals produce DNA damage and accumulated damages lead to somatic mutations and malignancy
   - Reactive oxygen species induce mutations and inhibit DNA repair mechanism which result in inactivation of tumor suppressor genes leading to cancer
   - Free radicals also trigger cell death and promote rapid growth of tumor cells.

j. Male infertility
   - Free radicals reduce sperm motility and viability.

k. Ageing
   - Free radicals play a pivotal role in degenerative brain disorders like Parkinsonism, Alzheimer's dementia and multiple sclerosis
   - Free radicals are closely associated with various biochemical and morphological changes occurring during normal aging.

**Application**

- Free radicals produced by X-ray destroy tumor tissue, thus radiation therapy is used in treatment of cancer.

## 17. Name subcellular organelles. Which are metabolic functions of cytosol?

Refer Question No. 7 Dec. 2012 (RS2).

## 18. Degradation of heme.

Refer Question No. 8 June 2007 (RS2).

## 19. Gout.

Refer Question No. 2 June 2007 (RS2).

## 20. What is polymerase chain reaction? Mention its application.

Refer Question No. 11 June 2006 (RS2).

## 21. What are metabolic roles of zinc and selenium?

**For Selenium**

Refer Question No. 11 June 2010 (RS2).

**For Zinc**

Refer Question No. 10 June 2006 (RS2).

## 22. Which are biologically important nucleotides? Mention their functions.

- Nucleotides are nitrogenous bases attached to pentose to which is attached a phosphate, i.e. Nucleotide = (base + pentose) + phosphate = Nucleoside + phosphate
- Thus nucleotides are nucleosides phosphates
- Purine nucleotides contain either adenine or guanine as nitrogenous base whereas pyramidine nucleotides contain either uridine or cytosine as nitrogenous base.



### Biologically Important Nucleotides and their Function

| | *Function* |
|---|---|
| **Adenosine nucleotides** | |
| a. Adenosine triphosphate (ATP) | • Providing energy for many endergonic processes<br>• Synthesis of many biological important compounds like creatinine phosphate, fatty acids, proteins and glucose<br>• Donating phosphate group in phosphotransferase reactions<br>• Muscle contraction, sperm motility, nerve impulse transmission, etc.<br>• Formation of active methionine and active sulfate |
| b. Adenosine monophosphate (AMP) | • Constituent of RNAs<br>• Activates the enzyme phosphofructokinase and inhibits fructose 1-6 diphosphatase and adenylosuccinate synthetase |
| c. Deoxyadenosine monophosphate (dAMP) | • Constituent of DNA |
| d. Cyclic AMP (cAMP) | • Acts as second messenger for various hormones |
| **Gaunosine nucleotides** | |
| a. Guanosine triphosphate (GTP) | • Required for protein synthesis<br>• Involved in oxidation of succinyl CoA in TCA cycle |
| b. Guanosine monophosphate (GMP) and deoxyguanosine monophosphate (dGMP) | • Integral part of RNA and DNA respectively |
| **Uridine nucleotides** | |
| a. Uridine triphosphate (UTP) | • Can be converted to CTP by glutamine<br>• Forms UDPG on reacting with glucose-6-phosphate |
| b. Uridine monophosphate (UMP) | • Constituent of RNAs<br>• Can be converted to UDP and UTP |
| c. Deoxyuridine monophosphate (dUMP) | • Constituent of DNA |
| d. Uridine diphosphoglucose (UDPG) | • Acts as intermediate between glucose and galactose interconversion<br>• Transfers glucose molecule to glycogen primer in glycogenesis |

*Contd...*

Contd...

| | *Function* |
|---|---|
| **Cytidine nucleotides** | |
| a. Deoxycytidine monophosphate (dCMP) | • Constituent of DNA |
| b. Cytidine monophosphate (CMP) | • Integral part of RNA<br>• CMP-acetyl neuraminic acid is important precursor of cell wall polysaccharides in bacteria<br>• CMP-sialic acid is present in salivary glands |
| c. Cytidine diphosphate (CDP) | CDP-choline, CDP-glycerol and CDP-ethanolamine are involved in biosynthesis of phospholipids |
| **Miscellaneous nucleotides** | |
| a. Phosphoadenosine phospho sulphate (PAPS) | • Donates $SO_4$ group to various molecules in:<br>– Heparin biosynthesis<br>– Chondroitin sulfate biosynthesis<br>– Keratosulphate synthesis<br>– Formation of sulfalipids |
| b. S-adenosyl methionine (SAM) | • Donates methyl group to various molecules in methylation reactions |
| c. $NAD^+$, $NADP^+$, FAD and FMN | • Involved in oxidation-reduction reactions helping in transfer of $H^+$ |

## Significance

- Thus nucleotides play important role in biochemical functions of body besides being an integral part of nucleic acids.

# MBBS PHASE I EXAMINATION
## DECEMBER 2005
### (Revised Scheme 2)

## LONG ESSAYS

### 1. Enumerate the compounds formed from glycine, giving their biological importance. Why glycine is nutritionally nonessential?

- Glycine is an aliphatic amino acid (α amino acetic acid)
- Simplest amino acid
- Glucogenic amino acid
- Nutritionally, nonessential because can be synthesized in body from serine, choline, glycoxylic acid and threonine.

#### Glycine Metabolism

*Synthesis of Glycine*

| | |
|---|---|
| a. From serine | Serine + Tetrahydrofolate ($FH_4$)<br>↓ PFP Serine hydroxymethyl transferase<br>Glycine + $N^{5,10}$ methylene tetrahydrofolate |
| b. From ammonia, $CO_2$ and $N^{5,10}$ methylene $FH_4$ (By glycine synthase complex) | $CO_2 + NH_3 + N^{5,10}$ Methylene $FH_4$ + NADH + $H^+$<br>↓ PLP Glycine cleavage system (glycine synthase complex)<br>Glycine + $FH_4$ + $NAD^+$ |
| c. From choline | Choline → Betaine → Dimethylglycine → Glycine |
| d. From glyoxylate | Glyoxylate + Alanine (or glutamate)<br>↕ PLP alanine glyoxylate aminotransferase<br>Glycine + Pyruvate (or α-ketoglutarate) |
| e. From threonine | Threonine<br>↓ Threonine aldolase<br>Acetaldehyde + Glycine |

#### Compounds Formed from Glycine (Metabolic Role)

a. Proteins and peptides
   - Glycine is richly present in collagen (in collagen, every third amino acid is glycine)

b. Creatine

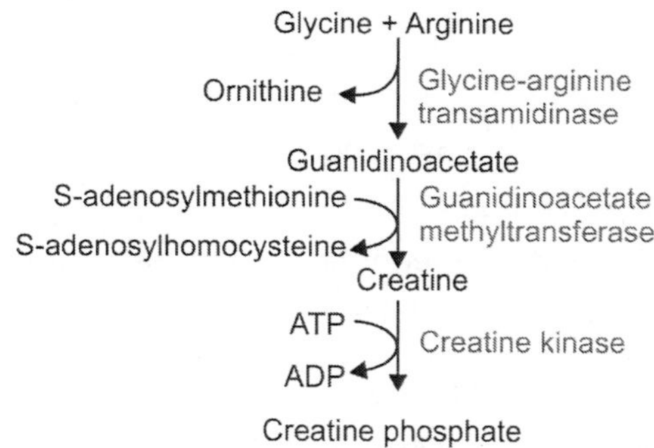


**Fig. 1:** Formation creatine

*Functions of creatine*

- Phosphorylated form of creatine storage form of high energy compound in muscle and heart
- Used to regenerate adenosine triphosphate (ATP) required during vigorous muscle contraction or cardiac contractility by donating phosphate for conversion of ADP to ATP by enzyme creatine kinase (Lohmann's reaction).

c. Glutathione

- Glutathione is a tripeptide containing glutamic acid, cysteine and glycine present widely in various tissues but highly concentrated in red blood cells (RBCs).

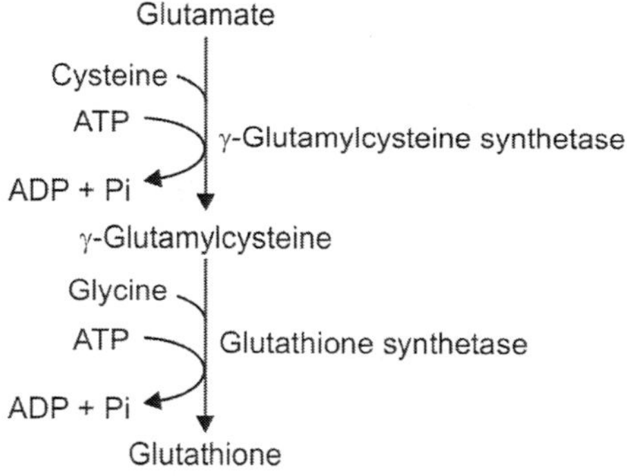


**Fig. 2:** Formation of glutathione

*Functions of glutathione (oxidation-reduction reactions)*

- Keeps enzymes in reduced state (active state)
- Suppresses oxidative stress in cell by converting $H_2O_2$ (oxidant) to $H_2O$ (antioxidant function)
- Reduced glutathione maintenance red cell membrane stability
- Reduced glutathione also prevents oxidation of hemoglobin to methemoglobin
- Helps in absorption of amino acids (gamma-glutamyl cycle).

d. Heme

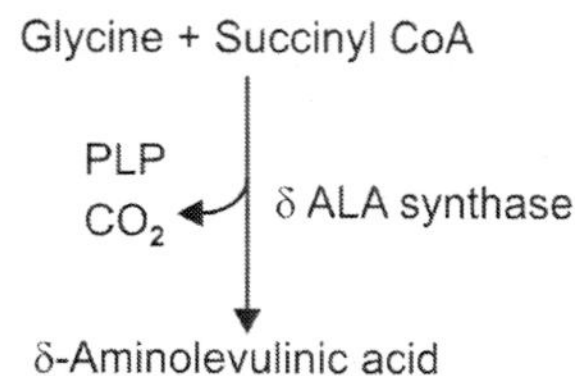


**Fig. 3:** Formation of ALA (precursor of heme)

*Functions of heme*

- Required for biosynthesis of hemoglobin, myoglobin and heme-containing enzymes such as cytochrome oxidase, catalase and peroxidise.

e. Bile acids

Cholyl CoA + Glycine —(Conjugation)→ Glycocholate

Chenodexycholyl CoA + Glycine —(Conjugation)→ Glycochenodeoxycholate

*Functions of bile acids*

– Sodium or potassium salts of bile acids are required for solubilization of cholesterol, excretion of cholesterol, digestion and absorption of triacylglycerols and fat-soluble vitamins.

f. Purine nucleotides (De novo synthesis)

– Glycine contributes C4, C5 and N-7 of purine ring

5-Phosphoribosylamine + Glycine + ATP —(Glycinamide ribose phosphate synthetase)→ Glycinamide ribose-5 phosphate + ADP + Pi

g. Serine

$N^{5\text{-}10}$ methylene $FH_4$ + Glycine —(Serine hydroxy methyl transferase)→ Serine + $FH_4$

h. Glucose

Glycine → Serine → Pyruvate → Glucose

i. Hippuric acid (detoxification of benzoic acid)

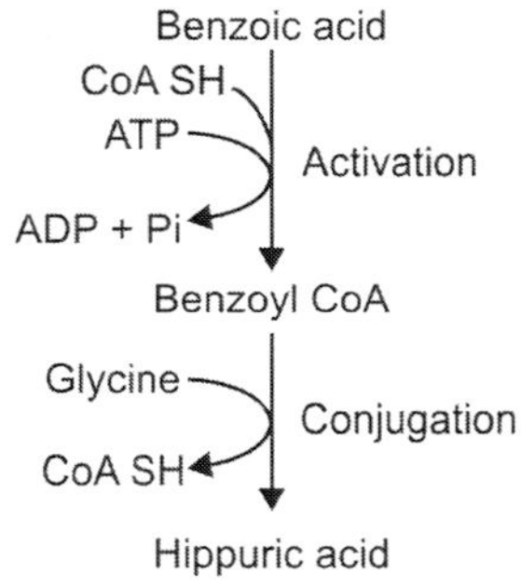


**Fig. 4:** Formation of hippuric acid

## Catabolism

| | |
|---|---|
| a. To glutamate (by transamination) | |
| b. To oxalate and formate | Glycine —(FAD → $FADH_2$, $NH_3$; Glycine oxidase)→ Glyoxylate; Glyoxylate —(Decarboxylation)→ Formate; Glyoxylate —(Oxidation)→ Oxalate<br>**Fig. 5:** Catabolism of oxalate and formate |
| c. To $N^{5,10}$ methylene $FH_4$ (by glycine cleavage system) | Glycine + $FH_4$ (tetrahydrofolate) + $NAD^+$ ⇌ (PLP; Glycine cleavage system) $CO_2$ + $NH_3$ + $N^{+5,10}$ methylene $FH_4$ + NADH + $H^+$<br>**Fig. 6:** Glycine of glycogen cleavage system |

## Disorders of Glycine Metabolism

a. Hyperglycemia
   – Rare inborn error due to defect in glycine cleavage system.

| *Inheritance* | *Deficiency enzyme* | *Clinical features* | *Biochemical findings* |
|---|---|---|---|
| Autosomal recessive | Glycine synthase | Mental retardation and seizures | ↑ blood glycine levels<br>Glycinuria |

b. Glycinuria

| *Inheritance* | *Defect* | *Features* |
|---|---|---|
| Autosomal recessive | Defective renal tubular reabsorption of glycine | Excretion of large amount of glycine and proline in urine |

c. Primary hyperoxaluria

| *Inheritance* | *Types (Defects)* | *Clinical features* |
|---|---|---|
| Autosomal recessive | 1. Type I hyperoxaluria<br>Defect in transamination of glyoxylate to glycine (due to deficiency of alanine glyoxylate aminotransferase<br>2. Type II hyperoxaluria<br>Defect in reduction of glyoxylate due to deficiency of D-glyceric acid dehydrogenase | • Seen in infancy<br>• Urolithiasis (urinary oxalate stone formation) and oxalosis (deposition of calcium oxalate stones in renal and extrarenal tissues)<br>• Renal stone formations leads to renal colic, renal hypertension and renal failure |

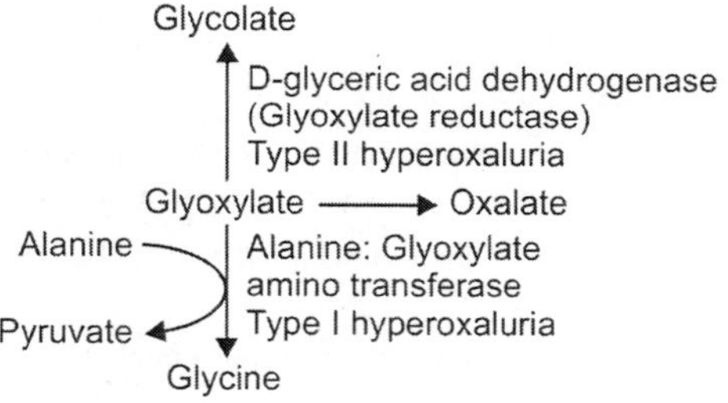


**Fig. 7:** Hyperoxaluria—types

### 2. Give an account of the chemistry, sources, daily requirement of vitamin C. Enumerate its biochemical functions and deficiency manifestations.

- Vitamin C or L-ascorbic acid is a water-soluble vitamin
- Also called antiscorbutic vitamin.

| *Chemistry* | *Sources* | *RDA* |
|---|---|---|
| • Enediol lactone of a hexuronic acid with a $C_2$–$C_3$ double bond with empirical formula $C_6H_8O_6$<br>• Pure vitamin C is a white, crystaline, odorless substance with acidic taste<br>• Highly water soluble and easily destroyed by heat, alkali and storage<br>• Has reducing action and can itself oxidize to dehydro-ascorbic acid | • Citrus fruits (oranges, lemon), tomatoes, strawberries, green vegetables, guava | • Children: 40 mg<br>• Adults: 60 mg<br>• Pregnancy: 70 mg<br>• Lactation: 95 mg |

## Coenzyme Forms

- Ascorbic acid (reduced form)
- Dehydro-ascorbic acid (oxidized form).

**Biochemical functions (based on reversible oxidation and reduction between two coenyzmes)**

| | |
|---|---|
| Collagen formation | Promotes collagen formation through its action on post-translational hydroxylation of proline and lysine residues; thus procollagen is transformed to mature collagen<br>*Protocollagen proline hydroxylase*<br>Proline → Hydroxylase<br>Vitamin C, $Fe^{++}$<br>mol. $O_2$<br>*Protocollagen lysine hydroxylase*<br>Lysine → Hydroxylase<br>Vitamin C, $Fe^{++}$<br>mol. $O_2$<br>**Fig. 8:** Hydroxylation of proline and lysine (in collagen maturation) |
| Bone formation | Essential for formation of bone matrix |
| Iron and Hb metabolism | • Enhances intestinal iron absorption by maintaining it in ferrous state<br>• Helps in reconversion of methemoglobin to hemoglobin |
| Tryptophan metabolism | Implicated in hydroxylation of tryptophan to serotonin |
| Tyrosine metabolism | Facilitates oxidation of parahydroxy phenyl pyruvate to homogentisic acid |
| Folic acid metabolism | Reduces folic acid to THFA, thus helps in maturation of RBCs |
| Corticosteroid synthesis | Plays a key role in biosynthesis of adrenal cortical hormones |
| Sparing action | • Has sparing action on other vitamins for oxidation like vitamin A, E and some B complex vitamins<br>• Stimulates growth of intestinal flora thus augments activities of vitamin B complex |
| Immunological action | Augments functions of reticuloendothelial system and has stimulating effect on phagocytic action of leukocytes and formation of antibodies |
| Prevention of cataracts | Reduces the risk of cataract formation (on regular intake) |
| Prevention of chronic diseases | As an antioxidant, it prevents cancer formation and inhibits formation of nitrosamines, a carcinogen |
| Cholesterol metabolism | Stimulates 7 alpha hydroxylase step in synthesis of bile acids from cholesterol |
| Carnitine synthesis | Required for biosynthesis of carnitine from lysine and methionine |



## Deficiency Manifestations

- Deficiency of vitamin C results in scurvy.

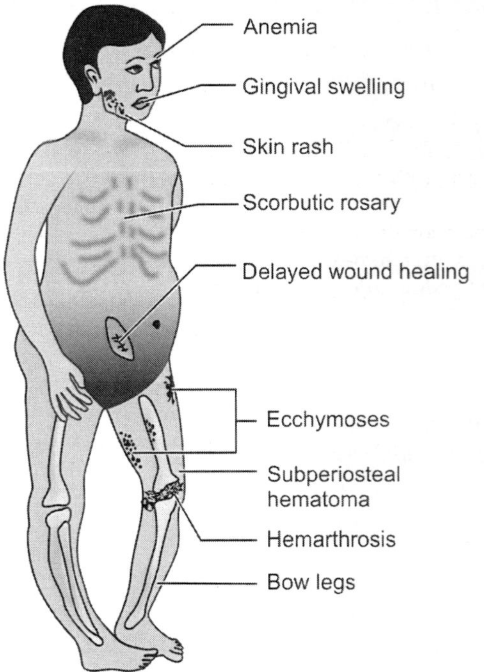


**Fig. 9:** Scurvy—manifestations

| *Causes* | *Features* | *Biochemical findings* |
|---|---|---|
| • Dietary deficiency<br>• Impaired absorption (celiac sprue)<br>• Increased demand (pregnancy, surgery, burns) | • Swollen and bleeding gums due to impaired osteoid tissue formation<br>• Petechial hemorrhages and ecchymoses due to rupture of capillaries, resulting from lack of intracellular substances<br>• Bleeding into bones and joints leads to subperiosteal hematoma and hemoarthrosis<br>• Arthritis due to impaired osteoid tissue formation<br>• Delayed wound healing due to impaired collagen formation<br>• Anemia—normochromic, normocytic (due to bleeding), megaloblastic (due to reduced erythropoiesis) and microcytic hypochromic anemia (due to impaired iron absorption and impaired heme synthesis)<br>• Fatigue, depression and susceptibility to infections | • Decreased plasma, platelet or leukocyte ascorbic acid levels<br>• Decreased vitamin C excretion in urine after a test dose of vitamin C |

## Significance

- Scurvy is first disease found to be associated with diet; first observed by James Lind in men at sea due to deficiency of fresh fruits in diet and their miraculous recovery following supply of lime.

## SHORT ESSAYS

### 3. Write steps of beta oxidation of fatty acids with energetics.

Refer Question No. 1 Dec. 2008 (RS2).

### 4. Give outline of gluconeogenesis and mention its significance.

Refer Question No. 1 June 2009 (RS2).

### 5. What are isoenzymes and give their clinical importance citing two examples.

Refer Question No. 1 Dec. 2007 (RS2).

### 6. What is P: O ratio? Which are inhibitors of electron transport chain?

Refer Question No. 5 June 2007 (RS2).

### 7. Write detail with examples reactions involved in detoxification.

- Detoxification refers to series of biochemical reaction occurring in body to convert endogenous or exogenous toxic compounds to nontoxic or less toxic compounds and more easily excretable forms
- Detoxification reactions generate more polar metabolites, that are readily excreted from body
- Liver plays the most important role.

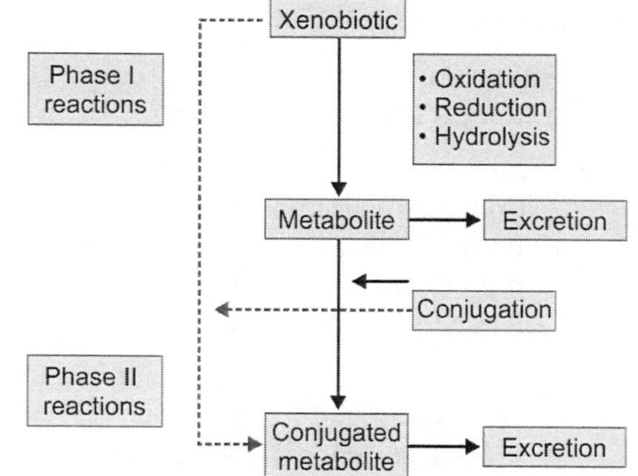


**Fig. 10:** Phases of detoxification

## Phases

- Phases I involving oxidation, reduction and hydrolysis
- Phase II involving conjugation reactions.

*Phase I Reactions*

a. Oxidation reactions (addition of oxygen or removal of hydrogen or electrons)
   - Enzymes involved are:
     - Microsomal oxidation system contains cytochrome P450 system

- Non-microsomal oxidoreductases include mitochondrial cytochrome P450 system, alcohol dehydrogenase (cytosol), aldehyde dehydrogenase (mitochondria) and mono amine oxidase
- Substances detoxified are alcohol aldehydes, amines, aromatic hydrocarbons and sulfur compounds
  i. Alcohols

| | | |
|---|---|---|
| $CH_3OH$ Methanol | → | HCOOH Formic acid |
| $C_2H_5OH$ Ethanol | → | $CH_3COOH$ Acetic acid |

  ii. Aldehydes

| | | |
|---|---|---|
| $C_6H$ CHO Benzaldehyde | → | $C_6H_5COOH$ Benzoic acid |
| $CH_3CHO$ Acetaldehyde | → | $CH_3COOH$ Acetic acid |

  iii. Amines and their derivatives

| | | |
|---|---|---|
| $RCH_2NH_2$ Aliphatic amine | → | $R - COOH + NH_2 - CO - NH_2$ Aliphatic acid + Urea |

  iv. Aromatic hydrocarbons
  Benzene → phenol
  v. Sulfur compounds
  * Organic sulfur is oxidized to sulfuric acid

b. Reduction reactions (removal of oxygen or addition of hydrogen or electrons)
  i. Acetaldehydes
  $CCI_3CHO \rightarrow CCI_3CH_2OH$
  ii. Aromatic nitro compounds

| | | |
|---|---|---|
| $C_6H_2OH(NO_2)_3$ Picric acid | → | $C_6H_2OH(NO_2)_2NH_2$ Picramic acid |
| Nitrobenzene | → | Aminobenzene |

c. Hydrolysis reaction (breakdown of compound using water)

| | | |
|---|---|---|
| Acetyl salicylic acid (Aspirin) | → | Salicyclic acid and Acetic acid |
| Acetanilide | → | Aniline + Acetic acid |
| Atropine | → | Tropic acid and Tropine |
| Procaine | → | p-Aminobenzoic acid + Diethylaminoethanol |

*Phase II Reactions*

- Conjugation reactions
  - Conjugation is process in which a foreign compound combines with a substance produced in body.

*Features*
- Conjugation is done by substances available in body or some of them are synthesized in body
- It principally occurs in liver but can also occur in kidneys also
- It produces less toxic and more water-soluble compounds
- It occurs independently or follows phase I reactions

*Types*
- Glucoronic acid
  - Most common detoxification reaction
  - Active form of glucoronic acid (UDP gluocoronic acid) transfers a molecule of glucoronic acid to convert a toxic molecule with hydroyl, carbonyl, sulfhydryl or amino group into a nontoxic compound

| | | |
|---|---|---|
| Bilirubin + UDP gluocoronic acid | → | Biliruibin monoglucoronide + UDP |
| Bilirubin monoglucoronide + UDP gluocoronic acid | → | Bilirubin diglucoronide + UDP |
| Phenol + UDP gluocoronic acid | → | Phenyl glucuronide |
| Benzoic acid + UDP gluocoronic acid | → | Benzoyl glucuronide + UDP |

- Glycine
  - Many aromatic carboxylic acids are detoxified by conjugation with glycine

| | | |
|---|---|---|
| Benzoyl CoA + Glycine | → | Hippuric acid |
| Phenylacetic acid + Glycine | → | Phenylaceturic acid |
| Cholic acid + Glycine | → | Glycocholic acid |

- Cysteine
  - Cystine is used for conjugation reactions of alkyl or aryl halides, alkenes, nitro compounds and epoxides
- Glutamine
  - Phenylacetic acid is conjugated with glutamine to form phenylacetyl glutamine
- Methyl group
  - Methyl group of SAM is frequently used to methylate certain xenobiotics
  - Example: Nicotinamide
- Sulfate
  - PAPS (3'phospho-adenosine 5 phosphosulfate), active form of sulfate is used in detoxification of several aliphatic and aromatic compounds

| | | |
|---|---|---|
| Phenol + PAPS | → | Phenoxyl sulfate |
| Indoxyl + PAPS | → | Indoxyl sulfate |

- Acetic acid
  - Acetyl CoA, active form of acetic acid also detoxifies many toxic substances
  - Example: Isoniazid, sulfanilamide
- Thiosulfate
  - Thiosulfate conjugates highly toxic cyanides.

### Significance

- Detoxification serves as an important defense mechanism in that toxic metabolites are converted into less harmful substances and substances that can be excreted from body
- Detoxification differ from biotransformation (modifications of xenobiotics occurring in body) as biotransformation deals with only exogenous toxic substances and not all reactions of biotransformation yield nontoxic metabolities.

## 8. What is normal serum calcium level? Explain its regulation.

Refer Question No. 2 June 2009 (RS2).

## 9. Name the clearance tests used to assess kidney function. Explain any one of the clearance tests and mention its significance.

- Clearance refers to plasma that is completely cleared of the substance (which appears in urine) in a unit time and expressed as mL/min
- Clearance tests are assess kidney function by measuring the glomerular filtration rate
- Measurement of glomerular filtration rate (GFR) provides the most useful general index for assessment of severity of renal damage.

### Clearance Tests to Assess Kidney Function

- Creatinine clearance tests (overestimates GFR)
  - Most commonly used clearance test to assess renal functioning

- Inulin clearance test (true measure of GFR)
  - Used as a reference method for the determination of GFR
  - Inulin is readily filtered by glomerulus, not reabsorbed by the tubules and not secreted by tubule
  - However, not used for routine diagnostic use since it is exogenous material and infusion requires monitoring for constant amount of inulin in plasma during the test.
- Urea clearance test (underestimates GFR)
  - Also an index of glomerular filtration and clearance is lower than inulin clearance since it is reabsorbed by the tubules
  - Not used for renal function test since it is subjected to variations due to changes in its production in disease states and enhanced reabsoption in prerenal failure.

## Creatinine Clearance Test

- Creatinine clearance is an endogenous cleareance test to asses glomerular function of kidney
- It is calculated by estimating serum and urine creatinine.

*Principle*

- Creatinine in glomerular filtrate is only minimally absorbed and not secreted by tubules
- Since its excretion rate is relatively constant and its production is independent of metabolism or hormonal factors; it is a good measure for renal glomerular function.

*Procedure*

- Give 500 mL of water to promote good urine flow
- After about 30 minutes empty the bladder and discard the urine
- Exactly after 60 minutes again void the bladder and collect the urine and note the volume
- At the same time, take a blood sample
- Creatinine level in blood and urine are tested by Jaffe's reaction
- Blood level is tested after removing the serum protein and then adsorbing creatinine on Lloyd's reagent and then reacting with alkaline picarate to give an orange color
- Urine is tested after dilution due to high creatinine concentration and then creatinine clearance is calculated.

*Calculations*

Uncorrected clearance = $(U/P) \times V$

where U = Urine creatinine concentration

P = Plasma creatinine concentration

V = Urine flow in mL/min

*Normal values*

- Males : 85–125 mL/min
- Females : 80–115 mL/min

## Significance

- A decreased creatinine clearance is a very sensitive indicator of reduced glomerular filtration rate due to acute or chronic damage
- Clearance value up to 75% of average normal value indicates adequate renal function
- Importance of creatinine clearance is in early detection of functional impairment of kidney without overt signs and symptoms
- It is very helpful in long-term monitoring of patients with renal insufficiency under a protein restricted diet.

**Advantages and disadvantages of creatinine clearance (as GFR marker)**

| *Advantages* | *Disadvantages* |
|---|---|
| • Extrarenal factors will rarely interfere<br>• Conversion of creatine phosphate to creatinine is spontaneous, nonenzymatic<br>• As production is continuous, blood levels will not fluctuate and blood may be collected at any time<br>• Not affected by diet or exercise | • Creatinine is filtered by glomeruli and actively excreted by tubules. Of total excretion, about 10% is tubular component. When GFR is reduced, the secretion component is increased and will viciate the results. Creatinine clearance is said to overestimate GFR by about 10–20 mL/mt<br>• When GFR is severely reduced, extrarenal excretion increases. Then the major route becomes the degradation by intestinal bacterial flora<br>• Very early stages of decrease in GFR may not be identified (creatinine blind area)<br>• Other prerenal, renal and postrenal causes will influence creatinine clearance |

## 10. Name the buffer system of body fluids. Explain any one of them.

Refer Question No. 2 June 2012 (RS2).

## 11. Give an account of salvage pathway.

- Salvage pathway is addition of ribose 5-phosphate to preformed purine bases or addition of phosphate to purine nucleosides.

### Sources of Purine Bases and Nucleosides

- From degradation of purine nucleotides (nucleotide turnover)
- From dietary sources (in smaller extent).

### Salvage Pathway

a. Synthesis of purine nucleotides from purine bases (salvage of purine bases)
   - Adenine is converted to AMP by the enzyme adenine phosphoribosyl transferase (APRT) using PRPP

| Adenosine + PRPP | → | Adenosine monophosphate + PPi |
|---|---|---|
| | APRT | |

   - Hypoxanthine-guanine phosphoribosyl transferase (HGPRT) transfers the phosphoribosyl group from PRPP to hypoxanthine, guanine or xanthine, converting them to IMP, GMP and XMP respectively

| Hypoxanthine + PRPP | → | Inosine monophosphate + PPi |
|---|---|---|
| | HGPRT | |

| Guanine + PRPP | → | Guanosine monophosphate + PPi |
|---|---|---|
| | HGPRT | |

   - These pathways are closely related to de novo synthesis as PRPP is substrate for both the pathways

b. Synthesis of purine nucleotides from purine nucleosides (salvage of purine nucleosides)
   - Adenosine kinase phosphorylates adenosine and deoxyadenosine with ATP to form AMP and dAMP

| Adenosine + ATP | → | AMP + ADP |
|---|---|---|
| | Adenosine kinase | |

| Deoxyadenosine + ATP | → | dAMP + ADP |
|---|---|---|
| | Adenosine kinase | |

   - Deoxycytidine kinase catalyzes addition of phosphate to deoxycytidine and deoxyguanosine

| Deoxycytidine + ATP | → | dCMP + ADP |
|---|---|---|
| | Deoxycytidine kinase | |

| Deoxyguanosine + ATP | → | dGMP + ADP |
|---|---|---|
| | Deoxycytidine kinase | |

   - This salvage and interconversion of purine nucleosides constitute purine salvage cycle

## Significance

- Salvage pathways provide a pathway for utilization of purine bases derived from diet (exogenous) and normal turnover of nucleic acids
- It is particularly important in certain tissues such as RBCs and brain where de novo synthesis of purine nucleotides does not takes place due to absence of PRPP amidotransferase
- It also economizes intracellular energy expenditure.

## Disorder

*Lesch-Nyhan Syndrome*

- Inherited disorder of salvage pathway of purine nucleotide synthesis

| *Inheritance* | *Deficient enzyme* | *Clinical feature* | *Treatment* |
|---|---|---|---|
| X-linked recessive | Hypoxanthine guanine phosphoribosyltransferase (HGPRT) | • Excessive uric acid production causing gouty arthritis and neurological abnormalities such as mental retardation, aggressive behavior and learning disabilities<br>• Patients have an urge for self mutilation by biting their own fingers and lips | Allopurinol to reduces uric acid formation (does not improve neurologic symptoms) |



### 12. Hemoglobinopathies.

Refer Question No. 2 Dec. 2013 (RS2).

## SHORT ANSWERS

### 13. Mention the significance of HMP shunt pathway.

Refer Question No. 4 Dec. 2013 (RS3).

### 14. Name essential fatty acids and mention their importance.

Refer Question No. 4 Dec. 2016 (RS2).

### 15. What is km value? Explain its importance.

Refer Question No. 6 Dec. 2010 (RS2).

### 16. Name three important growth factors and mention their function.

- Growth factors are substances which stimulate cell proliferation and regulate cell division by transmitting the message across plasma membrane to cell interior
- They cause mitoses or differentiation of target cells

| *Growth factor* | *Source* | *Function* |
|---|---|---|
| a. Platelet derived growth factor (PDGF) | • $\alpha$ granules of platelets<br>• Activated macrophages, endothelium and smooth muscles<br>• Certain tumor cells | • Stimulates growth of mesenchymal cells and glial cells<br>• Causes migration and proliferation of fibroblasts, smooth muscle cells and monocytes<br>• Promotes wound healing in vivo |
| b. Epidermal growth factor (EGF) | • Fibroblasts, submaxillary gland | • Stimulates growth of epidermal and epithelial cells |
| c. Fibroblast growth factor (FGFs) | • Activated macrophages (basic FGFs)<br>• Neural tissue (acidic FGFs) | • Binds to heparin and cause fibroblast proliferation and neovascularization |
| d. Transforming growth factor-$\alpha$ (TGF-$\alpha$) | • Epithelial cells | • Stimulates growth of epidermal and epithelial cells |

*Contd...*

*Contd...*

| *Growth factor* | *Source* | *Function* |
|---|---|---|
| e. Transforming growth factor-β (TGF-β) | • Platelets, kidney, placenta<br>• T cells<br>• Endothelium and macrophages | • Inhibits growth of most cells except fibroblasts<br>• Inhibits collagen degradation<br>• Deactivates macrophages<br>• Favors fibrogenesis in that stimulates fibroblast chemotaxis and collagen production |
| f. Erythropoietin (EP) | Renal non-tubular mesangial cells | Stimulates erythropoietic cells to proliferate and mature into erythrocytes |
| g. Nerve growth factor (NGF) | Salivary glands | Stimulates growth of sensory and sympathetic neurons |
| h. Insulin like growth factors (IGFI and II) | Serum | • Stimulates incorporation of sulfates in to cartilage<br>• Exerts insulin like action on certain cells<br>• Mitogenic for chondrocytes |
| i. Tumor necrosis factor-α (TNF-α) | Monocytes | • Necrosis of tumor cells, proliferation of leukocytes |
| j. Granulocyte monocyte colony stimulating factor (GM-CSF) | • Endothelial cells<br>• T cells<br>• Fibroblasts<br>• Keratinocytes | • Activates granulocytes, monocytes and megakaryocytes<br>• Stimulates hemopoietic progenitor cells of multiple lineage |
| k. Granulocyte colony stimulating factor (G-CSF) | • Endothelial cells<br>• Fibroblasts | • Stimulates granulocytes<br>• Activates neutrophils |
| l. Monocyte colony stimulating factor (M-CSF) | • Endothelial cells<br>• Monocytes<br>• Fibroblasts | • Activates monocytes<br>• Stimulates macrophage colony formation |
| m. Interleukin 1 (IL-1) | • Monocytes, leukocytes<br>• Macrophages<br>• Endothelium<br>• Glial cells | • Stimulates T lymphocytes to produce IL-2<br>• Stimulates mesenchymal cells to produce CSFs<br>• Chemotactic for fibroblasts and increases collagen synthesis |
| n. Interleukin 2 (IL – 2) | Activated T lymphocytes | • Stimulates growth of T lymphocytes<br>• Co-stimulates B-cells and monocyte differentiation<br>• Activates and promotes growth of NK cells |

## Significance

- Growth factors are usually polypeptides
- Can initiate cell migration, differentiation and tissue remodeling
- May be involved in various stages of wound healing
- Can affect many different types of cells, viz. hemopoietic cells, epithelial tissues, nervous system and mesenchymal tissues
- Play a major role in regulating differentiation of stem cells to form various types of mature cells
- Are mitogenic to target cells
- Products of several oncogenes are either growth factors or parts of receptors for growth factors
- Some growth factors may be inhibitory to growth of certain cells, e.g. TGF-β
- Chronic exposure of target cells to increased amounts of a growth factor or to decreased amounts of a growth inhibitory factor may alter the balance of cellular growth (growth autonomy).

## 17. Explain troponin as a marker for myocardial infarction.

Refer Question No. 5 Dec. 2014 (RS2).

## 18. What is Bence-Jones proteins? Mention its significance.

- Bence-Jones proteins are free monoclonal light chain immunoglobulins (κ or λ) of smaller molecular weight (Mol weight of 20,000–40,000)

| *Cause* | *Pathogenesis* | *Features* | *Electrophoresis* |
|---|---|---|---|
| They are overproduced in multiple myeloma (plasma cell tumor) wherein it is excreted in urine | This is due to asynchronous production of H and L chains or due to deletion of portions of L chains, so that they cannot combine with H chains | • Precipitate on heating urine to 45°C, maximally precipitated at 60°C but start redissolving at 60°C and forms a clear solution at 100°C<br>• Precipitate reforms on cooling | Serum protein electrophoresis shows presence of prominent M band in α2 to γ globulin region |

## Significance

- Presence of Bence-Jones proteins in urine is diagnostic and prognostic of multiple myeloma
- Bence-Jones proteinuria is detected by heat test, Bradshaw's test and electrophoresis
- Excretion and deposition of these proteins damage the renal tubules.

## 19. Name bacterial DNA polymerases. Mention its significance.

- A DNA polymerase is chief enzyme involved in DNA replication (DNA repair and DNA polymerization).

## Prokaryotic DNA Polymerase (in Bacteria)

| *Bacterial DNA polymerases* | *Significance* |
|---|---|
| Pol I<br>Kornberg's enzyme [named after it discoverer Arthur Kornberg (Nobel prize, 1959)] | Implicated in DNA repair and has both 5'->3' (Nick translation) and 3'->5' (Proof-reading) exonuclease activity |
| Pol II | Involved in replication of damaged DNA and has both 5'->3'chain extension ability and 3'->5' exonuclease activity |
| Pol III<br>(Main replication enzyme) | • Main polymerase in bacteria (elongates in DNA replication), as such it has 3'->5' exonuclease proofreading ability<br>• Has beta, gamma, delta and delta dash units |

## Significance

- DNA polymerase of prokaryotes has diverse functional variety, specially DNA Pol I though it does not possess DNA repair function
- Taq DNA polymerase obtained from thermophilic bacteria *Thermus aquaticus*, being heat resistant is used in PCR.

(**Note:** Eukaryotic DNA polymerase has five types, namely α, β, γ, δ and ε)

| *Bacterial DNA polymerases* | *Eukaryotic DNA polymerase* | *Functions* |
|---|---|---|
| Pol I | α | Gap filling and synthesis of lagging strand |
| Pol II | ε | Proof-reading of DNA and repair |
| — | β | DNA repair |
| — | γ | Required for mitochondrial DNA synthesis |
| Pol III | δ | Helps in leading strand synthesis |

## 20. Distinguish between RNA and DNA.

| *Points of difference* | *DNA* | *RNA* |
|---|---|---|
| • Bases present | Adenine, guanine, cytocine and thymine | Adenine, guanine, cytosine and uracil |
| • Bases absent | Uracil | Thymine |
| • Pentose sugar | Deoxyribose | Ribose |
| • Intracellular location | Nucleus, mitochondria but never in cytoplasm | Nucleus and cytoplasm |
| • Number of strands | Double stranded (helical) | Single stranded |
| • Function | Genetic information (transcription, replication) | Gene expression (translation) |

*Contd...*

*Contd...*

| *Points of difference* | *DNA* | *RNA* |
|---|---|---|
| • Types | A, B, C, D and E | t-RNA, m-RNA, r-RNA, hn-RNA and Sn RNA |
| • Size | Large molecules<br>>100,000 base pairs | Only hn, m and r-RNA are large molecules<br>60-20,000 base pairs |
| • Genetic information | One strand 3′-5′ carries genetic information | m-RNA transcribed from DNA carries genetic information |
| • Synthesis of RNA or DNA | DNA can form RNA by transcription | Under normal circumstances RNA can never form DNA (only possible by enzyme reverse transcriptase which is absent in humans) |
| • Purine and pyramidine content | Almost equal<br>(Guanine content equal to cytosine and adenosine is equal to uracil) | Not equal<br>(Guanine content not equal to cytosine and adenosine is not equal to uracil) |
| • Alkali hydrolysis | Alkali resistant | Gives 2′-3′ cyclic mononucleotides |

## 21. What is gene therapy? Name vectors used for gene therapy.

Refer Question No. 12 Dec. 2007 (RS2).

## 22. Nutritional deficiency anemias.

- Anemia is clinical condition characterized by hemoglobin concentration below lower limit of normal range for age and sex of individual
- In an adult, lower extreme of normal hemoglobin for males is taken as 13 g/dL and for females as 11.5 g/dL.

### Nutritional Deficiency Anemias

- Anemia produced due to deficiency of important nutrients which are essential for proper erythropoiesis are collectively termed nutritional anemia.

| *Nutrient* | *Anemia* | *Remarks* |
|---|---|---|
| • Iron (iron deficiency anemia)<br>• Copper and pyridoxine | Microcytic anemia | • Reduced RBC size<br>• Most common |
| • Folic acid and vitamin $B_{12}$ (megaloblastic anemia) | Macrocytic anemia | Large, immature RBCs |
| • Proteins | Normocytic anemia | Normal size RBCs but low RBC count |

# MBBS PHASE I EXAMINATION
## JUNE 2006
## (Revised Scheme 2)

### LONG ESSAYS

**1. Discuss the significance of multienzyme complexes with respect to carbohydrate and lipid metabolism.**

- Multienzyme complexes are complexes of enzyme which collectively catalyze a single reaction in association with co-enzymes or co-factors which aid this process.

*Examples*

| Metabolic pathway | Carbohydrate metabolism | Integrated metabolism | Lipid metabolism |
|---|---|---|---|
| Example | Pyruvate dehydrogenase complex | Alpha ketoglutarate dehydrogenase complex | Fatty acid synthase complex |
| Seen in | Oxidation of pyruvate | TCA cycle | Fatty acid biosynthesis |
| Subcellular site | Mitochondria | Mitochondria | Cytosol |
| Structure | Monomer | Monomer | Dimer of 2 identical units |
| Reaction catalyzed | Oxidation reaction | Oxidation reaction | Synthetic reaction (reduction/ dehydration) |
| Components | 3 enzymes + cofactor | 3 enzymes + cofactor | 3 enzymes + carrier protein |

### Advantages of Multienzyme Complex

- Intermediates of reaction can easily interact with active sites of the enzymes
- One gene codes all enzymes, so all enzymes are in equimolecular concentrations
- Efficiency of process is enhanced.

### Pyruvate Dehydrogenase Complex

- Mitchondrial multienzyme complex catalaysing oxidative decarboxylation of pyruvate to acetyl CoA
- Highly concentrated in cardiac muscles and kidneys.

*Components*

| *3 enzymes* | *Co-factors* |
|---|---|
| • 29 molecules of pyruvate dehydrogenase<br>• 1 molecule of dihydrolipoyl trans acetylase<br>• 8 molecules of flavoprotein containing dihydrolipoyl dehydrogenase | • Thiamine pyrophosphate (TPP)<br>• Lipoic acid (thioctic acid) has 2 sulphur atoms and 8 carbon atoms and accepts or donates hydrogen atoms<br>• CoA-SH<br>• FAD<br>• $NAD^+$ |

*Sequence of Reaction*

i. Pyruvate is decarboxylated to a hydroxymethyl derivative of thiazole ring of enzyme bound TPP
ii. Which in turn, reacts with oxidized lipoamide to form 'acetyl lipoamide'
iii. In presence of dihydrolipoyl transacetylase, acetyl lipoamide reacts with CoA.SH to form 'acetyl CoA' and reduced lipoamide
iv. Latter is reoxidized by a flavoprotein in presence of dihydrolipoyl dehydrogenase
v. Finally, reduced flavoprotein is oxidized by $NAD^+$, which in turn, transfers reducing equivalents to respiratory chain.

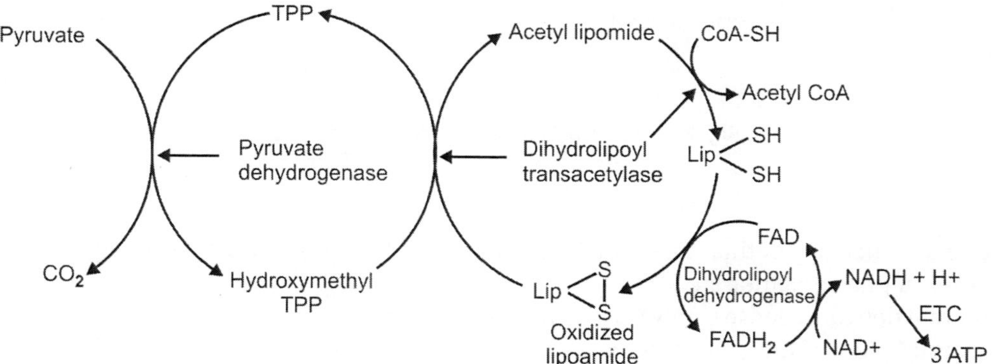


**Fig. 1:** Pyruvate dehydragenase complex

*Significance*

- Lack of TPP due to deficiency of thiamine inhibits activity of PDH resulting in accumulation of pyruvate
- In thiamine deficient alcoholics, pyruvate is rapidly converted to lactate resulting in lactic acidosis
- Lactic acidosis is commonly seen in after glucose load in patients with inherited deficiency of PDH
- PDH catalyzes an irreversible reaction, therefore, though glucose can be used for fatty acid synthesis (through acetyl CoA) but fatty acids cannot be used for gluconeogenesis
- Arsenic and mercuric ions inhibit PDH activity by binding to –SH group of lipoic acid.

## Alpha Ketoglutarate Dehydrogenase Complex

- Mitchondrial multienzyme complex catalayzing oxidative decarboxylation of alpha ketoglutarate to succinyl CoA in TCA cycle.

*Components*

| *3 enzymes* | *Co-factors* |
|---|---|
| • Alpha ketoglutarate dehydrogenase<br>• Dihydrolipoyl trans succinylase<br>• Flavo protein containing dihydrolipoyl dehydrogenase | • Thiamine pyrophosphate (TPP)<br>• Lipoic acid (thioctic acid) has 2 sulphur atoms and 8 carbon atoms and accepts or donates hydrogen atoms<br>• CoA-SH<br>• FAD<br>• $NAD^+$ |

*Sequence of Reaction*

i. Alpha ketoglutarate is decarboxylated to a hydroxysuccinyl derivative of thiazole ring of enzyme bound TPP
ii. Which in turn, reacts with oxidized lipoamide to form 'succinyl lipoamide'
iii. In presence of dihydrolipoyl transsuccinylase, succinyl lipoamide reacts with CoA.SH to form 'succinyl CoA' and reduced lipoamide
iv. Latter is reoxidized by a flavoprotein in presence of dihydrolipoyl dehydrogenase
v. Finally, reduced flavoprotein is oxidized by $NAD^+$, which in turn, transfers reducing equivalents to respiratory chain.

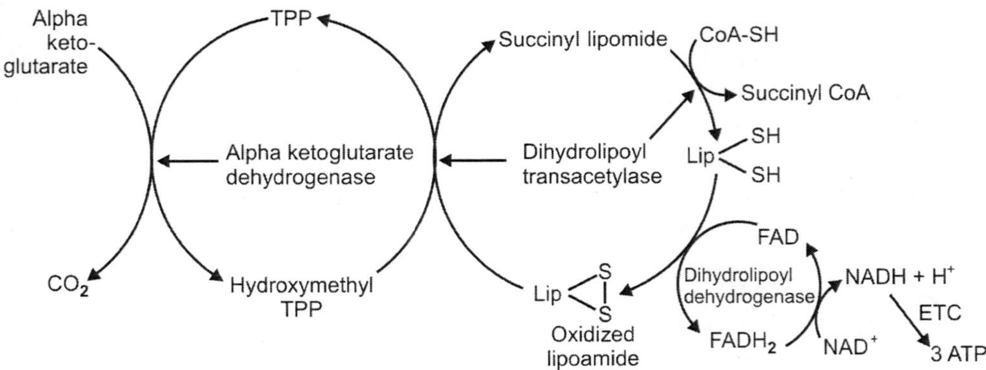


**Fig. 2:** Alpha ketoglutarate dehydrogenase complex

*Significance*

- Lack of TPP due to deficiency of thiamine inhibits activity of alpha ketoglutarate dehydrogenase complex resulting in accumulation of alpha ketoglutarate
- Alpha ketoglutarate dehydrogenase catalyzes an irreversible reaction
- Arsenic and mercuric ions inhibit alpha ketoglutarate dehydrogenase complex activity by binding to -SH group of lipoic acid.



## Fatty Acid Synthase Complex

- Cytosolic enzyme complex made up of a dimmer composed of two identical subunits.

*Structure*

- Each monomer has molecular weight of 240,000 and lies antiparallel to each other linked by -SH group of phosphopantetheine of one subunit with-SH group of cysteine residue of ketoacyl synthase of other subunit.

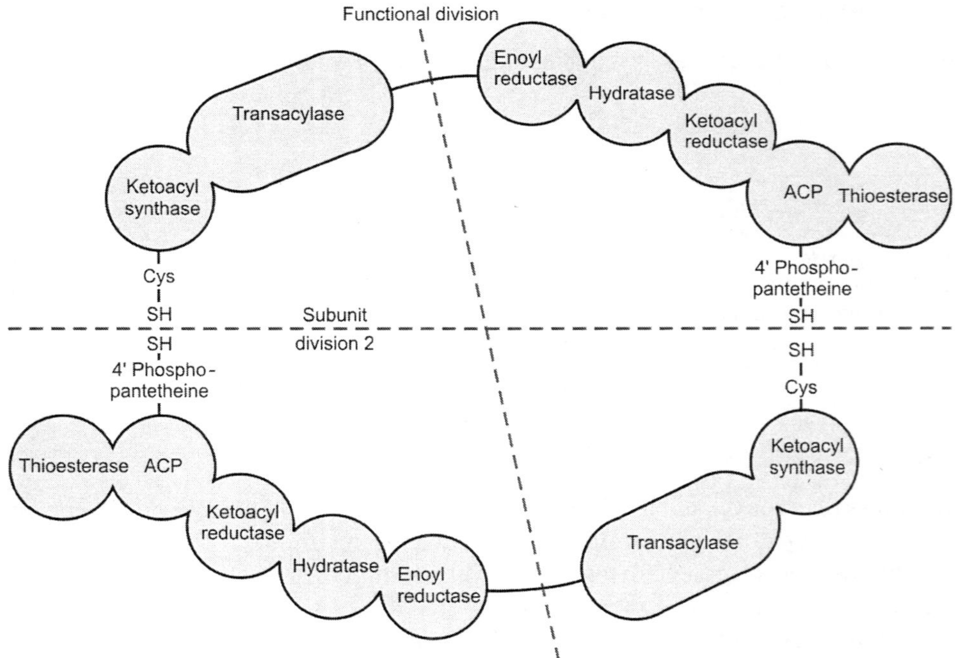


**Fig. 3:** Structure of fatty acid synthase complex

*Components of Each Monomer (3 Domains Joined by Flexible Regions)*

| *First domain (condensing unit)* | *Second domain (reduction unit)* | *Third domain (releasing unit)* |
|---|---|---|
| • Acetyl transferase<br>• Malonyl trans acylase<br>• Beta-keto acyl synthase or condensing enzyme | • Acyl carrier protein<br>• Beta-keto acyl reductase<br>• Dehydratase<br>• Enoyl reductase | • Thioesterase or deacylase |

*Sequence of Reaction*

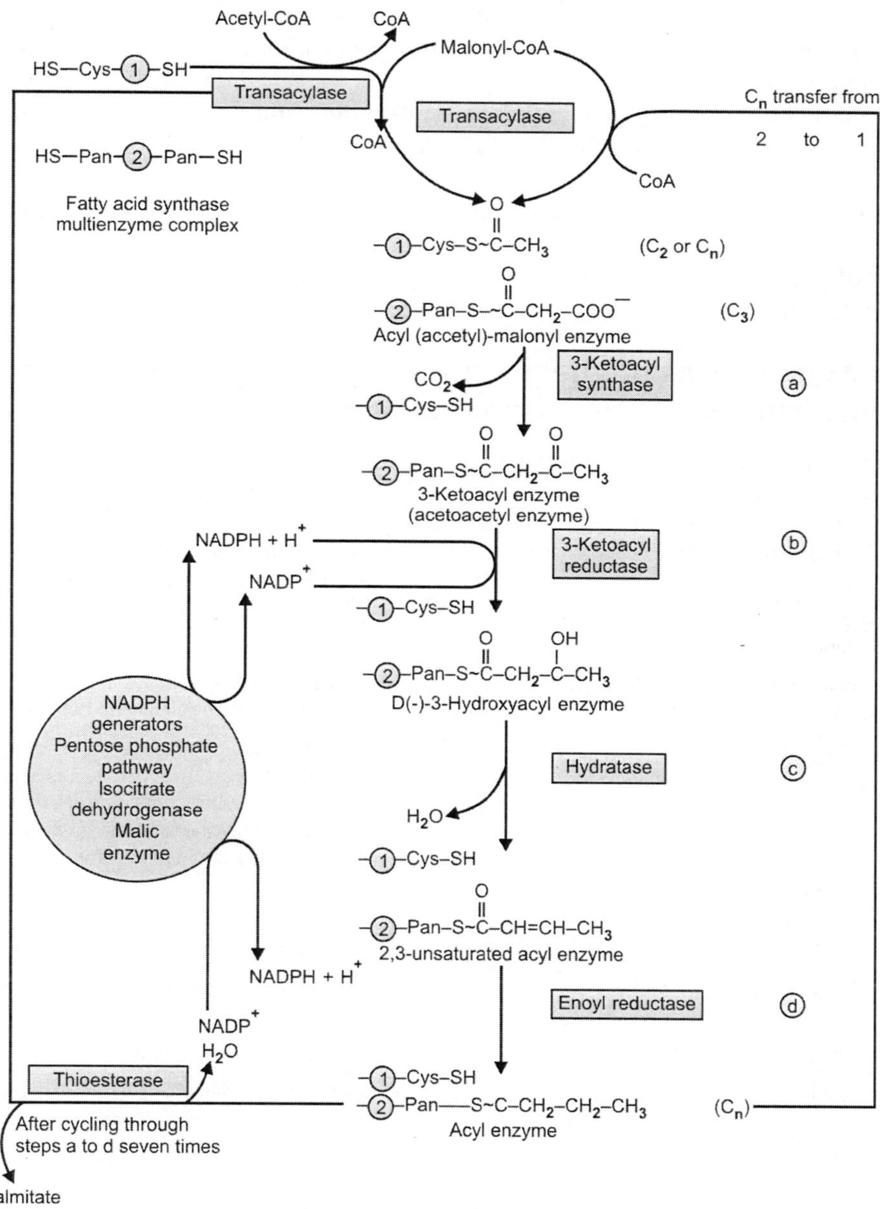


**Fig. 4:** Reaction of fatty acid synthase complex

i. 2 carbon fragments of acetyl CoA are transferred to ACP of fatty acid synthese, catalyzed by acetyl CoA-ACP transacetylase thus transferring acetyl unit from ACP to cysteine residue of enzyme
ii. Enzyme malonyl CoA-ACP transacylase transfers malonate from malonyl CoA to bind to ACP
iii. Acetyl unit attached to cysteine is transferred to malonyl group which loses $CO_2$ catalyzed by beta ketoacyl ACP synthase releasing energy which is required for reaction to proceed further

iv. Beta ketoacyl ACP reductase reduces ketoacyl group to hydroxyacyl group, reducing equivalents supplied by NADPH
v. Beta hydroxyacyl ACP undergoes dehydration thus introducing a double bond between $\alpha$ and $\beta$ carbons
vi. 2nd NADPH dependent reduction, catalyzed by enoyl-ACP reductase occurs to produce acyl-ACP
  - Reaction ii-vi are repeated 6 more times and each time fatty acid chain is lengthened by a 2 carbon unit and at end of 7th cycle, fatty acid synthesis is complete and a 16 carbon fully saturated fatty acid namely palmitate is formed
vii. Enzyme palmitoyl thioesterase separates palmitate from fatty acid synthase thus completing synthesis of palmitate.

## Significance

- Though each subunit of enzyme complex contains all enzymes, it is not active at a monomer because functional unit consists of ½ of each subunit interacting with complementary ½ of other, i.e. fatty acid synthase complex has a subunit division and a functional division
- However, 2 functional subunits of fatty acid synthase operate independently synthesizing 2 fatty acids simultaneously
- Fatty acid synthase complex offers great efficiency that is free from interference of other cellular reactions for synthesis of fatty acids
- Since entire process of metabolic pathway is confined to complex, there are no permeability barriers for various intermediates
- Multienzyme polypeptide complex is coded by a single gene. Thus there is a good coordination in synthesis of all enzyme of fatty acid synthase complex.



## 2. Name the coenzyme forms of vitamin involved in amino acid metabolism. Discuss the biochemical functions and deficiency manifestations of this vitamin.

- Coenzyme forms of vitamin involved in amino acid metabolism

| *Vitamin* | *Coenzyme form* | *Involvement in amino acid metabolism* |
|---|---|---|
| Vitamin $B_1$ (Thiamine) | Thiamine pyrophosphate (TPP) | • Decarboxylation steps in degradation of alpha ketobutyrate and alpha keto derivatives of branched chain amino acids |
| Vitamin $B_2$ (Riboflavin) | • Flavin mononucleotide (FMN)<br>• Flavin adenine dinucleotide (FAD) | • Amino acid oxidation |
| Niacin | • Nicotinamide adenine dinucleotide ($NAD^+$)<br>• Nicotinamide adenine dinucleotide phosphate ($NADP^+$) | • Glycine cleavage system<br>• Conversion of phenylalanine to tyrosine |
| Vitamin $B_6$ (Pyridoxine) | Pyridoxal phosphate (PLP) | • Transamination<br>• Decarboxylation<br>• Metabolism of sulfur-containing amino acids<br>• Conversion of glycine to serine<br>• Non-oxidative deamination of hydroxy amino acids |
| Pantothenic acid | Coenzyme A (CoA) | • Conversion of alanine and glucogenic amino acids and leucine and ketogenic amino acid to acetyl CoA<br>• Conversion of threonine, valine, isoleucine to succinyl CoA |
| Biotin | Biotin | • In leucin metabolism, beta methyl crotonyl CoA is catalyzed to beta methyl glutaconyl CoA |
| Folic acid | 5,6,7,8-tetrahydrofolic acid (THFA) | • Synthesis of active methionine |
| Vitamin $B_{12}$ | Methyl cobalamin | • Metabolism of valine, isoleucine, methionine and threonine<br>• Synthesis of active methionine |
| Vitamin C | Ascorbic acid | • Hydroxylation of proline and lysine<br>• Hydroxylation of tryptophan to serotonin<br>• Oxidation of parahydroxy phenyl pyruvate to homogentisic acid in tyrosine metabolism |

## Pyridoxine (Vitamin $B_6$)

- Pyridoxine is a water-soluble vitamin
- It is the major vitamin involved in amino acid metabolism

| *Sources* | *RDA* |
|---|---|
| Rich sources—whole grain cereals, organ meats, eggs and legumes | • Adults—2 mg/day<br>• Pregnancy and lactation—2.5 mg/day |

## Coenzyme

- Pyridoxal phosphate (PLP); acts as a coenzyme principally in amino acid metabolism.

### *Biochemical Function*

- In transamination
  - Reversible reaction taking place in liver, heart, kidney, heart and brain
  - Here α-$NH_2$ group of an amino acid is transferred to a α-keto acid resulting in formation of a new amino acid and a new keto acid
  - These reactions are catalyzed by transaminase enzyme and PLP acts as a coenzyme

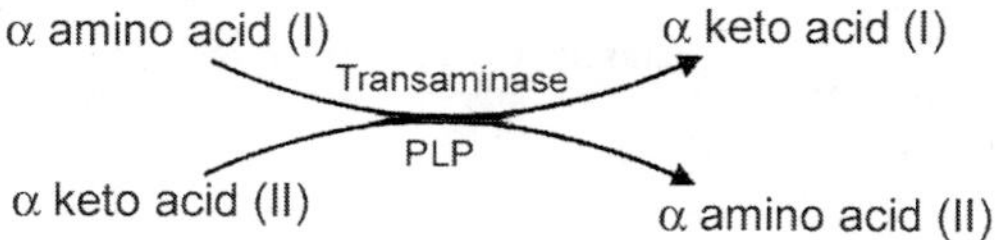


**Fig. 5:** Transamination reaction

  - Generally transaminases are specific to one of amino acid and other substrate is always α ketoglutarate which is converted to glutamate.

  *Significance*
  - Responsible for synthesis of nonessential amino acids from other amino acids
  - Helps in catabolism of amino acids
  - Overall tries to maintain a proper concentration of various amino acids in body
- In decarboxylation
  - Amino acid undergoes alpha decarboxylation to form corresponding amine catalyzed by alpha decarboxylase using PLP as a coenzyme

COOH
CHNH ——Alpha decarboxylase——→ $CH_2NH_2$
R                                                    R

  *Example*
  - Glutamate → GABA (an inhibitory neurotransmitter)

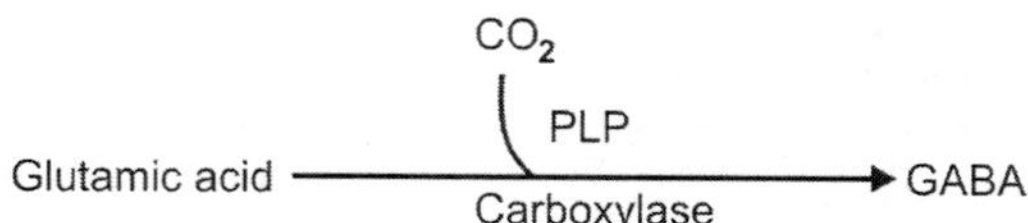


  - Histidine → Histamine (mediator of allergy and anaphylaxis)
  - 5-hydroxy tryptophan → Serotonin (neurotransmitter)
  - Cysteine → Taurine
  - Serine → Ethanolamine
- Nonoxidative deamination of -OH amino acids viz. serine, threonine, etc.
- Coenzyme for kynureninase in tryptophan metabolism

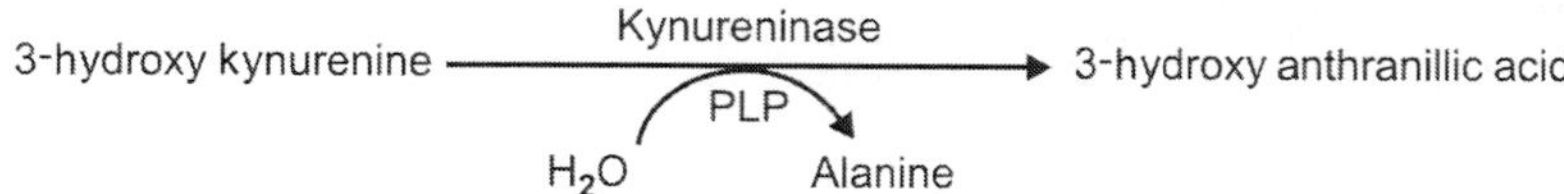

- Transulfuration
  - PLP takes part in transulfuration reactions involving transfer of -SH groups

$$\text{Homocysteine + serine} \xrightarrow{\text{PLP}} \text{homoserine + cysteine}$$

- Coenzyme for desulfhydrases which catalyzes nonoxidative deamination of cysteine
- In interconversion of glycine and serine by serine hydroxymethyl transferase
- Coenzyme for biosynthesis of arachidonic acid from linoleic acid
- Synthesis of sphingomyelin from serine
- Coenzyme for amino acid racemases

$$\text{D - Glutamic acid} \rightarrow \text{L Glutamic acid}$$

- Coenzyme for condensing enzyme for chain elongation of fatty acid
- Active transport of amino acids through cell membrane intestinal absorption of amino acids
- Constituent of muscle phosphorylase
- Transport of $K^+$ from exterior to interior across cell membrane
- Coenzyme for amino acetone synthase

$$\text{Glycine + Acetyl CoA} \xrightarrow[\text{PLP}]{\text{Amino acetone synthase}} \text{Aminoacetone}$$

- Synthesis of coenzyme A from pantothenic acid
- Porphyrin synthesis.

$$\alpha \text{ amino } \beta \text{ keto adipic acid} \xrightarrow[\text{ALA synthase}]{CO_2 \text{ PLP}} \delta \text{ ALA}$$

## Deficiency

| *Causes* | *Clinical features* | *Biochemical findings* |
|---|---|---|
| • Decreased dietary intake<br>• Alcoholism<br>• Impaired absorption (small intestine diseases)<br>• Antivitamins (chronic administration of drugs such as isoniazid and penicillamine) | *Neurological*<br>• Very common because pyrodoxine deficiency leads to inadequate production of neurotransmitters (serotonin, epinephrine, noradrenaline and GABA)<br>• In children: Convulsions d' to ↓ formation of GABA<br>• Adults: Peripheral neuritis because of demyelination of nerves due to ↓ synthesis of sphingolipids and associated with synovial swelling and tenderness<br>*Dermatological*<br>• Pellagra may manifested as pyrodoxine is involved in synthesis of niacin from tryptophan<br>*Hematological*<br>• Hypochromic microcytic anemia due to inhibition of heme biosynthesis and impaired antibody formation | • Decreased levels of plasma pyridoxine and PLP<br>• Decreased levels of plasma transaminase (AST, ALT)<br>• Increased excretion of xanthurenic acid after tryptophan load (tryptophan load test)<br>– Due to impairment in conversion of tryptophan to niacin and increased amounts of metabolites (xanthurenic acid) formed from alternate pathways are excreted in urine |

## SHORT ESSAYS

### 3. How is ammonia detoxified in the body?

Refer Question No. 1 Dec. 2011 (RS2).

### 4. Mechanism of oxidative phosphorylation.

Refer Question No. 1 June 2010 (RS2).

### 5. Ketogenesis.

Refer Question No. 1 June 2011 (RS2).

### 6. Gluconeogenesis.

Refer Question No. 1 June 2009 (RS2).

### 7. Conjugation in detoxification.

Refer Question No. 7 Dec. 2005 (RS2).

### 8. Clearance tests.

Refer Question No. 9 Dec. 2005 (RS2).

### 9. Blood buffers and their role in acid-base balance.

Refer Question No. 2 June 2012 (RS2).

### 10. Biological role of zinc in the body.

- Zinc is an essential trace element mainly present intracellularly

| *Total body content* | *Body tissue rich in zinc* | *RDA* | *Sources* |
|---|---|---|---|
| 2 g | Hippocampus, choroids of eye, liver, prostate gland and prostate fluid | 10 mg/day | Grains, beans, nuts, meat, green leafy vegetables and fruits |

#### Biological Role of Zinc

- Regulation of body function as essential component of >300 metalloenzymes
  Example: Carbonic anhydrase (acid-base balance), alkaline phosphatase (bone remodeling), lactate dehydrogenase (glycolysis, gluconeogenesis), alcohol dehydrogenase (alcohol metabolism), glutamate dehydrogenase (amino acid metabolism), RNA polymerase (transcription), carboxypeptidase (protein digestion), superoxide dismutase (control of oxidative stress), etc.
- Protein biosynthesis as a content of RNA polymerase enzyme
- Antioxidant as extracellular superoxide dismutase is zinc dependent
- Helps in synthesis of retinol binding protein thus maintains normal vitamin A levels in serum and stimulates release of stored vitamin A from liver
- Necessary for normal immunological function
- Necessary for storage and secretion of insulin from pancreatic β cells
- Important for taste sensation as component of Gusten (zinc containing salivary protein)
- Maintain integrity of skin and is required for wound healing
- Essential for growth and reproduction; proper action of steroid hormones, spermatogenesis.

#### Clinical Significance

- Zinc supplementation in mother improves birth weight of babies
- Zinc supplementation is useful in controlling acute diarrhea.

| *Decreased plasma zinc levels* | *Increased plasma zinc levels* |
|---|---|
| Chronic alcoholism, malabsorption due to conditions such as regional ileitis, nephrotic syndrome, infections and myocardial infarction | Exposure to excess zinc (as in welder) |

### 11. Polymerase chain reaction.

- Polymerase chain reaction (PCR) refers to in vitro amplification of DNA (up to 100,000 fold) using multiple cycles of DNA elongation reaction
- It is a test tube method which amplifies a select segment of DNA fragment which may be either animal, plant, bacterium and virus permitting synthesis of million of copies of specific DNA sequence in a few hours

## Principle

- Based on knowing the nucleic acid sequence for a region which for a diagnostic application is produced in large amount in vitro.

## Materials Required

- Target DNA (100–35,000 bp in length) to be amplified from any source either leukocytes, tissues or single cells
- Two synthetic oligonucleotide primers (17–30 nucleotide length) complementary to ends of each strand of target DNA
- Heat stable Taq DNA polymerase (obtained bacterial Thermus aquaticus)
- Four deoxyribonucleotides (dATP, dCTP, dGTP and dTTP).

## Procedure (Involves multiple cycles of denaturation of DNA followed by annealing using a thermal cycler)

a. Melting of DNA
   - Double stranded DNA is dissociated to a single stranded DNA at a denaturing temperature of 94°C.

b. Annealing/renaturation (hybridization of primers to target DNA)
   - Reaction mixture is cooled to an anenealing temperature of about 50–65°C for about 1–3 minutes [usually about 2–3°C below Tm (melting temperature)]
   - The oligonucleotide primers hybridise to target DNA.

c. Extension (DNA synthesis)
   - Synthesis of DNA is carried out at a polymerization temperature of 75°C using heat resistant Taq DNA polymerase derived from *Thermus aquaticus* in presence of deoxynucleotide triphosphate resulting in duplication of starting material
   - It starts at 3'-hydroxyl end of each primer and primers are extended by joining the bases complementary to DNA strands
   - Synthetic process in PCR is quite comparable to DNA replication of leading strand.

d. Melting products of DNA duplexes and repeating these cycles of heating and cooling, typically 20–30 or more times an exponential increase in amount of target DNA occurs.

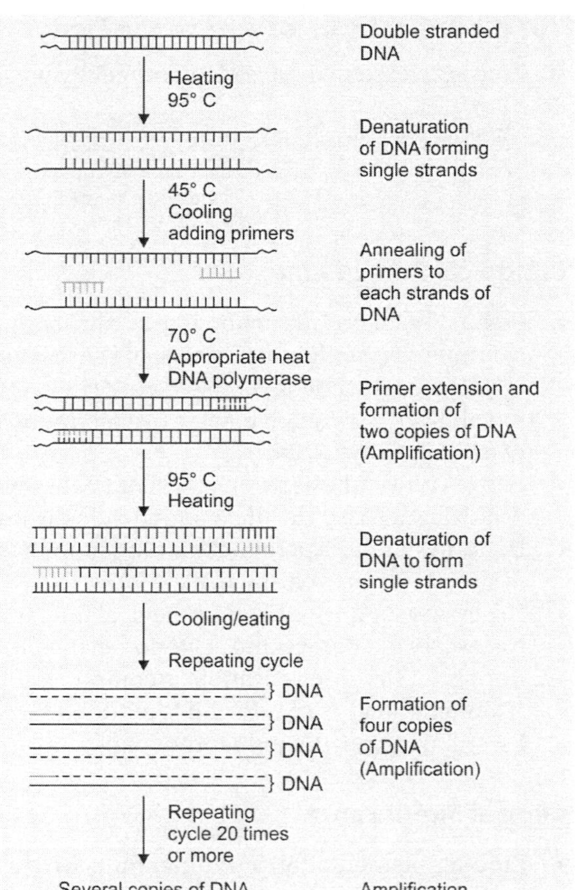


**Fig. 6:** Procedure of polymerase chain reaction

## Application

a. Molecular diagnostics
   - PCR provides extremely rapid analysis, ease of automation, relative economy and 100% efficiency
   - It is used for diagnosis of:
     - Infectious diseases such as tuberculosis and AIDS:
     - Genetic diseases such as alpha-1-antitrypsin deficiency, muscular dystrophy and hemophilia A
     - Malignant conditions such as retinoblastoma, chronic and myeloid leukemia.

b. Synthesis of cDNA
   - cDNA is synthesized with reverse transcriptase followed by amplification of cDNA.

c. Synthesis of single stranded DNA
   - By altering the ratio of oligonucleotide primers, single stranded DNA can be synthesized.

d. Detection of nucleotide sequence of infections agents

| | |
|---|---|
| Bacteria | *H. pylori, M. tuberculosis, C. trachomatis* |
| Viruses | Coxsackievirus, cytomegalovirus, herpes simplex virus, hepatiti B and C virus, HIV |
| Fungi | *Candida albicans* |
| Protozoa | *T. gondii, Pneumocystis carinii, T. cruzi* |

e. Research applications (genetic engeering)
   – Recombinant DNA construction, mutagenesis of cloned DNA and detection of rare nucleotide sequence.

f. Forensic application
   – Identification of DNA of accused using blood, hair or semen.

g. In prenatal diagnosis
   – Especially useful for prenatal diagnosis of inherited diseases, where cells obtained from fetus by amniocentesis are very few.

h. Fossil studies
   – DNA isolated from fossil is amplified by PCR to study evolution by comparing sequences in extinct and living organisms.

## 12. Basal metabolic rate.

- Basal metabolic rate (BMR) is amount of energy produced by a person at complete physical and mental rest, lying supine, comfortably awake in a thermoneutral environment (20–25°C) and in postabsorptive state (12 hours after food)
- It is the minimum energy required to maintain life or sustain vital functions
- It is expressed as calories/square meter body surface/hour

| *Measurements* | *Calculations* | *Normal values (temperate climate)* |
|---|---|---|
| • Directly<br>– By heat evolved<br>• Indirectly<br>– By measuring volume of $O_2$ consumed and $CO_2$ evolved per unit time using either Benedict–Roth spirometer or Knipping spirometer | • Energy consumption from $O_2$ consumption<br>– Oxygen consumed per hour (in liters) × 4.825 calories (because one liter of $O_2$ consumption is equivalent to 4.825 calories when RQ of diet is 0.82)<br>• Calculation of body surface area<br>– Body surface area (sq.m)<br>= Height 0.725 (in cm) × Weight 0.425 (in kg) × 71.84/10000<br>Average body surface area for Indian males is 1.62 sqm and for females it is 1.4 sqm | • Infant—53 Cal/m²/hr<br>• Adolescent :<br>– Boy—42 Cal/m²/hr<br>– Girl—38 Cal/m²/hr<br>• 25 years<br>– Man—40 Cal/m²/hr<br>– Woman—36 Cal/m²/hr<br>• 40 years<br>– Man—38 Cal/m²/hr<br>– Woman—34 Cal/m²/hr |

### Factors Affecting BMR

| | |
|---|---|
| • Body surface area | More the surface area, more the BMR |
| • Age | BMR decreases as age progress being highest for infant |
| • Sex | Females of same age group have BMR less by 3–5 cal/m²/hr |
| • Nutrition | Starvation decreases BMR |
| • Body temperature | • BMR increases during fever<br>• There is 10% rise in BMR for every 1°C rise in temperature |
| • Climate | Cold increases BMR to keep body warm |
| • Muscular work | Raises BMR by increasing the metabolism |
| • Sleep | Slows BMR |
| • Thyroxine | BMR is increased in thyrotoxicosis and decreases in myxedema |
| • Adrenaline | Increases BMR |
| • Pregnancy | 5% rise in BMR in first two trimester and 12% in last trimester |
| • Diseases | • BMR is elevated in various infections, leukemias, polycythemia, cardiac failure, hypertension, etc.<br>• BMR is lowered in Addison's disease (adrenal insufficiency) |
| • Race | BMR of Eskimo's is higher |

### Importance of BMR

- As a diagnostic aid especially for thyroid function tests
- For calculation of caloric requirement
- To note effect of drugs and foods on BMR.

## SHORT ANSWERS

### 13. Carnitine cycle.

Refer Question No. 1 Dec. 2008 (RS2).

### 14. Biologically active peptides.

- Peptides are secondary derived proteins composed of less than 10 amino acids joined by peptide bonds.

#### Biologically Important Peptides

| *Features* | *Functions* |
|---|---|
| a. Glutathione<br>– Tripeptide, chemically known as γ-glutamyl-cysteinyl-glycine | • Destroys $H_2O_2$ and other peroxides under action of glutathione peroxidase by donating $H_2$<br>• Acts as coenzymes for many enzymes like glutathione-insulin transhydrogenase, formaldehyde dehydrogenase, glyoxylase, maleyl-acetoacetate isomerase<br>• Along with glutathione transhydrogenase help to cause reductive cleavage of S-S linkage in thyroglobulin glycoprotein<br>• Protects many –SH group containing enzymes against oxidation, e.g. glyceraldehyde 3 P-dehydrogenase<br>• Takes part in γ- glutamyl cycle for absorption of amino acids from intestine<br>• Reduced (G–SH ) glutathione is required for:<br>– Conversion of dopa-quinone to glutathione<br>– Prostaglandin synthesis by cyclooxygenase pathway as coenzyme<br>– Activation of methionine to S-adenosyl methionine |
| b. Thyrotropine releasing hormone (TRH)<br>– Tripeptide secreted by hypothalamus | Stimulates pituitary gland to release thyrotropic hormone |
| c. Oxytocin<br>– Nova peptide synthesized by paraventricular nucleus of hypothalamus | • Brings about ejection of milk from mammary glands<br>• Causes contraction of smooth muscles of uterus and quickens process of labor<br>• Facilitates transport of sperms through female genital tract |
| d. Vasopressin (ADH)<br>– Nova peptide synthesized by supraoptic nucleus of hypothalamus<br>– Also known as antidiuretic hormone | • Increases water reabsorption from distal convoluted tubules and collecting ducts<br>• Increases urea absorption from collecting ducts<br>• Promotes $Na^+$ reabsorption from thick ascending limb of loop of Henle<br>• Causes vasoconstriction and rise in blood pressure |
| e. Angiotensins<br>– Angiotensin I is a decapeptide which is converted to angiotensin II, a octapeptide | • Angiotensin has hypertensive effect<br>• Angiotensin II stimulates release of aldosterone from adrenal gland |
| f. Methionine enkephalin<br>– Pentapeptide formed in brain and has opiate like function | Inhibits sense of pain |
| g. Bradykinin and kallidin<br>– Nona and decapeptides respectively | Powerful vasodilators |
| h. Peptide antibiotics<br>– Gramicidin, bacitracin, tyrocidin and actinomycin are peptide in nature | Antibiotics |
| i. Substance P<br>– Decapeptide | Neurotransmitter |
| j. Gastrointestinal hormone<br>– Gastrin, secretin, etc. | Gastrointestinal peptides which act as local hormones |

### 15. Glycosaminoglycans.

Refer Question No. 5 Dec. 2015 (RS2).

### 16. Vitamin E.

- Vitamin E is fat soluble vitamin, chemically known as tocopherol.

| *Chemistry* | *Sources* | *RDA* |
|---|---|---|
| • Vitamin E consists of a chroman structure with a hydrocarbon chain<br>• α tocopherol has widest distribution, predominant in diet and high biological activity | • Rich sources: Vegetable oils (Wheat germ oil, sunflower oil, cotton seed oil, palm oil)<br>• Meat, milk, butter and eggs | • Children—7 mg<br>• Males—10 mg<br>• Females—8 mg<br>• Pregnancy—10 mg<br>• Lactation—12 mg |

## Biochemical Functions

- Antioxidant (most powerful, naturally occurring)
  - Vitamin E is a chain breaking antioxidant which interferes with chain propagation
  - It prevents oxidation of easily oxidisable lipids such as vitamin A and PUFA (in cell membrane phospholipids)
  - It blocks lipid peroxidation chain; converts peroxy free radicals to hydroperoxy radicals through transfer of its phenolic hydrogen atom to a peroxy free radical
  - It acts as a first line of defence against oxidative stress
  - This action is aided by selenium (second line of defence against oxidative stress)
  - In presence of oxidising agents such as $H_2O_2$ or high concentration of $O_2$, double bond in such lipids may undergo oxidative cleavage reaction (involving production of free radicals) which not only destroys lipids but which may produce toxic end products that can damage adjacent molecules within the cell membrane causing cell lysis
  - Products from oxidation of fat solutions may be carcinogenic or may bring about degenerative changes in RBC, muscles and lungs
- Preserves vegetable oils
  - Vitamin E present in vegetable oils inhibits development of peroxidative cleavage and rancidity
- Anti-sterility vitamin
  - Vitamin E prevents sterility in lower animals like rodents by preserving and maintaining germinal epithelium of gonads

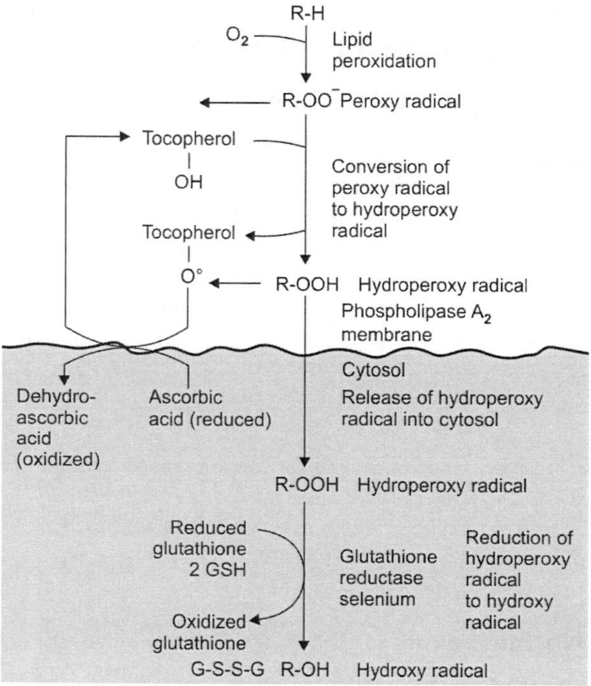


**Fig. 7:** Biochemical functions of vitamin E

- Other actions
  - Increases heme synthesis by enhancing activity of enzymes 6-aminolevulinic acid (ALA) synthase and ALA dehydratase
  - Required for cellular respiration through electron transport chain (stabilize coenzyme Q)
  - Required for proper storage of creatine in skeletal muscle
  - Needed for optimal absorption of amino acids from intestine
  - Involved in proper synthesis o f nucleic acids
  - Protects liver from toxic compounds such as carbon tetrachloride
  - Delays onset of cataract (by working in association with v tamins A, C and β-carotene)

## Deficiency Manifestations

| *Causes* | *Clinical features* |
|---|---|
| • Premature infants (since transfer of vitamin E from maternal sources occurring during last few weeks of pregnancy)<br>• Impaired absorption (fat malabsorption, obstructive jaundice, celiac sprue)<br>• Genetic vitamin E deficiency (absence of vitamin E transport protein) | • Hemolytic anemia (due to oxidative stress on RBCs)<br>• Muscle weakness and proteinuria<br>• Spinocerebellar ataxia, impaired vision, retinopathy (due to increased lipid peroxidation of nervous tissue and oxidation of PUFA present in outer rods of retina) |

## Clinical Significance

- Oxygen free radical (oxidative stress) are implicated in aging as well as various disease processes including cancer and atherosclerosis and vitamin E is used clinically as an antioxidant to protect against these oxidative stress.

## 17. Methanol poisoning can be alleviated by ethanol, justify.

- Ethyl alcohol (ethanol) has structural similarity to methyl alcohol (methanol)
- Due to this structural similarity, ethanol competitively competes with methanol to saturate (inhibit) alcohol dehydrogenase enzyme and retards metabolism of methanol
- Thus rate of production of formaldehyde, a toxic metabolite of methyl alcohol is reduced
- Therefore, methanol poisoning can be alleviated by ethanol.

## 18. 2,3 bisphosphoglycerate.

- 2,3 bisphosphoglycerate (2,3 BPG) is a intermediate of Rapaport-Leubering cycle operational in red blood cells (RBCs).

## Synthesis

- From 1,3 bisphosphoglycerate by enzyme 2,3 bisphosphoglycerate mutase.

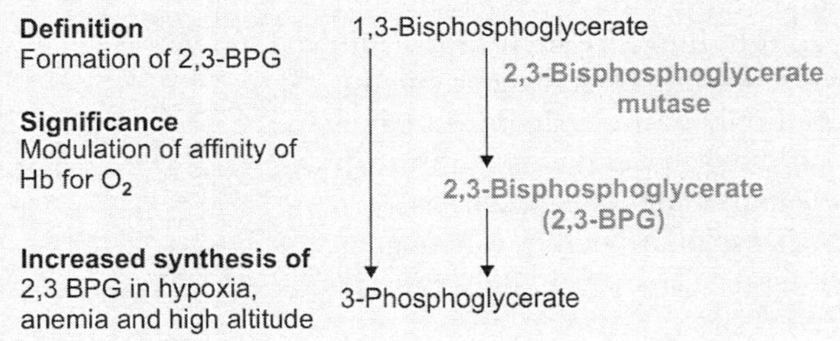


**Fig. 8:** Synthesis of 2,3-bisphosphoglycerate



## Normal Level

- 15 + 1.5 mg/g Hb
- Concentration higher in young children compared to elderly.

## Significance (Functions)

- Production of 2,3 BPG allows glycolysis to proceed without synthesis of ATP
- 2,3 BPG combines with hemoglobin and reduces affinity of hemoglobin to oxygen thus it favors unloading of oxygen to tissues (allosteric effector)
  - It binds to one molecule of deoxyhemoglobin in central cavity of four subunits thus stabilizing it.

| *Increased 2,3 BPG levels* | *Decreased 2,3 BPG levels* |
|---|---|
| • Hypoxia, anemia, high altitude, fetal tissue<br>• Pyruvate kinase deficiency | • Hexokinase deficiency, acidosis<br>• Stoppage of blood |
| $O_2$ dissociation curve shifts to right | $O_2$ dissociation curve shifts to left |
| Enhances oxygenation of tissues | Reduces oxygen delivery to tissues |

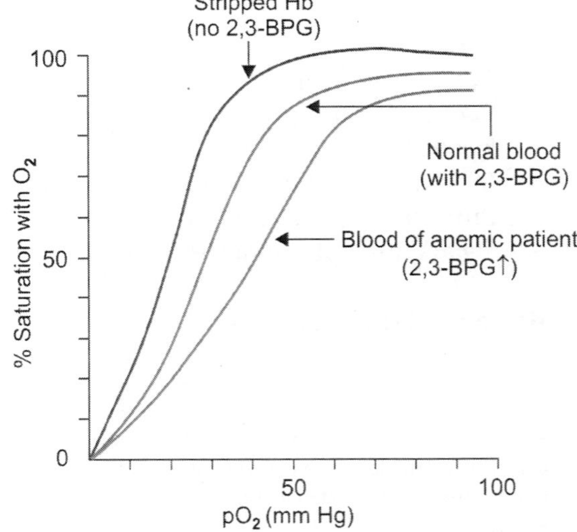


**Fig. 9:** Functions of 2,3-bisphosphoglycerate

- Glycolysis in RBCs is linked with 2,3BPG production and oxygen transport
  - In deficiency of enzyme hexokinase, glucose is not phosphorylated hence synthesis and concentration of 2.3 BPG are low in RBCs and such patients exhibit high oxygen deficiency
  - On other hand, patients with pyruvate kinase deficiency, levels of 2,3 BPG in erythrocytes is high resulting in low oxygen affinity.

## 19. Cyclic nucleotides.

- Cyclic nucleotides are nucleotide with phosphodiester linkage between 3' and 5' positions of ribose group, hence forming a cyclic ring
- This cyclic conformation allows them to bind to proteins to which other nucleotides cannot.

| *Functional groups* | *Examples* | *Functions* |
|---|---|---|
| • Nitrogenous aromatic base (adenine or guanine)<br>• Sugar (ribose)<br>• Phosphate | • Cyclic AMP<br>• Cyclic GMP<br>• Cyclic ADP ribose | • Act as second messengers playing a key role in many vital processes and some diseases<br>• In brain, cAMP and possibly cGMP are critical in formation of both long-term and short-term memory<br>• In liver, cAMP coordinates function of many metabolic enzymes to control level of glucose and other nutrients in bloodstream |

## 20. Intracellular insulin receptor.

- Intracellular insulin receptor is a glycoprotein with 4 subunits, 2 alpha and 2 beta subunits held together by disulfide linkage
- These subunits are in glycosylated forms.

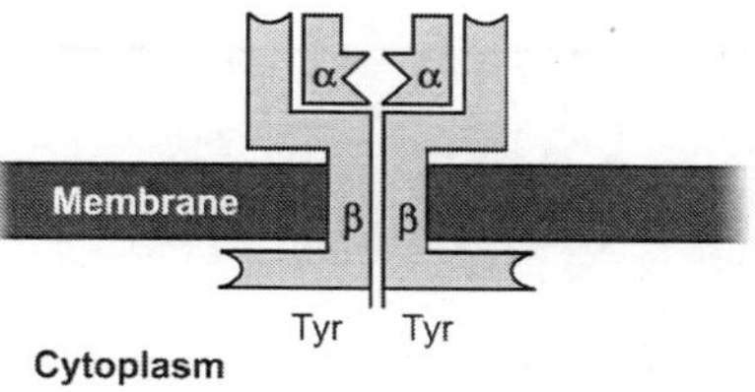


**Fig. 10:** Intacellular insulin receptor

### Components

| *Unit* | *Mol weight* | *Location* | *Function* |
|---|---|---|---|
| a. Alpha subunit | 135,000 | Extracellularly | Contains insulin binding site |
| b. Beta subunit | 95,000 | Transmembrane protein (activated by insulin) | Possess tyrosine kinase activity (cytoplasmic domain) |

- Insulin receptors are synthesized as a single polypeptide and cleaved to alpha and beta subunits which are then reassembled
- There are about 20,000 receptors per mammalian cell and each has half life of 6–12 hours

### Clinical Significance

- Decrease in insulin receptors on insulin responsive (target) cells is mechanism involved in NIDDM or type II diabetes mellitus (especially in obesity).

## 21. How bilirubin is made water soluble?

Refer Question No. 8 June 2007 (RS2).

## 22. Bence-Jones proteins.

Refer Question No. 18 Dec. 2005 (RS2).

# MBBS PHASE I EXAMINATION
## DECEMBER 2006
### (Revised Scheme 2)

## LONG ESSAYS

**1. Explain the influence of various factors on enzyme activity.**

Refer Question No. 1 June 2013 (RS2).

**2. Write in detail about the distribution of calcium in body, its function and regulation of serum levels.**

Refer Question No. 2 June 2009 (RS2).

## SHORT ESSAYS

**3. Urea formation in liver.**

Refer Question No. 1 Dec. 2011 (RS2).

**4. Glycogen storage diseases.**

- Glycogen storage diseases are genetic disease characterized by deposition of abnormal type or abnormal quantity of glycogen in tissue
- Classified into different types of depending on deficient enzyme
- Most are autosomal recessive except type VIII which a sex-linked recessive trait.

| Glycogen storage diseases |
|---|
| 1. **V**o **P**hysics **C**hemistry **AND M**aths mei **H**oshiyar **T**ha<br>✓ **V**on Gierke's<br>✓ **P**ompe's<br>✓ **C**ori's<br>✓ **AND**erson<br>✓ **M**c Ardle<br>✓ **H**er's<br>✓ **T**auri's<br>2. Anderson's (IV) vs. Cori's (III) enzyme defect—**ABCD**<br>**A**nderson's = **B**ranching enzyme<br>**C**ori's = **D**ebranching enzyme<br>3. **Type 1** = one (**Von**)—Von Giereke's disease<br>4. **Pompe's disease: "Police = Po + lys"**<br>**PO**mpe's disease - **LYS**osomal storage disease (alpha 1,4 glucosidase) |

| *Deficient enzyme* | *Inheritance* | *Glycogen structure* | *Organs affected* | *Clinical features* |
|---|---|---|---|---|
| **Type 0** | | | | |
| Glycogen synthase | | | Liver | • Deficiency of glycogen rather that its accumulation<br>• Transient hyperglycemia after meals and hypoglycermia between meals |

*Contd...*

*Contd...*

| *Deficient enzyme* | *Inheritance* | *Glycogen structure* | *Organs affected* | *Clinical features* |
|---|---|---|---|---|
| **Type Ia: Von Gierke's disease (most common)** | | | | |
| Glucose-6-phosphatase | Autosomal recessive | Normal | Liver, kidney, intestine (muscles not affected enzyme absent in them) | • Hypoglycemia, ketosis and acidosis, lactic acid and uric acid, massive hepatomegaly, enlarged kidney<br>• Hyperlipidemia, hyperuricemia<br>• Short stature, protuberant abdomen<br>• Doll like facies with fat cheeks<br>• Relatively thin extremities |
| **Type Ib** | | | | |
| Endoplasmic reticulum glucose-6-phosphate transporter (GLUT-7) | | | | • As type Ia + neutropenia<br>• Recurrent bacterial infection, inflammatory bowel disease |
| **Type II: Pompe's disease** | | | | |
| Lysosomal a (1-4) (1-6) glucosidase (acid maltase) | Autosomal recessive | Normal | Liver, heart, smooth and striated muscles (lysosomes) | • Cardiomegaly, muscle hypotonia<br>• Usually infants die before 9 months of age due to cardiac failure and bronchopneumonia |
| **Type III: Forbe's/ Cori's disease (limit dextrinosis)** | | | | |
| Debranching enzyme | Autosomal recessive | Abnormal short outer chains (limit dextrin type) | Liver, heart and muscles | • Fasting hypoglycemia, acidosis, myopathy, hepatomegaly<br>• Accumulation of characteristic branched polysaccharides (limit dextrin)<br>• Patients survive well to adult life |
| **Type IV: Anderson's disease (amylopectinosis)** | | | | |
| Branching enzyme | Not known | Abnormal long outer chains (amylopectin type) | Liver, heart, muscle, RE system | • Moderate hypoglycemia, hepatosplenomegaly, ascites, nodular cirrhosis of liver, hepatic failure<br>• Accumulation of polysaccharides with few branch points<br>• Prognosis fatal |
| **Type V: Mac Ardle's disease** | | | | |
| Muscle glycogen phosphorylase | Autosomal recessive | Normal | Muscles | • Muscle cramps on exercise, pain in muscles, weakness and stiffness of muscles<br>• Muscle glycogen abnormally high<br>• Affects children and adults |
| **Type VI: Her's disease** | | | | |
| Liver glycogen phosphorylase | Autosomal dominant | Normal | Liver | Hypoglycemia, mild-to-moderate acidosis, hepatomegaly |
| **Type VII: Tarui's disease** | | | | |
| Muscle and erythrocyte phosphofructokinase 1 | | Normal | Muscles and RBCs | Hemolytic anemia, rise in muscle glycogen, reduced capacity for muscular work, low blood lactate and muscle cramps |
| **Type VIII: X-linked phosphorylase kinase deficiency** | | | | |
| Phosphoylase kinase | Sex-linked recessive | | Liver | Mild hypoglycemia, rise in liver glycogen level and hepatomegaly |
| **Type IX: Autosomal phosphorylase kinase deficiency** | | | | |
| Phosphoylase kinase | Autosomal recessive | | Liver and muscles | |
| **Type X** | | | | |
| Protein kinase A | | | Liver | Hepatomegaly |

## 5. Name any five products formed from glycine.

Refer Question No. 1 Dec. 2005 (RS2).

## 6. Fatty liver and lipotrophic factors.

- Fatty liver is excess deposition of triacylglycerol in liver cells
- Usually associated with fibrotic changes and cirrhosis.

| *Etiology (causes)* | *Pathogenesis (net accumulation of fat in liver due to three reasons)* |
|---|---|
| i. Increased synthesis of triacylglycerols<br>ii. Impaired lipoprotein synthesis<br>iii. Deficiency of lipotrophic factors | i. Blood concentration dependent hepatic uptake of fatty acids<br>ii. Limited capacity of liver to dispose fatty acids by oxidation<br>iii. Limited capacity of liver to secrete VLDL |

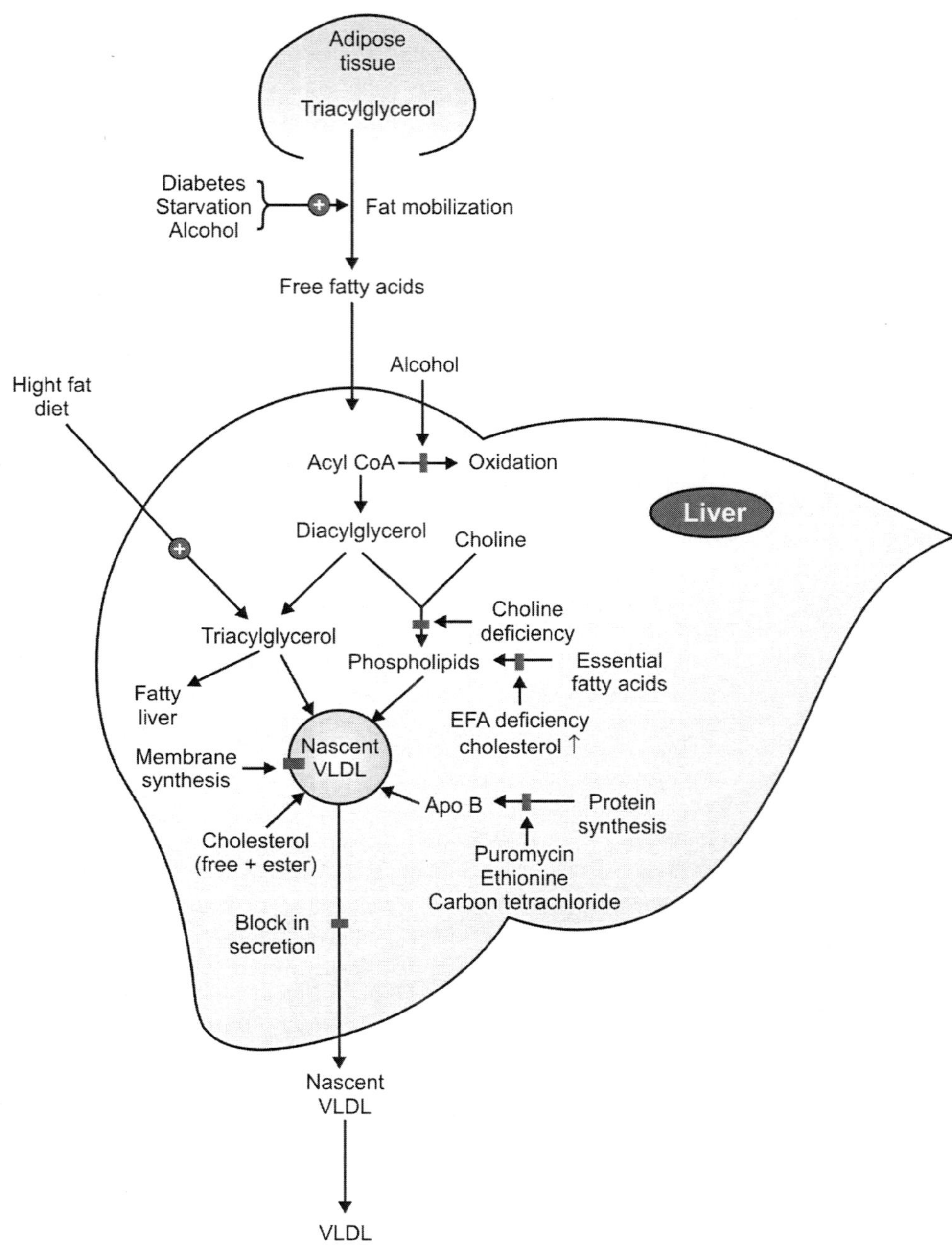


**Fig. 1:** Fatty liver

| ↑ synthesis of triacylglycerols | Impaired lipoprotein synthesis | Deficiency of lipotrophic factors |
|---|---|---|
| • Seen in diabetes mellitus, starvation, alcoholism and high fat diet<br>↑ mobilization of free fatty acids from adipose tissue into liver<br>⇓<br>Over production of triacylglycerols<br>⇓<br>Accumulation of TGs in liver | • Liver is major organ synthesising VLDL<br>• VLDL synthesis requires phospholipids and apoprotein B<br>*Factors cause fatty liver*<br>i. Defect in phospholipid synthesis<br>– Usually due to dietary deficiency of lipotrophic factors or essential fatty acids<br>ii. Block in apoprotein formation<br>– Usually caused by certain chemicals like $CCl_4$, chloroform, lead, etc.<br>iii. Failure in formation and secretion of lipoproteins<br>– Due to reduced level of ATP required for synthesis and secretion of VLDL<br>– ATP levels are reduced in pyridoxine and pantothenic acid deficiency as well as by ethionine | • Lipotrophic factors are agents required for normal mobilization of fat from liver<br>• Example: Choline, lecithin, betaine, methionine and inositol<br>*Mechanism of action*<br>• Choline and inositol are components of phospholipids and hence are required for their synthesis<br>• Other lipotropic factors are involved in transmethylation reaction and thus directly or indirectly in choline synthesis<br>• Deficiency of choline thus produce fatty liver by:<br>– Decreased phospholipid synthesis<br>– Impaired formation of lipoprotein membrane<br>– Reduced synthesis of carnitine due to insufficient supply of methyl groups<br>– Impairment in fatty acid oxidation |

## 7. Purine salvage pathways.

Refer Question No. 11 Dec. 2005 (RS2).

## 8. Chemistry, sources and daily requirement of folic acid.

Refer Question No. 2 Dec. 2016 (RS2).

## 9. Renal mechanism in acid-base balance.

Refer Question No. 2 June 2012 (RS2).

## 10. Transcription.

- Transcription is synthesis of RNA (all forms) from DNA.

### Factors Required

i. DNA strand (as template)
ii. Enzymes (RNA polymerases or DNA dependent RNA polymerase)

| RNA polymerases | Intracellular location | RNA synthesized |
|---|---|---|
| RNA polymerase I | Nucleolus | Ribosomal RNA (rRNA) |
| RNA polymerase II | Nucleoplasm | Messenger RNA (mRNA) |
| RNA polymerase III | Nucleoplasm | Transfer RNA (tRNA) |

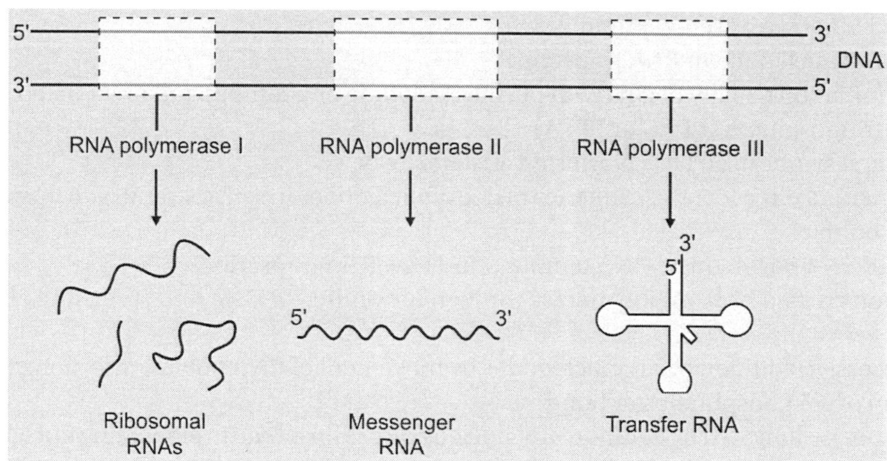


**Fig. 2:** RNA polymerases

iii. ATP, GTP, CTP and UTP
iv. Transcription factors (proteins that bind to specific sequence elements and determine rate of transcription)
  - TFllD, TFllA, TFllB, TFllF, TFllE, TFIIH
v. Termination factors

## Steps

a. Initiation
  i. Formation of transcription initiation complex
    - Most of the DNA in a cell does not code for proteins; but a segment of the DNA acts as a template for RNA is called a gene
    - Hence, recognition of this correct sequence of DNA sequence for transcription requires interaction of RNA polymerase with DNA at the promoter region
    - This requires the transcription factor which identifies two specific base sequences (gene promoter sequence) which are:

| | *Base sequence* | *Location* |
|---|---|---|
| Hogness box (TATA box) | ATATAA | 25 bases upstream on left from starting point |
| CAAT box | CGCCAATC | 70–80 bases upstream on left from starting point |

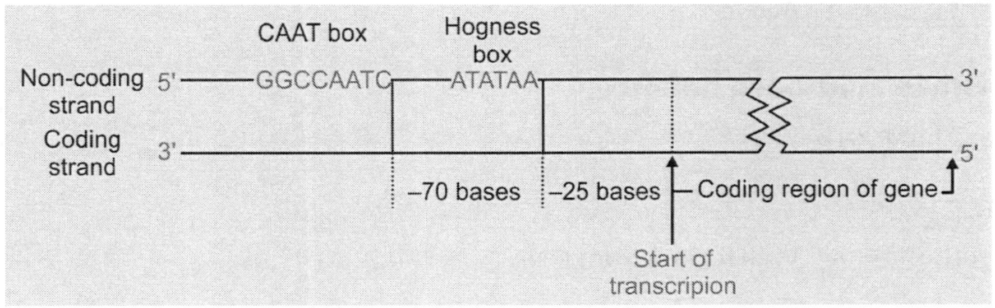


**Fig. 3:** Specific base sequence of transcription

    - These sequences bind transcription factors and transcription factors link RNA polymerase to promoter to form a transcription initiation complex.
  ii. Unwinding of DNA
    - Binding of RNA polymerase is followed by unwinding and separation of DNA strand for a short length
    - One DNA strand serves as a template strand or antisense strand and used as template to which nucleotides base pair for RNA synthesis
    - Other strand is known as sense strand.
  iii. Formation of first nucleotide in RNA transcript
    - RNA chain initiation usually begins with purines (adenine or guanine) and first nucleotide is incorporated as nucleoside triphosphates (PPPG or PPPA)
    - Position of first synthesized base is referred as start site or +1
    - RNA sequence is a direct copy of sequence of deoxynucleotides in sense strand with insertion of U in place of T.
  iv. Transcription bubble
    - A complex of RNA polymerase, DNA template and new RNA transcript
    - It has a region created by RNA polymerase through unwinding of DNA and spreading of DNA strands apart.

b. Elongation
  – Occurs by successive addition of ribonucleotides by movement of RNA polymerase along DNA
    i. Formation of 3′5 phosphodiester bond
      * RNA chain is elongated by addition of 5′ nucleoside triphosphate to elongating nucleotides of RNA through the formation of 3′5′ phosphodiester bond

ii. Base pairing
   * Nucleotides are added in a base pairing manner between newly-formed RNA and the DNA template.
iii. Elongation in 5′ → 3′ direction
   * Elongation of RNA occurs in 5′-3′ direction by movement of RNA polymerase along with template in 3′–5′ direction

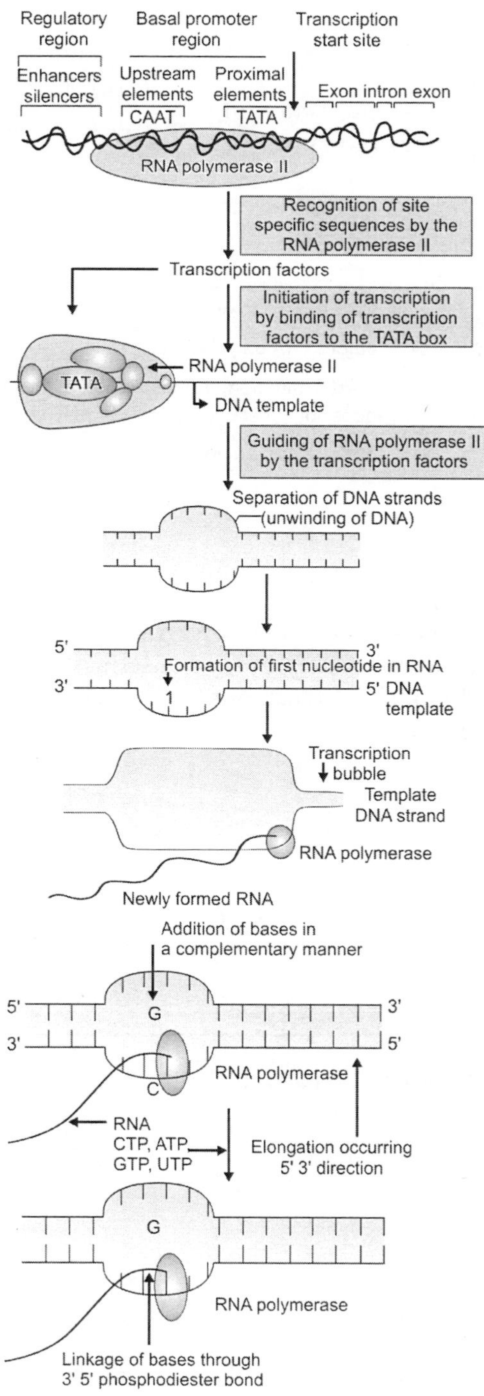


**Fig. 4:** Steps of transcription

c. Termination
   i. Chain termination by secondary structure of RNA
      - Presence of an hairpin structure followed by several uracil residues signals dissociation of RNA from DNA as well as RNA polymerase.
   ii. Protein factor dependent termination (in eukaryotes)
      - Termination of transcription by termination factors.

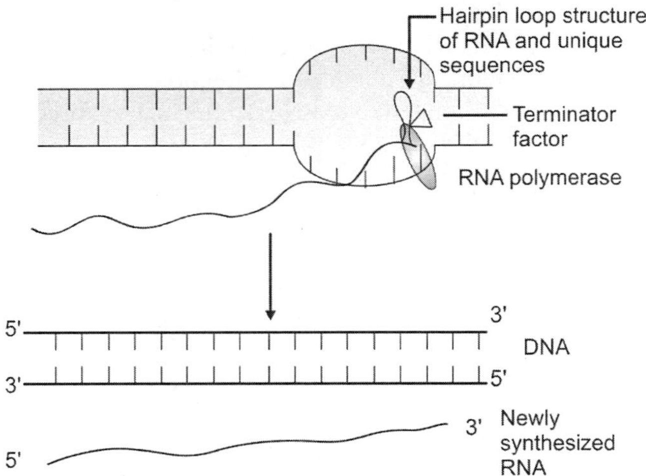


**Fig. 5:** Termination of transcription

## Regulation

- Availability of DNA for transcription
- Regulation of transcriptional initiation ← interaction of transcription factors with gene regulatory (enhancer or silencer) sequences.

## Inhibitors

| | |
|---|---|
| • Actinomycin | Binds to DNA template and blocks movement of all forms of RNA |
| • α-amanitin (from mushroom *Amanita phylloids*) | Inhibits RNA polymerase II |
| • Rifampicin, tetracycline | Inhibits initiation of transcription by binding to β subunit of prokaryotic RNA polymerase (does not affect eukaryotic RNA polymerase) |
| • Daunomycin | Intercalates with double-stranded DNA |

## Significance

- Transcription of mRNA is essential for expression of genotype to phenotype, i.e. conversion of genetic information into body proteins which exhibit the phenotype
- Transcription is selective, i.e. only a selected region of DNA is transcripted
- Products formed in transcription is referred to as primary transcript and most often, primary RNA transcripts are inactive which undergo post-transcriptional modifications (splicing, terminal additions, base modifications, etc.) to produce functionally active RNA molecules.

Revised Scheme 2

### 11. Genetic code.

Refer Question No. 2 June 2011 (RS2).

### 12. Catabolism of purines.

Refer Question No. 2 June 2007 (RS2).

## SHORT ANSWERS

### 13. Mechanism of oxidative phosphorylation.

Refer Question No. 1 June 2010 (RS2).

### 14. Functions of prostaglandins.

Refer Question No. 15 Dec. 2014 (RS2).

### 15. Oncogenes.

Refer Question No. 3 Dec. 2010 (RS2).

### 16. Mutarotation.

- Mutarotation is change in optical rotation of α and β anomeric forms of monosaccharides

- When kept in solution α and β anomeric forms finally attain specific optical rotation characteristic of that sugar.

| *Causes* | *Mechanism* |
|---|---|
| Alkalies, acids, heat and enzyme mutarotase | When sugar is kept in solution, the open form is formed in small amounts that is converted to one of anomeric ring forms |

Example:

**Mutarotation of glucose**

**α-D-Glucose** (+ 112.2°)
**D-Glucose** (Aldehyde form)
**β-D-Glucose** (+ 18.7°)

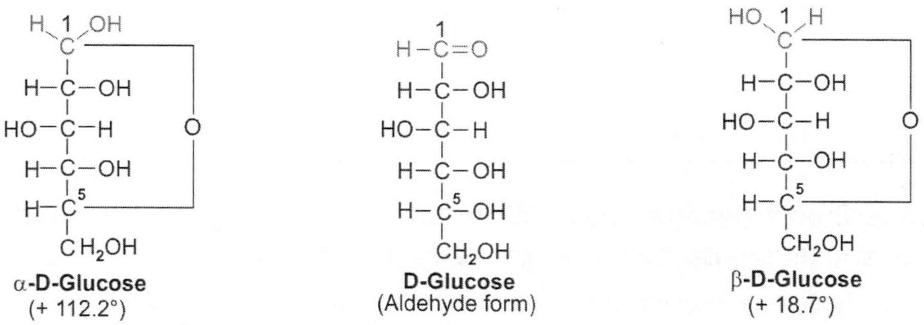

**Fig. 6:** Mutarotation of glucose

| In cold water (4°C) | | At room temperature | | In boiling water or in pyridine solution |
|---|---|---|---|---|
| α-D-glucose | ↔ | Equilibrium mixture | ↔ | β-D-glucose |
| +112.2° | | +52.7° | | +18.7° |

- Equilibrium mixture contains 63% β-anomers and 36% α-anomers of glucose with 1% open chain form.

## Significance

- Phenomenon of mutarotation provides evidence for ring structure of sugars
- Mutarotation is also exhibited by fructose (optical rotation – 92°C at equilibrium).

## 17. Antioxidants.

Refer Question No. 6 June 2008 (RS2).

## 18. Clearance tests.

Refer Question No. 9 Dec. 2005 (RS2).

## 19. Functions of albumin.

Refer Question No. 8 Dec. 2012 (RS2).

## 20. Catabolism of heme.

Refer Question No. 2 Dec. 2013 (RS2).

## 21. Trace elements.

Refer Question No. 22 Dec. 2008 (RS2).

## 22. Mention the normal levels of serum protein, urea and creatinine.

| | *Normal level* |
|---|---|
| Serum protein | 6–8 g/dL |
| Urea | 15–40 mg/dL |
| Creatinine | 0.5–1.5 mg/dL |

# MBBS PHASE I EXAMINATION
## JUNE 2007
## (Revised Scheme 2)

## LONG ESSAYS

### 1. Define glycogenesis and glycogenolysis. Write the reactions of glycogenesis and glycogenolysis in liver. How are these two pathway reciprocally regulated?

- Glycogen is a homopolysaccharide of glucose and is the storage form of glucose in animals
- Excess glucose in body is converted to glycogen (glycogenesis) for storage especially in liver and muscles and whenever required, it is broken down to glucose (glycogenolysis).

### Biomedical Importance of Glycogen

- Glycogen is storage form of glucose in animals
- Stored primarily in liver and muscles in ratio of about 1 : 3
- Liver glycogen helps maintain blood glucose level during fasting whereas muscle glycogen serves as fuel reserve for ATP supply during muscle contraction.

### Metabolism of Glycogen

a. Synthetic phase: Formation of glycogen—glycogenesis
b. Catabolic phase: Breakdown of glycogen—glycogenolysis.

### Glycogenesis

- Glycogenesis is biosynthesis of glycogen by polymerization of glucose
- About 10% of glucose is used for glycogenesis.

| *Tissue site* | *Intracellular site* | *Substrate* | *Product* |
|---|---|---|---|
| • Liver and muscles (main sites)<br>• Other tissues except mature RBCs, brain and kidney | • Cytosol (Smooth ER) | • Glucose | • Glycogen |

*Steps*

- Glucose can only be transferred to a small fragment of pre-existing glycogen called as primer or a specific protein called glycogenin
- UDP-glucose is the carrier of glucose which is formed from glucose-1-P and UTP in a reaction catalyzed by UDP-glucose pyrophosphorylase (activation of glucose)
- Glucose from UDP-G is attached at nonreducing end of glucose molecule of glycogen primer by enzyme glycogen synthase forming a $\alpha$ (1-4) glycosidic linkage so that chain is lengthened
- When chain is lengthened to about 11 glucose residue, branching enzyme transfers at least 7 glucose residue portion from one chain to neighboring chain to form $\alpha$ (1-6) linkage thus establishing a branch point.

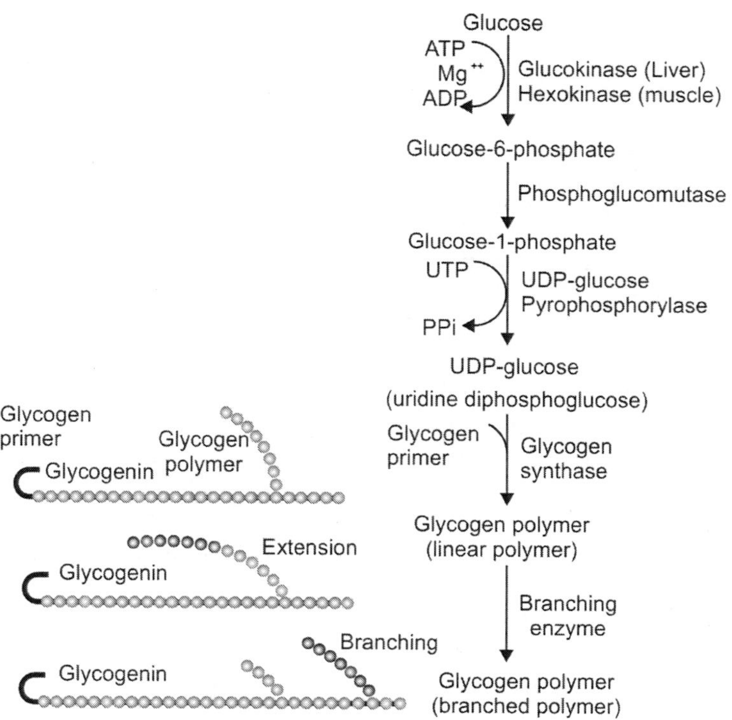


**Fig. 1:** Steps of glycogenesis

**Energetics (for incorporating 1 glucose molecule into glycogen)**

| *Reaction* | *Enzyme* | *Energy source* | *Energy expenditure* |
|---|---|---|---|
| Glucose → Glucose-1-P | Glucokinase/Hexokinase | ATP | –1 |
| Glucose-1-P → UDPG | Glucose-1-P uridyltransferase | UTP | –2 |
| UDPG → Amylose | | UTP | +1 |
| | | **Total** | **–2 ATPs** |

## Glycogenolysis

- Glycogenolysis is breakdown of glycogen into glucose or glucose-6-phoshate.

| *Tissues sites* | *Intracellular site* | *Substrate* | *Products* |
|---|---|---|---|
| • Liver and muscles<br>• Brain, kidney and intestine (minor) | • Cytosol | • Glycogen | • Glucose (liver glycogenolysis)<br>• Glucose-6-phosphate (muscle glycogenolysis)—d' to absence of G-6-phosphatase |

### *Steps*

- Glycogen phosphorylase phosphorlytically splits α-1, 4 glycoside bonds from outermost chains of glycogen until 4 glucose residue remain on either side of 1, 6 branch point
- These smaller glycogen polymers are metabolized into individual glucose molecules by debranching enzyme, which is a bifunctional enzyme
- α-1, 4 glucan transferase component—transfers α-3 glucose residue portion from one side chain to other thus exposing α-1, 6 branch point
- α-1,6 glucosidase component—splits α-1, 6 linkages hydrolytically
- Thus action of these enzymes produces free glucose molecules with removal of a branch

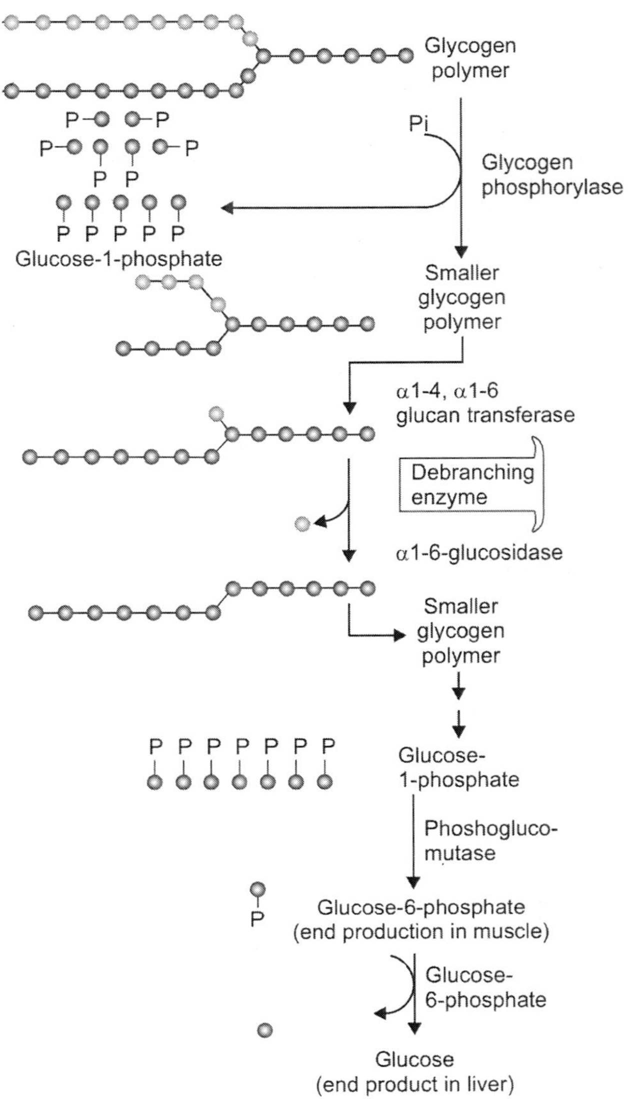


**Fig. 2:** Steps of glycogenolysis

- Further action produces mainly glucose-1-phosphate and few glucose molecules
- Glucose-1-phoshate is isomerized into glucoze-6-phosphate by enzyme phosphoglucomutase
- In muscles, it is the end stage of glycogenolysis and the glucose-6-phosphate is converted into lactate via Cori's cycle
- In liver, enzyme glucose-6-phosphatase hydrolytically cleaves the phosphate molecule releasing glucose molecule as end product.

*Regulation*

- Glycogenesis and glycogenolysis are reciprocally regulated pathways to maintain blood glucose level, i.e. when one pathway is operational, other is inhibited and vice versa
- The substances (glucose-6-P) which activate glycogenetic enzyme inhibit glycolytic enzyme and likewise hormones stimulates one enzyme inhibit other enzyme thus reciprocally regulating both cycles together to minimize energy wastage.

| *Key enzymes* | *Type of regulation* | *Activated by* | *Inhibited by* |
|---|---|---|---|
| • Glycogen synthase (glycogenesis) | Allosteric | Glucose-6-P | — |
| | Hormonal through phosphorylation and dephosphorylation mediated via cAMP (covalent modification) 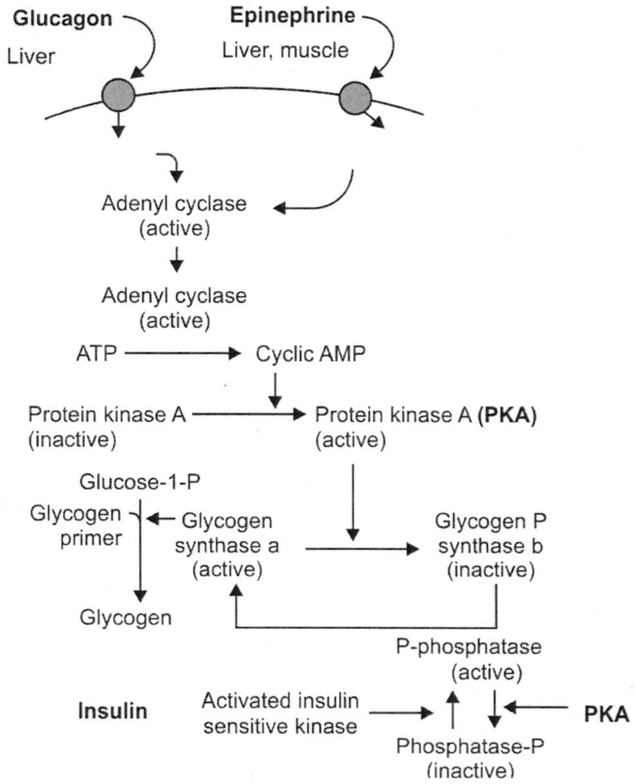<br>**Glucagon** Liver<br>**Epinephrine** Liver, muscle<br>Adenyl cyclase (active)<br>Adenyl cyclase (active)<br>ATP → Cyclic AMP<br>Protein kinase A (inactive) → Protein kinase A **(PKA)** (active)<br>Glucose-1-P<br>Glycogen primer ← Glycogen synthase a (active) → Glycogen P synthase b (inactive)<br>Glycogen<br>P-phosphatase (active)<br>**Insulin** Activated insulin sensitive kinase → ↑ ↓ ← **PKA**<br>Phosphatase-P (inactive)<br>**Fig. 3:** Regulation of glycogen synthase | Insulin | Glucagon (in liver)<br>Epinephrine (in liver and muscle) |
| • Glycogen phosphorylase (glycogenolysis) | Allosteric | AMP and $Ca^{2+}$ (muscle) | Glucose-6-P (liver and muscle)<br>ATP (muscle)<br>Glucose (liver) |
| | Hormonal through phosphorylation and dephosphorylation mediated via cAMP (covalent modification) 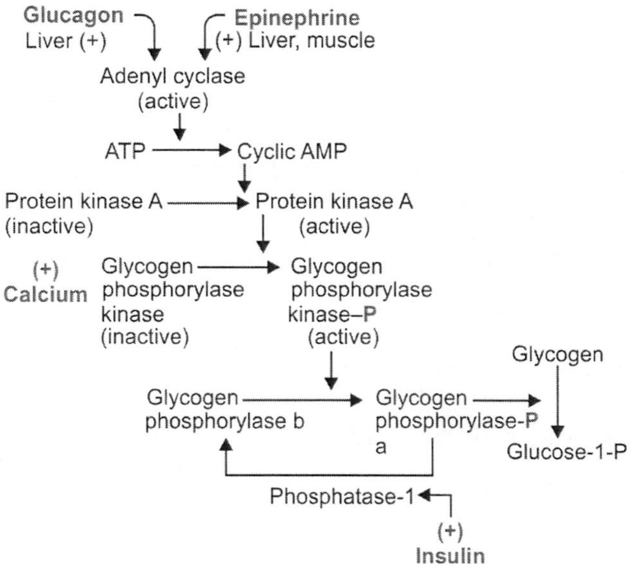<br>**Glucagon** Liver (+)<br>**Epinephrine** (+) Liver, muscle<br>Adenyl cyclase (active)<br>ATP → Cyclic AMP<br>Protein kinase A (inactive) → Protein kinase A (active)<br>(+) **Calcium** Glycogen phosphorylase kinase (inactive) → Glycogen phosphorylase kinase–P (active)<br>Glycogen phosphorylase b → Glycogen phosphorylase-P a → Glycogen → Glucose-1-P<br>Phosphatase-1 ← (+) **Insulin**<br>**Fig. 4:** Regulation of glycogen phosphorylase | Glucagon (liver)<br>Epinephrine (liver and muscle) | Insulin |

*Reciprocal Regulation*

- Glycogenenesis and glycogenolysis are reciprocally regulated to prevent futile cycles
- Phosphorylated form of glycogen phosphorylase is active; but glycogen synthase becomes inactive on phosphorylation
- Covalently modified phosphorylase is active even without AMP
- Active (dephosphorylated) glycogen synthase is responsive to action of glucose-6-phosphate
- Covalent modification modulates effect of allosteric regulators
- Hormonal control by covalent modification and allosteric regulation are interrelated
- These hormones act through a second messenger, cyclic AMP (cAMP)
- Covalent modification of glycogen phosphorylase and synthase is by a cyclic AMP mediated cascade
- Specific protein kinases bring about phosphorylation and protein phosphatases cause dephosphorylation.

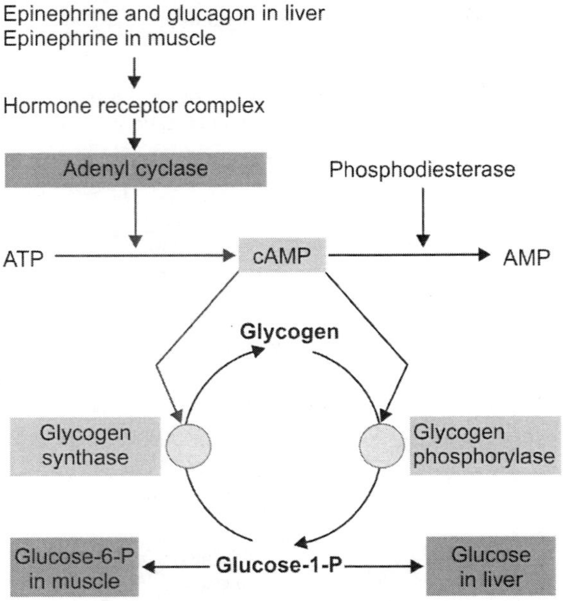

**Fig. 5:** Reciprocal regulation of glycogenesis and glycogenolysis

*Significance*

- Both the pathways (glycogenesis and glycogenolysis) are nonreversible and are controlled by end products and hormones at substrate level
- They are both different and are carried out by different sets of enzymes from each other
- Whenever glycogenesis occurs, glycogenolysis does not take place and vice versa
- Glycogen metabolism in liver differs from that in muscle as follows.

| *Glycogen metabolism* | *In liver* | *In muscle* |
|---|---|---|
| • Amount stored | 5% | 1% |
| • Source of glucose | • Blood glucose<br>• Galactose<br>• Fructose | Blood glucose |
| • Enzyme converting glucose to glucose-6-P | Glucokinase | Hexokinase |
| • End product of glycogenolysis | Glucose (because of presence of G-6-phosphatase) | Glucose-6-phosphate (because of absence of G-6-phosphatase) |
| • Effect of glucagon | Stimulates glycogenolysis and inhibits glycogenesis | No effect |
| • Metabolic significance | Regulation of blood glucose | Provision of energy for muscle contraction (Cori's cycle) |
| • Inherited disorders | Von Geirke's disease | McArdle's disease |

**2. What are nucleotides? Explain the catabolism of purine nucleotides. Write briefly on metabolic disorders associated with purine metabolism.**

- Nucleotides are nitrogenous bases attached to pentose to which is attached a phosphate, i.e. nucleotide = base + pentose + phosphate = nucleoside + phosphate.

*Example*

- Adenosine triphosphate (ATP) = Adenosine base + ribose sugar + triphosphate.

## Metabolim of Purine Nucleotides (Synthesis of Uric Acid)

- Catabolism of purines yields uric acid as follows:

*Reactions*

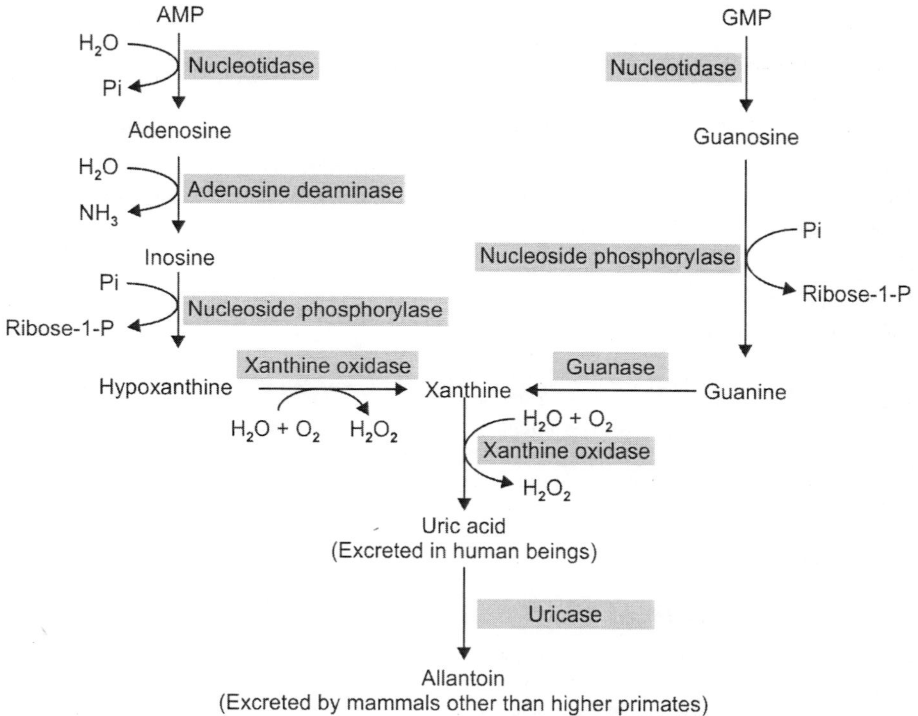


**Fig. 6:** Synthesis of uric acid (catabolism of purine nucleotides)

*Disorders*

a. Hyperuricemia (gout)
 – Gout is abnormal rise in plasma uric acid levels (hyperuricemia).

*Causes*

| *Increased production of uric acid* | | *Decreased renal excretion of uric acid* |
|---|---|---|
| *Primary* | *Secondary* | |
| • ↑ activity of PRPP synthetase<br>• ↑ activity of PRPP amidotransferase<br>• HGPRT deficiency (Lesch-Nyhan syndrome)<br>• Glucose-6-phosphatase deficiency (von Gierke's disease) | • Malignancy (↑ nucleic acid turnover)<br>• Alcoholism (↑ production) | • Renal failure<br>• Inhibition of uric acid secretion by drugs and substances (thiazides, diuretics, lactic acid and ketone bodies) |

| *Biochemical defect* | *Clinical features* | *Diagnosis* |
|---|---|---|
| • Accumulation of uric acid in body → formation uric acid crystals in joints (tophi)<br>• Excretion of uric acid in urine → formation of uric acid crystals in urine | • Deposition of uric acid crystals (sodium urate crystals) in single joints (especially great toe), connective tissue (tophi) and later several joints at late stages<br>• Renal stones or uric acid stones due to solubility of uric acid in urine | • Significant elevation in plasma uric acid levels (>7 mg/dL)<br>• Sodium urate crystals in tissue and synovial fluids |

*Treatment*

| *Acute gout (Sudden onset of severe inflammation in small joints due to precipitation of urate crystals in joint space)* | *Chronic gout (Manifests as persistence of pain and stiffness in joint between attacks)* |
|---|---|
| • Nonsteroidal anti-inflammatory drugs (NSAIDs) and steroids (inhibition of cyclooxygenase, phospholipase A2)<br>• Cochicine (blocks engulfing of urate crystals of leukocytes) | • Allopurinol (competitive inhibitor of xanthine oxidase)—first choice drug<br>• Uricosuric drugs (increases uric acid excretion)—adjuvant drug<br>  – Probenecid and sulfinpyrazone<br>• NSAIDs (inhibition of cyclooxygenase, phospholipase A2)<br>• Acetazolamide and soda carb (alkalinizes urine) |

b. Severe combined immune deficiency disease

| *Cause* | *Inheritance* | *Deficient enzyme* |
|---|---|---|
| • Several defect in metabolism of lymphocytes | • Autosomal recessive | • Adenosine deaminase |

| *Biochemical defect* | *Clinical features* | *Treatment* |
|---|---|---|
| • Impaired deoxyadenosine and adenosine → accumulation of dATP → inhibition of ribonucleotide reductase → decreased DNA synthesis → impaired lymphocyte proliferation | • Affects both T and B cells<br>• Recurrent and chronic infection | • Bone transplantation<br>• Enzyme replacement<br>• Gene therapy |

c. Purine nucleoside phosphorylase deficiency
   – Inborn error of purine metabolism.

| *Deficient enzyme* | *Biochemical defect* | *Clinical features* | *Treatment* |
|---|---|---|---|
| • Purine nucleoside phosphorylase | • Accumulation of dGTP → inhibition of ribonucleotide reductase → decreased DNA synthesis → impaired lymphocyte proliferation | • Affects T cells<br>• Recurrent or chronic infections | • Bone transplantation |

d. Xanthine oxidase deficiency
   – Inborn error of purine metabolism.

| *Deficient enzyme* | *Biochemical defect* | *Clinical features* |
|---|---|---|
| • Xanthine oxidase | • Accumulation of hypoxanthine and xanthine → increased excretion of hypoxanthine and xanthine in urine and decreased plasma uric acid levels | • Renal stones of hypoxanthine and xanthine |



## SHORT ESSAYS

### 3. Explain competitive and noncompetitive inhibition. Mention significance of competitive inhibition.

- Competitive and noncompetitive enzyme inhibition is a type of reversible enzyme inhibition where the inhibitor binds noncovalantly to enzyme and inhibition can be reversed once inhibitor is removed.

| | *Competitive inhibition (substrate analog inhibition)* | *Noncompetitive inhibition* | *Uncompetitive inhibition* |
|---|---|---|---|
| | • A type of reversible enzyme inhibition<br>• So called because inhibitor bears a close structural resemblance with substrate and thus competes with substrate for active site on enzyme | • A type of reversible inhibition<br>• Here inhibitor neither bears a structural resemblance to substrate nor does it compete with substrate for attaching at active site | • An uncommon type of reversible inhibition |
| | **Fig. 7A:** Competitive inhibition | **Fig. 7B:** Noncompetitive inhibition | |
| Type of inhibition | • Reversible but competitive | • Reversible but noncompetitive | • Reversible but un-competitive |

*Contd...*

*Contd...*

| | *Competitive inhibition (substrate analog inhibition)* | *Noncompetitive inhibition* | *Uncompetitive inhibition* |
|---|---|---|---|
| Inhibitor has affinity to | • Enzyme | • Enzyme | • Enzyme-substrate complex |
| Structural similarity to substrate | • Present | • Absent | • Absent |
| Mechanism | • Inhibitor (I) binds with binding group of enzyme (E) to form an enzyme inhibitor complex (EI). Thus substrate affinity of enzyme is lowered progressively with rise in inhibitor concentration<br>• Degree of inhibition depends; therefore, on relative concentration of substrate and inhibitor and also on relative affinities of enzyme for the two | • Inhibition is brought about by conformational changes in enzyme structure by binding at a different site<br>• Inhibitor has strong affinity for enzyme and also it does not interfere with enzyme-substrate complex formation | • Inhibitor does not have affinity for free enzyme but binds with enzyme substrate complex |
| Properties | | | |
| → $K_m$ | • Increased (decrease in affinity of enzyme towards substrate) | • Unaltered | • Decreased |
| → $V_{max}$ | • Unaltered (high substrate concentration overcomes inhibition by forcing out inhibitor from its combination with enzyme) | • Decreased | • Decreased |
| Examples | • Malonate and glutarate competitively inhibit enzyme succinate dehydrogenase which oxidizes succinate to fumarate due to their structural similarity to succinate<br>• In methanol poisoning ethanol is used due to structural similarity for causing inhibition of alcohol dehydrogenase and thus prevents formation formaldehyde, a toxic compound | • Trypsin inhibitors of Ascaris or soybean attaches to trypsin and inactivate it. Because of this ascaris worms are not digested in human intestine<br>• Heavy metal ions ($Ag^+$, $Hg^{2+}$, $Pb^{2+}$) noncomparatively inhibit enzyme by binding with cysteinyl sulfhydryl group | |

## Clinical Significance

- Certain compounds due to their property of competitive enzyme inhibition are widely used as drugs
- They inhibit a specific enzyme in a metabolic pathway; hence, also called antimetabolites.

a. Sulfonamides
   - Sulfonilamide has structural similarity to PABA (paraamino benzoic acid), which is essential for biosynthesis of folic acid in bacteria
   - Thus it acts as a competitive inhibitor of the enzyme, dihydropteroate synthetase thus blocking conversion of PABA to folic acid thus causing death of bacteria (bacteriocidal)
   - Sulfonamides are used to treat respiratory and urinary tract infections.

b. Allopurinol
   - Allopurinol is a structural analog of hypoxanthine
   - It acts as a competitive inhibitor of xanthine oxidase, an enzyme catalyzing conversion of hypoxanthine to xanthine and xanthine to uric acid
   - Allopurinol blocks formation of uric acid (from degradation of purine nucleotides)
   - Allopurinol is used in the treatment of gout (an arthritic condition characterized by increased plasma uric acid levels).

c. Methotrexate
   - Methotrexate is a folic acid analog
   - It competitively inhibit dihydrofolate reducatse, thus blocking the regeneration of tetrahydrofolate from dihydrofolate
   - Impaired regeneration of tetrahydrofolate leads to impaired synthesis of dTMP, thus leading to defective DNA synthesis
   - It is used in treatment of cancer such as leukemia and choriocarcinoma.

d. Dicumarol and warfarin
   - Dicumarol and warfarin have structurally similarity to vitamin K

- They competitively inhibit vitamin K epoxide reductase and vitamin K quinone reductase and block regeneration of active form of vitamin K
- They are used as oral anticoagulants in treatment of thrombotic conditions such as thrombosis occurring after myocardial infarction or surgery.

e. Statins
- Statins are competitive inhibitors of HMG CoA reductase and decrease cholesterol synthesis in liver
- They are used to lower blood cholesterol levels.

## 4. What is fatty liver? Explain its causes.

Refer Question No. 6 Dec. 2006 (RS2).

## 5. Give an account on organization of electron transport chain (ETC).

- Electron transport chain is a complex of mitochondrial proteins involved in transport of electrons
- Also called respiratory chain

| *Location* | *Components* | |
|---|---|---|
| | *Enzyme complexes* | *Free electron carriers* |
| • Mitochondria | • Complex I (NADH dehydrogenase complex)<br>• Complex II (succinate dehydrogenase)<br>• Complex III (ubiquinol cytochrome oxidoreductase)<br>• Complex IV (cytochrome oxidase) | • Coenzyme Q<br>• Cytochrome C |

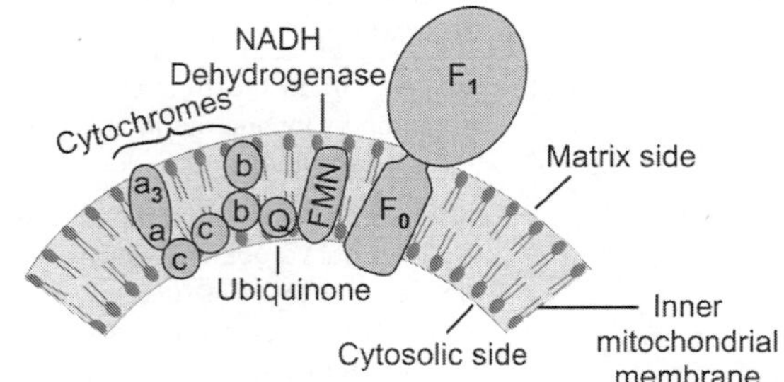


**Fig. 8:** Electron transport chain—location and components

### Organization

a. Complex I (NADH dehydrogenase complex)
- A multisubunit protein containing NADH dehydrogenase FMN and iron-sulfur clusters
- Iron cycles between reduced and oxidized states.

b. Complex II (succinate dehydrogenase complex)
- A multisubunit protein containing FAD dehydrogenase and iron-sulfur clusters
- Iron cycles between reduced and oxidized states.

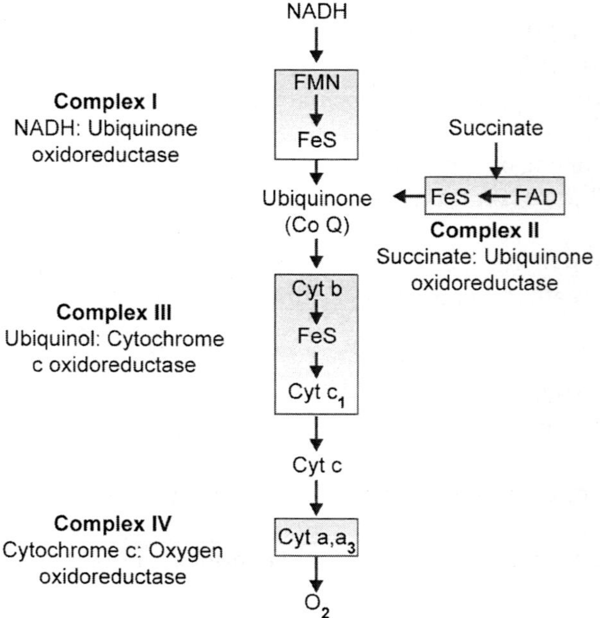


**Fig. 9:** Electron transport chain—organization

c. Coenzyme Q
   - Lipid-soluble isoprene compound
   - Coenzyme Q cycles between reduced quinol form and oxidized quinone form.

d. Complex III (cytochrome reductase complex)
   - A multisubunit protein containing iron-sulfur proteins, cytochrome b and cytochrome $c_1$.

e. Complex IV (cytochrome oxidase)
   - A multisubunit protein containing 2 copper atoms and 2 heme groups (cytochrome a and $a_3$).

## Sources of Electrons

| | |
|---|---|
| a. NADH | • Enters electron chain through complex I |
| b. $FADH_2$ | • Enters electron chain through complex II |

## Flow of Electrons

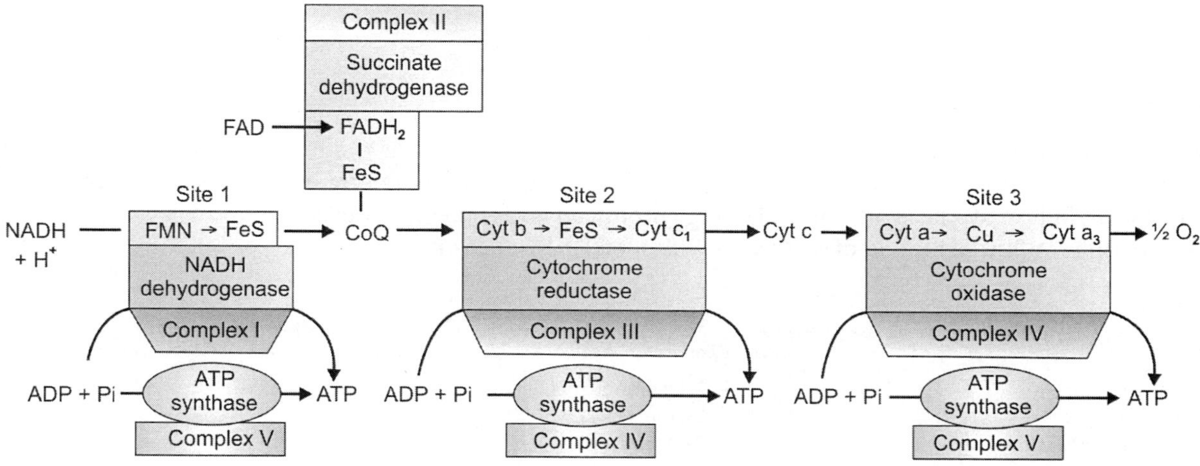


**Fig. 10:** Flow of electrons

- Electron transport chain is involved in transfer of hydrogen and electron from a number of substrates through its components, finally to $O_2$
- Chain is initiated by action of specific dehydrogenase reducing coenzyme NAD to NADH + $H^+$ which transfers reducing equivalents to flavoproteins (FP) which gets reduced to $FPH_2$
- In this way every member undergo reduction and oxidation
- Up to stage of CoQ, hydrogen is transferred and thereafter only electrons are transferred.

## Function

- Transfer of electron along respiratory chain releases energy trapped in substrate and this energy is utilized to bond an ADP with phosphate to produce ATP by oxidative phosphorylation.

## Sites of ATP Synthesis (Coupling of ETC to Oxidative Phosphorylation)

| *Site* | *Proton pumps* | *Transfer of electron between* | *Energy released* |
|---|---|---|---|
| a. Site I | Complex I | NADH to CoQ | 12 kcal/mol |
| b. Site II | Complex III | Cyt b to Cyt $c_1$ | 10 kcal/mol |
| c. Site III | Complex IV | Cyt $_{aa3}$ to $O_2$ | 24 kcal/mol |

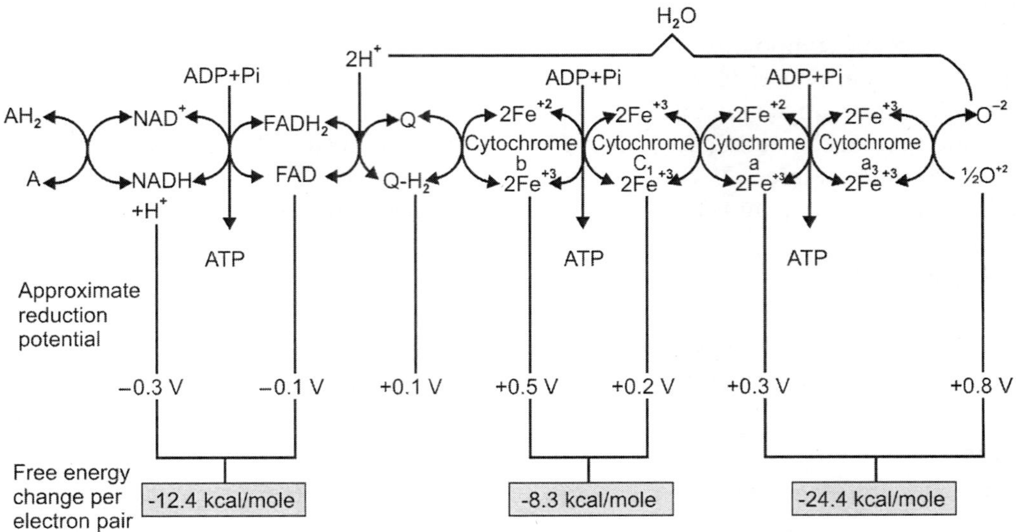


**Fig. 11:** Sites of ATP synthesis



## Uncouplers

- Electron flow in electron transport chain and oxidative phosphorylation proceed simultaneously but certain compounds uncouple or delink this symbiosis by increasing permeability of inner mitochondrial membrane to protons
- This results in failure of ATP synthesis and energy produced is dissipated as heat
- Thus uncouplers allow oxidation of substrates without ATP production.

*Examples*

| *Physiological* | *Chemical* |
|---|---|
| • Thermogenin<br>• Thyroxine<br>• Long chain free fatty acids | • 2,4 dinitrophenol<br>• Dinitrocresol<br>• Pentachlorophenol<br>• Triflurocarbonylcyanide phenylhydrazone (FCCP)<br>• Aspirin (in high doses) |

## Inhibitors

- Compounds which binds to one of components of ETC and block transport of electron causing accumulation of reduced components before inhibitor blockade step and oxidized components after that step
- These inhibitors are site specific, i.e. they inhibit sites of ATP synthesis.

*Examples*

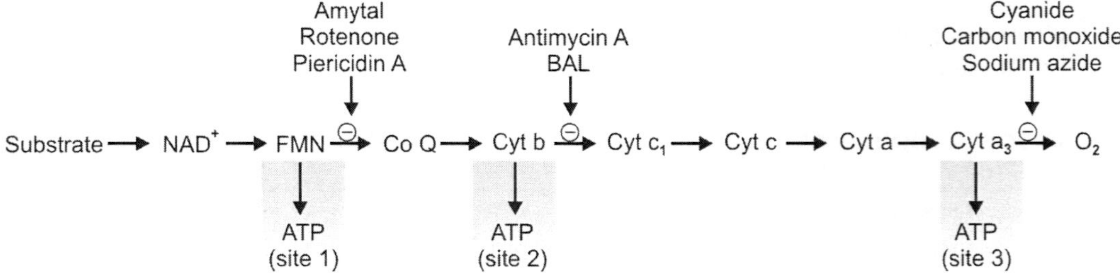


**Fig. 12:** Inhibitors of electron transport chain

| Complexes | ATP synthesis site | Inhibitors |
|---|---|---|
| a. Complex I | Site I (between NADH and CoQ) | • Alkylguanides (a hypotensive drug)<br>• Rotenone (fish poison)<br>• Chlorpromazine (tranquilizer)<br>• Barbiturate (sedative)<br>• Progesterone (steroid hormone)<br>• Piercidin (antibiotic) |
| b. Complex II | — | • Malonate<br>• Carboxin |
| c. Complex III | Site II (between cyt b and $c_1$) | • Antimycin C (antibiotic)<br>• British Anti Lewisite (chelating agent)<br>• Biguanides (hypoglycemic drug)<br>• Naphthoquinone<br>• Hydroxyquinoline |
| d. Complex IV | Site 3 (inhibitor of cytochrome oxidase) | • Carbon dioxide<br>• Cyanide<br>• Hydrogen sulphide<br>• Azide |

## Significance

*P : O Ratio*

- P : O ratio is number of inorganic phosphate molecules incorporated into ATP for every atom of oxygen consumed
- In other words, it is ratio of phosphate utilized to atoms of oxygen consumed in oxidation
- It represents number of ATP molecules synthesized per pair of electrons carried through electron transport chain
- P : O ratio of oxidation of NADH is 3 and that of $FADH_2$ is 2
- But recent studies on isolated mitochondria indicate it to be 2.5 for NADH and 1.5 for $FADH_2$.

## 6. Tumor markers.

- Tumour markers are biological substances synthesized and released by cancer cells or produced by host in response to cancerous substance and are used to monitor or identify presence of a cancerous growth.

## Characteristics of Tumor Markers

- Tumor marker is a specific marker for the tumor
- Level of tumor marker is increased in plasma, urine, other biological fluids and tissues
- Concentration of tumor marker in plasma of healthy subjects is very low compared to cancerous state
- Stoichiometric correlation occurs between plasma level and tumor mass
- Quantitation of tumor marker is easy and inexpensive
- Tumor marker suggests the low and high risk for cancer
- Level of tumor marker changes as status of tumor is altered
- Tumor marker is useful both for prediction of presence of tumor and recurrence of tumor.

## Classification (Examples)

| Tumor marker | Features | Associated tumor |
|---|---|---|
| a. Oncofetal antigens | • Proteins synthesized during fetal life<br>• Serum levels are markedly lower after birth; however, these proteins reappear with onset of cancer, indicating reactivation of genes during malignant transformation of tumor | |
| i. Alpha fetoprotein | Oncofetal glycoprotein<br>• Sources—liver and yolk sac (embryonic life)<br>• Normal serum level—<10 µg/L | • Hepatocellular carcinoma, non-seminomatous germ cell tumor of testis (high rise >400 µg/L)<br>• Benign hepatic disorders, pregnancy (moderate rise) |

*Contd...*

*Contd...*

| *Tumor marker* | *Features* | *Associated tumor* |
|---|---|---|
| ii. Carcinoembryonic antigen | • Glycoprotein<br>• Source: Fetal gastrointestinal tract | Cancer of bowel, pancreas and breast |
| b. Cytoplasmic proteins | | |
| i. Immunoglobulins | • Globular protein<br>• Sources: Plasma cell | Multiple myeloma, other gammapathies |
| ii. Prostate-specific antigen | • Extracellular protease<br>• Source: Prostate gland<br>• Normal serum level: 0 to 4.5 µg/L | Prostatic carcinoma |
| c. Enzymes | | |
| i. Acid phosphatase | • Sources: Prostate and erythrocytes; bone, leukocytes and platelets<br>• Normal serum level: 2–12 IU/L | Prostatic carcinoma and hemolytic anemia |
| ii. Alkaline phosphatase | • Sources: Liver (epithelial cells of biliary canaliculi) bone, intestine, kidney and placenta<br>• Normal serum level: 30–115 U/L | Primary liver cancer or secondary metastatic tumors in liver<br>Bony metastasis |
| d. Hormones | | |
| i. Human chorionic gonadotropin | • Glycoprotein<br>• Source: Trophoblastic tissues of placenta and testes<br>• Normal serum level: <5 IU/L | Trophoblastic tumors, germ cell tumors of testis |
| ii. Calcitonin | • Polypeptide<br>• Source: C cells of thyroid<br>• Normal serum level: <8.8 ng/L | Medullary carcinoma of thyroid |
| iii. Catecholamines and vanillyl mandelic acid | | Neuroblastoma, pheochromocytoma |
| iv. Ectopic hormone production | Increased production of hormones by a non-endocrine tissues | Paraneoplastic syndrome |
| e. Secreted cancer antigens (carbohydrate antigens) | • Antigens present on surface of tumor cells or antigens secreted by tumor cells<br>• Detected by monoclonal antibodies developed against these antigens<br>• More specific than either enzymes or hormones | |
| i. CA-125 | • Glycoprotein antigen<br>• Recognized by monoclonal antibody OC-125<br>• Source: Ocular tissues and respiratory tract and female reproductive system<br>• Normal serum level: 35 kU/L (35 µg/mL) | • Ovarian and endometrial cancer (high rise)<br>• Menstrual cycle and cirrhosis of liver (moderate rise) |
| ii. CA-19.9 | • Glycoprotein antigen<br>• Sources: Colon cancer cell and pancreatic cancer<br>• Normal serum level: 40 U/mL | • Intra-abdominal adenocarcinomas such as pancreatic tumor, gastric cancer and colon cancer<br>• Adenocarcinoma of lung |

## Clinical Significance (Application of Tumor Markers)

- For screening of cancer in asymptomatic population
- For diagnosis of cancer in asymptomatic patients
- As a prognostic indicator
- As an aid in clinical staging of cancer
- For monitoring patient under treatment
- For early detection of relapse and recurrence of cancerous process.

## 7. Explain the steps of urea cycle and mention the names of its disorders.

Refer Question No. 1 Dec. 2011 (RS2).

## 8. How bilirubin is formed and detoxified in the body?

- Bilirubin is a bile pigment which is toxic and water insoluble
- It is primarily derived from metabolism of heme component of hemoglobin.

### Sources of Bilirubin (250–300 mg/day)

| *Major source (85%)* | *Minor source (15%)* |
|---|---|
| • Heme from degradation of Hb released from aged RBCs in RE system of liver, spleen and bone marrow | • Heme released from ineffective erythropoiesis in bone marrow<br>• Catabolism of other heme containing compounds in liver and other tissues (catabolism of myoglobin in muscles and cytochromes in liver) |

### Bilirubin Metabolism

*Formation of Unconjugated Bilirubin (Metabolism of Hemoglobin)*

| *Site* | *Substrate* | *Products* |
|---|---|---|
| Reticuloendothelial system | Hemoglobin | • Heme (metabolized to biliverdin and then to bilirubin)<br>• Globin (hydrolyzed to amino acids that enter amino acid pool) |

*Steps*

i. Formation of biliverdin
   - Heme is converted to biliverdin, carbon monoxide and ferric iron in a reaction catalyzed by microsomal heme oxygenase (enzyme requires NADPH and oxygen).

ii. Formation of bilirubin
   - Biliverdin is reduced to form bilirubin in a reaction catalyzed by biliverdin reductase (enzyme is NADPH dependent).

### Bilirubin Transport

- Bilirubin from reticuloendothelial system enters into plasma where it binds to albumin and is transported to liver
- One molecule of albumin takes 2 molecules of bilirubin and 100 mL of plasma can transport 25 mg of bilirubin.

### Bilirubin Catabolism (Bilirubin Detoxification)

a. Hepatic metabolism
   i. Hepatic uptake of bilirubin
      - In liver, bilirubin dissociates from albumin and enters to hepatocytes through carrier mediated transport
      - Inside hepatocytes, bilirubin is reversibly bound to ligandins (cytosolic proteins called Y proteins) which prevent entry of bilirubin back to plasma
   ii. Conjugation of bilirubin
      - Unconjugated bilirubin is conjugated in hepatic microsomes to form water-soluble bilirubin diglucuronide in a 2 step reaction catalyzed by bilirubin UDP-glucuronyl transferase

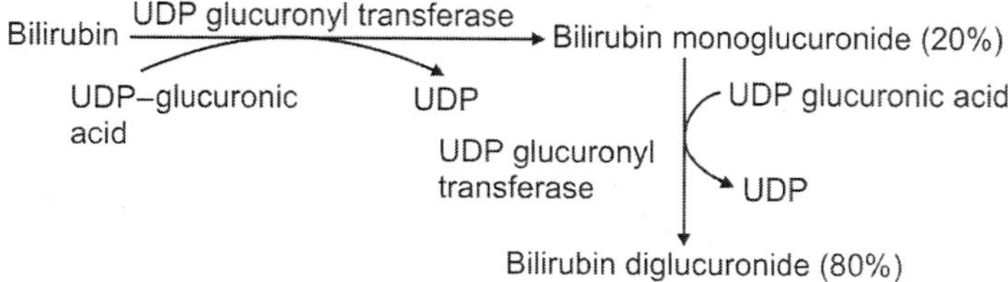

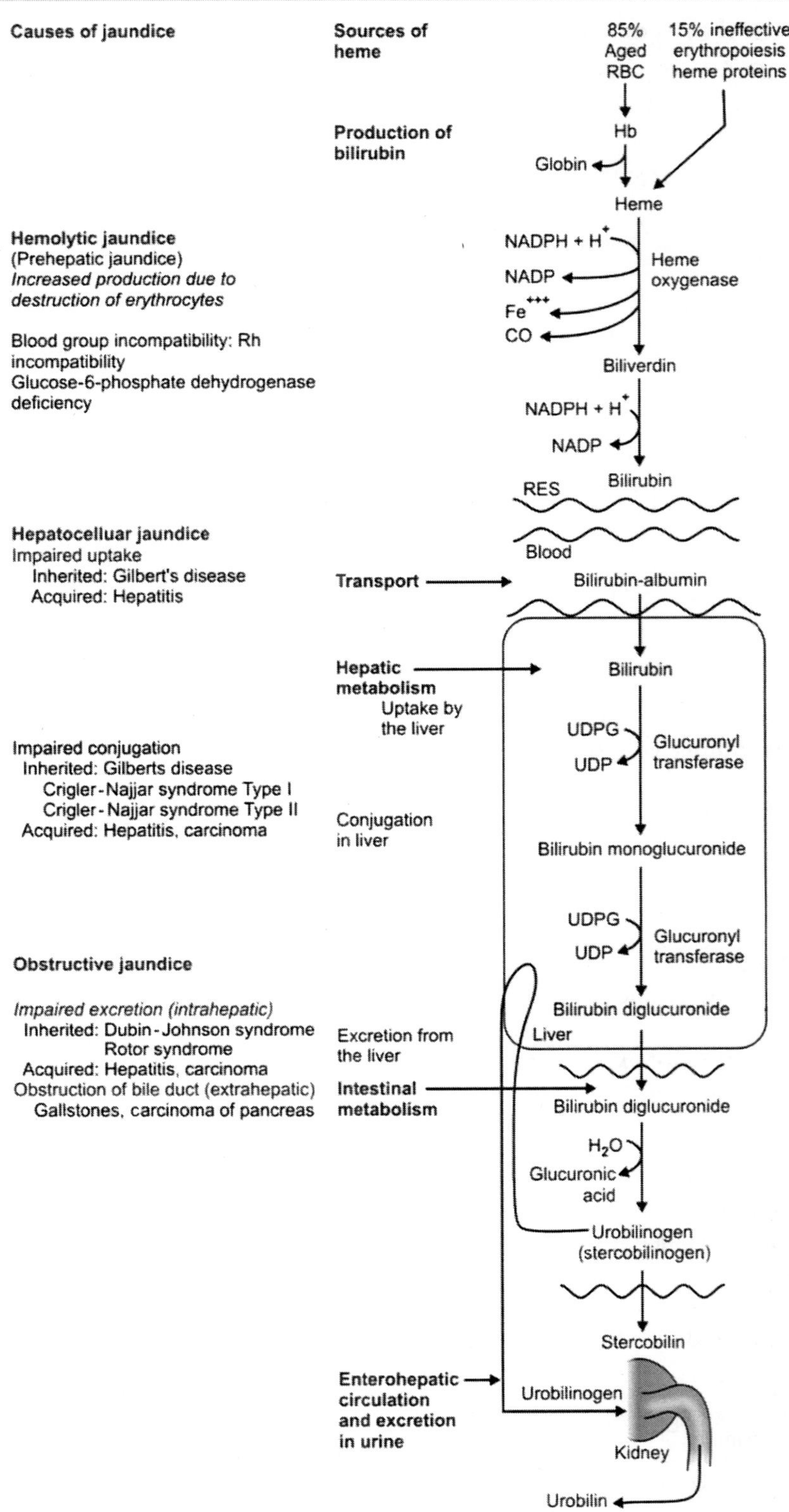


**Fig. 13:** Bilirubin medabolism

iii. Excretion of conjugated bilirubin to bile
- This conjugated bilirubin is excreted into bile by an energy dependent active transport process at biliary canaliculi membrane.

b. Intestinal metabolism
   i. Formation of urobilinogens in intestine
      - Conjugated bilirubin is transported through biliary ducts into duodenum where it is hydrolyzed by intestinal and bacterial β glucuronidase to form unconjugated bilirubin
      - Unconjugated bilirubin is reduced by intestinal bacteria to form a group of compounds called urobilinogens (also called stercobilinogens).

## Excretion (of Urobilinogens)

a. Excretion in feces
   – About 80% of urobilinogens are excreted in feces as urobilins or stercobilins (formed by oxidation of urobilinogen lower intestinal tract or in excreta) which constitute the major pigment (orange brown) in stool imparting brown color to feces
b. Excretion in urine (enterohepatic circulation)
   – 20% of urobilinogen in intestinal lumen is reabsorbed and most of it is taken up by liver and re-excreted in bile (enterohepatic circulation)
   – A small amount enters general circulation and appears in urine (<4 mg/day).

## Anomalies Associated with Bilirubin Metabolism

| | *Pathogenesis* | *Inherited cause* | *Acquired cause* |
|---|---|---|---|
| Hepatocellular jaundice | Impaired intake | • Gilbert's disease | • Hepatitis |
| | Impaired conjugation | • Gilbert's disease<br>• Crigler-Najjar syndrome (Type I and II) | • Hepatitis<br>• Hepatic carcinoma |
| Obstructive jaundice | Impaired excretion (intrahepatic) | • Dubin-Johnson syndrome<br>• Rotor syndrome | • Hepatitis<br>• Hepatic carcinoma |
| | Obstruction of bile duct (extrahepatic) | — | • Gallstones<br>• Carcinoma of pancreas |

## Clinical Significance

- Bilirubin is displaced from its binding sites on albumin by drugs like aspirin, sulpha, penicillin, etc. Therefore, care should be taken while administrating these drugs to the newborn babies to avoid kernicterus
- Drugs like primaquin, chloramphenicol, androgen and pregnanediol may interfere with conjugation process of bilirubin thus causing jaundice
- Drugs like barbiturates induce conjugating enzyme system thus enhancing excretion of bilirubin.

# 9. Explain metabolic role of calcitriol.

- Calcitriol is active form of vitamin D; a fat-soluble vitamin.

## Chemistry

- Vitamin D is structurally a sterol
- Vitamin $D_3$ or cholecalciferol is form of vitamin D found in animals.

| *Provitamin (precursor) form* | *Active form* | *Sources* | *RDA* |
|---|---|---|---|
| • 7-dehydrocholesterol (an intermediate of cholesterol metabolism found in skin) | • Calcitriol (1, 25 dihydroxy cholecalciferol) | *Dietary sources*<br>• Fatty fish, fish liver oil, egg yolk<br>*In vivo sources*<br>• Provitamin D3 (7-dehydrocholesterol) is partly synthesized in skin or intestinal mucosa | • 200–400 IU or 5–10 mg of cholecalciferol |

Activation of vitamin D (formation of calcitriol or activation of cholecalciferol)

7-dehydrocholesteol —(Skin, UV rays)→ Secosterol (cis) ——→ Cholecalciferol (trans)

- Cholecalciferol is first transported to liver where 25 hydroxylation occurs followed by transportation of 25 hydroxycholecalciferol in plasma (bound to alpha globulin) to kidney where it is further hydroxylated at 1st position to give calcitriol

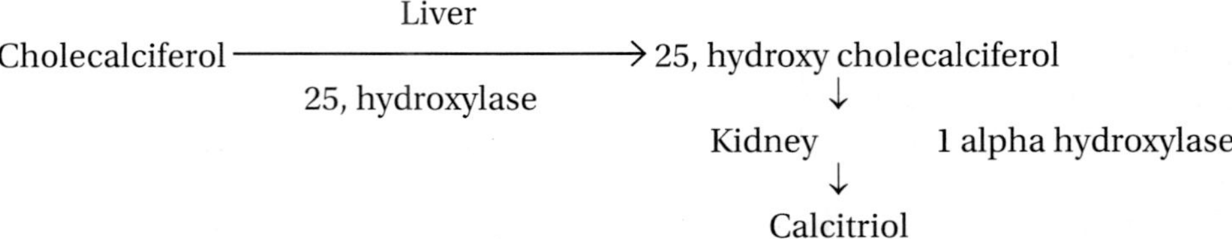


## Regulation of Synthesis of Calcitriol (Regulated by Serum $Ca^{2+}$ Level)

- Low serum $Ca^{2+}$ stimulates parathyroid glands to release parathyroid hormones (PTH) → increases 1α-hydroxylase in kidney
- Excess calcitriol decreases 1α-hydroxylase activity.

## Mechanism of Action

- Mechanism of action of calcitriol is typical of steroid hormones
- It enters intestinal cells and binds to a cytoplasmic receptor and then vitamin $D_3$-receptor complex moves into nucleus to interact with DNA
- This results in synthesis of mRNA which in turn forms a calcium binding protein
- Calcium binding protein thus produced, increases absorption of $Ca^{2+}$
- Therefore, calcitriol or vitamin $D_3$ can also be called as a hormone.

## Metabolic Role/Biochemical Role (Function)

| *Regulation of plasma calcium and phosphate levels (calcium homeostasis)* | *Other effects* |
|---|---|
| • Increase blood calcium level by:<br>– Increasing absorption of $Ca^{2+}$ and phosphate from small intestine<br>– Causing removal of $Ca^{2+}$ from bone (bone resorption)<br>– Minimizing excretion $Ca^{2+}$ and phosphate through kidney by decreasing their excretion and increasing reabsorption | • Inhibition of proliferation of keratinocytes<br>• Stimulate differentiation of kertainocytes<br>• Induce monocyte maturation to macrophages |

## Deficiency Disorders

- Less common due to in vivo synthesis in body

| *Causes* | *Clinical forms* | |
|---|---|---|
| | *Rickets (Eng. Wrickken—to twist)* | *Osteomolacia (Gr. Osteon—bone and malkia—softness)* |
| • Insufficient exposure to sun (due to geographical location—northern latitudes or social customs—purdah system in Muslim women)<br>• Dietary deficiency (strict vegetarians)<br>• Chronic alcoholics<br>• Liver or kidney disorders<br>• Fat malabsorption syndrome | • Seen in children between 4 months to 2 years<br>*Clinical features*<br>• Delayed milestones<br>• Soft and pliable bone (due insufficient mineralization)<br>• Delay in teeth eruption<br>• Bow legs, knock knee<br>• Rickety rosary and pigeon chest<br>• Harrison sulcus<br>• Craniotabes (softening of skull on pressure)<br>• Bossing of frontal bones | • Seen in adults<br>*Clinical features*<br>• Soft and pliable bone more liable to fracture (due to demineralization)<br>• Bone aches and pains |

*Contd...*

Contd...

| | | |
|---|---|---|
| | *Biochemical findings*<br>• Plasma calcium level ↓<br>• Plasma phosphate level ↓<br>• Plasma alkaline phosphatase level 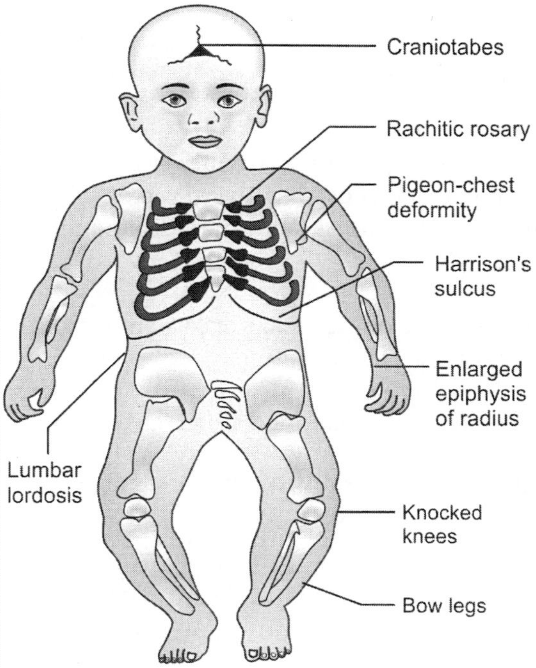 ↑<br><br>Craniotabes<br>Rachitic rosary<br>Pigeon-chest deformity<br>Harrison's sulcus<br>Enlarged epiphysis of radius<br>Lumbar lordosis<br>Knocked knees<br>Bow legs<br><br>**Fig. 14:** Rickets—clinical manifestations | |

## Toxicity

| *Causes* | *Clinical features* |
|---|---|
| • Overingestion of vitamin D preparations | • Hypercalcemia<br>• Metastatic calcification |



## 10. What is plasmid? What is its application in recombinant DNA technology?

- Plasmids are small, extrachromosomal, independent circular double stranded, self-replicating DNA molecules
- Can be easily separated from host bacteria and DNA sequence restriction maps of many plasmids are known
- Once established in bacterial cell, they undergo autonomous replication and they are passed on to successive generations as bacteria undergo cell division.

*Example*

i. pBR322
   - A plasmid of *E. coli* discovered by Bolivar and Rodriguez is most popular and widely used plasmid vector.

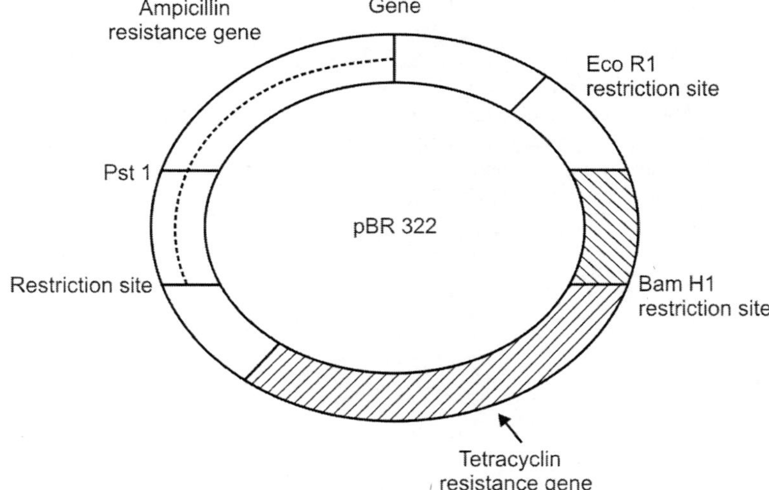


**Fig. 15:** Plasmid

## Uses

- For incorporation of foreign target DNA and they can accept DNA fragments of length 6,000–10,000 nucleotide base sequence
- Well suited for cDNA cloning
- Plasmids transfer gene for antibiotic resistance in bacteria.

## Application in Recombinant DNA Technology

a. Synthesis of peptide hormones for medications
   - Selected segment of DNA which codes for peptide hormones such as insulin, growth hormone and oxytocin is incorporated into the plasmid and bacteria is used as a viral vector, which is encouraged to reproduce so as to recapitulate altered DNA within other cells it infects and increase amount of cells with recombinant DNA present within them.

b. Gene therapy
   - In gene therapy, related viruses are used as cloning vectors or carriers to transport and pass on genes in recombinant DNA through viral reproduction throughout organism.

c. Copying genes
   - Plasmids are used in genetic and biochemistry laboratories to make copies of or express particular gene.



## 11. Give an account of storage and transport of iron.

- Iron is an essential trace element.

| *Dietary sources* | *Daily requirement* |
|---|---|
| • Rich sources: Organ meats like liver, heart, kidney<br>• Good sources: Leafy vegetables, pulses, cereals, fish, apples, dried fruits<br>• Poor sources: Milk, wheat, polished rice | • Children: 20–30 mg<br>• Adult male: 20 mg<br>• Adult female: 30 mg<br>• Pregnancy and lactation: 40 mg |

## Absorption

| *Site of absorption* | *Absorption form* |
|---|---|
| • Upper part of duodenum | • Ferrous form (as it is readily soluble)<br>• Ferric form is converted (reduced) to ferrous form by ferric reductase enzymes present on surface of intestinal cells, vitamin C, cysteine and gastric HCl |

## Factors Affecting Absorption

| *Factors promoting* | *Factors inhibiting* |
|---|---|
| • Ferrous form of iron<br>• Ascorbic acid (by favoring reduction of ferric form to ferrous form)<br>• Cysteine (reduces ferric form to ferrous form)<br>• HCl (by facilitating reduction of ferric form to ferrous form)<br>• Iron deficiency state (due to low ferritin levels) | • Phytates and phosphates (form complexes with iron)<br>• Antacid ingestion, achlorohydria or gastric surgery (due to deficiency of HCl)<br>• Gastrointestinal diseases (infections or muscosal damages) |

## Mechanism

- Dietary iron is present in 3 forms, which are absorbed by different mechanisms

| *Ferrous form* | *Ferric form* | *Heme form* | |
|---|---|---|---|
| • Major form of absorption<br>• Taken up by mucosal cells which is dependent upon proton coupled divalent metal transporter 1 (DMT-1)<br>• Inside mucosal cell cytoplasm, ferrous iron ($Fe^{2+}$) is converted back into ferric iron ($Fe^{3+}$) which either combines with apoferritin to form ferritin or is transported to circulation<br>• Transport of iron from basolateral surface of mucosal cell into circulation requires a transport protein, ferroprotein I or iron regulatory protein I which interacts with hephaestin (an substance with ferroxidase activity, i.e. catalyzes conversion of ferrous iron to ferric iron) | • Majority converted (reduced) to ferrous form by reducing agents like ferric reductase, vitamin C, cysteine and gastric HCl<br>• Some amount absorbed as it is by a transport carrier called integrin<br>• Inside mucosal cell cytoplasm, ferric form combines with mobilferrin, another protein<br>• This ferric-mobilferrin complex wither transfers iron to apoferritin or to basolateral surface of cell | • Absorbed into mucosal cell through transport protein called heme transporter<br>• Inside mucosal cell, heme is acted upon by heme oxygenase which releases ferrous iron from heme | 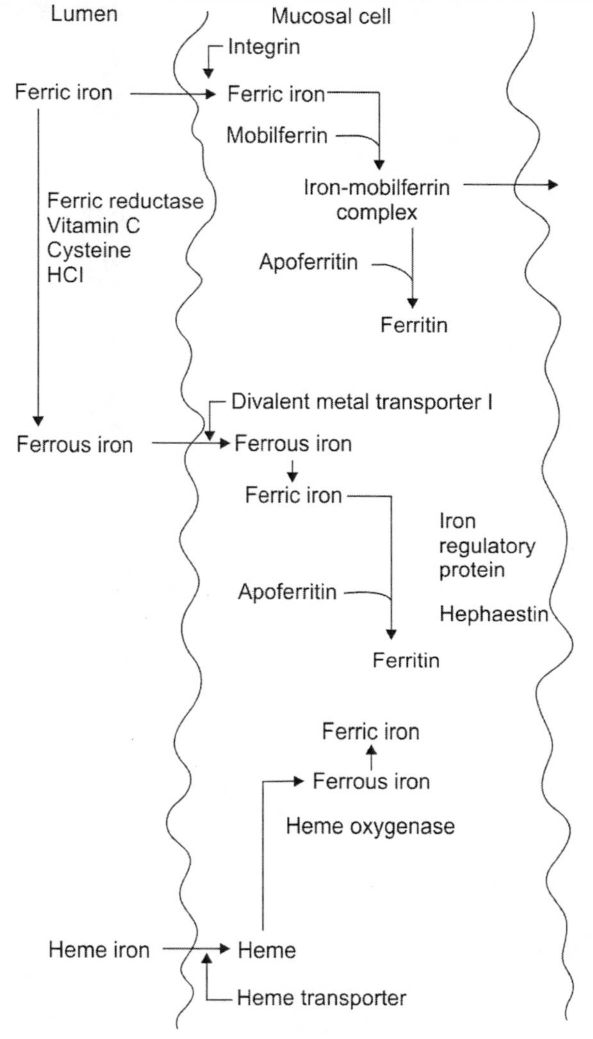 <br>**Fig. 16:** Absorption of iron |

## Regulation

- Iron metabolism is unique because homeostasis is maintained by regulation at level of absorption and not at excretion
- When iron stores in body are depleted, absorption is enhanced and when adequate quantity of iron is stored absorption is decreased
- Ferritin content of intestinal mucosal cell (indicates endogenous iron status) regulates iron absorption.

  *Mucosal block theory (blocking of iron absorption when mucosal iron content is more)*
  - Excess ferritin content of mucosal cells, blocks absorption of iron and vice versa.

  *Mechanism*
  - Regulation of iron absorption mainly occurs at translational level of gene expression for apoferritin
  - Expression of this gene is regulated by iron responsive element located on 5′ end of mRNA for apoferrtin
  - When intracellular iron levels are low, regulatory protein binds to iron responsive element and blocks the mRNA to be utilized for protein synthesis
  - As a result, less iron is incorporated to form ferritin and more iron available for its entry into circulation.

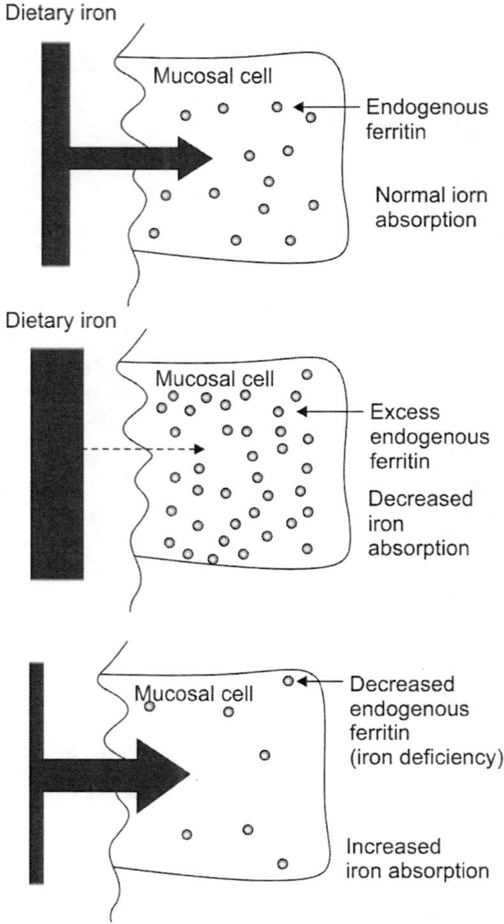


**Fig. 17:** Mucosal block theory



## Transport

- Iron enters mucosal cell in ferrous form which is reconverted into ferric form by ceruloplasmin
- Ferric iron is then incorporated into a glycoprotein, transferrin
- This transferrin binds to specific receptors on target cells like RBCs, spleen cells or liver cells and release iron after internalisation (receptor mediated endocytosis)
- Later the apotransferrin is released back into plasma.

*Transport Form*

- Transferrin, a β globulin and glycoprotein is iron transport protein in plasma
- A single molecule of transferrin binds 2 molecules of ferric iron
- Synthesized by liver
- Transports iron to storage sites (liver), RBC and processing sites (bone marrow).

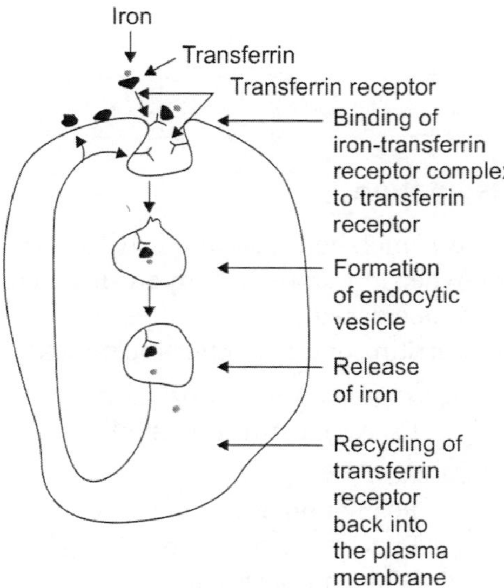


**Fig. 18:** Transport of iron

## Storage

| *Sites* | *Storage form* |
|---|---|
| Liver, spleen, bone marrow and intestine | • Ferritin and hemosiderosis are storage form of iron<br>• Ferritin and hemosiderosis are complexes of iron and apoprotein<br>• Under normal conditions, iron is stored as ferritin and when iron is excess, it is stored as hemosiderin |

## Biochemical Function

- Iron in necessary for synthesis of certain proteins
- Iron-containing proteins are of two types—heme protein and non-heme proteins.

| *Iron compounds* | *Function* |
|---|---|
| a. Heme proteins | |
| – Hemoglobin | 70% of body iron is in form of Hb<br>Present RBC and helps in transport of respiratory gases<br>Also acts buffer |
| – Myoglobin | Storage site of $O_2$ and releases it when required<br>Accounts for 5% of total body iron |
| – Catalase and peroxidase | Helps in decomposition of $H_2O_2$ |
| – Cytocromes b, $C_1$, $C_a$, $C_{a3}$ | Components of respiratory chain, where transports electron producing ATP from NADPH and NADH |
| – Tryptophan pyrolase | Enzyme taking part in tryptophan metabolism |
| – Glutathione peroxidase | Catalyzes conversion of $H_2O_2$ using reduced glutathione |
| b. Non-heme proteins | |
| – Ferritin and hemosiderin | Storage form of iron in body<br>Present in liver, spleen and bone<br>Comprises 15% of total body iron |
| – Transferrin | Iron transport protein in blood |
| – Iron sulfur protein | Involved in electron transport |
| – Succinate dehydrogenase | Catalyzes conversion of succinate to fumarate (citric acid cycle) |
| – Xanthine oxidase | Conversion of hypoxanthine to xanthine and xanthine to uric acid (purine nucleotide catabolism) |

## 12. Explain metabolic and respiratory acidosis.

| *Metabolic acidosis* | *Respiratory acidosis* |
|---|---|
| Primary bicarbonate, $HCO_3^-$ deficit | Primary carbonic acid excess |
| ↓ $HCO_3^-$ = pH ↓<br>$H_2CO_3$ | $HCO_3^-$ = pH ↓<br>↑ $H_2CO_3$ |
| Causes | |
| • Abnormal ↑ in anions other than $HCO_3^-$ (acid gain acidosis)<br>– Endogenous production of acid ions<br>- Diabetes acidosis<br>- Starvation<br>- High fever<br>- Violent exercise<br>- Lactic acidosis d' shock and hemorrhage<br>– Ingestion of acidifying salts<br>– Renal insufficiency (acid retention)<br>• Abnormal loss of $HCO_3^-$<br>– Severe diarrhea<br>– Fistulas | • Depression/suppression of respiration<br>– Damage to CNS<br>- Brain damage (trauma, inflammation, compression), convulsions<br>- Drug poisoning (morphine, barbiturates)<br>- Excessive anesthesia<br>- Bulbar polio<br>– Loss of ventilatory function<br>- Tension pneumothorax, mediastinal tumor, emphysema<br>– Pain due to pleurisy<br>• Impairment of diffusion of $CO_2$ across alveolar membrane<br>– Reduction of respiratory surface<br>- Emphysema, pneumonia, pulmonary fibrosis, pulmonary edema, etc. |

*Contd...*

*Contd...*

| *Metabolic acidosis* | *Respiratory acidosis* |
|---|---|
| | • Obstruction to escape of $CO_2$ from alveoli<br>– Obstruction to respiratory tract<br>– Rebreathing from a closed space<br>• Insufficient pulmonary blood flow<br>– Congenital heart diseases, Ayerza's disease |
| In uncompensated phase | |
| $HCO_3^-$: Disproportionate ↓<br>$H_2CO_3$: ↓<br>$pCO_2$: ↓<br>Total $CO_2$: ↓<br>Ratio: ↓ | $HCO_3^-$: Disproportionate<br>$H_2CO_3$: ↑<br>$pCO_2$: ↑<br>Total $CO_2$: ↑<br>Ratio: ↑ |
| Fully compensated phase | |
| Total $CO_2$: ↓<br>$HCO_3^-$ and $H_2CO_3$: Proportionate ↓<br>Ratio: 20:1 | Total $CO_2$: ↑<br>$HCO_3^-$ and $H_2CO_3$: Proportionate ↑<br>Ratio: 20:1 |
| Compensatory mechanism | |
| Primary: Respiratory<br>Stimulation of respiratory centers → hyperventilation and $H_2CO_3^-$ | • Primary: Renal<br>↑ $H^+$–$Na^+$ exchange<br>↑ $HCO_3^-$ reabsorption<br>↑ $NH_3$ formation |
| • Secondary: Renal<br>↑ $H^+$–$Na^+$ exchange<br>↑ $HCO_3^-$ reabsorption<br>↑ $NH_3$ formation | • Secondary: Respiratory (partial)<br>Low pH and high $CO_2$ induces hyperventilation<br>But $CO_2$ elimination is partial |
| • Urinary findings<br>pH: Acidic<br>↑ excretion of $NH_4Cl$ and $NaH_2PO_4$<br>↑ titrable acidity | • Urinary findings<br>pH: Acidic<br>↑ excretion of $NH_4Cl$ and $NaH_2PO_4$<br>↑ titrable acidity |

## SHORT ANSWERS

### 13. Explain enzyme profile in myocardial infarction.

Refer Question No. 5 Dec. 2014 (RS2).

### 14. What is normal serum level of cholesterol? Name its four biological functions?

Refer Question No. 1 June 2016 (RS2).

### 15. What are antioxidants? Name chain breaking and preventive antioxidants.

Refer Question No. 6 June 2008 (RS2).

### 16. Give metabolic functions of endoplasmic reticulum and mitochondria.

Refer Question No. 7 Dec. 2012 (RS2).

### 17. Explain detoxification by conjugation with two examples.

Refer Question No. 7 Dec. 2005 (RS2).

### 18. Which are inhibitors of protein synthesis?

Refer Question No. 2 Dec. 2008 (RS2).

## 19. Protein calorie malnutrition.

Refer Question No. 9 June 2010 (RS2).

## 20. Significance of nonprotein nitrogenous substances.

- Nitrogen is usually present in body in form of protein but in some body fluids, it is present in nonprotein forms called as nonprotein nitrogenous substances.

*Examples*

- Urea and uric acid
- Creatine, creatinine
- Ammonia
- Purine and pyrimidines
- Histamine

| NPN substances: PUNCH |
|---|
| ✓ **P**urine and pyrimidines |
| ✓ **U**rea and uric acid |
| ✓ **N**$H_3$ (ammonia) |
| ✓ **C**reatine, creatinine |
| ✓ **H**istamine |

*Normal level*

| NPN substance | Blood level |
|---|---|
| a. Total NPN | 20–40 mg/dL |
| Important Components | |
| b. Urea | 15–40 mg/dL |
| c. Creatinine | 0.5–1.5 mg/dL |
| d. Uric acid | 4–8 mg/dL |

### Significance

- Estimation of nonprotein nitrogenous substances is helpful in assessing renal function
- Increase in the blood levels of nonprotein nitrogen (NPN) is referred to as azotemia and is hallmark of renal failure
- Nonprotein nitrogen concentration can be used as an alternative to blood urea level as follows:
  - Molecular weight of urea is 60 and about half of it (28) is contributed by 2 nitrogen atoms
  - Thus, if blood urea concentration is 60 mg, then about half of it (28 mg) is blood urea nitrogen (BUN)
  - Therefore, BUN = ½ NPN OR NPN = 2 BUN.

## 21. Functions of pyridoxal phosphate.

Refer Question No. 2 June 2006 (RS2).

## 22. Types of RNA and their functions.

Refer Question No. 8 June 2013 (RS2).

# MBBS PHASE I EXAMINATION
## DECEMBER 2007
## (Revised Scheme 2)

## LONG ESSAYS

### 1. Define isoenzymes. Mention the principles used for separation of isoenzymes. Write about the clinical importance of isoenzymes.

- Isoenzymes are multiple molecular forms of same enzyme catalyzing the same reaction and differ from each other structurally (amino acid and carbohydrate composition), chemical and physical properties, electrophoretically and immunologically.

### Formation

| *Types* | *Mechanism* | *Examples* |
|---|---|---|
| a. Oligomeric Isoenzyme | In multimeric protein, arrangement of subunits arising from two different genes or loci in different combinations (most common) | Lactate dehydrogenase (LDH) |
| b. Monomeric isoenzyme | Single subunit protein may be coded by different genes and have different primary amino acid sequences | Asparate amino transferase (SAT) |
| c. Genetic variation | Occurrence of different allelic forms in an individual | Alcohol dehydrogenase |
| d. Post-translational modifications | Post-translational modifications | Alkaline phosphatase |

### Separation of Isoenzymes

*Principle*

- Isoenzymes are present in different body tissues and are different from each other physically and chemically different.

*Methods*

- Acid phosphatase of red cells can be differentiated from that of prostate as acid phosphatase of prostate is extremely heat labile and can be inhibited by ethanol while acid phosphatase of red cells is inactivated by 20% neutral formaldehyde
- Alkaline phosphatase isoenzyme of placental origin is extremely heat stable
- Some isoenzymes like lactate dehydrogenase, creatinine phosphokinase can be separated by electrophoresis as they differ in their mobility due to different electric charge due to difference in contents of acidic and basic amino acids
- Some enzymes like creatinine phosphokinase can be separated by chromatography
- Creatinine kinase can also be separated using antibodies against one of the isoenzyme form.

## Isoenzymes

| | *Isoenzymes* | *Clinical significance (diagnosis and prognosis of)* |
|---|---|---|
| A. Lactate dehydrogenase (LDH) [A tetramer of 2 types subunits; Heart type (H) and muscle type (M)] | a. LDH1 – H4 (Heart): Fastest electrophoretic mobility, heat stable<br>b. LDH2 – H3M (RBC): Heat stable<br>c. LDH3 – H2M2 (Brain)<br>d. LDH4 – HM3 (Liver): Heat labile<br>e. LDH5 – M4 (Muscles): Slowest electrophoretic mobility, heat labile | Normal level: 60–200 IU/L<br>Myocardial infarction<br>• LDH1 levels are increased after 12–24 hours and peak increase seen on 2nd day |
| B. Creatinine phosphokinase (CPK) [A dimer of 2 subunits; muscle type (M) and brain type (B)] | a. CPK1 – BB (Brain): Slowest electrophoretic mobility<br>b. CPK2 – MB (Heart)<br>c. CPK3 – MM (Skeletal muscles): Fastest electrophoretic mobility | Normal level: 20–80 IU/L<br>Myocardial infarction<br>• CKMB levels are increased within 6–18 hours<br>Muscular dystrophies<br>• CKMM significantly increased |
| C. Alkaline phosphatase (ALP) | a. Bone form: Heat labile but pre-beta in electrophoresis<br>b. Liver form: Heat labile but alpha-electrophoretic mobility<br>c. Intestinal form: Inhibited by phenylalanine<br>d. Placental form: Heat-stable | Normal level: 2–13 KA units/dL<br>Bone isoform<br>• Increased in bone diseases<br>Liver isoform<br>• Increased in obstructive jaundice<br>Intestinal isoform<br>• Increased in intestinal diseases<br>Placental isoform<br>• Increased in normal pregnancy<br>Regan isoenzyme (resembles placental isoform)<br>• Increased in malignancies such as carcinoma of liver |
| D. Acid phosphatase (ACP) | a. Erythrocyte isoform (not inhibited by tartarate)<br>b. Prostate isoform (inhibited by tartarate) | Normal level: 0.5–4 KA units/dL<br>Prostatic isoform<br>• Increased in prostatic carcinoma |

## Biomedical Importance of Isoenzymes

a. Metabolic Significance
   - Though isoenzymes catalyze same reaction, they may have different kinetic and regulatory properties
   - Example: LDH in muscle preferentially catalyzes Pyruvate → Lactate whereas in liver it preferentially catalyzes Lactate → Pyruvate

b. Diagnosis and monitoring of diseases
   - Detection and quantification of isoenzyme in serum is used clinically for diagnostic purposes and assessment of prognosis of diseases which is more sensitive than determination of total enzyme activities
   - Example: In myocardial infarction, significant increase occurs in CKMB isoenzyme form of CK and LDH1 isoform of LDH.

### 2. What is the importance of maintaining acid-base balance in the body? Write in detail how kidney helps in maintaining acid-base balance.

Refer Question No. 2 June 2012 (RS2).

## SHORT ESSAYS

### 3. List the important products formed from tyrosine and write the metabolic pathways leading to the formation of any two of them.

Refer Question No. 1 Dec. 2010 (RS2).

### 4. Mechanism of action of glucagon.

- Glucagon is a hyperglycemic hormone.

| *Chemistry* | *Source* |
|---|---|
| Linear polypeptide containing 29 amino acids and molecular weight 3495 | • α cells of pancreatic islets<br>• Produced as proglucagon and released by exocytosis |

## Mechanism of Action

- Glucagon acts by activating intracellular enzyme system and formation of second messenger cyclic AMP which exerts effect of glucagon
- When glucagon binds to a specific membrane receptor, a series of events takes place mediated by G-proteins
- Steps in cAMP formation are:
  - Hormone binds to specific membrane receptor, which in turn, stimulates associated G protein
  - G protein is a trimer consisting of α, β and γ subunits; where α subunit is in a bound form to a GDP
  - Hormone receptor complex causes exchange of GDP with GTP on this α subunit and dissociates it from rest of 2 subunits. This GTP bound α subunit of G protein stimulates adenyl cyclase enzyme
  - Activated adenyl cyclase coverts ATP to cAMP
  - GTP is hydrolyzed to GDP and a subunit bound to GTP returns to combine with β and γ subunits to form original G protein
- Once formed, cAMP activates protein kinase A, a heterotetramer consisting of 2 regulatory subunits (R) and 2 catalytic subunits (C)
- Activation is brought about by dissociation of R and C subunits

$$4\text{ cAMP} + R_2C_2 \rightarrow R_2\text{ (4cAMP)} + 2C\text{ (Active)}$$

- Active subunit (C) catalyzes phosphorylation of protein and it is phosphoprotein that causes desired biochemical effect.

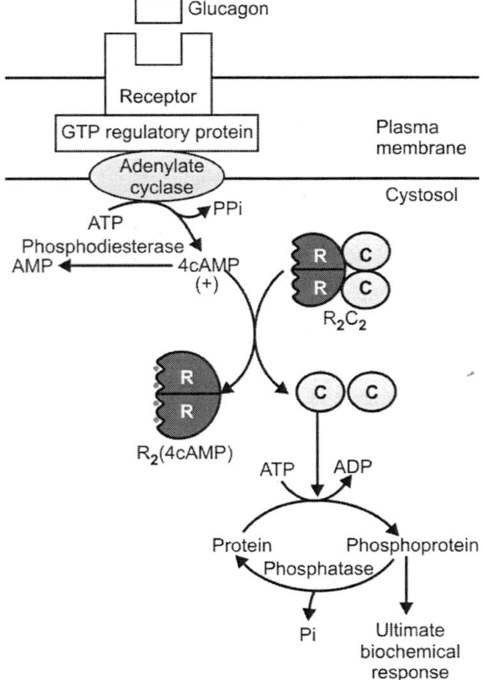


**Fig. 1:** Glucagon—mechanism of action

## Metabolic Effects (Functions)

a. Effect on carbohydrate metabolism
   - Increases blood glucose level by following ways:
     - Stimulates glycogenolysis in liver but not in muscles by inhibiting glycogen synthetase and activation of phosphorylase enzyme
     - Activates phospholipase C and resultant increase in intracellular $Ca^{2+}$ also stimulates glycogenolysis
     - Promotes gluconeogenesis in liver by activating key enzymes and increasing deamination and transport of amino acid into liver cells.

b. Effect on lipid metabolism
   - Increases release of free fatty acids from adipose tissue and in turn promotes ketogenesis.

c. Effect on protein metabolism
   - Increases deamination of amino acids for gluconeogenesis.

d. Effect on other hormones
   - Stimulates secretion of growth hormone, insulin and pancreatic somatostatin.

e. On heart
   - Large doses of exogenous glucagon exerts a positively ionotropic effect on heart and it also accelerates AV conduction.

## 5. Single electron carrier components of respiratory chain.

Refer Question No. 5 June 2007 (RS2).

## 6. Mechanism of pyruvate dehydrogenase enzyme action and its biochemical importance.

Refer Question No. 1 June 2006 (RS2).

## 7. List various types of fatty acid oxidation. Write about activation of fatty acids for oxidation.

Refer Question No. 1 Dec. 2008 (RS2).

## 8. Replication of lagging strand.

Refer Question No. 2 June 2010 (RS2).

## 9. List metabolic functions of ascorbic acid. How do you detect its deficiency? What is the daily requirement?

Refer Question No. 2 Dec. 2005 (RS2).

## 10. Basal metabolic rate (BMR).

Refer Question No. 12 June 2006 (RS2).

## 11. Degradation of heme.

Refer Question No. 2 Dec. 2013 (RS2).

## 12. Gene therapy.

- Gene therapy refers to introduction of functional genetic material into target cells to replace or supplement defective genes or to modify target cells so as to achieve therapeutic goals.

### Procedure

- In gene therapy, a corrected gene is inserted into genome to replace an abnormal, disease causing gene
- A carrier called a vector must be used to deliver therapeutic gene to patient's target cells
- Most common vectors are genetically altered viruses and target cells such as patient's liver or lung cells are infected with these vectors
- Vectors unload their genetic material containing therapeutic human gene into target cell and generation of a functional protein product from therapeutic gene restores target cell to a normal state.

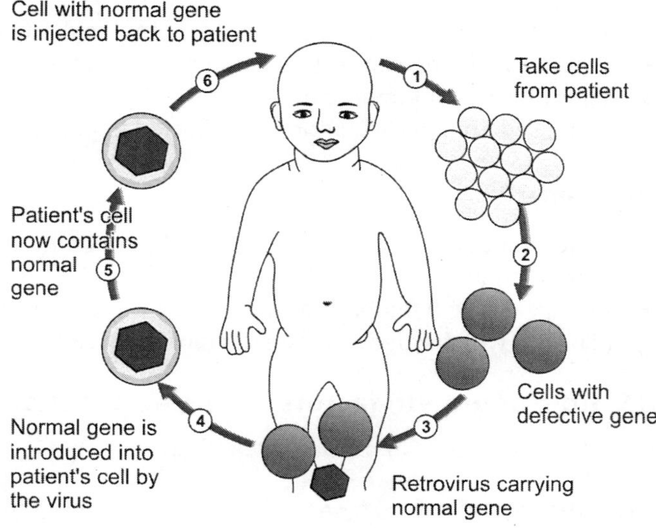


**Fig. 2:** Gene therapy

### Types of Gene Therapy

| *Germ line gene therapy* | *Somatic cell gene therapy* |
|---|---|
| • Germ cells, i.e. sperms or eggs, are modified by introduction of functional genes, which are ordinarily integrated into their genomes<br>• Thus inducing inheritable change that would be passed on to later generations<br>• Prohibited for application in human beings, for technical and ethical reasons | • Gene is introduced only in somatic cells, especially of these tissues in which expression of concerned gene is critical for health<br>• Expression of introduced gene relieves/eliminates symptoms of disorder, but this effect is not inheritable as it does not involve germ line |

### Vectors

| *Plasmids* | *Bacteriophage (virus)* | *Cosmids* |
|---|---|---|
| • Small, independent circular double stranded DNA, conferring antibiotic resistance to a bacteria<br>• Can be easily separated from host bacteria and DNA sequence restriction maps of many plasmids is known<br>• Useful for incorporation of foreign target DNA<br>• Can accept DNA fragments of length 6,000–10,000 nucleotide base sequence | • Linear DNA molecules, containing several restriction enzymes sites<br>• Can accept DNA fragments of length 10,000–20,000 nucleotide base sequences | • Specialized plasmids containing DNA sequence namely Co sites<br>• Can accept DNA fragments of length 20,000-50,000 nucleotide base sequence |

### Applications

- Used in treatment of cystic fibrosis, growth hormone deficiency, Lesch Nyhan syndrome, familial hypercholesterolemia, etc.

## SHORT ANSWERS

### 13. Functions of plasma membrane.

Refer Question No. 4 Dec. 2009 (RS2).

### 14. Lipid peroxidation—clinical importance.

- Lipid peroxidation is a chain reaction of oxidation of double bonds in unsaturated fatty acids of triacyglycerols initiated by free radicals which provides a continuous supply of other free radicals which initiate further peroxidation
- In vitro, it leads to rancidity of fats and oils and in vivo damages integrity of plasma membrane
- It is increased by heat, light, moisture and air.

### Clinical Importance

- Lipid peroxidation leads to production of ketones, aldehydes and peroxy radicals (free radicals)
- These free radicals cause damage to biomolecules in cell
- This peroxidation can be prevented by antioxidants like vitamin E or tocopherols
- Thus dietary supplement of these antioxidants is very important to prevent lipid peroxidation in vivo
- Increased lipid peroxidation is implicated in pathogenesis of Alzheimer's disease.

### Assessment

- Malondialdehyde is a product of lipid peroxidation is used as a biochemical marker for the assessment of lipid peroxidation
- MDA reacts with thiobarbituric acid and produce red-colored products namely thiobarbituric acid reactive substances (TBARS) which can be measured colorimetrically.



### 15. Role of growth factors in carcinogenesis.

Refer Question No. 16 Dec. 2005 (RS2).

### 16. Glucose-6-phosphate dehydrogenase deficiency.

- Glucose 6 phosphate dehydrogenase (G-6-PD) is a dimer with identical subunits and is an important enzyme in HMP pathway of glucose metabolism.

### Glucose-6-Phosphate Dehydrogenase Deficiency

- Most commonly encountered enzyme deficiency in clinical practice.

### Inheritance

- X-linked recessive trait.

| *Precipitating conditions* | *Clinical features* | *Diagnosis* | *Treatment* |
|---|---|---|---|
| Usually asymptomatic but manifest on exposure of patient to oxidative stress such as infections, oxidants drugs like antimalarials (primaquine), sulpha drugs, or fava beans (favism) | • Drug-induced hemolytic anemia (nonspherocytic)<br>• Hemolysis is caused decreased NADPH levels which reduce glutathione levels thus making red cell membrane instable which rupture under oxidative stress<br>• This hemolysis leads to jaundice, anemia and blackening of urine<br>• Hemolytic jaundice may be seen in neonatal period | • ↓ G-6-PD level in RBCs | • Avoidance of oxidative stress<br>• Symptomatic management |

### Clinical Importance

- This condition provides immunity from *Plasmodium* infection as there is unavailability of reduced glutathione required by the parasite
- It also shows a close linkage with color blindness.

## 17. Functional classification of proteins.

Refer Question No. 7 June 2013 (RS2).

## 18. Iodine metabolism.

- Iodine is an important trace element.

| *Source* | *RDA* | *Distribution* |
|---|---|---|
| Sea foods, eggs, dairy products and iodized salt | 150 micrograms/day | Total body iodine content—50 mg<br>15 mg present in thyroid gland |

### Iodine Metabolism

i. Uptake of iodine
   - Iodine is taken up by thyroid cells by active transport against the concentration gradient.

ii. Oxidation of iodine
   - For incorporation into thyroid hormone, iodine has to be activated by oxidation which can be done only by thyroid gland
   - The enzyme thyroperoxidase oxidizes iodine in presence of $H_2O_2$ which is converted to $H_2O$.

iii. Iodination of thyroglobulin
   - Active iodine is incorporated into thyroglobulin to form mono iodotyrosine.

### Function

- Iodine is essential for synthesis of thyroid hormones.

## 19. Importance of base pairing.

Refer Question No. 19 June 2013 (RS2).

## 20. Molecular defect and consequences of sickle cell disease.

- Sickle cell disease is the most common hemoglobinopathy characterized by presence of sickle cell hemoglobin (HbS) instead of normal HbA.

### Etiology

- Single gene disorder arising from point mutation of in DNA causing substitution of thymine for adenine.

### Inheritance

- Autosomal recessive
  - Homozygous inheritance (HbSS): Sickle cell anemia
  - Heterozygous inheritance (Hb AS): Sickle cell trait (50% Hb is normal).

### Molecular Basis

- Sickle cell hemoglobin (HbS) occurs due to substitution of valine in place of glutamic acid in 6th position of β chain of normal adult Hb
- Hydrophobic valine residue in HbS is on surface which adheres to a complementary site on surface of deoxyhemoglobin (formation of sticky ends) which leads to polymerisation of Hb

- Hemoglobin S has decreased solubility in deoxygenated state which results in formation of a gelatinous network of fibrous polymers called tactoids
- Tactoids become stiff and distort RBCs and produce rigid erythrocytes (sickled erythrocytes): This phenomenon is called sickling
- These rigid erythrocytes traverse small blood vessel with great difficulty or cause obstruction of small blood vessels resulting in repeated infarctions of organs, leading to sickle cell crisis
- Sickling and distortion of erythrocytes also results in hemolytic anemia
- Sickling can be reversed on oxygenation, however, once it occurs then a vicious cycle starts.

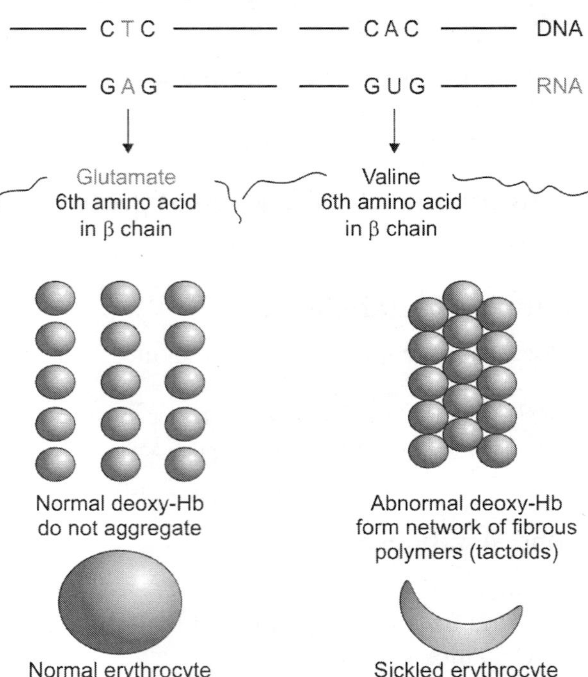

**Fig. 3:** Molecular defect and consequences of sickle cell disease

## Precipitating Factors

- Infections, hypoxia, dehydration, cold and acidosis.

## Clinical Features (Consequences)

- Chronic hemolytic anemia—pallor of mucous membranes, fatigue, dyspnea, jaundice and gallstone formation
- Impairment of growth and development
- Increased susceptibility to infection
- Vaso-occlusive or painful crisis of varying severity and frequency manifest as which manifest as pain and swelling of joints and bony pains due to infarction and sequestration
- Leg ulcers, priapism (painful penile erection), repeated episodes of pulmonary infarction, pulmonary hypertension, hematuria, stroke and aseptic necrosis of bone.

## Laboratory Diagnosis

- Microcytic hypochromic anemia
- Sickling test: Demonstration of sickled RBC in a blood smear exposed to low oxygen tension in presence of a reducing agent (sodium metabisulfite)
- Sickle cell solubility test: Turbid appearance of Hb solution due to precipitation of HbS in presence of reducing agents (sodium dithionate)
- Electrophoresis: Shows a slower moving band of HbS than HbA at alkaline pH
- Molecular diagnosis: DNA analysis using RFLP.

## Treatment

- Avoidance of oxidative stress
- Hydroxyurea and bone marrow transplantation.

## Clinical Significance

- Sickle cell trait has a protective effect on *Plasmodium falciparum* infection; it reduces severity of infection.

### 21. Sources and beneficial effects of dietary fiber.

Refer Question No. 10 Dec. 2014 (RS2).

## 22. What is reference range? How is it calculated?

- Reference range or normal range or normal value is a set of values of some measurement that are used to interpret a set of results for a particular test or finding.
- A reference range for a particular test or measurement, is usually defined as values that 95% (or 2 standard deviations) of population fall into.

### Calculations

- In an ideal situation, where the distribution is normal, reference range can be obtained by simply measuring a population and taking 2 standard deviations either side of mean
- If a normal population shows a bimodal distribution, then 2 reference ranges can be established for 2 different groups of people. For example, different reference range for males and females.

# MBBS PHASE I EXAMINATION

## JUNE 2008

## (Revised Scheme 2)

## LONG ESSAYS

### 1. Describe TCA cycle. Discuss in detail its energetics, regulation and its role.

- TCA (Tri carboxylic acid) cycle is final common metabolic pathway for oxidation of carbohydrates, fatty acids and amino acids
- Also called Kreb's cycle or citric acid cycle
- Oxalaoacetate used in first step is regenerated in last step hence called cycle.

| *Principal organs* | *Subcellular site* | *Substrate* | *Product* |
|---|---|---|---|
| • All tissues except erythrocytes | • Mitochondrial matrix | Primary substrate<br>• Acetyl CoA formed from pyruvate (carbohydrate), fatty acids and amino acids | • $CO_2$, $H_2O$ and energy (in form of ATP bonds) |

**Steps**

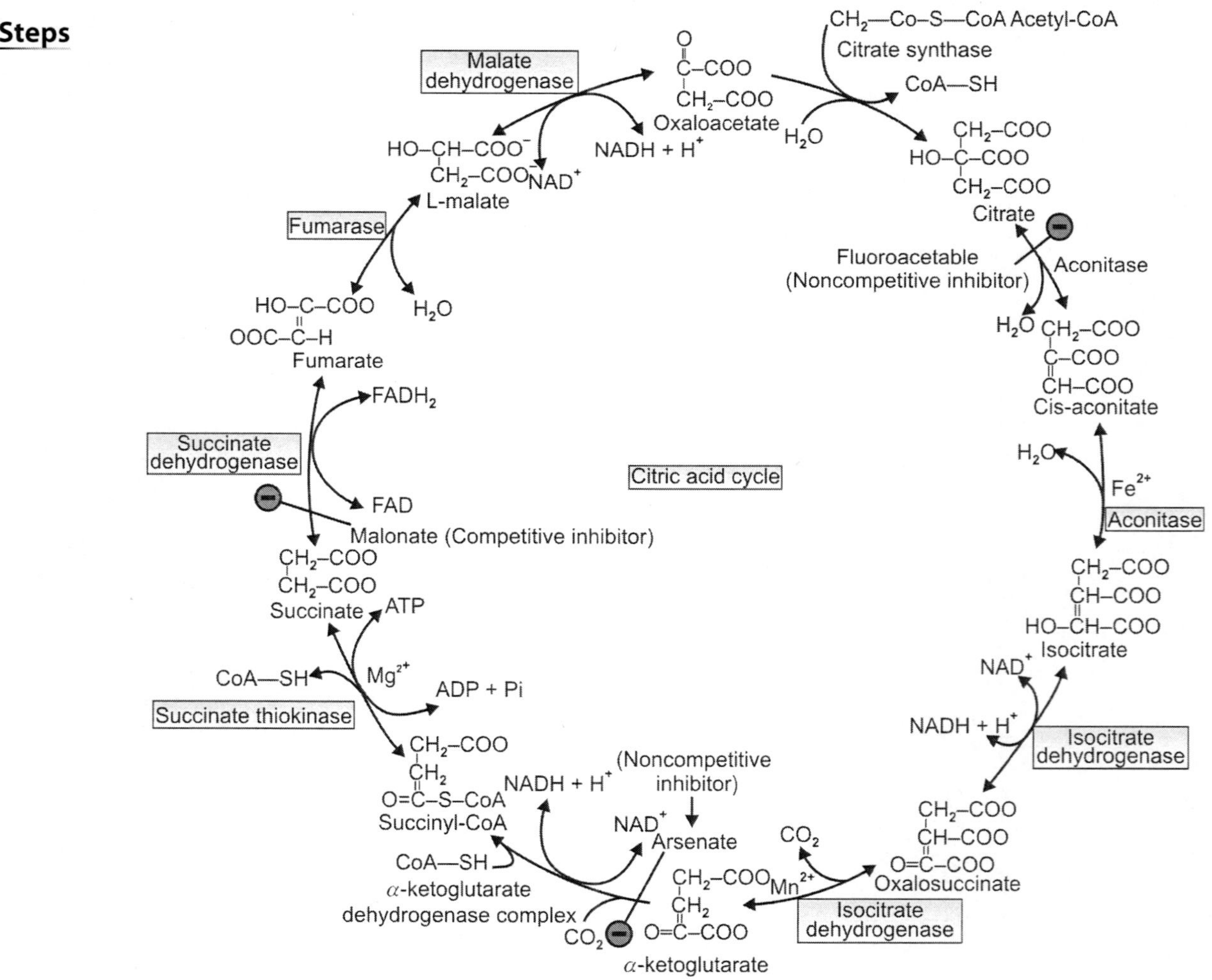


**Fig. 1:** Steps of TCA cycle

## Energetics

| *Reaction* | *Enzyme* | *Mode of phosphorylation* | *Reduced coenzyme* | *ATP produced* |
|---|---|---|---|---|
| Isocitrate → α-ketoglutarate | Isocitrate dehydrogenase | Oxidative | NADH+H$^+$ | 2.5 ATP |
| α-ketoglutarate → Succinyl CoA | α-ketoglutarate dehydrogenase | Oxidative | NADH+H$^+$ | 2.5 ATP |
| Succinyl CoA → Succinate | Succinate thiokinase | Substrate level | — | 1 ATP |
| Succinate → Fumarate | Succinate dehydrogenase | Oxidative | $FADH_2$ | 1.5 ATP |
| Malate → Oxaloacetate | Malate dehydrogenase | Oxidative | NADH+H$^+$ | 2.5 ATP |
| | | | **Total** | **10 ATP** |
| | | | **Per glucose molecule** | **20 ATP** |

## Regulation

| *Key enzyme* | *Modulation* | *Stimulator* | *Inhibitor* |
|---|---|---|---|
| • Isocitrate dehydrogenase (rate limiting enzyme) | Allosteric | ADP, calcium, isocitrate | ATP, NADH |
| • Citrate synthase | Feedback inhibition | Acetyl CoA, oxaloacetate | NADH, ATP, succinyl CoA, citrate |
| • α-ketoglutarate dehydrogenase | — | $Ca^{2+}$, AMP, ADP | ATP, NADH, succinyl CoA |

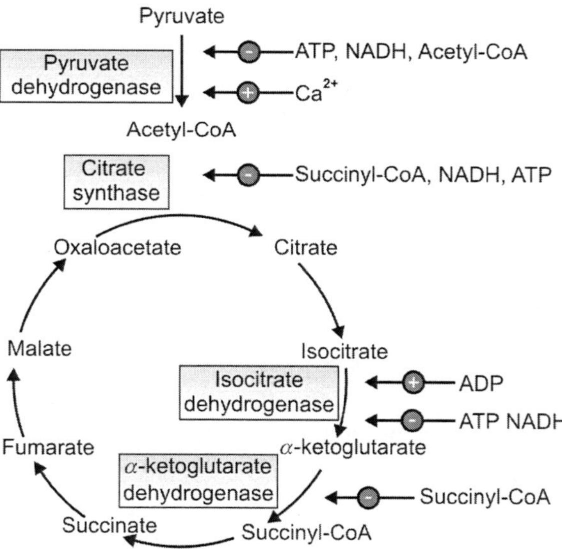


**Fig. 2:** Regulation of TCA cycle

## Inhibitors

- Fluoroacetate: Suicide inhibition of aconitase
- Arsenate: Irreversible inhibition of α-ketoglutarate dehydrogenase
- Malonate: Competitive inhibition of succinate dehydrogenase.

## Significance

a. Amphibolic pathway
   - TCA cycle is amphibolic in nature, i.e. it has both catabolic and anabolic functions.

| *Catabolic function* | *Anabolic functions* |
|---|---|
| • Final common pathway for oxidation of acetyl of CoA derived from carbohydrates, fatty acids and certain amino acids | • Provides precursors for porphyrins, amino acids, fatty acids, and steroids<br>– Oxaloacetate and α-ketoglutarate → asparate and glutamate respectively<br>– Succinyl CoA → heme<br>– Glucose (gluconeogenesis)<br>– Acetyl CoA → fatty acids, steroids |
| 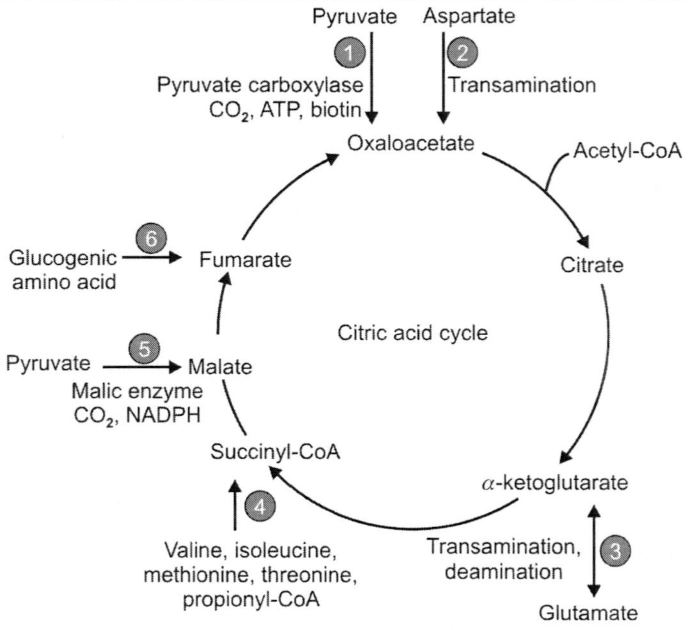 **Fig. 3A:** Catabolic functions of TCA cycle | 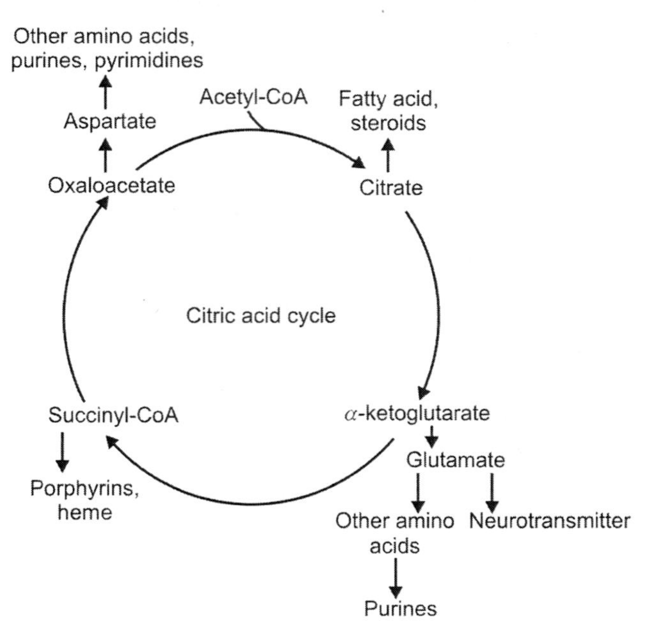 **Fig. 3B:** Anabolic functions of TCA cycle |

b. Energy production
   – One cycle of TCA cycle provides 12 ATPs (10 ATPs as per new concept)
c. Anaplerotic reactions
   – Reactions which supply intermediates back to TCA cycle
   – (Gr. Anaplerosis = fill up)
   – These reactions keep TCA cycle running, providing continuous energy.

   *Example*

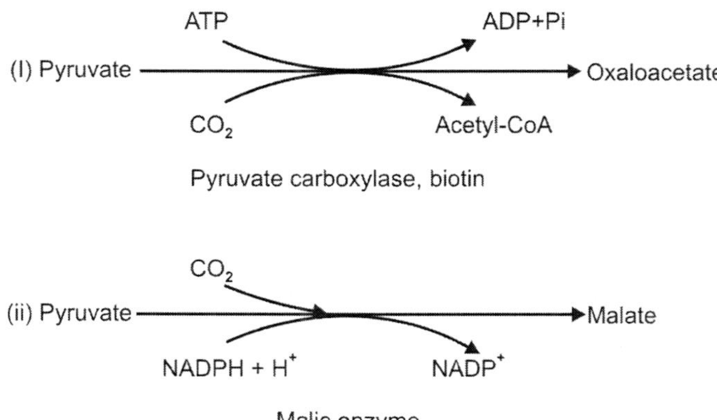


**Fig. 4:** Anaplerotic reaction of TCA cycle

d. Final common pathway for food oxidation
   – TCA cycle is final common cycle in metabolism of carbohydrates, lipids and amino acids

- These nutrients enter TCA cycle as follows:
  i. Carbohydrates

| Substrates | Enzyme | Products |
|---|---|---|
| Pyruvate + NAD$^+$ + CoA–SH | Pyruvate dehydrogenase → | Acetyl CoA + NADH + H$^+$ + $CO_2$ |
| Pyruvate + $CO_2$ + ATP | Pyruvate carboxylase → | Oxaloacetate + ADP + Pi |
| Pyruvate + NADPH + H$^+$ | Malic enzyme → | Malate + NADP+ + $H_2O$ |

  ii. Lipids

| Substrates | Enzyme | Products |
|---|---|---|
| Even chain fatty acids | β oxidation → | n acetyl CoA |
| Odd chain fatty acids | β oxidation → | n acetyl CoA + succinyl CoA |

  iii. Proteins (amino acids)

| Substrates | Enzyme | Products |
|---|---|---|
| Aspartate + α oxoglutarate | Aspartate transaminase → | Oxaloacetate + glutamate |
| Alanine + α oxoglutarate | Alanine transaminase → | Pyruvate + glutamate |
| Glutamate + NADP + $H_2O$ | Glutamate dehydrogenase → | α ketoglutarate + NADPH + H$^+$ + $NH_4^+$ |

## 2. Discuss in detail recombinant DNA technology and its clinical application.

- Recombinant DNA technology is genetic manipulations in laboratory involving isolation and cloning of specific DNA
- Also called genetic engineering
- Resulting DNA is called recombinant DNA (rDNA).



### Steps

a. Isolation of desired DNA fragment
   - Desired DNA fragment is isolated by digestion of cell membrane exposing nucleic acids, followed by their separation from other organelles and then isolating nucleic acid in pure form

b. Fragmentation of DNA (restriction fragments) by restriction endonuclease enzyme
   - Isolated DNA is cut to obtain desired DNA fragment by enzyme restriction endonuclease and which also separates it from large nucleic acids

c. Isolation of specific DNA by electrophoresis or HPLC
   - Fragments obtained are further segregated by gel electrophoresis or high performance liquid chromatography

d. Cutting of vector
   - Vectors are DNA molecules into which desired foreign DNA fragments can be inserted to form rDNA, e.g. plasmids, bacteriophage, cosmids, etc.
   - Vectors are cut with same restriction endonuclease enzyme so as to enables matching ends of target DNA and vector DNA and reanneal with each other

e. Insertion of isolated DNA into vector to form chimeric or hybrid DNA—annealing
   - Selected DNA fragment is then inserted into vector to produce chimeric DNA by process called annealing

f. Joining of two different cut DNAs by DNA ligase
   - Desired DNA fragment and vector DNA strands are joined by using an enzyme called DNA ligase

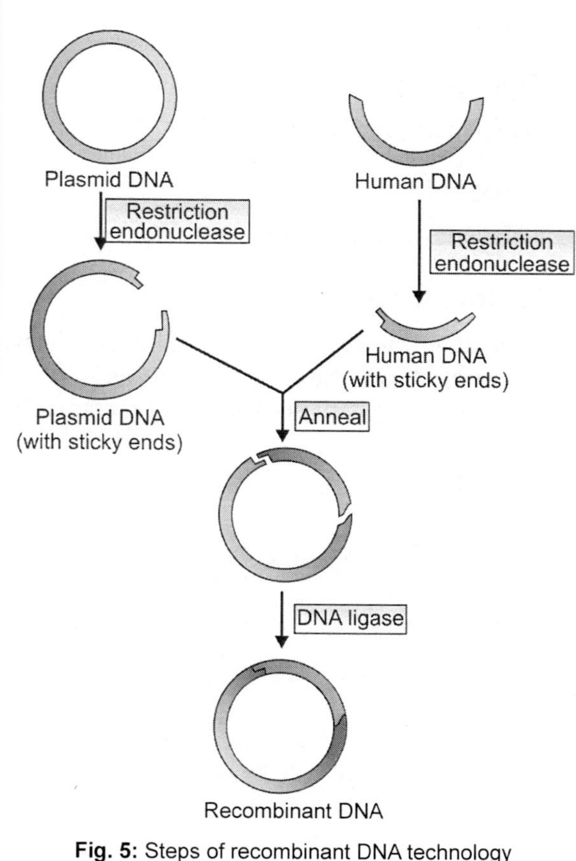


**Fig. 5:** Steps of recombinant DNA technology

## Clinical Applications

a. Productions of proteins/hormones
   - Several proteins and hormones can be produced in abundance for therapeutic purposes
   - Example: Insulin, growth hormone, erythropoietin, interferons, clotting factors, vaccines and superoxide dismutase.

b. Molecular analysis of disease
   - To understand molecular basis of diseases such as sickle cell anemia, thalassemias, etc.

c. Gene therapy (most potential application)
   - Direct treatment of diseases by introduction of functional genes into individuals that carry gene mutations interfering with normal gene expression
   - Can be used in cases of sickle cell anemia, thalassemias, enzyme deficiencies, etc.

d. Laboratory diagnostic applications
   - Diagnosis of many diseases like AIDS has become simple and rapid.

e. Prenatal diagnosis of disease
   - DNA probes can be used for predicting risk of genetic disorders like sickle cell anemia by using DNA collected from amniotic fluid.

f. Application in forensic medicine
   - For identification of criminals or deciding paternity by techniques like DNA finger printing or southern blot.

g. Transgenesis
   - Refers to transfer of genes into fertilized ovum which will be found in somatic as well as germ cells and passed on to successive generations.



## SHORT ESSAYS

### 3. Secondary structure of proteins.

Refer Question No. 4 Dec. 2011 (RS2).

### 4. Glycogenesis.

Refer Question No. 1 June 2007 (RS2).

### 5. Serotonin.

Refer Question No. 17 June 2012 (RS2).

### 6. Antioxidants.

- Antioxidants are substances significantly delaying or inhibiting oxidation of a substrate
- Considered scavengers of free radicals
- Control and prevent peroxidation and rancidity.

## Classification

| *Enzymatic antioxidants* | *Nonenzymatic antioxidants* | | *Synthetic* |
|---|---|---|---|
| | *Nutrients antioxidants* | *Metabolic antioxidants* | |
| • Superoxide dismutase<br>• Catalase<br>• Glutathione peroxidase<br>• Glutathione reductase | • Carotenoids (vitamin A)<br>• α-tocopherols (vitamin E)<br>• Ascorbic acid (vitamin C)<br>• Selenium | • Glutathione<br>• Ceruloplasmin<br>• Albumin<br>• Bilirubin<br>• Transferring<br>• Ferritin | • Proply gallate<br>• Butylated hydroxy anisol (BHA)<br>• Butylated hydroxy toluene (BHT) |

## Mechanism of Action

| *Preventive antioxidants* | *Chain breaking antioxidants* |
|---|---|
| • Reduction of rate of chain initiation, i.e. blocking initial production of free radicals<br>• Example: Catalase, peroxidase | • Interference with chain prolongation, i.e. inhibit propagative phase of lipid peroxidation<br>• Example: Superoxide dismutase, urate, vitamin E |

## Significance

- Antioxidants are used commercially in food products to enhance their shelf life
- Also used in treatment of oxidative stress.

# 7. General mechanism of action of steroid hormones.

- Steroid hormones bind to intracellular receptors to form receptor hormone complexes through which biochemical functions are mediated (group I hormones).

## Mechanism of Action

- Steroid hormones are lipophilic and easily pass through plasma membrane
- Inside a cell, hormone binds with receptor located either in cytoplasm or nucleus forming a receptor hormone complex which is transported towards DNA
- Binding of receptors hormone complex to steroid responsive element of DNA causing increased expression of specific gene
- This increases transcription of mRNA which activates ribosomes to produce large quantities of proteins
- These newly synthesized proteins produce physiological response in target cells.

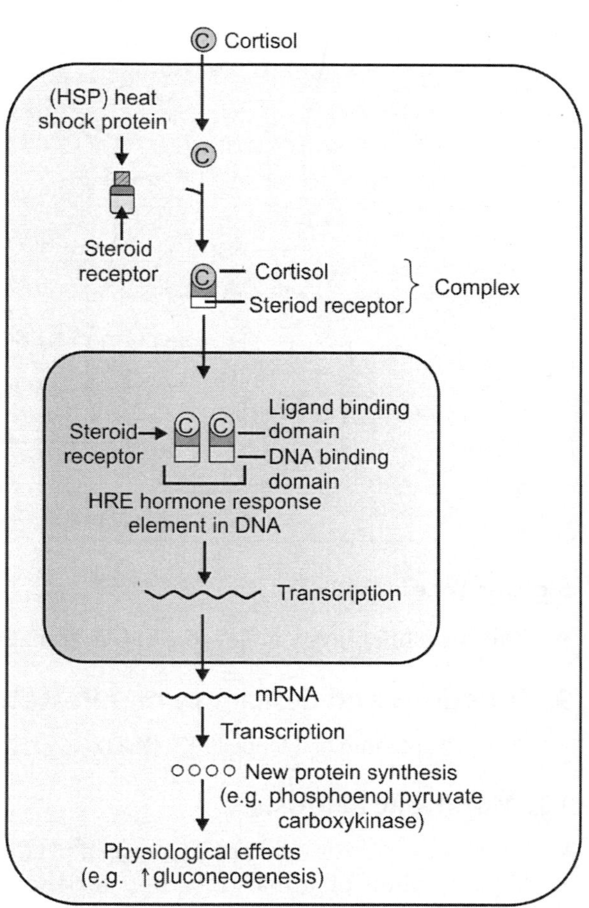


**Fig. 6:** Mechanism of action of steroid hormone

# 8. Chloride shift.

- Chloride shift is an important mechanism helping in $CO_2$ transport in body
- Also called Hamburger phenomenon.

## Mechanism

| | *Chloride shift* | *Reverse chloride shift* |
|---|---|---|
| Occurs at | • Tissue level | • Lungs |
| Mechanism | • $CO_2$ combines with water in presence of carbonic anhydrase in RBCs, it produces $H^+$ and $HCO_3^-$<br>• Bicarbonate ions thus formed move out of RBCs<br>• To maintain electrolytic equilibrium inside RBCs, Cl- from plasma move into RBCs | • Bicarbonates move back into RBCs making chloride move out |

*Contd...*

Contd...

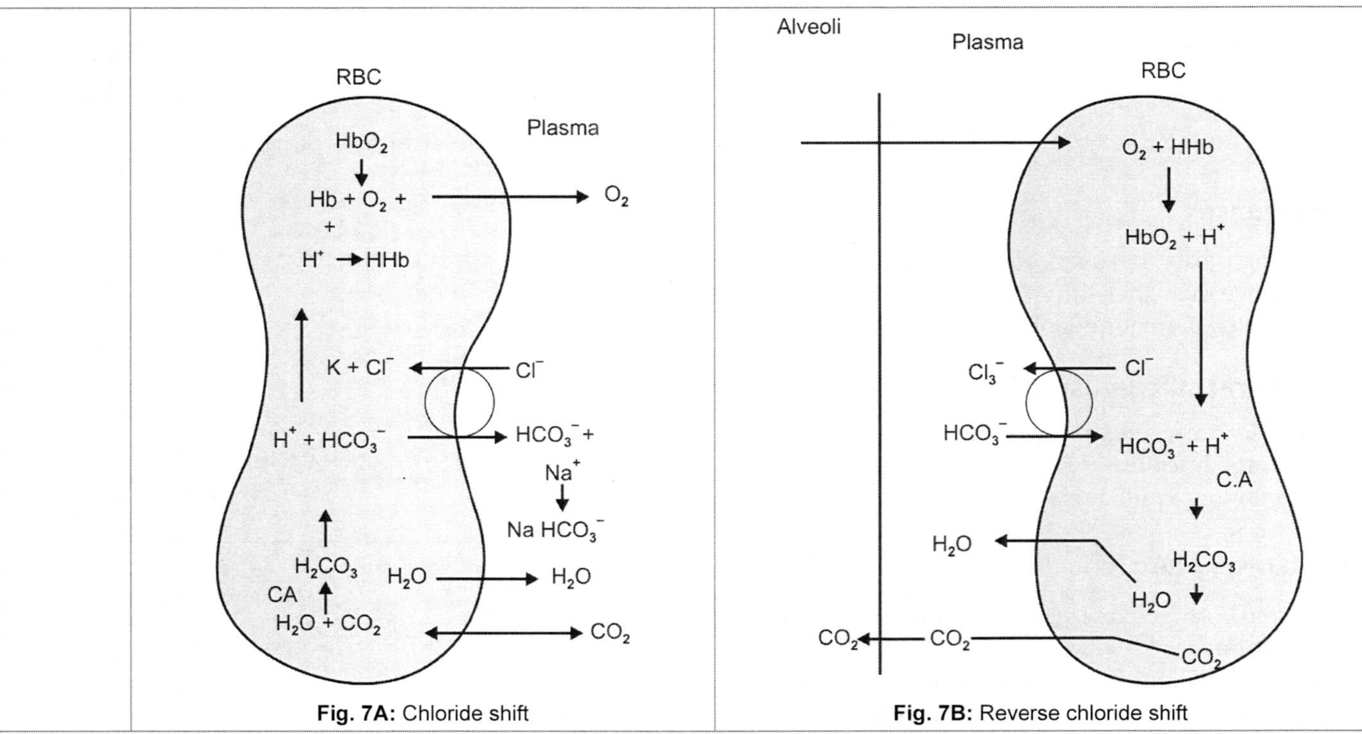


**Fig. 7A:** Chloride shift

**Fig. 7B:** Reverse chloride shift

## Significance

- Chloride shift plays a major role in $CO_2$ transport as 63% of $CO_2$ is transported in the form of bicarbonate.

## 9. Functions and deficiency manifestations of vitamin C.

Refer Question No. 2 Dec. 2005 (RS2).

## 10. Metabolic acidosis.

- Metabolic acidosis refers to decrease in pH due to causes other than increased $CO_2$
- It is a condition of primary bicarbonate deficiency resulting from excessive removal of bicarbonate into urine in order to buffer extra acids of body
- Also called primary alkali deficit.

### Causes

| *Increased acid production* | *Excessive bicarbonate loss* | *Reduced acid elimination* |
|---|---|---|
| • Increased production of organic acids like acetoacetic acid, β hydroxybutyric acid (diabetic ketoacidosis, starvation, lactic acidosis)<br>• Lactic acid production due to anerobic glycolysis (severe exercise)<br>• Methyl alcohol, salicylate and ethylene glycol poisoning (oxidation of these compounds produce organic acids) | • Decreased reclamation of bicarbonate from renal tubules due to its decreased reabsorption (renal tubular acidosis)<br>• Excessive loss of bicarbonate from duodenal fluid (acute diarrhea, pancreatitis, intestinal fistula) | • Reduction in elimination of $H^+$ (renal failure, distal renal tubular acidosis) |

### Types

| *High anion gap acidosis* | *Normal (low) anion gap acidosis* |
|---|---|
| • Increased production of unmeasured anions such as lactate and β-hydroxybutyrate<br>• Seen in lactic acidosisand ketoacidosis | • Increased accumulation of anions or decreased levels of cations in plasma<br>• Seen in diarrhea and renal tubular acidosis |

## Clinical Features

- Deep sighing respiration (Kaussmaul's breathing or air hunger)—in severe cases
- Peripheral vasodilatation and fall in cardiac output—fall in blood pressure
- Drowsiness, confusion and coma.

## Compensatory Mechanisms

| *Respiratory compensation (primary)* | *Renal compensation* |
|---|---|
| With decrease in $HCO_3^-/pCO_2$ ratio, pH falls which stimulates respiration causing hyperventilation which leads to wash out of $CO_2$ from blood producing drop in $pCO_2$, restoring pH | Increased acid excretion, ammonia formation and reclamation of bicarbonate ions |

## Biochemical Findings (Features)

| | Uncompensated | Partially compensated | Fully compensated |
|---|---|---|---|
| • pH | ↓↓ | ↓ | Normal |
| • $pCO_2$ | Normal | ↓ | ↓ |
| • $HCO_3^-$ | ↓↓ | ↓ | ↓ |
| • $HCO_3^-/H_2CO_3$ | ↓ | ↓ | Normal |
| • Ammonia in urine | Normal | ↑ | ↑ |

## 11. Degradation of pyrimidines.

- Pyrimidines are six membered nitrogenous ring compounds
- Pyrimidine nucleotides undergo dephosphorylation, deamination and cleavage of glycosidic bond (similar to degradation of purine nucleotides to liberate nitrogenous bases, cytosine, uracil and thymine.

| *Substrates* | *Products* |
|---|---|
| Pyramidines (Cytosine, uracil, thymine) | • $CO_2$<br>• $NH_3$<br>• β-alanine → acetyl CoA → TCA cycle<br>• β-aminoisobutyrate → methylmaonate semialdehyde (transamination) → methyl malonyl CoA → succinyl CoA → TCA cycle |

## Reactions

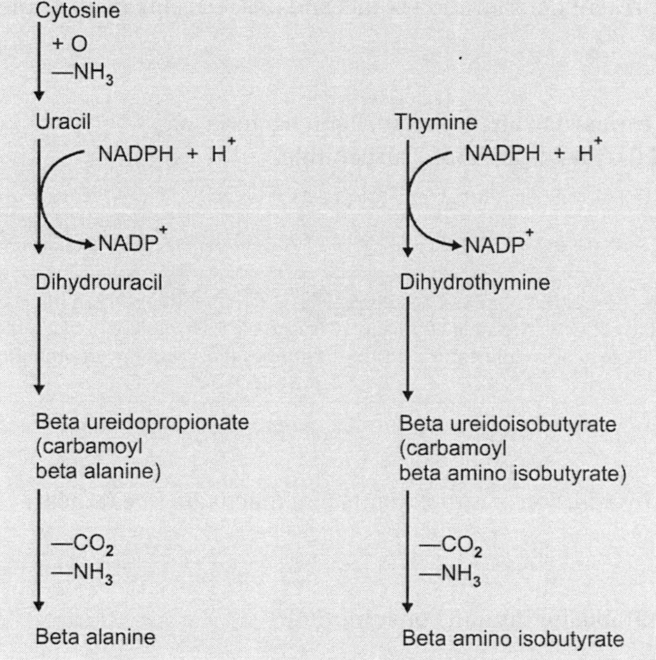


**Fig. 8:** Degradation

## Clinical Significance

- β amino isobutyric acid is formed exclusively from deoxythymidine is not further metabolized and excreted as it is
- Urinary excretion of β amino isobutyric acid is significantly increased during chemotherapy and radiotherapy and hence urinary excretion of β amino isobutyric acid is used as an index of tumor burden.

### 12. Salient features of genetic code.

Refer Question No. 2 June 2011 (RS2).

## SHORT ANSWERS

### 13. Prostate-specific antigen (SPA).

Refer Question No. 10 Dec. 2012 (RS2).

### 14. Uncouplers of oxidative phosphorylation.

Refer Question No. 1 June 2010 (RS2).

### 15. Refsum's disease.

- Refsum's disease is a rare but severe neurological disorder due to defect in α oxidation fatty acids.

| *Deficient enzyme* | *Mechanism (pathogenesis)* | *Clinical features* | *Treatment* |
|---|---|---|---|
| Phytanic acid α oxidase (α hydroxylase) | • Due to accumulation of phytanic acid (unusual fatty acid present in green leafy vegetables, milk, etc.)<br>• In Refsum's disease, phyatic acid cannot be metabolized by initial a oxidation (which is essential to render it capable of β oxidation) | • Cerebral ataxia<br>• Peripheral neuropathy<br>• Motor weakness<br>• Retinitis pigmentosa<br>• Nerve deafness | Dietary restrictions of food rich in phytanic acid (green leafy vegetables, milk, meat) |

### 16. Significance of HMP pathway.

Refer Question No. 4 Dec. 2013 (RS2).

### 17. Rancidity.

- Rancidity is term used to represent deterioration of fats and oils resulting in an unpleasant taste.

## Mechanism

- Occurs when fat and oil are exposed to air, moisture, light, bacteria, etc.
- Fats containing unsaturated fatty acids are more susceptible.

## Types

| *Oxidative rancidity (most common)* | *Hydrolytic rancidity* |
|---|---|
| Due to partial oxidation of unsaturated fatty acids with resultant formation of epoxides and peroxidase of small molecular weight fatty acids by peroxidase and free radicals | Due to partial hydrolysis of triacyl glycerol molecules by traces of hydrolytic enzymes (lipases) of microorganisms present in naturally occurring fats and oils |

## Prevention

- Rancidity can be prevented by addition of antioxidants that inactivate free radicals.

## Significance

- Rancid fats and oils are unsuitable for human consumption.

## 18. Carboxyhemoglobin.

- Carboxyhemoglobin (COHb) is a hemoglobin derivative that is bound to carbon monoxide.

| *Normal level* | *Detection* |
|---|---|
| 0.16% | COHb shows a green band (535 nm) and a yellow band (570 nm) when examined using spectroscope |

### Significance

- Increased levels of COHb causes weakness, irritability, breathlessness, nausea, vomiting, dizziness, headache, chest pain, cyanosis (>30%) or coma and death (>50%)
- Affinity of CO is 200 times more than $O_2$ thus presence of CO in blood impairs formation of oxyhemoglobin
- Administration of hyperbaric oxygen will dissociate CO from Hb.

## 19. Fluorosis.

- Fluorosis is a clinical condition produced due to excessive consumption of fluoride
- Fluoride is a cumulative toxin, and ingested fluoride gets accumulated in bones.

### Types

| | *Dental fluorosis* | *Skeletal fluorosis* |
|---|---|---|
| Etiology | Consumption of water with fluoride concentration above 2 ppm; particularly 5 ppm | Consumption of water with fluoride concentration above 20 ppm |
| Features | • Characterized by mottling of enamel and discoloration of teeth<br>• Teeth become weak and rough with characteristic brown or yellow patches on their surface<br>• Chronic intestinal upset, gastroenteritis, loss of appetite and loss of weight | • Characterized by pathological changes in bone in form of hypercalcification and increased bone density<br>• Even ligaments of spine and collagen of bones get calcified<br>• Alternate areas of osteoporosis and osteosclerosis, with brittle bones<br>• Genu valgum is characteristic feature |

### Diagnosis

- Blood fluoride concentration about 50 μg/dL (normal value 4 μg/dL)
- Urinary excretion of hydroxyl proline due to increased breakdown of bone matrix.

### Prevention

- Provide fluoride free water, restriction of intake of jowar, supplementation of vitamin C and regulation of fluoride containing toothpaste.

### Significance

- Fluorosis is more dangerous than caries; and it is a important public health problem.

## 20. Immunoelectrophoresis.

- Electrophoresis is movement of charged particles or ions in an electric field resulting in their migration towards oppositely charged electrodes.

### Immunoelectrophoresis

- A type of electrophoresis where electrophoretic separation is followed by antigen-antibody reaction.

| *Principle* | *Procedure* |
|---|---|
| Involves combination of electrophoresis with immunological reactions | • Complex biological proteins are subjected to electrophoresis<br>• Then antibodies to one or more of these proteins is applied in trough parallel to electrophoretic separation<br>• Antibodies diffuse and form arc-shaped precipitin bands when come in contact with antigen |

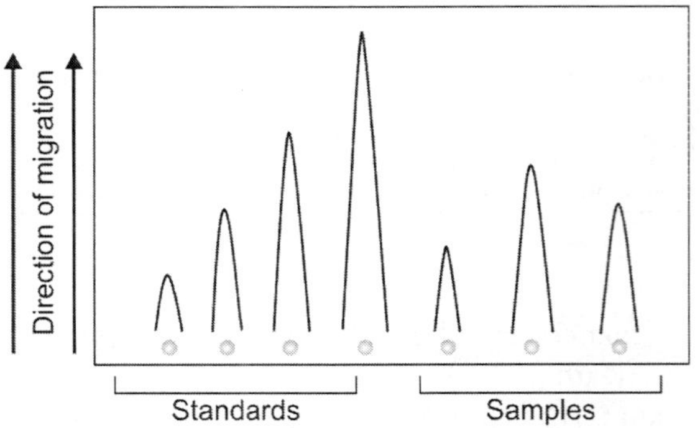


**Fig. 9:** Immunoelectrophoresis

| *Advantage* | *Applications* |
|---|---|
| • More sensitive and specific than ordinary electrophoresis<br>• Size of precipitin bands allow semiquantitative estimation of proteins | • For analysis of complex mixture of antigen and antibodies<br>• For semiquantitative estimation of proteins<br>• For detection of abnormal proteins (M protein in multiple myeloma) |



## 21. Anticoagulants.

- Anticoagulants are substances which inhibit process of blood clotting.

### Mechanism of Action

- Most of these substances act by forming complex with $Ca^{++}$ and decreases ionic calcium levels which is essential for coagulation cascade
- Heparin inhibits conversion of prothrombin to thrombin (ideal anticoagulant).

### Examples (Classification)

| *Natural anticoagulants (in vitro)* | *Used in blood bank* | *Used in laboratory* | *Therapeutic anticoagulants (in vivo)* |
|---|---|---|---|
| • Endothelium<br>• Antithrombin III<br>• Fibrinolytic system (plasmin)<br>• Protein 'C'<br>• Protein 'S'<br>• Heparin<br>• Thrombomodulin | • Acid citrate dextrose (ACO)<br>• Citrate phosphate dextrose (CPD) | • Ethylene diamine tetra acetate (EDTA)<br>• Oxalates<br>• Citrates (sodium, potassium or ammonium salts of citrate)<br>• Sodium flouride | • Heparin<br>• Coumarin derivatives (dicoumoral and warfarin) |

### Significance

- In diagnostic medicine, anticoagulants are essential for transport and storage of blood so that blood does not clot
- Anticoagulants are also used as therapeutic agents in patients with clotting disorders
- Sodium fluoride is preferred for blood glucose estimation.

## 22. Limiting amino acid.

- Essential amino acids that are deficient in particular dietary protein are called limiting amino acid of that protein.

*Example*

| *Dietary protein* | *Limiting amino acid* |
|---|---|
| • Rice and wheat proteins | • Lysine and threonine |
| • Maize protein | • Tryptophan |
| • Bengal gram protein | • Methionine and cystine |

## Significance

- Most of proteins have some limiting amino acids; however, egg protein has no limiting amino acids
- Limiting amino acids are used for calculating chemical score of a protein (ratio between content of most limiting amino acid in a protein to content of same amino acid in egg protein expressed as a percentage)
- Feeding of a particular proteins with limiting amino acid as only source of proteins results in failure of growth.

# MBBS PHASE I EXAMINATION
## DECEMBER 2008
(Revised Scheme 2)

## LONG ESSAYS

### 1. Explain in detail the β oxidation of palmitic acid with its energetic.

#### Oxidation of Fatty Acids

- Fatty acids are oxidized in 3 ways, namely α oxidation, β oxidation and ω oxidation based upon carbon atom oxidized.

*Types*

| | *α oxidation* | *β oxidation* | *ω oxidation* |
|---|---|---|---|
| | Minor pathway for fatty acids possessing methyl group at β carbon atoms preventing its β oxidation | Major pathway | • Minor pathway<br>• Important when β oxidation becomes defective |
| Principle organs | Brain | All tissues except brain, erythrocytes and adrenals | Brain |
| Subcellular site | Endoplasmic reticulum | Mitochondria | Microsomes |
| Mechanism | Removal of carbon atom one at time by oxidation of α carbon atom from the carboxyl end | Sequential removal of a 2 carbon fragment, acetyl CoA by oxidation of β carbon atom till end product is $CO_2$ and acetyl CoA (propionyl CoA in case of odd chain fatty acids) | Hydroxynation ($CH_3$ converted to $CH_2OH$) followed by oxidation with help of $NAD^+$ to a COOH at ω carbon present as a methyl group at other end of fatty acid producing a diacarboxylic acid, which is then subjected to β oxidation to form successively smaller dicarboxylic acids |
| Special requirement | None | Prior activation with CoA | Cytochrome $P_{450}$, NADPH and $O_2$ |
| Energy produced | Nil | 129 ATPs (from 16 carbon palmitic acid) | |

#### Beta Oxidation of Fatty Acids

- β oxidation is most common method of metabolism of lipids by oxidation of fatty acid at β carbon atom with successive removal of 2 carbon atoms as acetyl CoA.

*Reactions*

| | *Activation of fatty acids* | *Transport of acyl CoA into mitochondria* | *β oxidation of fatty acids* |
|---|---|---|---|
| Principle organs | — | — | All tissues except brain, erythrocytes and adrenals |
| Intracellular site | Cytosol (membranes of ER, mitochondria and perosxysomes) | — | Mitochondria |
| Substrate | Long chain fatty acids | — | Acyl CoA |
| Product | Acyl CoA | — | Acetyl CoA (even chain fatty acids like palmitic acid)<br>Propionyl CoA (odd chain fatty acids) |

a. Activation of long chain fatty acids

**Intracellular site**

- Cytosol (membranes of ER, mitochondria and perosxysomes).

*Steps*

Fatty acid
Thiokinase
ATP
$Mg^{++}$ CoA SH
AMP + PPi
Acyl CoA

b. Transport into mitochondria (role of carnitine in β oxidation)

- Activated fatty acyl CoA is transported across mitochondrial wall by a carrier protein called carnitine
- Carnitine or β-hydroxy-γ-trimethyl ammonium butyrate is a carrier protein located on mitochondrial wall
- Synthesized from lysine mainly in liver and supplied to other tissues.

*Steps*

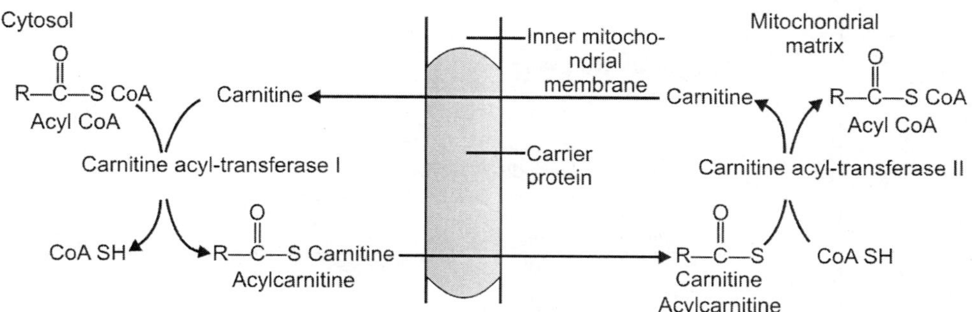


**Fig. 1:** Carnitine cycle

- Carnitine acyl transferase I, located on cytoplasmic surface of inner membrane transfers acyl group from cytoplasmic acyl CoA to carnitine forming acylcarnitine and free coenzyme A
- An inner membrane protein, called carnitine acyl carnitine translocase then transports acylcarnitine across membrane into mitochondria in exchange of carnitine transported out from mitochondria
- Reaching mitochondrial matrix, acylcarnitine donates its acyl group to coenzyme A under action of carnitine acyl transferase II located on matrix surface of inner membrane producing acyl CoA and free carnitine in matrix
- Carnitine is translocated back to cytoplasm in exchange of another acylcarnitine molecule brought into mitochondrial matrix.

c. Beta oxidation of fatty acids

- β-oxidation pathway is a repeating sequence of four reactions namely oxidation, hydration, oxidation and thiolytic cleavage and at end of each cycle, one acetyl CoA is split off
- It continues till an even chain fatty acid is broken down to acetyl CoA (2C) or an odd chain fatty acid is broken down to propionyl CoA (3C)

| *Intracellular site* | *Substrate* | *Product* |
|---|---|---|
| • Mitochondria | • Fatty acids (palmitic acid) | • Acetyl CoA (even chain fatty acids like palmitic acid)<br>• Propionyl CoA (odd chain fatty acids) |

*Steps*

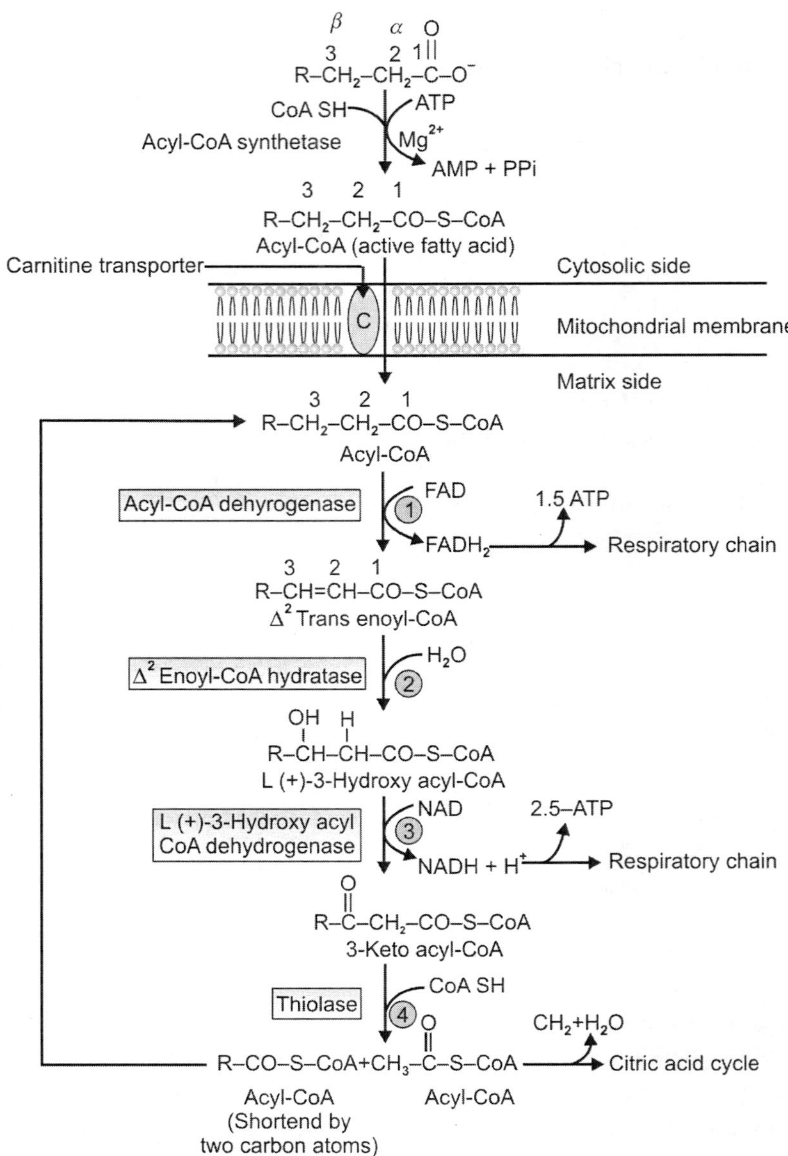


**Fig. 2:** Steps of beta oxidation of fatty acids

– This cycle continues till end product is acetyl CoA (2C).

## Energetics

| *Reactions* | *Reduced coenzyme* | *ATPs generated* |
|---|---|---|
| **For activation of fatty acid** | | |
| • Fatty acid → Fatty acyl CoA | — | - 2 ATP |
| **From 1 cycle of β oxidation** | | |
| • Fatty acyl CoA → Trans Δ2 enoyl CoA | $FADH_2$ | 1.5 ATP |
| • 3-L hydroxyacyl CoA → 3 ketoacyl CoA | NADH-$H^+$ | 2.5 ATP |
| | **Total** | **4 ATPs** |
| **From oxidation of acetyl CoA by TCA cycle** | | |
| • Isocitrate → α-ketoglutarate | NADH+$H^+$ | 2.5 ATP |
| • α- ketoglutarate → Succinyl CoA | NADH+$H^+$ | 2.5 ATP |
| • Succinyl CoA → Succinate | — | 1 ATP |
| • Succinate → Fumarate | $FADH_2$ | 1.5 ATP |
| • Malate → Oxaloacetate | NADH+$H^+$ | 2.5 ATPs |
| | **Total** | **10 ATPs** |

**For palmitic acid**

– 1 molecule of palmitic acid ($C_{16}$) undergoes 7 cycles of β oxidation producing 8 molecules of acetyl CoA.

| *Source* | *ATPs generated* |
|---|---|
| Activation of fatty acid | – 2 ATP |
| 7 cycles of β oxidation | 7 × 4 = 28 ATP |
| 8 acetyl CoA (TCA cycle) | 8 × 10 = 80 ATP |
| **Total** | **106 ATPs** |

**Regulation**

| *By fatty acid availability* | | *By inhibiting fatty acid transfer* |
|---|---|---|
| *Glucagon and epinephrine* | *Insulin* | *Excess glucose* |
| Stimulates adipose tissue lipolysis ⇓ ↑ fatty acids availability ⇓ β-oxidation promoted | Inhibits adipose tissue lipolysis ⇓ ↓ fatty acids availability ⇓ β-oxidation inhibited | Blocks carnitine acyl transferase I by malonyl CoA (derived from glucose) thus inhibits mitochondrial transfrer |

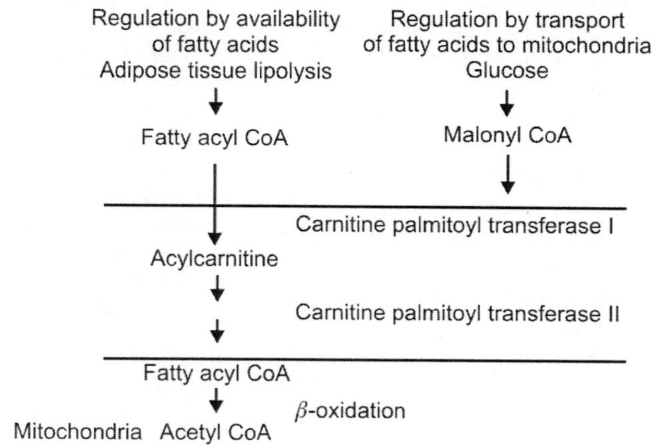


**Fig. 3:** Regulation of β-oxidation



## Significance

- A major pathway of energy production fulfilling 20–30% energy requirement of cell
- Provides ketone bodies for energy production to peripheral tissues like muscles, kidney in conditions of glucose deficit
- Provides acetyl CoA for biosynthesis of several molecules like acetylcholine, cholesterol, etc.

### 2. Describe in detail biosynthesis of protein and discuss its regulation.

Refer Question No. 2 June 2005 (RS2).

## SHORT ESSAYS

### 3. Function of carbohydrates.

- Carbohydrates are polyhydroxyaldehydes or ketones or compounds which produce them on hydrolysis.

## Function (Significance)

- Most abundant dietary source of energy (glucose, starch, lactose, etc.) and only source of energy for RBCs and brain
- Serve as storage form of energy (glycogen) to meet immediate energy demands

- Precursors for many organic compounds like fat, amino acids
- Component of cell membrane and other important biological molecules like DNA, RNA, glycoproteins, etc.
- Participate in cellular functions like cell growth, adhesion, lubrication, intercellular communication, immunity and fertilization
- Nondigestable carbohydrates serve as dietary fibers.

## 4. Competitive inhibition and its importance in medicine.

Refer Question No. 3 June 2007 (RS2).

## 5. Metabolic changes in diabetes mellitus.

- Diabetes is metabolic disorder of carbohydrate metabolism due to deficiency of insulin characterized by hyperglycermia.

### Types

| *Type 1 diabetes mellitus [Insulin dependent diabetes mellitus (IDDM)]* | *Type 2 diabetes mellitus [Noninsulin dependent diabetes mellitus (NIDDM)]* | *Diabetes prone states* | *Diabetes mellitus secondary to other causes (secondary diabetes mellitus)* |
|---|---|---|---|
| **Etiopathogenesis**<br>• Total absence of circulating insulin due to damage to islet of pancreas by autoantibodies or infection or toxic insult<br>• Autoantibodies against islet cells of pancreas detected in 85% of cases<br>• Strongly associated with HLA-DR3 or HLA-DR4<br>**Clinical features**<br>• Most common in children but also seen in adults<br>• Associated with ketosis if untreated<br>**Treatment**<br>• Insulin administration | **Etiopathogenesis**<br>• Defect in uptake of circulating insulin because of defective or deficiency in insulin receptors<br>• Displays strong genetic predisposition<br>**Clinical features**<br>• More common in adults<br>• Not associated with high incidence of ketosis<br>**Treatment**<br>• Diet, exercise and oral hypoglycemic drugs | i. Gestational diabetes mellitus<br>– Glucose intolerance in 1st trimester pregnancy<br>ii. Impaired glucose tolerance<br>– Fasting glucose is less than those required for diagnosis of diabetes mellitus<br>iii. Impaired fasting glycemia<br>– Fasting glucose is level is between normal and diabetic individual | i. Pancreatic disorders<br>– Chronic pancreatitis in alcoholics<br>ii. Hormonal causes<br>– Pheochromocytoma, acromegaly, Cushing's syndrome, steroid therapy<br>iii. Genetic syndromes<br>– Lipodystrophies, myotonic dystrophia, ataxia telengectasia<br>iv. Drug induced |

### Metabolic Adaptation

| *Organ* | *Increased* | *Decreased or impaired* |
|---|---|---|
| • Liver | ↑ gluconeogenesis<br>↑ lipolysis<br>↑ VLDL synthesis<br>↑ fatty acid oxidation<br>↑ ketogenesis | ↓ glucose oxidation<br>↓ glycogenolysis |
| • Muscle | ↑ proteolysis<br>↑ ketone bodies utilization | Impaired glucose uptake<br>Negative nitrogen balance |
| • Adipose tissue | ↑ lipolysis<br>↑ ketone bodies utilization | ↓ lipogenesis |
| • Brain | Adaptation to ketone bodies utilization | — |
| • Kidney | ↑ gluconeogenesis<br>↑ synthesis of glutaminase →↑ ammonia formation<br>↑ ketone bodies utilization | — |

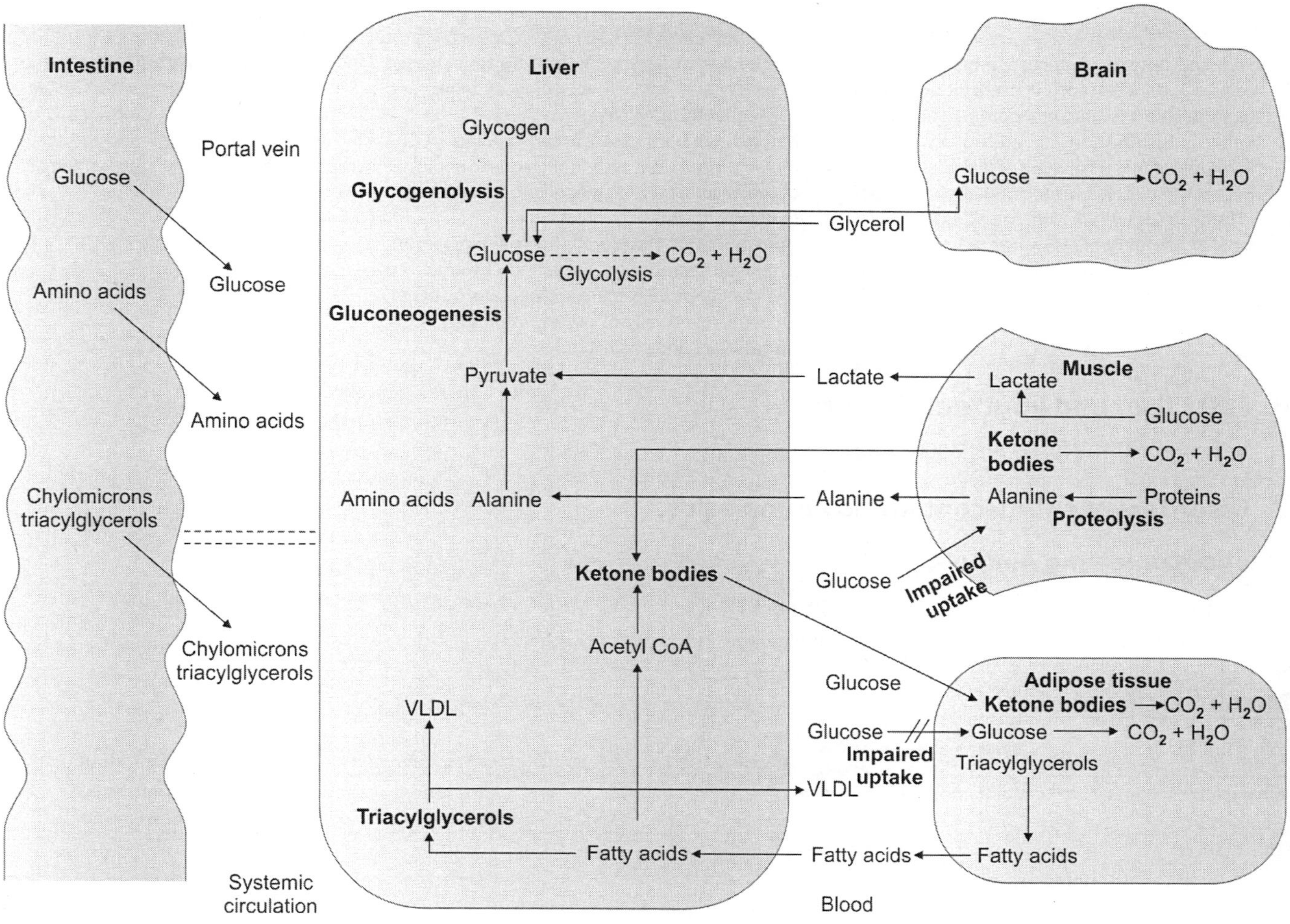

**Fig. 4:** Metabolic adaptation in diabetes mellitus

## Biochemical Changes

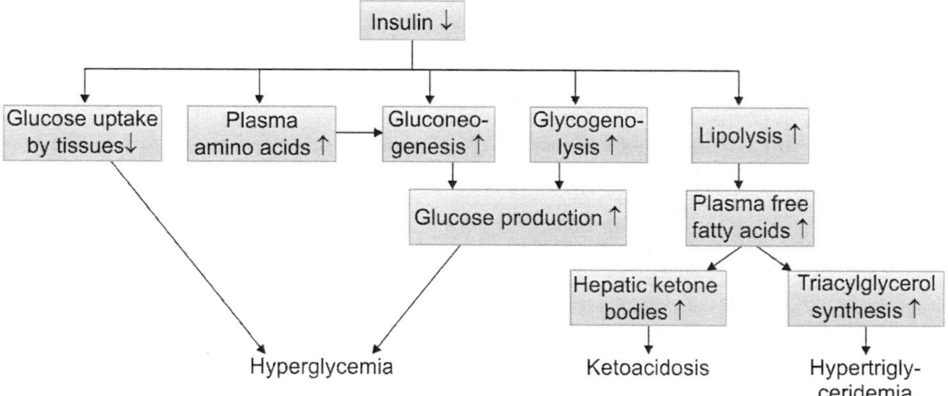


**Fig. 5:** Biochemical changes of diabetes mellitus

| *On carbohydrate metabolism* | *On lipid metabolism* | *On protein metabolism* | *On general metabolism* |
|---|---|---|---|
| • Reduced uptake of glucose, inhibition of glycolysis and increased glucose production due to stimulation of gluconeogenesis and glycogenolysis resulting in elevated glucose levels (hyperglycemia)—hallmark of diabetes mellitus<br>• Hyperglycemia leads to accumulation of sorbitol in body tissues (retina, lens, nervous tissues and renal glomeruli) which because of its osmotic effect causes deleterious effects (retinopathy, cataract, neuropathy and nephropathy respectively) | • Breakdown of fatty acids, leading to increased free fatty acid levels (hypertriglyceridemia) and consequently fatty liver<br>• Ketogenesis from excess acetyl CoA (acetyl CoA metabolism via TCA cycle limited due to depletion of oxaloacetate during gluconeogenesis) leading to ketoacidosis<br>• Conversion of fatty acids to triacylglycerols, increased secretion of VLDL and chylomicrons and low lipoprotein lipase activity causing hyperlipidemia especially of nonessential fatty acids, triglycerides and cholesterol | Increased breakdown of proteins and amino acids for providing substrates for gluconeogenesis is responsible for muscle wasting | Increased oxidation occurs because of autooxidation of glucose and indirect effects of dyslipidemia |

## 6. Fatty liver and lipotropic factors.

Refer Question No. 6 Dec. 2006 (RS2).

## 7. Disorders of sulfur-containing amino acids.

### Sulphar-containing Amino Acids

a. Cysteine — Nonessential amino acid
b. Methionine — Essential amino acid

### Metabolic Disorders

| | *Homocystinurias* | *Cystathioninuria* | *Methylmalonic aciduria* |
|---|---|---|---|
| Characterized by | Excretion of homocysteine in urine | Excretion of cyationine in urine | Inborn error of methionine, valine and isoleucine metabolism |
| Inheritance | Autosomal recessive | Autosomal recessive | Autosomal recessive |
| Cause (types) | **Homocystinuria type I**<br>• Cystathionine β synthase deficiency (causes ↑ plasma level of methionine and homocysteine d' to block in catabolism of homocysteine)<br>**Homocystinuria type II**<br>• N methylene $FH_4$ reductase deficiency (↓ methionine synthesis)<br>**Homocystinuria type III**<br>• Defective biosynthesis of cobalamin (required as coenzyme for enzyme $N^5$ methyl-THF- homocysteine-methyl transferase) 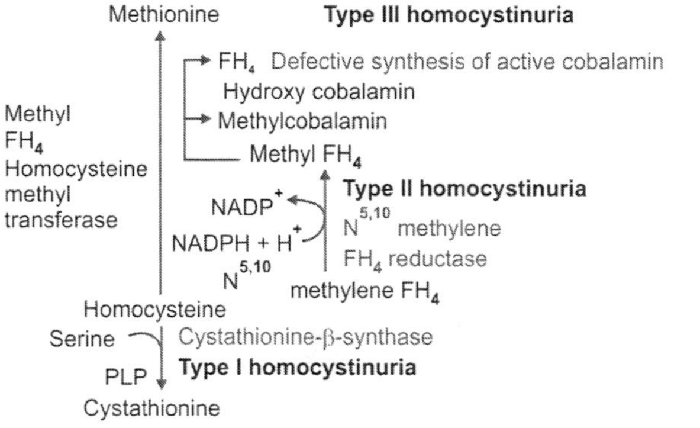<br>Methionine — **Type III homocystinuria**<br>$FH_4$ Defective synthesis of active cobalamin<br>Hydroxy cobalamin<br>Methylcobalamin<br>Methyl $FH_4$<br>Methyl $FH_4$ Homocysteine methyl transferase<br>**Type II homocystinuria**<br>$NADP^+$<br>$NADPH + H^+$<br>$N^{5,10}$ methylene $FH_4$ reductase<br>$N^{5,10}$ methylene $FH_4$<br>Homocysteine<br>Serine — Cystathionine-β-synthase<br>PLP — **Type I homocystinuria**<br>Cystathionine<br>**Fig. 6:** Homocystinuria—types | Deficiency of enzyme cystathioninase | Deficiency of L-methylmalonyl CoA mutase |
| Clinical features | • Mental retardation, growth failure, flat foot, Charlie Chaplin gait, kyphosis, scoliosis, ectopia lentis, myopia, glaucoma<br>• Life-threatening vascular thrombosis or cerebrovascular accidents d' ↑ platelet adhesiveness<br>• ↑ blood homocysteine and methionine levels | Mental retardation, anemia, thrombocytopenia, anomalies of ear and endocrinopathies | Mental retardation |

## 8. Name five heme proteins and their functions.

- Heme is a complex of iron (ferrous form) and protoporphyrin III.

### Heme Structure

- Made of ferrous iron ($Fe^{2+}$) and porphyrin ring (protoporphyrin IX) which contains four pyrrole rings
- Ferrous iron forms 6 coordinate bonds (ligand bonds)
  - 4 for binding to protoporphyrin IX
  - 5th bound to proximal histidine residue in F helix (β 92 or α 87 histidine)
  - 6th between oxygen molecule interposed between iron and distal histidine in E helix (β 63 and α 58 histidine) on distal side of porphyrin ring.

### Heme Synthesis

| *Principle organs* | *Intracellular site* | *Substrate* | *Product* |
|---|---|---|---|
| • Mostly in liver and bone marrow<br>• Almost all tissue except RBCs | Mitochondria (1st and last 3 reactions) and cytosol | Glycine + Succinyl CoA | Heme |

*Steps*

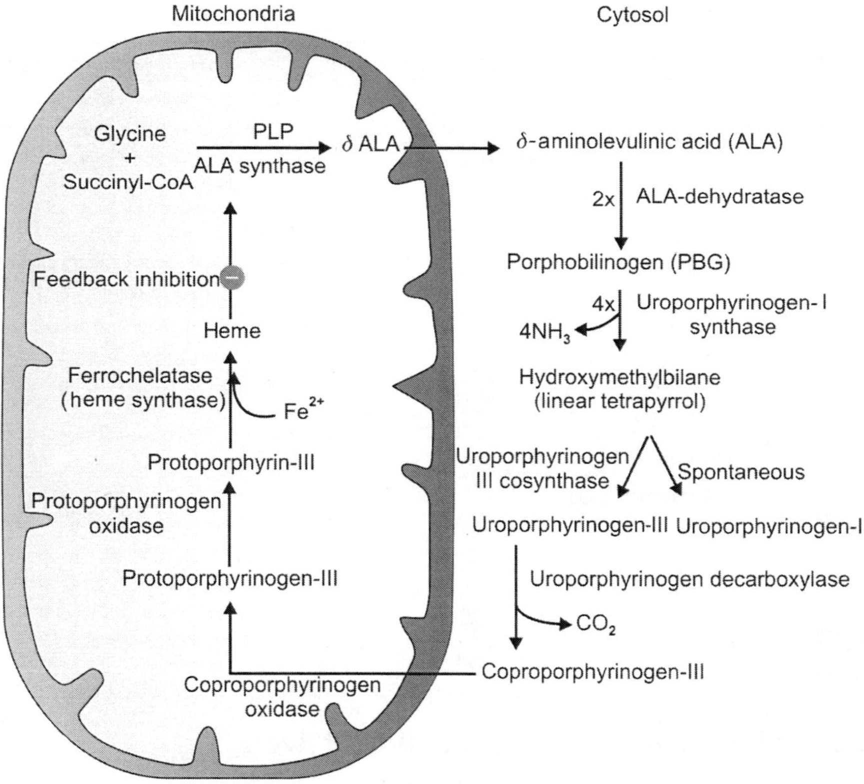


**Fig. 7:** Steps of heme synthesis

### Regulation

| *Enzyme* | *Inhibitors* | *Stimulators* |
|---|---|---|
| a. ALA synthase (an inducible enzyme)<br>– Rate limiting enzyme<br>– In liver | • Heme (inhibits synthesis of ALA synthase by feedback inhibition)<br>• Hematin (allosterically inhibits ALA synthase and inhibits translocation of ALA synthase from cytoplasm into mitochondria)<br>• Heavy metals like lead<br>• Drugs like INH<br>• Cellular glucose concentration | • Rate of globin synthesis<br>• Drugs requiring heme containing cytochrome p450 for their metabolism (barbiturates)<br>• Hormones like estradiol (permissive action) |
| b. Uroporphyrinogen synthase and ferrochelatase<br>– In bone marrow | — | • Cellular uptake of iron<br>• Activity of erythroid specific transcription factors |

## Functions

- Heme is component of various proteins a prosthetic group

| *Heme protein* | *Functions* |
|---|---|
| a. Hemoglobin | Transport of respiratory gases ($O_2$ and $CO_2$) |
| b. Myoglobin | Oxygen storage in muscles |
| c. Cytochromes (a, $a_3$, b, $c_1$) | Electron transport |
| d. Cytochrome p450 | Drug metabolism, steroid metabolism |
| e. Catalase | Degradation of $H_2O_2$ |
| f. Glutathione peroxidase | Degradation of $H_2O_2$ |
| g. Tryptophan pyrrolase | Oxidation of tryptophan |

## 9. Unconjugated hyperbilirubinemia.

- Unconjugated hyperbilirubinemia is increased level of unconjugated bilirubin either due to increased production of unconjugated bilirubin or impaired conjugation
- Characterized by absence of bilirubin in urine.

## Causes

| *Increased bilirubin production (hemolytic jaundice)* | *Decreased hepatic uptake* | *Decreased bilirubin conjugation (hepatic jaundice)* |
|---|---|---|
| • Intra- and extravascular hemolysis<br>– ABO or Rh incompatibility, hemoglobinopathies, G6PD dehydrogenase deficiency<br>• Ineffective erythropoiesis | • Drugs<br>• Prolonged starvation<br>• Sepsis | i. Hereditary disorders<br>– Gilbert's syndrome<br>– Crigler-Najjar syndrome<br>ii. Acquired defects<br>– Drugs<br>– Viral hepatitis<br>– Primary biliary cirrhosis<br>iii. Neonatal jaundice |

## Laboratory Diagnosis

| *Blood* | | *Urine* | |
|---|---|---|---|
| • Total bilirubin | Increased | • Bilirubin | Absent |
| • Unconjugated bilirubin | Markedly increased | • Urobilinogen | Increased |
| • Conjugated bilirubin | Normal or increased | | |
| • Liver function tests | Normal | | |

## 10. Lesch-Nyhan syndrome.

Refer Question No. 10 June 2005 (RS2).

## 11. Tests based on metabolic and excretory function of liver.

- Liver plays a central role in different metabolic processes.

## Indications

- Jaundice (differential diagnosis)
- Alcoholic liver disease
- Suspected liver metastasis
- Assessment of severity and progress of liver disease
- Any undiagnosed chronic illness
- Annual check up of diabetic patients

- Coagulation disorders
- Therapy with statins to check hepatotoxicity.

## Classification

| *Old nomenclature (based on function of liver)* | *Current clinical nomenclature* |
|---|---|
| • Excretory function<br>– Serum bilirubin estimation<br>– Urine bilirubin estimation<br>– Urine and fecal urobilinogen estimation<br>– Urine bile salts estimation<br>– Dye excretion tests<br>- Indocyanine green (ICG) or cyanine<br>- Bromosulphophthalein (BSP) dye tests<br>• Metabolic function<br>– Metabolism of carbohydrates<br>- Galactose tolerance test<br>– Metabolism of lipids<br>- Serum cholesterol level and ratio of free to esterified cholesterol<br>– Metabolism of amino acids<br>- Serum protein estimation<br>- Serum ammonia estimation<br>- Amino acid in urine<br>• Synthetic function<br>– Estimation of total proteins<br>– Estimation of albumin and AG ratio<br>– Prothrombin time<br>• Detoxification<br>– Blood, ammonia and bilirubin levels<br>– Hippuric acid test<br>• Secretory<br>– Estimation of serum enzymes—AST, ALT, ALP, GGT | • Tests to detect hepatic injury<br>– To detect the disease, whether mild or severe; whether acute or chronic<br>– To assess the nature of liver injury; hepatocellular (Group II) or cholestasis (Group III)<br>• Tests to assess hepatic function (Group I)<br>*Examples*<br>• Group I: Markers of liver dysfunction<br>– Serum bilirubin, total, conjugated<br>– Urine: Bile pigments, bile salts and UBG<br>– Total protein, serum albumin and A/G ratio<br>– Prothrombin time<br>– Blood ammonia, when indicated<br>• Group II: Markers of hepatocellular injury<br>– Alanine amino transferase (ALT)<br>– Aspartate amino transferase (AST)<br>• Group III: Markers of cholestasis<br>– Alkaline phosphatase<br>– Gamma glutamyl transferase |

## Tests Based on Excretory Functions

a. Determination of serum bilirubin
   - Bilirubin exists in the serum in two forms
     - Unconjugated or indirect bilirubin—water insoluble
     - Conjugated or direct bilirubin—water soluble.

   **Van den Berg's diazo reaction**

   *Principle*
   - Based on the formation of a reddish purple azo-bilirubin compound due to coupling of diazotised sulphanilic acid and bilirubin if present in serum.

   *Reagent*
   - Freshly prepared Ehrlich's diazo-reagent = 10 mL of solution A + 0.8 mL of solution B
     - Solution A: Contains sulphanilic acid in concentration of HCl.
     - Solution B: Sodium nitrite in water.

   *Procedure*
   - Take 0.3 mL of serum in 2 small tubes and add 0.3 mL of distilled water to one (Control tube) and 0.3 mL of freshly prepared diazo-reagent into 2nd tube (test tube)
   - Mix both and observe any color changes
   - Color developed is compared with a standard solution of bilirubin similarly treated.

*Observations*

| | | |
|---|---|---|
| • Immediate direct reaction | Immediate development of color proceeding rapidly to a maximum | Detects conjugated bilirubin |
| • Delayed direct reaction | Color only begins to appear after 5–30 minutes and develops slowly to a maximum | Detects conjugated bilirubin |
| • Indirect reaction | No direct reaction is obtained; color develops after addition of methanol | Detects unconjugated bilirubin |

b. Urine bilirubin
  - Presence of bilirubin indicates some pathologic condition of liver or biliary system
  - Bilirubinuria is always conjugated (water soluble).

**Fouchet's test**

*Procedure*

  - Add 2 mL of barium chloride solution to 10 mL of urine in a test tube and filter the urine
  - Dry the filtrate on a filter paper and add a drop of Fouchet's reagent (25 g TCA + 10 mL ferric chloride + 100 mL water) on filtrate.

*Inference*

  - A greenish color due an oxidation product of bilirubin is obtained if bilirubin is present.

c. Fecal urobilinogen
  - Amount of fecal urobilinogen depends primarily on amount of bilirubin entering intestine
  - In feces, excretion of urobilinogen is assessed by visual inspection of stools
  - Stool becomes pale or clay colored with decreasing amounts of pigment.

d. Urine urobilinogen
  - Amount of urobilinogen present in urine depends both on amount of bilirubin entering the intestine and on ability of liver to excrete urobilinogen coming to it from intestine.

**Clinical interpretation**

| | *Serum bilirubin* | | *Urine urobilinogen* | *Urine bilirubin* | *Faecal urobilinogen* |
|---|---|---|---|---|---|
| | *Direct (Conjugated)* | *Indirect (Unconjugated)* | | | |
| Normal | 0.1–0.4 mg/mL | 0.2–0.7 mg/mL | 0.4 mg/24 hr | Absent | 40–280 mg/24 hr |
| Hemolytic/prehepatic jaundice | Normal | Increased | Increased | Absent | Increased |
| Hepatic jaundice | Increased | Increased | Decreased if microobstruction to bile ductules occurs | Present if microobstruction to bile ductules occurs | Decreased |
| Obstructive/ posthepatic jaundice | Increased | Normal | Absent | Present | Traces to absent |

e. Bromosulphophthalein (BSP) excretion test
  - A 5% solution of BSP is injected intravenously in dose of 5 mg/kg body weight and a sample of blood is tested 45 minutes later for percentage of injected dye remaining in blood

$$\text{\% retained at 45 minutes} = \frac{\text{Serum concentration at 45 minutes}}{\text{Initial serum concentration}} \times 100$$

**Clinical interpretation**

  - In normal individuals, retention of BSP at 45 minutes is <5%
  - Impairment of liver cell function causes an increase in BSP retention

## Tests Based on Metabolic Function

a. Galactose tolerance test
  - Galactose is almost exclusively metabolized by liver and rate of utilization of galactose is proportional to functional liver cell mass
  - In patients with hepatic disease, ability to convert galactose to glucose is defective.

**Procedure**

- 25–30% solution of galactose in dose of 350 mg/kg body weight is given intravenously within 3 minutes
- Capillary blood is collected at 10 minutes interval for 1 hour.

**Clinical interpretation**

- Normally half life of galactose in blood is about 10–15 minutes
- It is markedly increased in cirrhosis and infective hepatitis but normal in patients with obstructive jaundice of brief duration.

b. Determination of serum total cholesterol and ratio of free to esterified cholesterol
  - Liver is involved in synthesis, esterification and excretion of cholesterol
  - In a normal individual, serum cholesterol level ranges between 150 and 250 mg/dL, approximately 70% of which is esterified.

**Clinical interpretation**

- Increase in total blood cholesterol is found in obstructive jaundice due to retention of cholesterol
- Normally, ester fraction predominates in plasma; but in liver damage it goes down
- In severe acute liver necrosis, total serum cholesterol value is usually low with a marked reduction in percentage of the esterified cholesterol.

c. Amino acids in urine (aminoaciduria)
  - Aminoaciduria is found in severe liver diseases with accompanying increase in plasma amino acids levels.

## Tests Based on Synthetic Function

a. Total proteins, albumin and globulin levels and AG ratio
  - Serum protein fractions are assessed by protein electrophoresis.

**Normal concentrations of serum proteins**

- Total serum protein = 6 to 8 g/dL
- Serum albumin = 3.5 to 5.5 g/dL
- Serum globulin = 2 to 3.5 g/dL
- Albumin/globulin ratio = 1.2:1 to 2.5:1.

**Clinical interpretation**

- Hypoalbuminemia may occur in cirrhosis
- Hyperglobulinemia may be present in chronic inflammatory disorders such as cirrhosis and in infectious hepatitis
- In advanced liver disease, albumin is decreased and globulins are increased, thus A/G ratio is reversed.

b. Prothrombin time
  - Various proteins participating in blood coagulation like fibrinogen, prothrombin (factor II) and factors V, VII, IX and X are synthesized in liver
  - Prothrombin time depends upon presence of prothrombin and factors V, VII and X
  - If any one of these factors is deficient, deficiency causes prolonged prothrombin time.

**Clinical interpretation**

- Increased prothrombin time indicates either
  - Deficiency of vitamin K (requires presence of bile salts for its absorption)
  - By damage to parenchymal cells.

## Tests Based on Detoxification Function

a. Hippuric acid test of Quick
  - Liver detoxifies benzoic acid by its detoxification by conjugation with glycine producing hippuric acid

**Principle**

- Amount of hippuric acid excreted in a fixed time is determined after a dose of sodium benzoate.

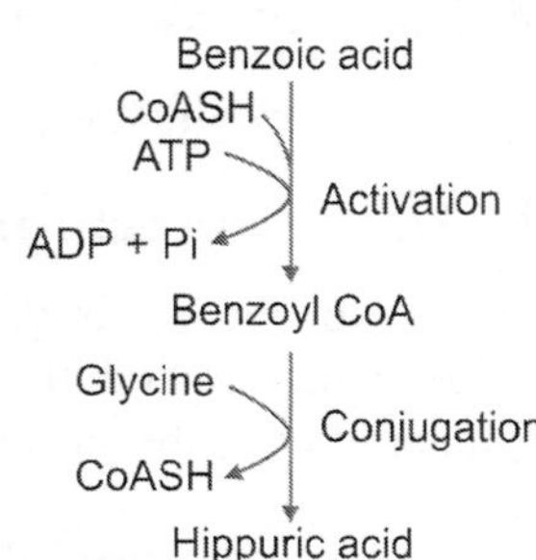


**Fig. 8:** Hippuric acid formation

**Procedure**

- After a oral dose of 6 g of sodium benzoate in 250 mL of water; bladder is voided at beginning of test
- After 4 hours, urine collected amount of hippuric acid in urine is estimated.

**Clinical interpretation**

- Normally 3–3.5 g of hippuric acid excreted in 4 hours period
- Decreased (<3 g) in hepatitis, tumors, cirrhosis and obstructive jaundice.

b. Determination of blood ammonia
   - Ammonia is detoxified to urea in liver which is impaired in liver diseases.

**Clinical interpretation**

- Normal blood ammonia level—40–70 µg/dL
- High blood ammonia levels found in acute hepatitis, cirrhosis and hepatic coma.

## Tests Based on Serum Enzymes

*Principle*

- Enzymes of diseased or damaged tissue may leak out into blood, when permeability of affected tissue is greatly enhanced thus significantly raising the activity of enzyme present in the affected tissue.

| *Enzyme* | *Tissues rich in* | *Normal level* | *Abnormal levels* |
|---|---|---|---|
| a. Alkaline phosphatase (ALP) | Liver, bones, small intestines, kidneys and placenta | 3–13 KA units/dL Or 40–140 IU/L | Levels above >35 KA units/dL in infectious hepatitis and post-hepatic (obstructive) jaundice—due to increased synthesis or regurgitation from bile |
| b. Alanine transaminase (ALT) | Liver (specific) | 3–15 IU/L | Rises rapidly in infective and toxic hepatitis, homologous serum jaundice and some forms of obstructive jaundice |
| c. Asparate transaminase (AST) | Heart, liver, skeletal muscles | 4–17 IU/L | Rises in infective hepatits |
| d. γ-glutamyl transferase (GGT) | Liver | 10–30 IU/L | Level increases both in liver disease and in cholestasis (marker) |

## Significance

- Liver is central organ for body metabolism and liver function tests (LFTs) are important tool in monitoring status of liver
- They are most widely performed biochemical tests in laboratory.

Revised Scheme 2

### 12. Applications of recombinant DNA technology.

Refer Question No. 2 June 2008 (RS2).

## SHORT ANSWERS

### 13. Mention two isotopes and mention their application in medicine.

Refer Question No. 22 Dec. 2013 (RS2).

### 14. Mention four tumor markers with their significance.

Refer Question No. 6 June 2007 (RS2).

### 15. Role of cytochrome $P_{450}$ in detoxification reaction.

- Cytochrome $P_{450}$ is a mono-oxygenase containing heme
- Also called mixed function oxidase
- 450 refers to absorption peak (at 450 nm) exhibited when exposed to carbon monoxide.

| *Location* | | *Role in detoxification reactions* |
|---|---|---|
| *Tissue* | *Subcellular* | Cytochrome P450 adds a hydroxyl group to aliphatic or aromatic compounds (hydroxylation) in presence of NADPH and $O_2$ $RH + O_2 + NADPH \rightarrow ROH + H_2O + NADP^+$ |
| Liver, kidney and brain | Endoplasmic retinaculum and mitochondria (adrenals) | |

## Significance

- Cytochrome P450 can be induced by alcohol and drugs like phenobarbitone.

## 16. Biologically important compounds derived from tyrosine.

Refer Question No. 1 Dec. 2010 (RS2).

## 17. What is reactive oxygen species (ROS)? How are they formed?

- Reactive oxygen species are oxygen derived molecules produced by gaining electrons to molecule oxygen
- Include both free radicals and non-free radicals.

| *Examples* | | *Characteristics* |
|---|---|---|
| *Free radicals* | *Non-free radicals* | |
| • Superoxide ion ($O_2^-$)<br>• Hydroxyl radical ($OH^-$)<br>• Peroxynitrate (ONOO)<br>• Hydroperoxy radical (HOO) | • Singlet oxygen ($^1O_2$)<br>• Hydrogen peroxide ($H_2O_2$) | • Highly reactive<br>• Very short half life<br>• Can generate new radicals by chain reaction<br>• Cause damage to biomolecules, cells and tissues |

## Formation

- Reactive oxygen species are derived from endogenous and exogenous sources.

a. Endogenous sources
   i. Mitochondrial leak
      - Due to leakage of free radical intermediates of electron transport chain, forming superoxide
   ii. Non-enzymatic reactions
      - Fenton reaction
        * Reaction of hydrogen peroxide with ferrous or cuprous ion to generate hydroxyl radical
          $Fe^{2+} + H_2O_2 \rightarrow Fe^{3+} + 2OH^-$
      - Haber Weiss reaction
        * Interaction of superoxide and hydrogen peroxide to form hydroxyl radicals
          $O_2^- + H_2O_2 \rightarrow O_2 + 2OH^-$
      - Lipid peroxidation.

Initialon  Lipid – H + OH $\longrightarrow$ Lipid + OH

Propagation  Lipid + $O_2$ $\longrightarrow$ Lipid OO
Pipid – OO + Lipid – H $\longrightarrow$ Lipid – OOH + Lipid

Degratation  Lipid–OOH + Lipid–H $\longrightarrow$ Lipid + Aldehydes
(Degraded lipid peroxide)

Termination  Lipid $\xrightarrow{\text{Vit E}}$ Lipid – H + Vitamin E

   iii. Enzymatic reactions

| | Xanthine oxidase | |
|---|---|---|
| Hypoxanthine + $H_2O$ + $O_2$ | → | Xanthine + $H_2O_2$ |

| | NADPH oxidase | |
|---|---|---|
| NADPH + $O_2$ | → | NADP+ + $O_2$ |

| | Superoxide dismutase | |
|---|---|---|
| O2 + $O_2$ + 2H | → | $H_2O_2$ + $O_2$ |

| | Myeloperoxidase | |
|---|---|---|
| $H_2O + Cl^-$ | → | HOCl |

December 2008 (RS2)

b. Exogenous sources
   – Cigarette smoke, pollutants, UV light, ionizing radiation and xenobiotics.

**Significance**

- Reactive oxygen species are double edged sword having both beneficial and harmful effects on human body
- They benefit body's immune system by phagocytic killing of bacteria
- Their harmful effects on human body include premature aging and causation of various diseases (cancer, diabetes, cataract infertility, etc.)
- They are best countered by antioxidants.

**18. What is the difference between endonuclease and restriction endonuclease? Give two examples of restriction endonuclease.**

Refer Question No. 8 Dec. 2015 (RS2).

**19. Deficiency manifestation of vitamin A.**

Refer Question No. 2 Dec. 2009 (RS2).

**20. Role of dietary fiber in the body.**

Refer Question No. 21 Dec. 2007 (RS2).

**21. Biochemical role of pyridoxine.**

Refer Question No. 2 June 2006 (RS2).

**22. Name the trace elements. Explain the biochemical role of any two trace elements.**

Refer Question No. 12 June 2017 (RS2).

# MBBS PHASE I EXAMINATION
## JUNE 2009
## (Revised Scheme 2)

### LONG ESSAYS

**1. Trace the pathway of gluconeogenesis starting from alanine. Mention the key enzymes and how they are regulated.**

- Gluconeogenesis is process by which new glucose is synthesized from noncarbohydrate precursors
- (Gluco = glucose, Neo = new, Genesis = synthesis).

| *Principle organs* | *Subcellular site* | *Substrates* | *Product* |
|---|---|---|---|
| • Liver, kidney, brain and small intestine | • Partly mitochondrial and partly cytoplasmic | • Pyruvate (most common)<br>• Lactate → pyruvate<br>• Glucogenic amino acids<br>– Glycine, alanine, serine, cysteine, glutamine, proline, glutamate, histidine, methionine, isoleucine, valine and aspartate<br>• Glycerol → dihydroxy acetone phosphate<br>• Propionic acid (in ruminents) | • Glucose |

**Steps**

a. Conversion of substrates into pyruvate or intermediates of TCA cycle or glycolysis
b. TCA cycle
c. Malate shuttle
d. Reversal of glycolysis (bypassing three irreversible steps)

| **Substrates for gluconeogenesis** |
|---|
| *"People Love Getting Girls Pregnant"*<br>✓ Pyruvate<br>✓ Lactate<br>✓ Glucogenic amino acids<br>✓ Glycerol<br>✓ Propionic acid |

a. Conversion of substrates into pyruvate or intermediates of TCA cycle or glycolysis
   i. Lactate

$$\text{Lactate} + NAD^+ \xrightarrow{\text{Lactate dehydrogenase}} \text{Pyruvate} + NADH + H^+$$

   ii. Glucogenic amino acids (Route of entry)

| ***Pyruvate (Sir Try All Three Glass Cups)*** | ***Oxaloacetate (As Per)*** | ***Fumarate (PT)*** | ***Sucinyl CoA (Most Voted Indian TV)*** | ***α-ketoglutarate (His 2 Guns Are Prolific)*** |
|---|---|---|---|---|
| • **S**erine<br>• **Try**ptophan<br>• **Al**anine<br>• **Three**onine<br>• **Gl**ycine<br>• **C**ysteine | • **As**pargine<br>• as**Per**tate | • **P**henylalanine<br>• **T**yrosine | • **M**ethionine<br>• **V**aline<br>• **I**soleucine<br>• **T**hreonine | • **His**tadine<br>• **G**lutamate<br>• **G**lutamine<br>• **Ar**ginine<br>• **Pro**line |

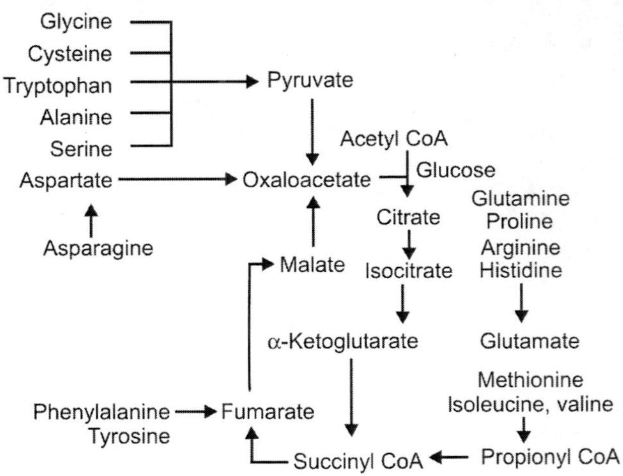


**Fig. 1:** Glucogenic amino acids

iii. Glycerol

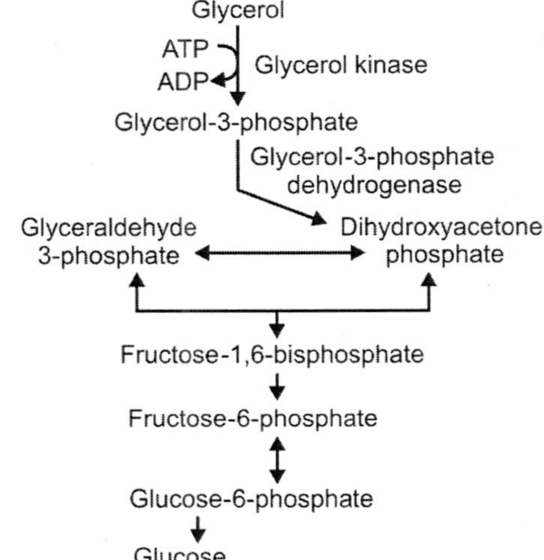


iv. Odd chain fatty acids

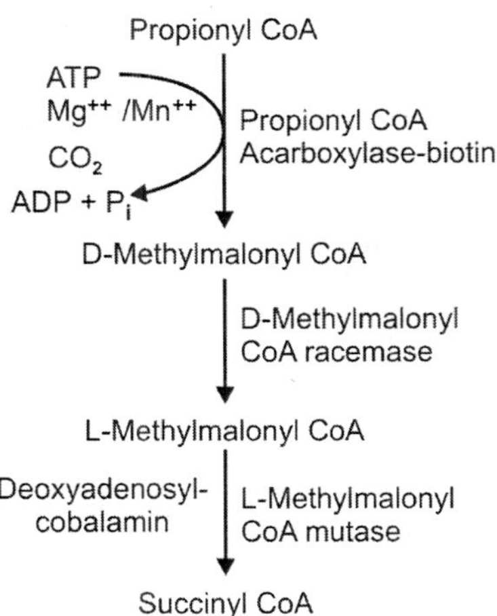


b. TCA cycle
  - After conversion of substrates into pyruvate or TCA cycle intermediates, TCA cycles continues till formation of oxaloacetate.

c. Malate shuttle
   – Oxaloacetate is impermeable through mitochondrial membrane thus it is reduced to malate which go out in cytoplasm and then get oxidized to oxaloacetate.
d. Reversal of glycolysis (bypassing three irreversible steps)
   i. Oxaloacetate is decarboxylated to form phosphophenol pyruvate (intermediate of glycolysis) and then steps of glycolysis are reversed till formation of glyceraldehyde 3-phosphate
   ii. One molecule of glyceraldehyde 3-phosphate is isomerized to dihydroxy acetone phosphate and then these two condense to give fructose-1,6-diphosphate
   iii. After a few reversible steps glucose-6-phosphate formed is thus converted to glucose.

## Summary

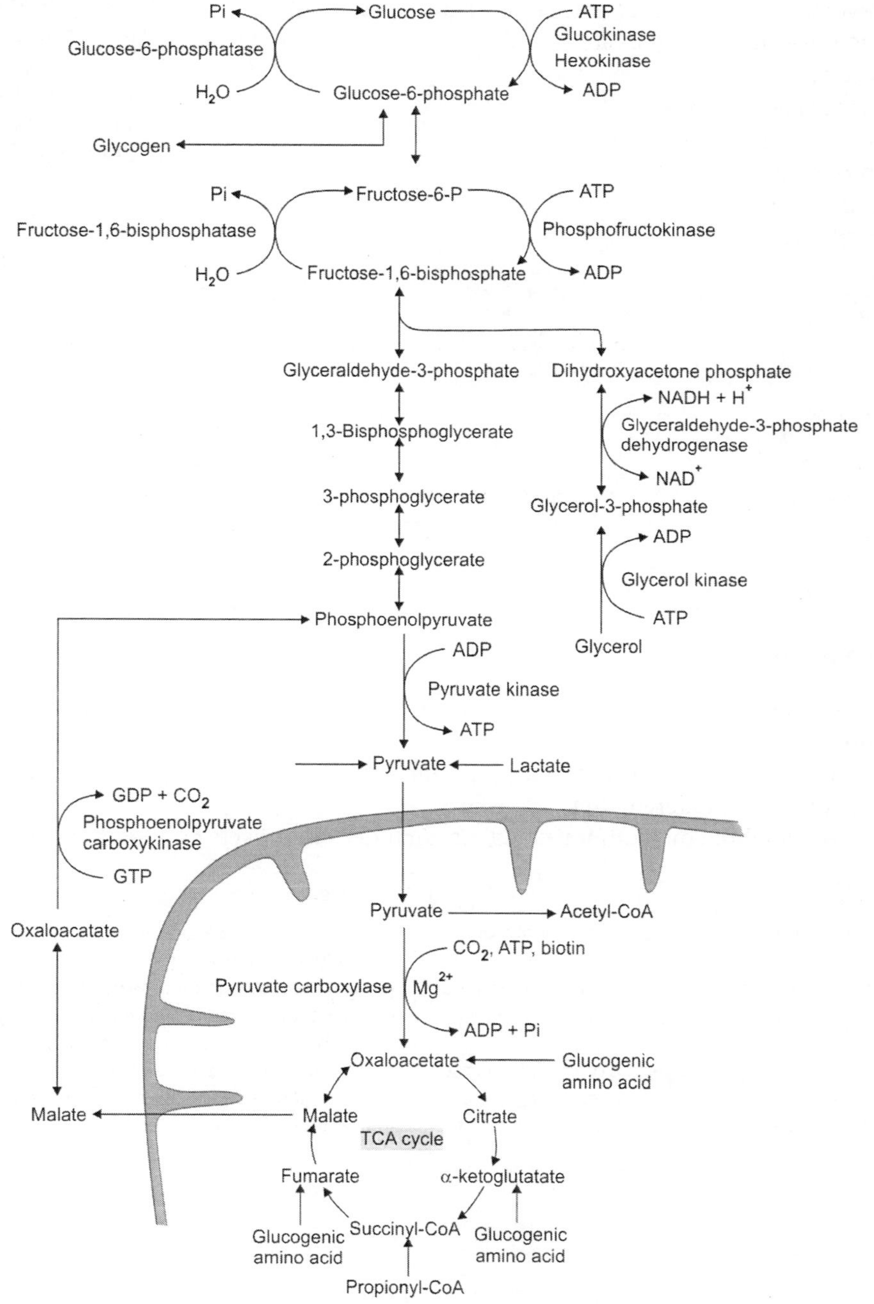


**Fig. 2:** Gluconeogenesis—reactions

## Energetics

| *Reaction* | *Enzyme* | *ATP utilized* |
|---|---|---|
| • Pyruvate → Oxaloacetate | Pyruvate carboxylase | – 1 ATP |
| • Oxaloacetate → Phosphoenol pyruvate | Phosphoenol pyruvate carboxykinase | 1 GTP = – 1 ATP |
| • 3 Phosphoglycerate →1, 3 bisphosphoglycerate | | – 1 ATP |
| Total | | – 3 ATPs |
| For every single glucose molecular ATPs used are | | – 6 ATPs |

## Regulation of Gluconeogenesis

Enzymes catalyzing reversal of three irreversible steps of glycolysis include:

a. Convert pyruvate to phosphoenol pyruvate
   - Pyruvate carboxylase
   - Phosphoenol pyruvate carboxykinase.

b. To bypass phosphofructokinase
   - Fructose-1,6-diphosphatase.

c. To bypass hexokinase step
   - Glucose-6-phosphatase.

**Key glucogenic enzymes**

*Pyar = Gulab Phool + Fruit and nut chocolate*

✓ **Py**ruvate carboxylase
✓ **G**lucose-6-phosphatase
✓ **Pho**sphoenol pyruvate carboxykinase
✓ **Fru**ctose-1,6-biphosphatase

| *Key enzyme* | *Regulation* | | | *Induction* | *Suppression* |
|---|---|---|---|---|---|
| | *Mechanism* | *Activator* | *Inhibitors* | | |
| • Pyruvate carboxylase | Allosteric | Acetyl CoA | — | Glucagon, cortisol, epinephrine | Insulin |
| • Phosphoenol pyruvate carboxykinase | — | — | — | Glucagon, cortisol, epinephrine | Insulin |
| • Fructose-1,6-biphosphatase | Allosteric | ATP, citrate | AMP, fructose 2,6-phosphate | Glucagon, cortisol, epinephrine | Insulin |
| • Glucose-6-phosphatase | — | — | — | Glucagon, cortisol, epinephrine | Insulin |

## Significance (Importance)

- Gluconeogenesis meets needs of body for glucose when carbohydrate is not available in sufficient amount from diet or during starvation
- It provides a continual supply of glucose necessary as a source of energy especially for brain, RBCs and skeletal muscles even when carbohydrate is not taken in diet
- It removes products of metabolism of other tissues, e.g. lactate from muscle and RBCs, glycerol from adipose tissue.

| *Glucose-alanine cycle* | *Cori's cycle* |
|---|---|
| • Alanine is a glycogenic amino acid and a major substrate for gluconeogenesis during starvation<br>• During starvation, muscle proteins are catabolized and alanine liberated is taken up by liver where it is transaminated to pyruvate by alanine transaminase<br>• Pyruvate thus generated undergoes gluconeogenesis producing glucose<br>• Glucose returns to skeletal muscle to supply quick energy by undergoing glycolysis to produce pyruvate which is transaminated to alanine by alanine transaminase | • During vigorous exercise, muscles metabolize glucoze anaerobically to produce lactate which is taken up by liver where it is converted to pyruvate and then to glucose by gluconeogenesis<br>• Glucose thus formed is used for glycogenolysis and stored in liver<br>• When required, glycogen is metabolized to glucose which is taken up by muscles and stored as glycogen<br>• During vigourous excercises, this glycogen is converted to glucose then into lactate |

*Contd...*

Contd...

- Thus transport of alanine from muscle to liver results in a reciprocal transfer of glucose to muscle
- This entire cyclic process is referred to as "glucose alanine cycle"

*Significance*

- Unlike Cori's cycle, glucose-alanine cycle plays a very important role during starvation providing energy for muscular activity
- Its importance is directly proportional to muscular activity of organism

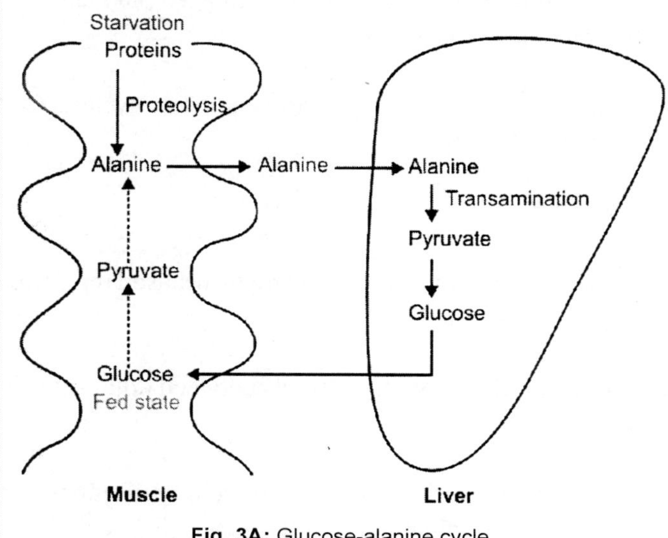


**Fig. 3A:** Glucose-alanine cycle

- This transport of glucose and lactate between liver and muscles is termed Cori cycle

*Significance*

- Cori cycle provides pathway for better utilization of lactate produced during vigorous exercise so that energy is not wasted

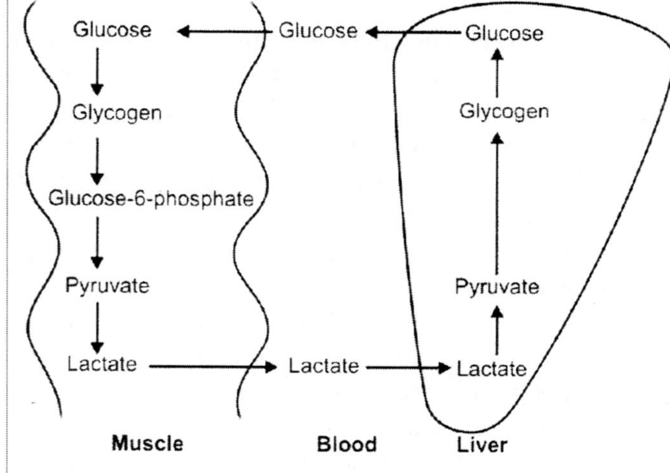


**Fig. 3B:** Cori's cycle

## 2. Describe in detail the sources, absorption, functions and factors regulating blood calcium level. Discuss about any clinical condition with abnormal blood calcium level.

- Calcium is a bulk mineral

| *Dietary sources* | *RDA* | *Distribution* |
|---|---|---|
| • Rich sources<br>– Milk and milk products<br>• Good sources:<br>– Meat, fish, green leafy vegetables, cereals and pulses | • Children<br>– 1 g/day<br>• Adults<br>– 0.5 g/day<br>• Pregnancy and lactation<br>– 1.5 g/day | • Total body calcium: 1–1.5 kg (2% of total body weight)<br>• Bones and teeth: 99%<br>• Muscles: 0.3%<br>• Other tissues: 1%<br>• Plasma calcium: 9–11 mg/dL |

## Absorption

| *Site* | *Mechanism (calcitriol mediated)* | *Factors affecting* | |
|---|---|---|---|
| | | *Enhanced by* | *Inhibited by* |
| • Upper small intestine | • Binding of calcitriol binds to vitamin D receptor and then with retinoic acid X receptor to form heterodimer complex<br>• Interaction of vitamin D-receptor complex with vitamin D responsive element in targeted DNA resulting in alteration in transcription of genes<br>• Increased synthesis of calcium binding protein<br>• Enhanced absorption of calcium across mucosal membrane<br>• Transport of calcium into blood | • Calcitriol<br>• Parathyroid hormone<br>• High protein diet<br>• Optimal $Ca^{2+}$ : $PO_4^-$ ratio in diet (0.5 : 2.0)<br>• Acidic pH<br>• Low calcium content in diet<br>• Bile salts | • Alkaline pH<br>• Phytates and oxalates<br>• Excess phosphate in diet<br>• Steatorrhea<br>• Vitamin D deficiency states |

## Functions

a. Constituent of bones and teeth
   - Principal mineral of bone matrix and enamel, dentin and cementum of teeth (99% of body calcium in present in bone and teeth)
   - Provides hardness, strength and concrete like elastic modules.

b. Blood coagulation
   - $Ca^{2+}$ ion gets chelated and helps prothrombin to anchor to phospholipid membranes of damaged platelets
   - Enhances activation of prothrombin to thrombin, thus helps in blood coagulation.

c. Enzyme action
   - Many enzymes such as phospholipase $A_2$, cAMP phosphodiesterase, glycogen synthase, guanylate cyclase, $Ca^{2+}$ ATPase, adenyl cylase, etc. are regulated through calmodulin $4Ca^{2+}$ complex.

d. Synaptic transmission
   - Helps in release of acetylcholine from presynaptic neurons.

e. Muscle contraction
   - Essential for both actin based regulation of skeletal and cardiac muscle contraction and myosin-based regulation of smooth muscle contraction.

f. Permeability of gap junctions
   - Fall in intracellular $Ca^{2+}$ level opens gap junctions (important communicating channels between adjacent cells of cardiac muscle, visceral smooth muscle, bone, lens and nerve tissue).

g. Membrane permeability
   - Reduces membrane permeability to ions and and water by binding with calmodulin of cell membranes and consequently changing conformation and hydration of membrane proteins.

h. Neuromuscular excitability
   - Reduces neuromuscular excitability by reducing membrane permeability.

i. Role in hormone action
   - Acts as either second or tertiary messenger to mediate cellular effects of many hormones such as vasopressin, catecholamines, dopamine, GnRH, gastrin and TRH.

j. Role in milk secretion
   - About 250–300 mg of calcium is secreted in daily milk output.

## Regulation of Serum Calcium

- Normal blood calcium level is 9–11 mg/dL
- Maintained within this level by three important hormones.

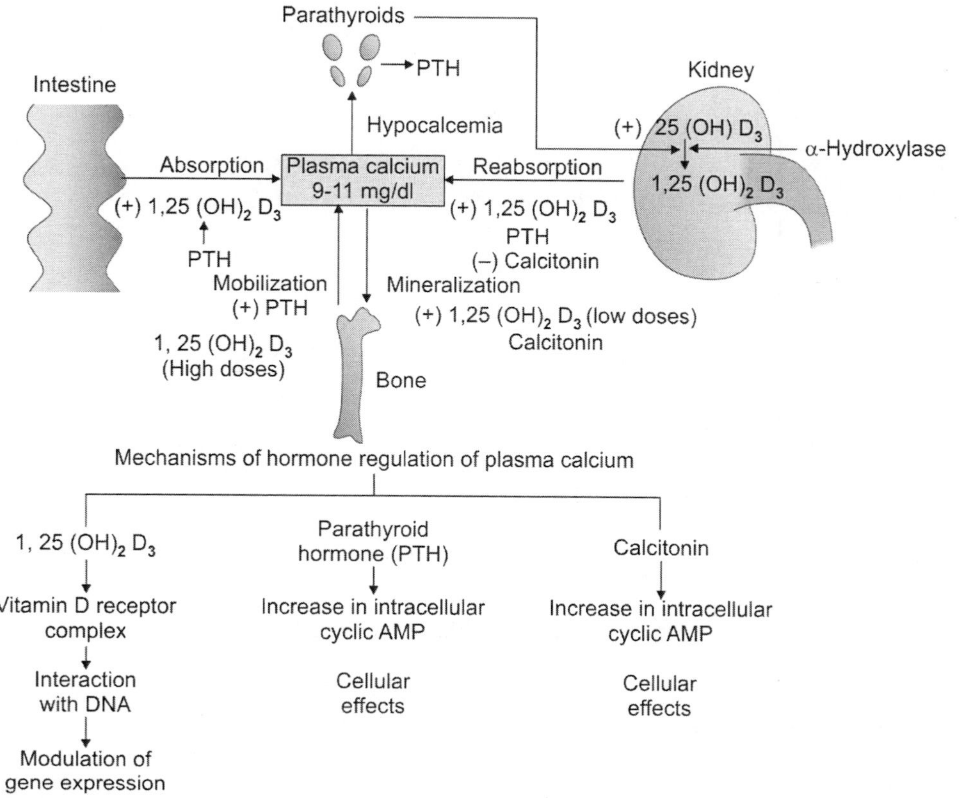


**Fig. 4:** Calcium homeostasis

| *Raise calcium level* | | *Reduce calcium level* |
|---|---|---|
| ***Parathormone*** | ***1, 25 dihydroxy cholecalciferol (Calcitriol)*** | ***Calcitonin*** |
| • Secreted by C-cells of parathyroid gland<br>• Acts mainly on kidney and bones<br>• Secretion stimulated by decreased calcium level | • Active form of vitamin D, synthesized in kidney by hydroxylation of 25 hydroxy cholecalciferol under influence of parathormone during hypocalcemia | • Secreted by parafollicular cells of thyroid gland |
| **Role in calcium metabolism** | | |
| • Raises blood calcium level | • Raises blood calcium level | • Reduces increased calcium level to normal |
| **Mechanism of action** | | |
| • Increasing synthesis of vitamin D<br>– ↑ activity of 1-hydroxylase in kidney which ↑synthesis of 1, 25 dihydroxy cholecalciferol and this in turn ↑absorption of $Ca^{2+}$ from GIT<br>• Regulating reabsorption of $Ca^{2+}$ from renal tubules<br>– ↑ reabsorption of $Ca^{2+}$ from glomerular filtrate in DCT by active process and inhibits reabsorption of $Ca^{2+}$ from PCT<br>– Former action is hypercalcemic and when this hypercalcemia is later amplified by outpouring of $Ca^{++}$ from bone under its own influence, later hypocalcemic action dominates<br>• Resorption of $Ca^{2+}$ from bones<br>– ↑ permeability of osetoclasts, osteocytes and osteoblasts to $Ca^{2+}$ causing osteoblasts to pump $Ca^{2+}$ into ECF | • Increasing intestinal absorption of $Ca^{2+}$<br>– Acts on nuclei of intestinal epithelial cells to ↑mRNA production which in turn ↑synthesis of a calcium binding protein<br>• Promoting bone resorption<br>– Acts directly on bones causing proliferation of osteoclasts which mobilize $Ca^{2+}$ from bones by increasing active transport of $Ca^{2+}$ out of osteoclasts into ECF<br>• ↑ reabsorption of $Ca^{2+}$ from renal tubules | • Inhibiting bone resorption and ↑deposition of $Ca^{2+}$ in bone<br>• Prevention of $Ca^{2+}$ reabsorption in renal tubules and ↑ excretion of $Ca^{2+}$<br>• ↓ renal formation of vitamin D<br>• Inhibiting intestinal absorption of $Ca^{2+}$ |

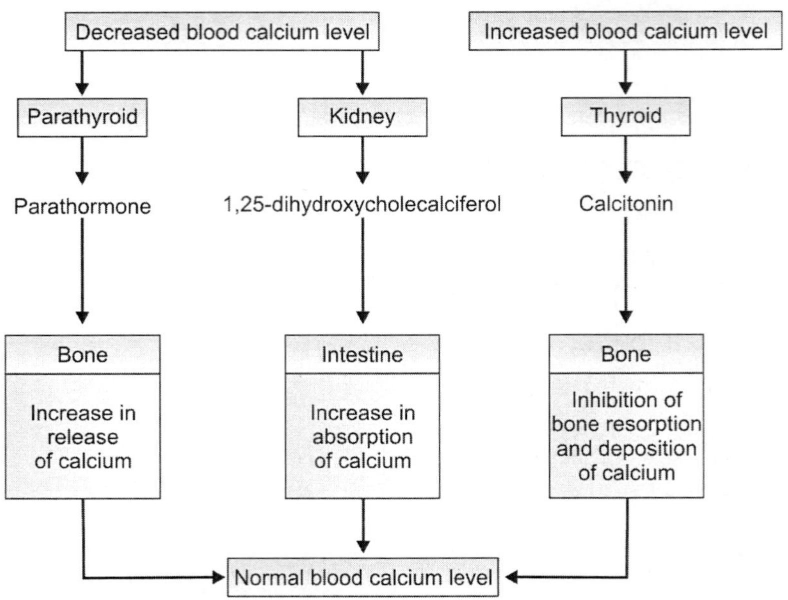


**Fig. 5:** Hormonal regulation of serum calcium



## Deficiency Disorder (Hypocalcemia)

| *Causes* | *Clinical features* | *Diagnosis* | *Treatment* |
|---|---|---|---|
| • Inadequate dietary intake<br>• Decreased absorption<br>– Vitamin D deficiency<br>– Small intestinal diseases<br>• Increased renal excretion<br>– Chronic renal failure<br>– Renal rickets<br>– Hypoparathyroidism<br>• Magnesium deficiency<br>• Acute pancreatitis | • Muscle cramps and tetany<br>– Laryngospasm and airway obstruction<br>– Chvostek's sign positive (contraction of facial muscles on tapping of facial nerve)<br>– Trousseau's sign positive (carpal spasm in response to brachial artery occlusion for 3 minutes)<br>– Convulsions<br>• Cardiac arrhythmias<br>– Prolonged QT interval (predisposes to ventricular arrhythmias)<br>– Heart block<br>• Cataract | • Estimation of total calcium level | • Calcium carbonate orally (in asymptomatic cases)<br>• Calcium gluconate intravenously (in severe cases) |

## SHORT ESSAYS

### 3. What are the biologically important compounds derived from cholesterol?

- Cholesterol is a sterol having 27 carbon atoms which is precursor for formation of some biologically important compounds.

## Compounds Derived from Cholesterol

a. Bile acids → Bile salts

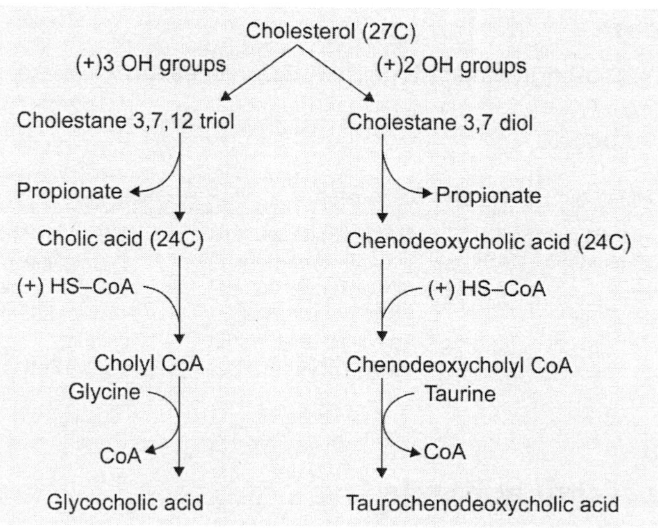


**Fig. 6:** Synthesis of bile acids

b. 7-Dehydrocholesterol → vitamin $D_3$
c. Steroid hormones
  - Adrenocortical hormones
  - Androgens
  - Estrogens
  - Progesterone.

## Biomedical Importance

| *Bile salts* | *Vitamin $D_3$* | *Aldosterone* |
|---|---|---|
| • Bile salts are sodium and potassium salts of bile acids<br>*Functions*<br>• Emulsification of fat by lowering of surface tension<br>• Accelerate pancreatic lipase action by shifting its optimal pH from 9.0 to 6.0 by colipase<br>• Help in absorption of water-insoluble lipids by formation of micelles<br>• Aid in adsorption of water-insoluble vitamins by forming water-soluble compounds with them<br>• Stimulation of intestinal motility<br>• Choleretic action on liver, i.e. stimulation of more bile secretion by liver<br>• Keep cholesterol in solution and prevent cholelithiasis | • 1, 25 cholecalciferol or calcitriol is active vitamin $D_3$ synthesized from 7-dehydrocholesterol, a catabolic product of cholesterol<br>*Functions*<br>• Regulation of serum calcium level by:<br>– ↑absorption of $Ca^{2+}$ from intestines by increasing formation of calcium binding proteins in intestinal epithelial cells<br>– ↑synthesis of calcium induced adenosine triphosphate in intestinal epithelium<br>– ↑synthesis of alkaline phosphate in intestinal epithelium<br>– ↑release of calcium from bone matrix<br>– ↑reabsorption of calcium and phosphate from renal tubules<br>• Regulation of serum phosphate level | • A mineralocorticoid synthesized in adrenal cortex from cholesterol<br>*Function*<br>• Effect on mineral metabolism<br>– ↓ $Na^+$ excretion by increasing rate of reabsorption of $Na^+$ by tubules especially distal tubules and collecting ducts<br>– Also ↓ elimination of $Na^+$ in saliva, sweat and gastric juice by promoting reabsorption from these secretions<br>– ↑ reabsorption of $Cl^-$ ions from tubules secondary to $Na^+$ reabsorption to maintain electrical potential gradient<br>– ↑ in loss of $K^+$ by renal distal tubules and collecting ducts in exchange for $Na^+$ by aldosterone induced sodium pump<br>• Effect on acid-base balance<br>– Causes excretion of $H^+$ ions in exchange of reabsorption of $Na^+$ ions thus elevating the body pH<br>• Effect on ECF and blood volume<br>– ↑ quantities of $Na^+$, $Cl^-$ and $HCO_3^-$ ions in ECF resulting in increase in ECF volume<br>– Blood volume also increases proportionally to ECF |

## 4. Prostaglandins.

Refer Question No. 15 Dec. 2014 (RS2).

## 5. Give four examples of transmethylation reactions.

Refer Question No. 4 June 2010 (RS2).

## 6. Maple syrup urine disease.

- Maple syrup urine disease is an inherited disorder hence, named because of characteristic smell of urine similar to burnt sugar or maple sugar
- Also called branched chain ketonuria.

| *Mechanism* | *Deficient enzyme* | *Clinical features* | *Diagnosis* | *Treatment* |
|---|---|---|---|---|
| • Deficient oxidative decarboxylation of branched chain keto acids into respective acyl CoA thioesters resulting in elevated levels of branched amino acids and their keto acids | • Branched chain α-keto acid dehydrogenase | • Starts in 1st week of life<br>• Convulsions, severe mental retardation, vomiting, acidosis<br>• Coma and death within 1st year of life | • Detection of branched chain amino acids and their keto acids (valine, leucine and isoleucine) in urine<br>• Positive Rothera's test (even with boiled and cooled urine) | • Dietary restrictions on branched chain amino acids<br>• High doses of thiamine for mild variant<br>• Hemodialysis or peritoneal dialysis<br>• Liver transplantation |

## 7. Energy releasing steps of citric acid cycle.

Refer Question No. 1 June 2008 (RS2).

## 8. What are the sources, functions and daily requirement of vitamin A?

Refer Question No. 2 Dec. 2009 (RS2).



## 9. Transport proteins of blood.

- Plasma proteins which serve as carriers of important biological products are called transport proteins of blood.

| *Transport protein* | *Compound transported* | *Significance* |
|---|---|---|
| • Albumin | Fatty acids, bilirubin, $Ca^{2+}$, thyroxine, heavy metals, drugs, etc. | • Aspirin competes with bilirubin for binding sites on albumin thus can precipitate kernicterus in neonatal jaundice |
| • Prealbumin | Steroid hormones, thryoxine, retinol | • Negative acute phase protein |
| • Retinal binding protein | Retinol | • Level indicates vitamin A status<br>• Useful to assess protein turnover rate |
| • Thyroxine binding globulin | Thyroxine | • Assessment of binding sites on TBG<br>• Important in studying thyroid function |
| • Transcortin (cortisol binding globulin) | Cortisol and corticosterone | • Increased in pregnancy<br>• Free unbound fraction of hormone is active |
| • Haptoglobin | Hemoglobin | • Low level indicate hemolysis<br>• Is an acute phase protein |
| • Transferrin | Iron | • Conserves iron by preventing iron loss through urine |
| • Hemopexin | Free heme | • Prevents loss of heme and iron from body |
| • HDL | Cholesterol and phospholipids | • Transports cholesterol from tissues to liver for metabolism<br>• Anti-atherogenic |
| • LDL | Cholesterol, phospholipids and triglycerides | • Transports cholesterol to tissues<br>• Predisposes to myocardial infarction |

### Significance

- Transport proteins are important constituents of blood helping transport of important biological compounds from site of synthesis to site of metabolism or action and even sometimes as reserve, preventing their loss from body.

## 10. Formation and fate of bilirubin in the body.

Refer Question No. 8 June 2007 (RS2).

## 11. Basal metabolic rate.

Refer Question No. 12 June 2006 (RS2).

## 12. Bicarbonate buffer system of blood.

Refer Question No. 2 June 2012 (RS2).

# SHORT ANSWERS

## 13. Name the two endopeptidases with their specifications.

- Endopeptidases are proteolytic enzymes which act on peptide bonds inside protein molecule, making proteins successively smaller and smaller units.

*Example*

| *Endopeptidases* | *Hydrolysis of bonds formed by carboxyl groups of:* |
|---|---|
| • Pepsin | Phenylalanine, tyrosine, tryptophan, methionine, glutamate, aspartate |
| • Trypsin | Arginine, lysine |
| • Chymotrypsin | Phenylalanine, tyrosine, tryptophan, valine, leucine, methionine |
| • Elastase | Alanine, glycine, serine |

## 14. What are functions of apolipoproteins?

- Apolipoprotein is protein part of lipoprotein which solubalises lipid.

### Functions

| *Type* | *Functions* |
|---|---|
| • Apo-A-I | • Activates lecithin cholesterol acyl transferase<br>• Acts as ligand for HDL receptor<br>• Anti-atherogenic |
| • Apo-B-100 | • Binds to LDL receptor on tissues |
| • Apo-B-48 | • Structural component of chylomicrons |
| • Apo-C-II | • Activates lipoprotein lipase |
| • Apo-E | • Cellular transport of lipids in CNS |

## 15. Give the significance of uronic acid pathway.

- Uronic acid pathway is an alternative oxidative pathway for glucose involved in formation of glucoronic acid and pentose sugars
- Also called glucuronic acid pathways
- Major function is to produce D-glucuronic acid and in this pathway energy is not produced.

| *Substrate* | *Products* |
|---|---|
| • Glucose | • Pentose sugars, UDP glucose, UDP-glucoronic acid<br>• Ascorbic acid (in lower animals) |

**Reactions**

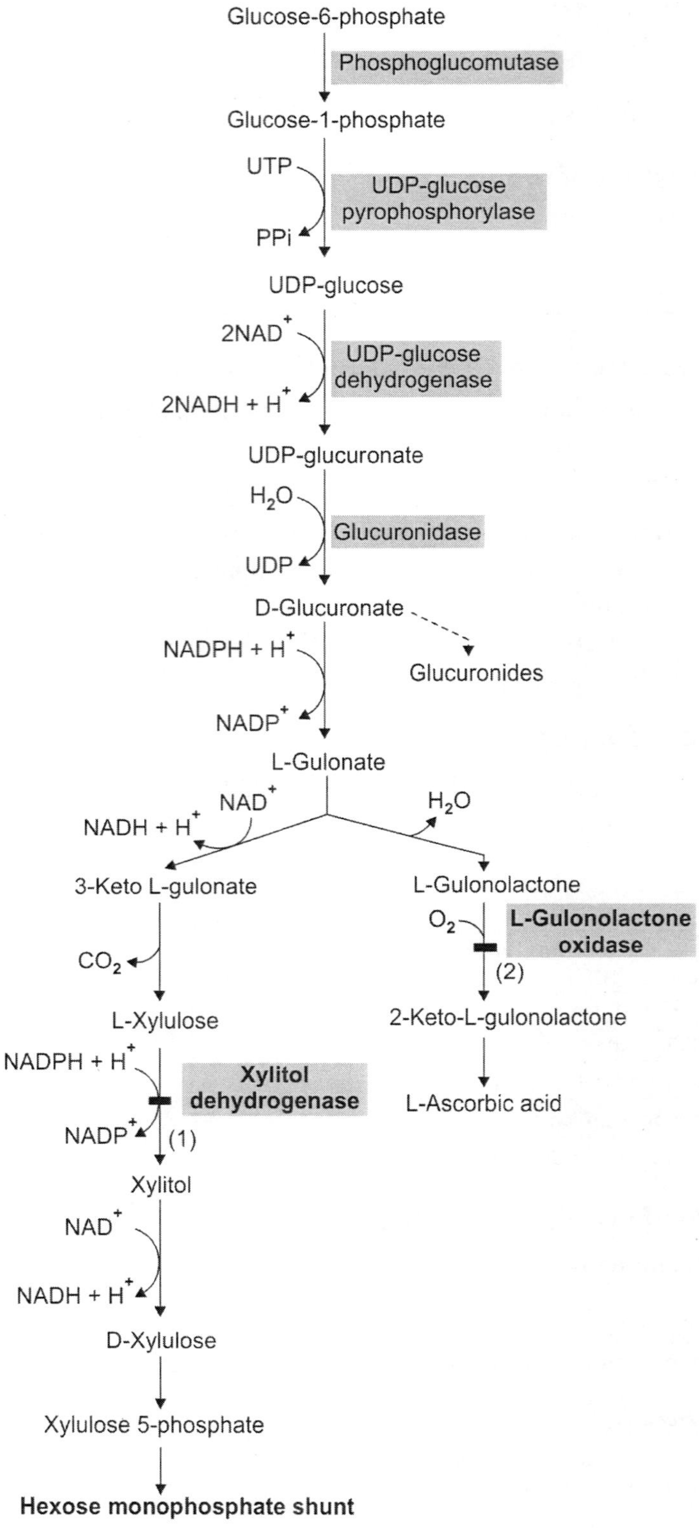


**Fig. 7:** Reactions of uronic acid pathway

**Significance (Function)**

a. Provides UDP-glucose which is required for:
   - Synthesis of glycogen
   - Metabolism of galactose
   - Lactose synthesis
   - Formation of UDP-glucuronic acid.

b. Provides UDP-glucuronic acid which is used for:
   - Detoxification reaction by conjugation (bilirubin, steroids and various drugs) rendering them water soluble
   - Synthesis of glycosaminoglycans and proteoglycans (hyaluronic acid, heparin)
   - Biosynthesis of L-iduronic acid which is component of glycosaminoglycans (heparin sulfate, dermatan sulfate).

c. Provides pentoses which enter pentose phosphate pathway.

d. Synthesizes ascorbic acid in lower animals.

## 16. Clinical importance of transamination.

Refer Question No. 2 June 2006 (RS2).

## 17. Detoxification of alcohol.

- Alcohol is detoxified in liver by two stages.

| *1st stage* | *2nd stages* |
|---|---|
| • Oxidation of alcohol into corresponding aldehyde by alcohol dehydrogenase | • Oxidation of aldehyde into corresponding acid by aldehyde dehydrogenase |
| Ethanol → Acetaldehyde | Acetaldehyde → Acetic acid |

**Significance**

- Knowledge about detoxification of alcohol is used in treatment of methyl alcohol poisoning, whose detoxified products are more toxic than methyl alcohol, i.e. formaldehye (x33 toxic) and formic acid (x6 toxic)
- Thus methyl alcohol poisoning is treated by inhibiting detoxification of methyl alcohol by competitive inhibition of alcohol dehydrogenase using ethyl alcohol.

## 18. Polymerase chain reaction.

Refer Question No. 11 June 2006 (RS2).

## 19. What is the daily requirement of thiamine, niacin and pyridoxine?

| | *Vitamin* | *RDA* |
|---|---|---|
| a. | Thiamine | 1–1.5 mg/day |
| b. | Niacin | 20 mg/day |
| c. | Pyridoxine | 1–2 mg/day |

## 20. Give enzyme defect in the following conditions:
## (a) Drug-induced hemolytic anemia
## (b) Criggler-Najjar syndrome

| | *Deficient enzyme* |
|---|---|
| (a) Drug-induced hemolytic anemia | Glucose-6-phosphate dehydrogenase |
| (b) Criggler-Najjar syndrome | UDP glucuronyl transferase |

## 21. Creatinine clearance test.

Refer Question No. 9 Dec. 2005 (RS2).

**22. Give the normal blood level of the following:**
**(a) Fasting blood glucose**
**(b) Total protein**
**(c) Urea**
**(d) Bicarbonate**
**(e) Sodium**
**(f) Potassium**

| | *Normal level* |
|---|---|
| (a) Fasting blood glucose | 70–110 mg/dL |
| (b) Total protein | 6–8 g/dL |
| (c) Urea | 20–40 mg/dL |
| (d) Bicarbonate | 22–26 mEq/L |
| (e) Sodium | 136–145 mE/L |
| (f) Potassium | 3.5–5 mEq/L |

# MBBS PHASE I EXAMINATION

## DECEMBER 2009

## (Revised Scheme 2)

### LONG ESSAYS

**1. What is the normal fasting blood glucose level? Why does it need to be regulated? Describe the various mechanisms of its regulation.**

- Glucose the main source of energy for body and glucose levels in body has to be in homeostasis to supply glucose to body tissues
- Normal blood glucose level varies between 80–100 mg/dL (Fasting) and 120–140 mg/dL (post-prandial).

#### Regulation of Blood Glucose Level

| *Sources of glucose* | *Utilization of glucose* |
|---|---|
| • Digestion and absorption of dietary carbohydrates<br>• Glycogen breakdown in liver (glycogenolysis)<br>• Glucose synthesis from non-carbohydrate substrates (gluconeogenesis)<br>• Metabolism of galactose and fructose | • Peripheral uptake of glucose<br>• Oxidation of glucose (glycolysis)—50%<br>• Glycogen synthesis (glycogenesis)—10%<br>• Conversion into fat (lipogenesis)—40% |

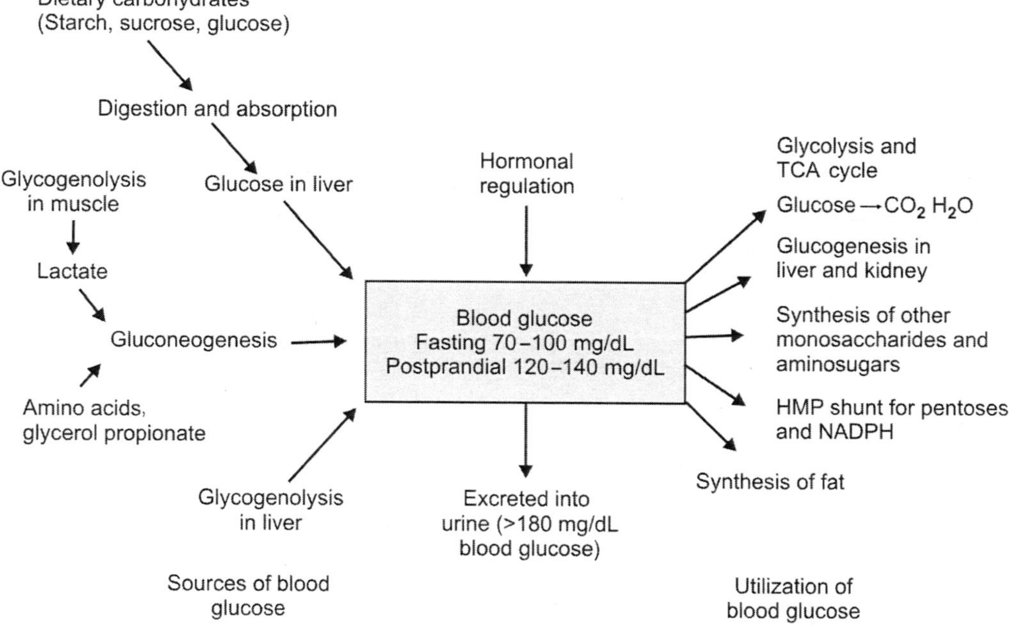


**Fig. 1:** Regulation of blood glucose level

## Hormonal Mechanism

- Various factors contribute to maintain this level within its physiological limits but hormones play a major role in regulation of blood glucose level.

| *Hormones* | *Action on glucose homeostasis* |
|---|---|
| **Hypoglycemic (antidiabetic) hormone** | **Decreases glucose level by** |
| • Insulin<br>– Only antidiabetic hormone<br>– Plays an important role in glucose homeostasis<br>– Secretion stimulated blood glucose level | • Inhibiting gluconeogenesis by suppressing enzymes<br>• Promoting glycogenesis by increasing formation of glycogen synthetase<br>• Increasing peripheral utilization of glucose<br>• Inhibiting glycogenolysis<br>• Promoting entry of glucose into cells<br>• Promoting lipogenesis and inhibiting lipogenolysis |

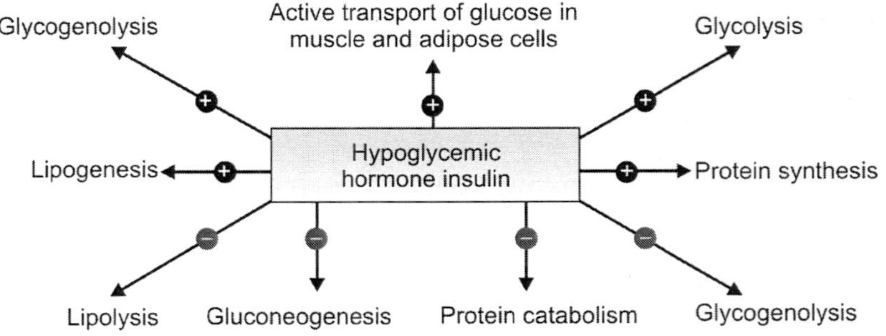


**Fig. 2:** Role of insulin in regulation of blood glucose level

| **Hyperglycemic (diabetic/anti-insulin) hormones** | **Increase glucose level by** |
|---|---|
| a. Glucagon<br>– Secreted by a cells of pancreas in response to ↓ blood glucose level | • Stimulating glycogenolysis and gluconeogenesis in liver |
| b. Growth hormone<br>– Secreted by acidophils of anterior pituitary | • Inhibiting glycolysis<br>• Opposing action of insulin in muscles<br>• Stimulating gluconeogenesis<br>• Preventing entry of glucose into cells |
| c. Cortisol<br>– Glucorticoid secreted by adrenal cortex | • Increasing muscle protein breakdown and liver gluconeogenesis<br>• Decreasing uptake of glucose by tissues |
| d. Epinephrine and norepinephrine<br>– Catecholamines secreted by adrenal medulla in response to hypoglycemia | • Stimulating glycogenolysis in liver and muscle |
| e. Thyroid hormones (T3 and T4)<br>– Secreted by thyroid hormones<br>– Increase blood glucose level but also increase glucose utilization by tissues | • Increasing glucose absorption from intestine<br>• Stimulating glycogenolysis and gluconeogenesis |
| f. ACTH<br>– A pituitary hormone | • Its action through cortisol |

- Thus regulation of blood glucose can be summarized as follows:

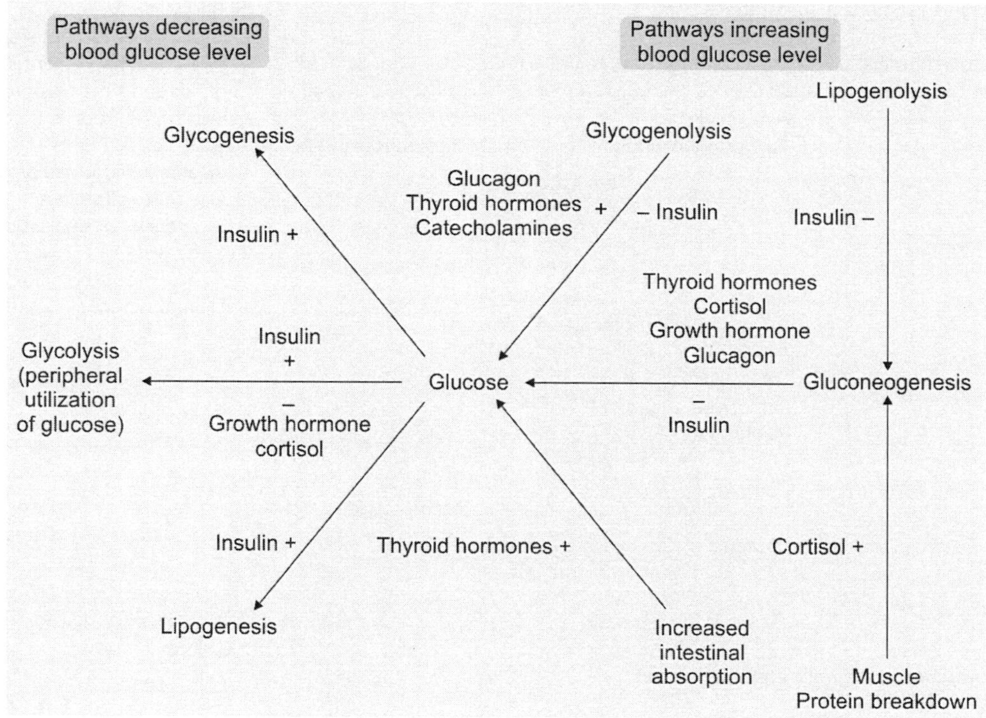


**Fig. 3:** Endocrine regulation of blood glucose level

## Significance

- Maintenance of glucose within its narrow normal limits is essential for health and any imbalance leads to hypoglycemia or hyperglycemia both of which are detrimental to health.

| *Hypoglycemia* | *Hyperglycemia* |
|---|---|
| • Reduced glucose levels<br>*Causes*<br>• Fasting hypoglycemia<br>– Administration of exogenous insulin or oral hypoglycemic drugs<br>– Insulinoma (insulin secreting tumor)<br>– Ketotic hypoglycemia in infants<br>– Alcohol<br>– Cirrhosis of liver<br>– Adrenal insufficiency<br>– Hypopituitarism<br>• Postprandial (reactive) hypoglycemia<br>– Alimentary hyperinsulinism (post-gastrectomy or idiopathic)<br>– Hereditary fructose intolerance<br>– Galactosemia<br>– Leucine insensitivity<br>*Significance*<br>• Dangerous because glucose is primary source of energy for brain and erythrocytes | • Increased glucose levels predisposes to numerous conditions collectively referred as diabetes mellitus<br>*Causes*<br>• Type 1 diabetes mellitus<br>– Congenital deficiency of insulin due to β cell destruction or antibodies against β cells<br>• Type 2 diabetes mellitus<br>– Insulin resistance<br>• Other types<br>– Gestational diabetes mellitus<br>– Impaired glucose tolerance<br>– Impaired fasting glycemia<br>– Pancreatic diseases (chronic pancreatitis)<br>– Hormonal imbalances (Cushing's syndrome, pheochromocytoma, acromegaly)<br>*Significance*<br>• Hyperglycemia has pathological impact on numerous organs resulting in nephropathy, retinopathy, neuropathy, etc. |

## 2. Describe the sources, functions, deficiency manifestations and daily requirement of vitamin A.

- Vitamin A is a fat-soluble vitamin.

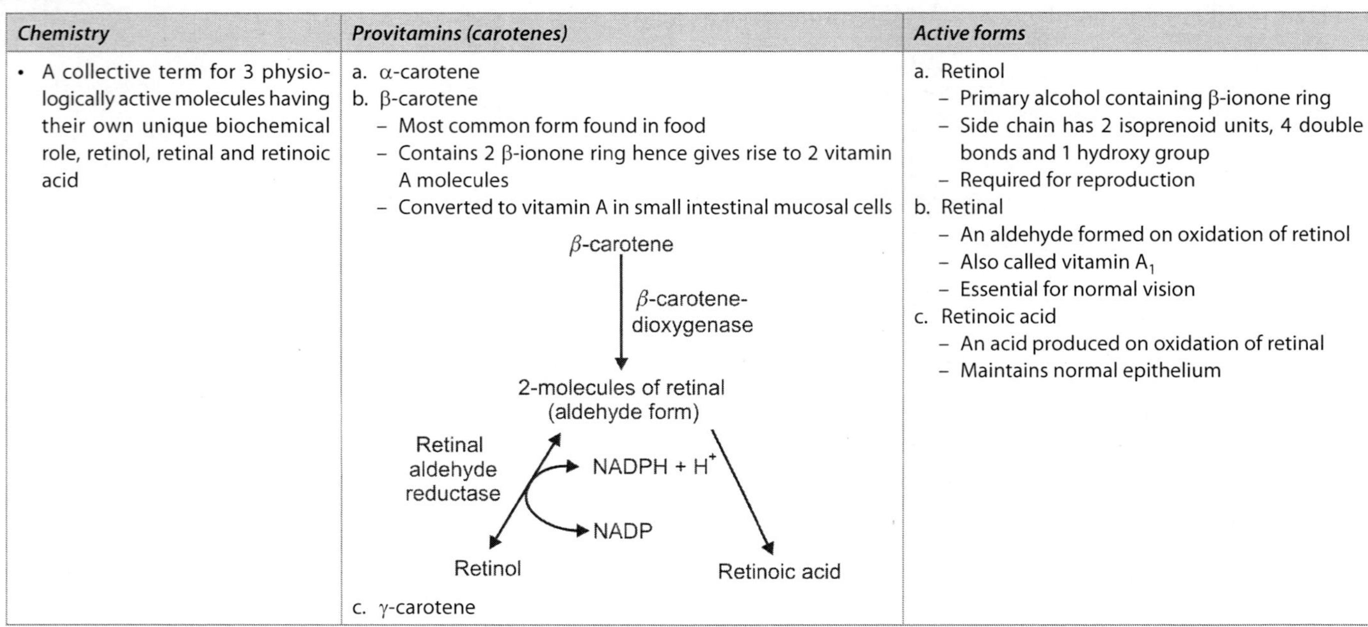

| *Chemistry* | *Provitamins (carotenes)* | *Active forms* |
|---|---|---|
| • A collective term for 3 physiologically active molecules having their own unique biochemical role, retinol, retinal and retinoic acid | a. α-carotene<br>b. β-carotene<br>– Most common form found in food<br>– Contains 2 β-ionone ring hence gives rise to 2 vitamin A molecules<br>– Converted to vitamin A in small intestinal mucosal cells<br>β-carotene<br>β-carotene-dioxygenase<br>2-molecules of retinal (aldehyde form)<br>Retinal aldehyde reductase<br>NADPH + $H^+$<br>NADP<br>Retinol<br>Retinoic acid<br>c. γ-carotene | a. Retinol<br>– Primary alcohol containing β-ionone ring<br>– Side chain has 2 isoprenoid units, 4 double bonds and 1 hydroxy group<br>– Required for reproduction<br>b. Retinal<br>– An aldehyde formed on oxidation of retinol<br>– Also called vitamin $A_1$<br>– Essential for normal vision<br>c. Retinoic acid<br>– An acid produced on oxidation of retinal<br>– Maintains normal epithelium |

| *Dietary sources* | *RDA* | |
|---|---|---|
| • Animal sources<br>– Milk, butter, cream, cheese, egg yolk, liver, cod liver oil<br>• Vegetable sources<br>– Carrot, papaya, mango, green leafy vegetables (spinach, amaranth)—contain β-carotene | • Children<br>• Male<br>• Female<br>• Pregnancy<br>• Lactation | 400–600 mg<br>1,000 mg<br>800 mg<br>800 mg<br>1,300 mg |

## Biochemical Role

| *Function* | *Active form* | |
|---|---|---|
| a. Role in vision (Wald's visual cycle) | Retinal | • Human retina contains two types of receptor cells, i.e. rods and cones<br>• Rods are responsible for vision in dim light, i.e. they are adopted to sensing low light intensities and are involved in night vision<br>• Cone are responsible for vision in bright light and also for color vision<br>• Rods contain rhodopsin or visual purple, a photo labile pigment which consists of a protein opsin and a non-protein part, 11 cis-retinal<br>• When exposed to light, following reactions take place in rhodopsin pigment<br>Light → Rhodopsin → Bathorhodopsin → Lumirhodopsin<br>Metarhodopsin I<br>Metarhodopsin II (active rhodopsin)<br>Dark<br>Scotopsin<br>All transretinal<br>Retinal isomerase<br>11 cis-retinal<br>Dehydrogenase + $NADH_2$<br>All transretinol (vitamin A)<br>Retinal isomerase<br>11 cis-retinal<br>**Fig. 4:** Wald's visual cycle |

*Contd...*

*Contd...*

| | | |
|---|---|---|
| | | • Dissociation of rhodopsin triggers a nerve impulse transmitted to optic area of brain via optic pathway<br>• All trans-retinal is reduced to all trans-retinol in retina and then transported to liver where it is isomerized to 11 cis-retinol which is transported back to retina where it is oxidized to 11 cis-retinal<br>• 11 cis-retinal spontaneously combines with opsin to form rhodopsin |
| b. Growth and differentiation | Retinoid acid | • Required for sulfation of mucopolysaccharides in matrix of bone and cartilage<br>• Also promotes growth and differentiation by regulating expression of genes required for growth and differentiation |
| c. Reproduction | Retinol | • Binds to specific cellular retinal binding protein and then this retinol-receptor complex binds to DNA to control of expression of certain genes<br>• Thus it acts like a steroid hormone |
| d. Glycoprotein synthesis | Retinoyl phosphate | • Acts as a donor of oligosaccharide unit across the lipid bilayer of cells involved in trans isomerization |
| e. Antioxidant | β-carotene | • Against peroxyl and free radicals trapped in tissue |
| f. Maintenance of epithelial integrity | Retinoic acid | • Essential for normal differentiation and mucus secretion of epithelial tissues |

***Deficiency disorder***

*Causes*

a. Inadequate intake
  - Nutritional or primary deficiency
b. Impaired absorption
  - Pancreatic diseases
  - Malabsorption syndrome
  - Obstructive jaundice.
c. Impaired storage and transport
  - Liver diseases like cirrhosis (deficiency of retinol binding protein)
d. Increased excretion
  - Nephritic syndrome

*Clinical features*

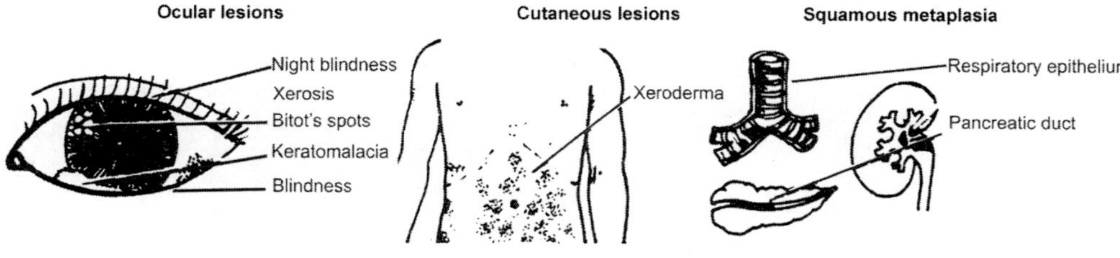


**Fig. 5:** Clinical features of vitamin A deficiency

a. Night blindness
  - Earliest sign
  - Due to failure of retina to adopt to dim light after exposure to bright light because of depletion of all visual purple
b. Xerophthalmia (severe deficiency)
  - Characterized by dryness of conjunctiva and cornea due to progressive keratinization
c. Bitot's spots
  - Small triangular grayish white spots on conjunctiva
d. Keratomalacia
  - Softening of cornea due to ulceration and necrosis leading to perforation, endophthalmitis and blindness
e. Keratinization of epithelial tissue
  - Lacrimal gland cells become keratinized and stop secreting tears
  - Keratinisation occurs in respiratory tract, genitourinary tract and alimentary tract leading to increased incidence of infectious diseases
  - Hyperkeratinization of skin leads to follicular hyperkeratosis of skin (skin appears like toad skin)
f. Anemia
  - Resembling iron deficiency anemia
g. Growth retardation
  - Retarded growth and skeletal abnormalities in children

***Toxicity (hypervitaminosis)***

a. Acute poisoning

  *Causes*
  - Accidental overingestion (after consumption of polar bear liver)

  *Clinical features*
  - Anorexia, nausea, vomiting, abdominal pain, headache, papilledema, diplopia, convulsions, delirium and coma
  - Rise in intracranial pressure, liver enlargement and shedding of skin
  - Infants show budging of frontenels
b. Chronic poisoning

  *Causes*
  - Excessive intake by children
  - Inappropriate therapy

  *Clinical features*
  - Anorexia, dry itching skin, loss of weight, increased irritability, low grade fever, alopecia, dependent edema with erythema and ecchymosis, bleeding, fissuring, refractory skin ulcers, anemia, increased intracranial tension, liver diseases and hepatomegaly
  - Headache and visual upsets are often seen. Joint pains, subcutaneous swellings and tenderness over long bones and bony exostoses
  - Premature closure of epiphysis and consequent growth retardation in children
  - Characteristic skin desquamation (major diagnostic point)

*Contd...*

*Contd...*

| | |
|---|---|
| *Diagnosis*<br>• Impaired dark adoption test<br>• Decreased vitamin A levels in plasma (<20 mg/dL)<br>• Decreased retinol binding protein in plasma<br>*Treatment*<br>• Oral vitamin A supplementation | |

## SHORT ESSAYS

### 3. Composition and function of any two phospholipids.

- Phospholipids are complex lipids containing phosphate as an additional group.

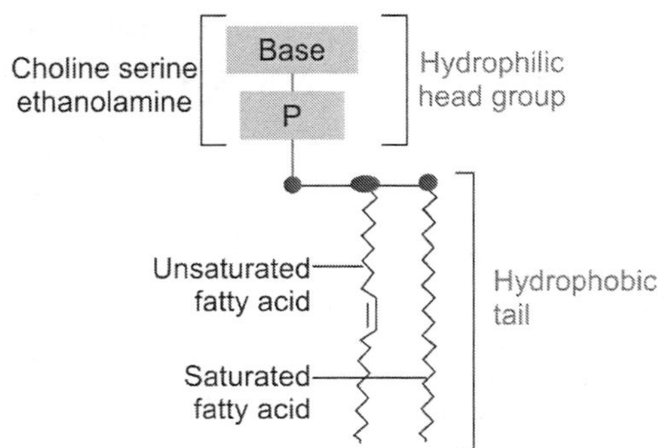


**Fig. 6:** Composition of phospholipids

#### Composition

- Fatty acids
- Phosphate
- Nitrogenous base (choline, serine, ethanolamine)
- Alcohol (glycerol, sphingosine).

#### Types (Based on Type of Alcohol Present)

| *Type* | *Composition* | *Source* | *Function* |
|---|---|---|---|
| **Glycerophospholipids (contain glycerol)** | | | |
| a. Phosphatidylcholine, (Lecithin) | Glycerol, fatty acids, phosphate, choline | Liver and brain | • Components of cell membranes<br>• Blood coagulation<br>• Pulmonary surfactant<br>• Digestion and absorption of fats<br>• Source of choline for acetylcholine<br>• Source of arachidonic acid<br>• Prevention of fatty liver<br>• Component of lipoproteins<br>• Activation of protein kinase C |
| b. Phosphatidyl-ethanolamine (Cephalin) | Fatty acids, glycerol, phosphate, ethanolamine. | All tissues | Similar to phosphatidylcholine (except synthesis of ACh) |
| c. Phosphatidylserine | Fatty acids, glycerol, phosphate, serine | All tissues (mainly in brain) | • Component of cell membrane<br>• Activation of PKC |
| d. Phosphatidylinositol | Fatty acids, glycerol, phosphate, inositol | Brain and nervous tissue | • Constituent of biomembranes<br>• Forms PIP2 which is involved in cell signalling |
| e. Cardiolipin | Diphosphatidylglycerol | Inner mitochondrial membranes | Component of pulmonary surfactant |
| f. Plasmalogens | Alkenyl ether lipids with either ethanolamine or choline | Myelin (Ethanolamine) Heart (Choline) | Components of cell membrane and myelin |
| g. Platelet-activating factor | 2-acetylglycerol-3 phosphocholine | Surface of leukocytes | Mediator of inflammatory reactions, aggregation of platelets |
| **Sphingophospholipid (contain sphingosine)** | | | |
| a. Sphingomyelin | Fatty acid, sphingosine, phosphate, choline | • Major component of nerve cell membrane<br>• Also present in other cell membranes | • Component of myelin<br>• Ceramide (released on degradation of sphingomyelin is an important regulator of cell function (inhibition of DNA synthesis and mediation of apoptosis) |

## Functions

a. Structural
   - Phospholipids participate in the lipoprotein complexes which are thought to constitute the matrix of cell walls and membranes, myelin sheath and of such structures as mitochondria and microsomes.

b. Role in enzyme action
   - Certain enzymes require tightly bound phospholipids for their actions, e.g. mitochondrial enzyme system involved in oxidative phosphorylation.

c. Role in blood coagulation
   - Phospholipids play an essential part in blood coagulation process (at stage of conversion of prothrombin to thrombin by active factorX and activation of factor VIII by activated factor IX).

d. Role in lipid absorption in intestine
   - Lecithin lowers surface tension of water and aids in emulsification of lipid water mixtures, a prerequisite in digestion and absorption of lipids from gastrointestinal tract.

e. Role in transport of lipids from intestines
   - Exogenous triglycerides are carried as lipoprotein complex, chylomicrons.

f. Role in transport of lipids from liver
   - Endogenous triglycerides are carried from liver to various tissues as lipoprotein complex pre-β-lipoprotein (VLDL)
   - Phospholipids are required for formation of lipoprotein complex.

g. Role in electron transport
   - Phospholipids help to couple oxidation with phosphorylation and maintain electron transport enzymes in active conformation and proper relative positions.

h. Lipotropic action of lecithin
   - Choline (in lecithin) acts as a lipotropic agent as it can prevent formation of fatty liver.

i. Membrane phospholipids as source of arachidonic acid
   - Phospholipids of membrane are hydrolyzed by phospholipase A2 to provide unsaturated fatty acid; arachidonic acid, which is utilized for synthesis of prostaglandins and leukotrienes.

j. Insulation
   - Phospholipids of myelin sheaths provide insulation around the nerve fibres.

k. Cofactor
   - Phospholipids are required as a cofactor for activity of the enzyme lipoprotein lipase and triacylglycerol lipase.

l. Role of phosphatidyl inositides metabolite in $Ca^{2+}$ dependent hormone action
   - Some signal must provide communication between hormone receptor on plasma membrane and intracellular $Ca^{2+}$ reservoirs (myo-inositol 1,4, 5-P3 and diacyl glycerol).

## Significance

- Decreased synthesis of pulmonary surfactant (dipalmitoyl lecithin) in newborn results in respiratory distress syndrome
- Decreased metabolism of sphingomyelin due to deficiency of sphinogmyelinase results in Niemann-Pick disease.

## 4. Cell membrane.

- Cell membrane is an limiting membrane surrounding the cells, required for cellular organization and integrity
- Also called plasma membrane.

## Structure (Fluid Mosaic Model)

- Best described by fluid mosaic model proposed by Singer and Nicolson.

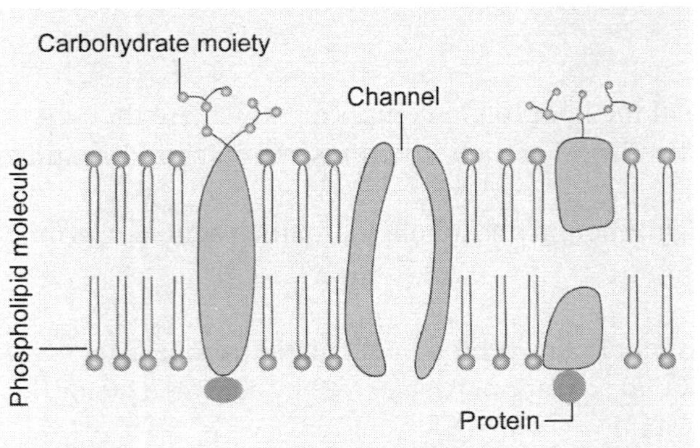


**Fig. 7:** Fluid mosaic model of cell membrane

## Salient Features

- Cell membrane is made up of lipid and protein subunits giving it a mosaic or ceramic tile appearance but unlike a fixed ceramic tile, membrane freely changes hence it is called fluid mosaic model
- Membrane is asymmetric due to irregular distribution of proteins and varies about 5–8 nm in thickness.

| *Arrangement of lipids* | *Arrangement of proteins* |
|---|---|
| • Lipids mainly phospholipids are arrangement is bilayer with hydrophobic tails facing each other in core of bilayer while hydrophilic head facing extra- or intracellularly<br>• Choline-rich phospholipids are located mainly in outer layer whereas inner layer contains phospholipids rich in ethanolamine and serine<br>• Each lipid layer is 2.4 nm thick, head portion accounting for 1 nm and tail portion 1.4 nm<br>• Lipid bilayer shows free lateral movement offering fluidity to membrane, however, inner to outer or outer to inner movement is restricted<br>• Fluidity of membrane is maintained by length of hydrocarbon chain, degree of unsaturation and nature of polar head group (more unsaturated cis fatty acid, more the fluidity) and cholesterol content alters fluidity of membrane (more cholesterol, less the fluidity)<br>• Fluidity enables membrane to perform endocytosis and exocytosis | • Proteins are also arranged in two sets, namely extrinsic (peripheral) and intrinsic (integral) proteins<br>• Peripheral proteins exist on surfaces of lipid bilayer and are loosely attached to polar head of phospholipids by ionic and polar bonds and can be easily removed<br>• Integral proteins are deeply embedded in bilayer and are attached by hydrophobic bonds or van der Waals forces and they require detergents or organic solvents to remove them<br>• Some integral proteins span entire lipid bilayer and are called trans-membrane proteins. They are anchored by embedding hydrophobic side chain of amino acid in hydrophobic central core of lipid bilayer. Such transmembrane proteins serves as receptors, tissue specific antigens, ion channels, membrane based enzymes, etc. |

## Functions

- Required for cellular organization and integrity of cell
- Poses as a barrier for free passage of compounds across it
- Proteins in plasma membrane help in transport of substances in and out of cell
- Transmembrane proteins acts as receptors for many biologically important substances like hormones
- Membrane proteins also play a role in cellular adhesions or cell-cell communications
- Membrane glycoproteins are involved in signaling and cellular regulation
- Aids in compartmentalization
- Plasma membrane is modified for specialized functions.

## 5. Essential amino acids.

- Essential amino acids are amino acids which cannot be synthesized by body and their need has to fulfilled from food
- Also called indispensable amino acids.

**Essential amino acids**

*Any Help In Learning These Little Molecules Proves Truly Valuable*

- ✓ **A**rginine
- ✓ **H**istadine
- ✓ **I**soleucine
- ✓ **L**eucine
- ✓ **T**ryptophan
- ✓ **L**ysine
- ✓ **M**ethionine
- ✓ **P**henylalanine
- ✓ **T**hreonine
- ✓ **V**aline

| Examples | Functions |
|---|---|
| • Arginine (semi-essential)<br>• HIstadine (semi-essential)<br>• Isoleucine<br>• Leucine<br>• Tryptophan<br>• Lysine<br>• Methionine<br>• Phenylalanine<br>• Threonine<br>• Valine | • Essential for normal growth and development<br>• Methionine is essential amino acid for initiating protein synthesis<br>• Methionine's active form SAM is essential for synthesis of creatine, epinephrine, choline and melatonin<br>• Histamine derived from histadine is important mediator of allergic reactions<br>• Phenylalanine is precursor for melanine, catecholamines and thyroxine<br>• Lysine is precursor of carnitine which is essential for β-oxidation of fatty acids<br>• Lysine is component of histone, a basic protein associated with nucleic acids<br>• Arginine is important intermediate of urea cycle<br>• Arginine is precursor of nitric oxide<br>• Tryptophan is precursor for serotonin, a neurotransmitter |

## Significance

- Carbon skeleton of these amino acids cannot be synthesized in humans and hence they need to be supplied through dietary sources
- However, arginine and histidine can be synthesized in adults but need to be supplied to children hence called semi-essential amino acids.

## 6. Enumerate ketone bodies. How they are formed?

Refer Question No. 1 June 2011 (RS2).

## 7. Phenylketonuria.

Refer Question No. 1 Dec. 2010 (RS2).

## 8. Regulation of blood calcium level.

Refer Question No. 2 June 2009 (RS2).

## 9. Catabolism of purines and related disorders.

Refer Question No. 2 June 2007 (RS2).

## 10. Post-transcriptional modifications.

- Post-transcriptional modifications are series of alterations in RNA formed from DNA during transcription (primary transcripts or heteronuclear mRNA or hnRNA) to make it mature.

## Intracellular Site

- Nucleoplasm

## Types

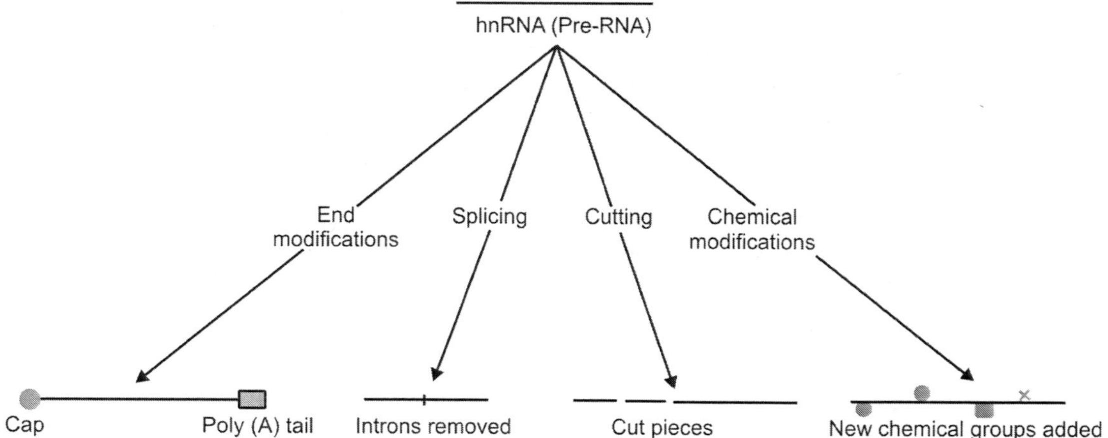


**Fig. 8:** Types of postranscriptional modifications

| Poly-A tailing at 3′ end | Capping at 5′ end | Methylations | Removal of introns |
|---|---|---|---|
| • Enzyme RNA endonuclease cleaves primary transcript at a position about 15 bases 3′ to a sequence AAUAAA which is a cleavage signal<br>• To this newly formed 3′ terminus, adenine nucleotides are added numbering about 20–250 which is called as poly-A tail which stabilizes mRNA and protects it from 3′ exonuclease | • 5′ end of mRNA is capped with 7-methyl guanosine triphosphate using an unusual 5′→ 5′ triphosphate linkage<br>• Helps in stablilizing mRNA and is required for translation | • Internal nucleotides of mRNA are methylated usually N6 of adenine residue and 2′-hydroxyl group of ribose | • A primary transcript consists of exons which posses genetic code and are responsible for protein biosynthesis interspersed with introns which do not code for any protein biosynthesis<br>• Junction of these exons-introns in hnRNA contain specific recognition areas called as consensus sequence which are cleaved by an energy consuming process called as splicing using small nuclear ribonucleoprotein particles (snRNPs) |

## Significance

- Post-transcriptional modification is an important step in nucleic acid metabolism as it stabilizes RNA and makes it worthy of acting as template for protein biosynthesis (gene expression).

## 11. Acute intermittent porphyria.

Refer Question No. 9 June 2015 (RS2).

## 12. Role of kidney in regulation of blood pH.

Refer Question No. 2 June 2012 (RS2).



## SHORT ANSWERS

## 13. Formation of ammonia and its toxicity in brain.

### Formation of Ammonia

a. From amino acids
   – Transdeamination (transamination followed by oxidative deamintion)
      - Major source of ammonia
      - Occurs in cytoplasm of hepatocytes
      - All amino acids are transaminated to glutamate followed by deamination by glutamate dehydrogenase
   – Nonoxidative deamination
      - Hydroxy amino acids like serine and threonine are undergo nonoxidative deamination by enzyme dehydratase to form corresponding keto acids and ammonia

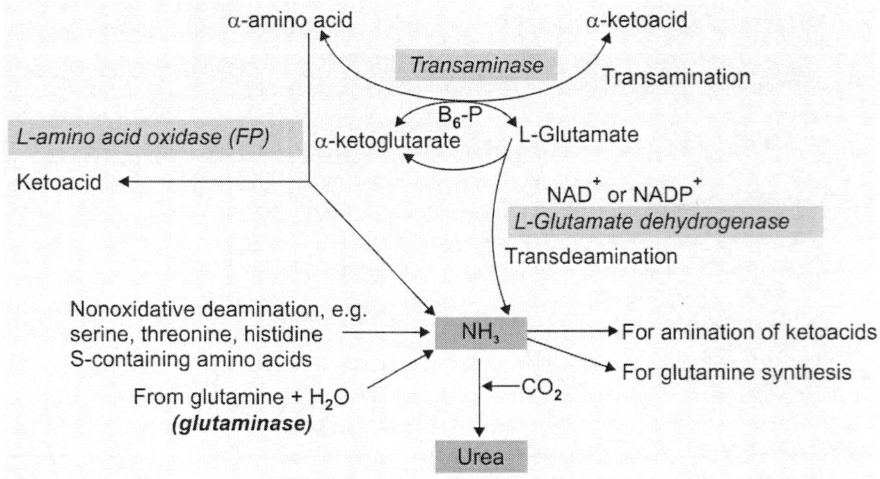


**Fig. 9:** Formation of ammonia

- Oxidation deamination
  - 2 enzymes D-amino acid oxides and L-amino acid oxides, oxidize amino acids to corresponding ketoacids and liberates free ammonia. They utilize FAD and FMN respectively

b. From pyramidine catabolism
c. Direct absorption from intestine
   - Considerable quantity of NH3 is produced in gut by intestinal bacterial flora, both from dietary proteins and from urea present in fluids secreted into GIT by action of enzyme urease.

## Ammonia Toxicity

- Normal blood level of NH3 is about 40–70 μg/dL
- Even marginal elevation in ammonia level is toxic to brain.

| *Effects* | *Mechanism* |
|---|---|
| • Slurring of speech<br>• Blurring of vision<br>• Flapping tremors<br>• Convulsions, coma and death | • Accumulation of ammonia results in more utilization α-ketoglutarate to form glutamate thus reducing levels of α-ketoglutarate (key intermediate of TCA cycle) resulting in impairment of TCA cycle leading to reduced ATP production<br>• Increased ammonia concentration enhances glutamine formation from glutamate thus reduces brain cell pool of glutamic acid; hence there is decreased formation of GABA (an inhibitory neurotransmitter)<br>• Rise in brain glutamine level enhances outflow of glutamine from brain cell using same co-transporter which imports tryphophan into brain thus leading to increased levels of tryptophan into brain cells causing increased synthesis of serotonin, a neurotransmitter |

## Fate of Ammonia

- Converted to urea (urea cycle)
- Formation of glutamine
- Amination of α-ketoacid to form α-amino acid.

## Significance

- In normal healthy person, liver promptly removes the ammonia from portal blood, so that blood leaving liver is virtually ammonia free
- This is essential since even small quantities of ammonia are toxic to CNS
- Hepatic encephalopathy is a complication of chronic liver disease due to ammonia.

## 14. What is zymogen? Give examples of zymogen.

- Zymogens are proenzymes which are converted to active form by some enzymatic activation by various proteolytic enzymes.

## Activation

- They are acted upon by proteolytic enzymes resulting in splitting of a single peptide bond or removal of a small polypeptide resulting in unmasking of active center on the enzyme.

*Examples*

| *Zymogen* | *Active enzyme* | *Activator* |
|---|---|---|
| • Pepsinogen | Pepsin | HCl |
| • Trypsinogen | Trypsin | Enteropeptidase |
| • Chymotrypsinogen | Chymotrypsin | Trypsin |
| • Procarboxypeptidase | Carboxypeptidase | Trypsin |
| • Proelastase | Elastase | Trypsin |

## Significance

- Most of proteolytic enzymes of GIT are secreted as zymogens to prevent autolysis of cellular structural proteins and activated in alimentary canal.

## 15. Diagrammatic representation of mitochondrial electron transport chain and location of ATP formation sites.

Refer Question No. 5 June 2007 (RS2).

## 16. Mechanism of carcinogenesis.

- Carcinogenesis means induction of cancer.

## Mechanism of Carcinogenesis

- Carcinogenesis is a complex interplay of various factors as shown below:

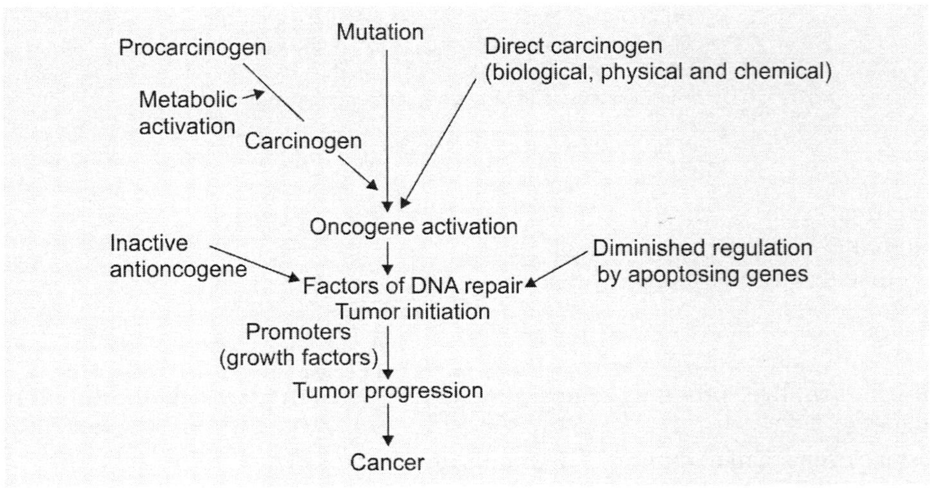


**Fig. 10:** Mechanism of carcinogenesis

## 17. Give two examples of detoxification by oxidation and reduction.

Refer Question No. 7 Dec. 2005 (RS2).

## 18. What is complete protein?

- Complete protein is protein containing all ten essential amino acids in required proportion by human body to promote growth
- Also called first class proteins
- Their biological value is high.

*Example*

- Egg albumin (biological value = 95)
- Milk casein (biological value = 75)

**19. Enumerate sources of atoms of purine ring by a diagrammatic representation.**

Refer Question No. 2 June 2013 (RS2).

**20. Give four characteristic feature of genetic code.**

Refer Question No. 2 June 2011 (RS2).

**21. What is recombinant DNA?**

Refer Question No. 2 June 2008 (RS2).

**22. Clinical interpretation of estimation of thyroid stimulating hormone (TSH) in blood.**

- Thyroid stimulating hormone is a regulatory hormone secreted by hypothalamus.

## Estimation of TSH in Blood

- Normal level is 1 mU/ml
- Levels are raised in primary hypothyroidism
- Levels are undetectable in hyperthyroidism.

# MBBS PHASE I EXAMINATION
## JUNE 2010
### (Revised Scheme 2)

## LONG ESSAYS

### 1. Discuss in detail oxidative phosphorylation and enumerate its inhibitors.

- Oxidative phosphorylation is production of ATP by combining ADP and Pi using energy produced by flow of electron from NADPH (or FAD) to molecular oxygen in electron transport chain of mitochondria.

#### Sites of Oxidative Phosphorylation (ATP Synthesis)

- Synthesis of a molecule of ATP requires about of 7.3 Kcal/mol and there are such 3 sites where energy produced is sufficient to bind a phosphate to ADP.

| *Site* | *Reaction* | *Energy* |
|---|---|---|
| Site I | NADH → CoQ | 12 Kcal/mol |
| Site II | Cyt B → Cyt C | 10 Kcal/mol |
| Site III | Cyt $aa_3$ → ½$O_2$ | 24 Kcal/mol |

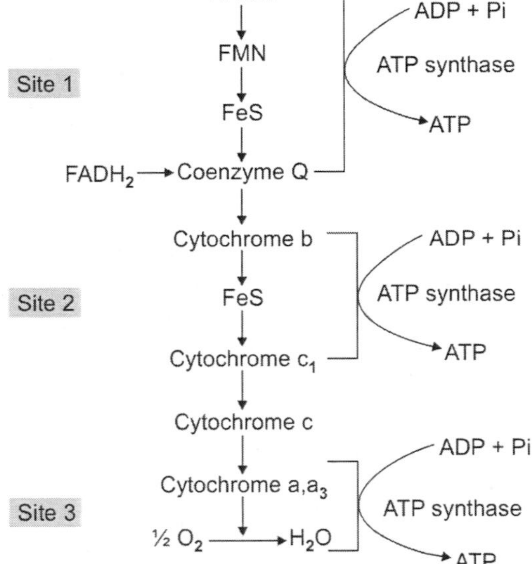

**Fig. 1:** Oxidative phosphorylation—sites

#### Mechanism (Chemiosmotic Theory)

- Mitchell's chemiosmotic theory best explains mechanism of oxidative phosphorylation.

#### Principle

- According to it, electron transfer in respiratory chain is coupled with phosphorylation of ADP provided
- Inner mitochondrial membrane is intact (so that protons can enter mitochondria by process coupled with ATP synthesis)
- Accumulation of high concentration of protons on outside of inner mitochondrial membrane (thus creating an electrochemical potential difference or proton gradient).

#### Process

- Enzyme complexes of respiratory chain, namely complex I, III and IV acts as a proton pump pumping 2, 1 and 2 protons for every 1 electron transported respectively
- This proton pumping is coupled with formation of ATP by ATP synthase (complex V), a membrane located enzyme
- This ATP synthase complex consist of:
  - Several proteins collectively known as Fi subunit which project into matrix and contain ATP synthase
  - A membrane protein subunit known as Fo which serves as a stalk for attachment of Fi and forms a channel for protons to move back into mitochondria
  - Oligomycin sensitivity conferring protein factor connecting Fo and Fi subunits.

## Steps

Passing of $H^+$ through Fo-Fi complex
↓
Translocation of $H^+$ into matrix by subunit Fo
↓
Conformational change in Fi subunit
↓
Coordination of Fo-Fi subunits couples disappearance of proton gradient with ATP synthesis
↓
ATP synthesis

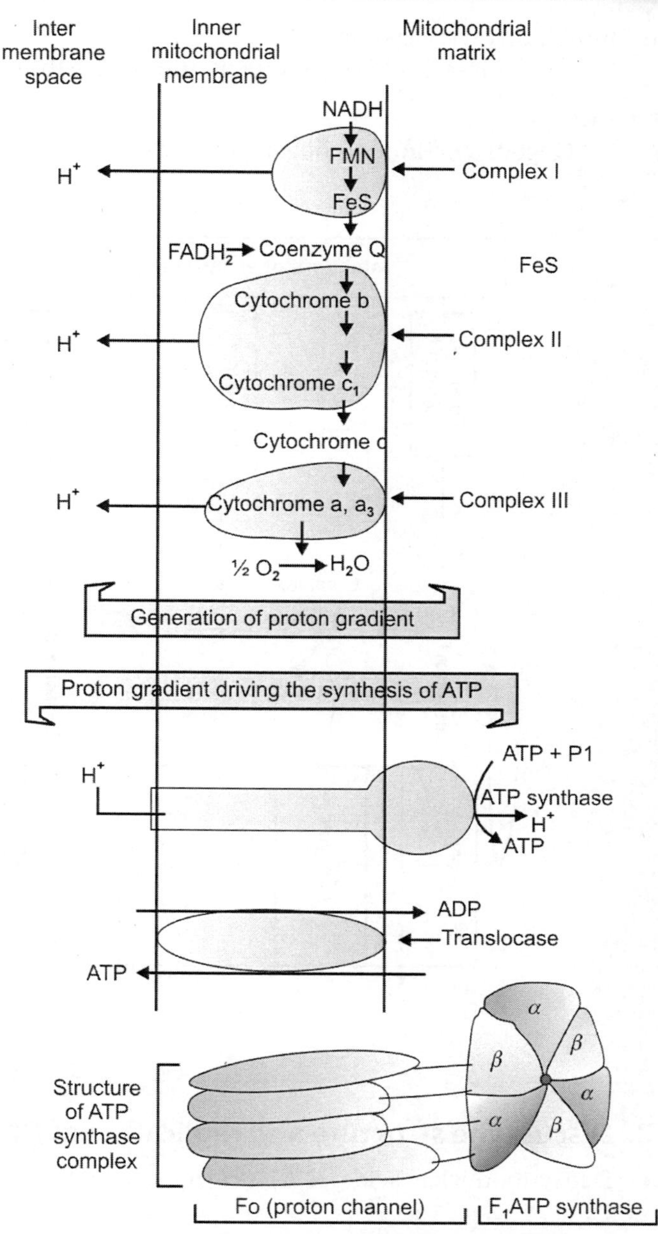


**Fig. 2:** Oxidative phosphorylation—mechanism (chemiosmotic theory)

## Inhibitors of Oxidative Phosphorylation

- Substances inhibiting synthesis of ATP.

## Types

a. Inhibitors of electron transport
b. Uncouplers
c. Inhibitors of ATP/ADP transport
d. Inhibitors of ATP synthase

a. Inhibitors of electron transport
   - Substances preventing transfer of electron in respiratory chain by inhibiting enzyme complexes.

*Examples*

| *Complexes* | *ATP synthesis site* | *Inhibitors* |
|---|---|---|
| i. Complex I | Site I (between NADH and CoQ) | • Rotenone (fish poison)<br>• Amytal (barbiturate) |
| ii. Complex III | Site II (Between cyt b and c1) | • Antimycin A (antibiotic)<br>• British Anti Lewisite (chelating agent) |
| iii. Complex IV | Site 3 (Inhibitor of cytochrome oxidase) | • Carbon dioxide<br>• Cyanide<br>• Hydrogen sulphide |

b. Uncouplers
   - Substances delinking symobiosis between oxidative phosphorylation and electron flow in electron.

*Examples*

| *Physiological* | *Chemical (acts as a transmembrane proton carrier thus collapsing proton gradient)* |
|---|---|
| • Thermogenin<br>• Thyroxine<br>• Long chain free fatty acids | • 2,4 dinitrophenol<br>• Dinitrocresol<br>• Pentachlorophenol<br>• Triflurocarbonylcyanide phenylhydrazone (FCCP)<br>• Valinomycin |

c. Inhibition of ATP/ADP transport system
   - Substances inhibiting ADP-ATP translocase

*Example*
   - Atractyloside.

June 2010 (RS2)

d. Inhibition of ATP synthase
   - Substances inhibiting flow of protons acting through a protein present in Fo-Fi stalk

   *Example*
   - Oligomycin (inhibits oligomycin sensitivity conferring protein factor).

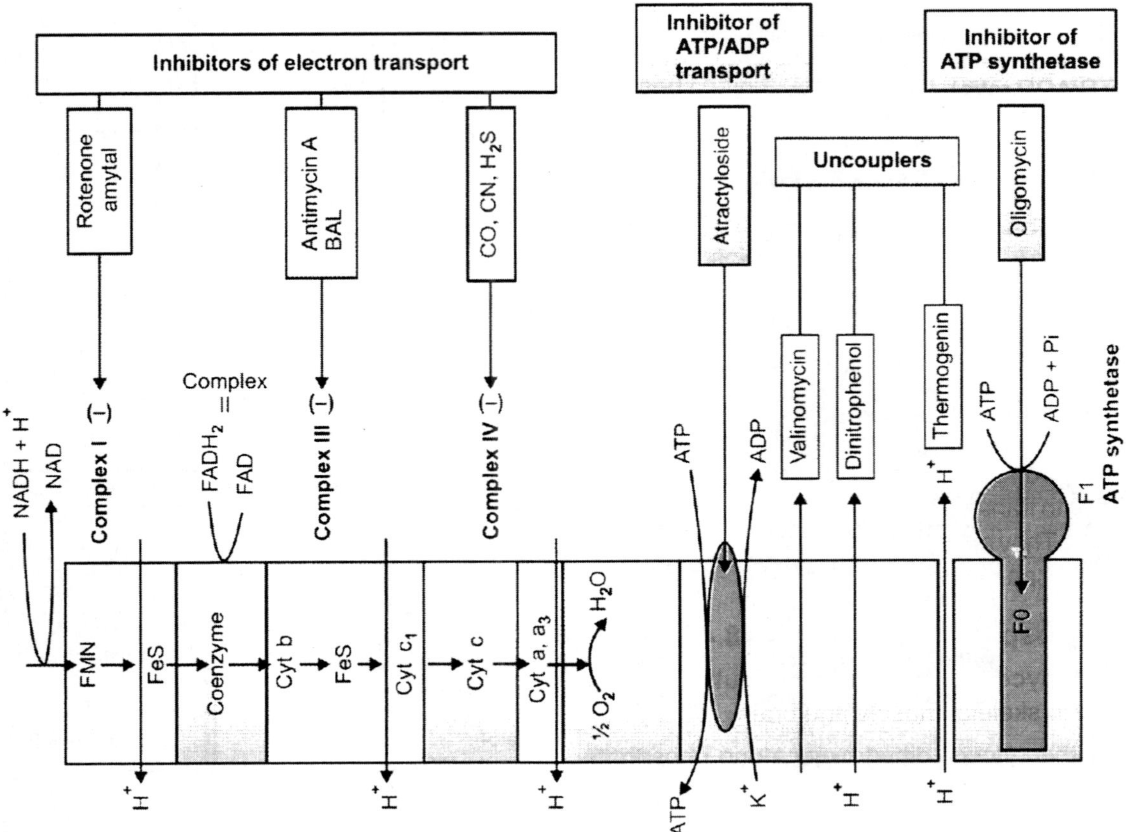


**Fig. 3:** Oxidative phosphorylation—inhibitors

## 2. Discuss the structure and replication of DNA.

- Deoxyribonucleic acid (DNA) is carrier of genetic information.

### Location

- Nucleus of all cells
- Mitochondria (in small quantity).

### Structure

| *Primary structure* | *Secondary structure (Watson Crick model, 1962)* |
|---|---|
| • Each DNA is a polymer of about four different types of deoxyribonucleotides namely:<br>– Adenine deoxyribonucleotide<br>– Thyamine deoxyribonucleotide<br>– Guanine deoxyribonucleotide<br>– Cytosine deoxyribonucleotide<br>• These deoxyribonucleotides are combined through 3′– 5′ phosphodiestic bonds to polymerise into a long chain | • DNA is in form of a right handed double helix formed by twisting of 2 polydeoxyribonucleotide chains held together by hydrogen bonds between bases (2 bonds between A and T and 3 bonds between C and G)<br>• Both strands are complementary to each other by maintaining base pairing rule, i.e. A bonds with T only by 2 hydrogen bonds and C bonds G with 3 hydrogen bonds<br>• Both strands run antiparallel direction, i.e. one strand runs in 5′– 3′ direction while other in 3′ – 5′ direction<br>• Spiral has a pitch of 3.4 nm per turn and each turn shows 10 base pairs<br>• Width of helix is 2 nm |

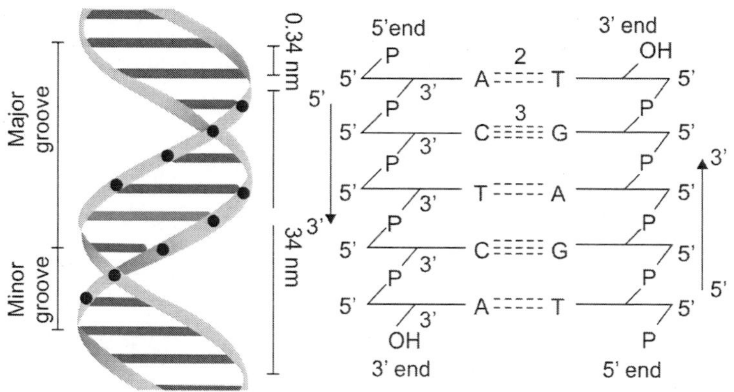


**Fig. 4:** Structure of DNA

## Functions

- Carrying genetic information from parents to offsprings
- Expression of genetic information by protein synthesis through mRNA synthesis.

## Replication (DNA Synthesis)

- An important aspect of inheritance and integral component of central dogma of life
- Called semi-conservative replication because a single strand of a double stranded DNA acts as template for synthesis of second strand resulting in formation of a double helical DNA molecules each of which is composed of a parental strand and newly synthesized daughter strand
- This is possible due to complementary nature of one DNA strand to another
- In eukaryotes, replication begins at a specific site along DNA helix called origin and then 2 strands unwind and separate forming a replication fork
- Then replication or DNA synthesis by insertion of deoxyribonucleotides in 5' → 3' direction (because DNA polymerase can add a nucleotide only to 3' end of a DNA strand).

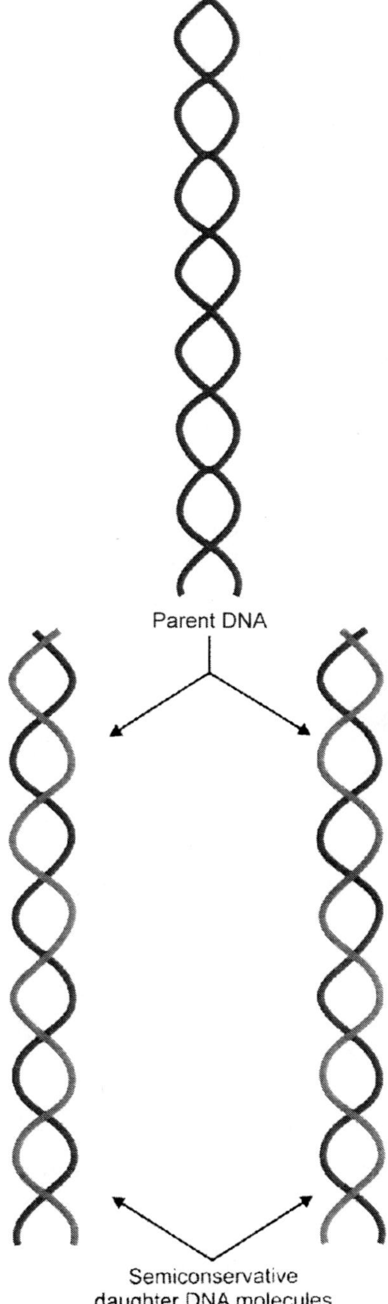


**Fig. 5:** Semiconservative replication of DNA

## Requirement

a. Template
   - Parental DNA strand
b. Nucleotides
   i. Deoxyribonucleotides (for complementary DNA synthesis)
      - dATP, dGTP, dCTP and dTTP
   ii. Ribonucleotides (for RNA primer synthesis)
      - ATP, GTP, CTP and UTP
c. Enzymes
   i. Helicase (catalyzes unwinding of DNA)
   ii. Topoisomerases (relieve torsion due to supercoiling by braking and resealing DNA strands)
      - Topoisomerase I
      - Topoisomerase II
   iii. DNA polymerases
      - DNA polymerase $\alpha$-multisubunit enzyme (synthesis of RNA primer and initiation of replication)

- DNA polymerase β (DNA repair)
- DNA polymerase γ (mitochondrial DNA replication and proofreading)
- DNA polymerase δ (proofreading and replication of lagging strand)
- DNA polymerase ε (proofreading and DNA repair)

iv. RNAse H1 (removal of RNA primer)
v. FEN-1 (removal of last ribonucleotide of RNA primer)
vi. DNA ligase (linking of nucleotides between 2 fragments)
vii. Telomerases (synthesis of telomere)

d. Accessory proteins
  i. RPA protein (maintenance of DNA in single strand)
  ii. PCNA (clumping of DNA polymerase δ to DNA during replication)
  iii. RFC (helps loading PCNA onto DNA)

**Steps**

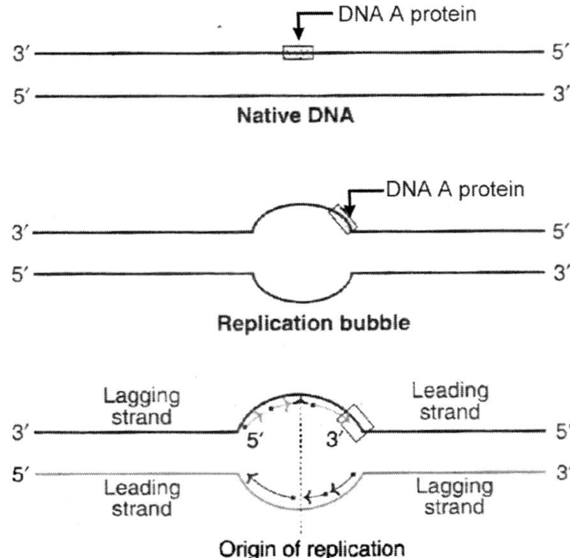


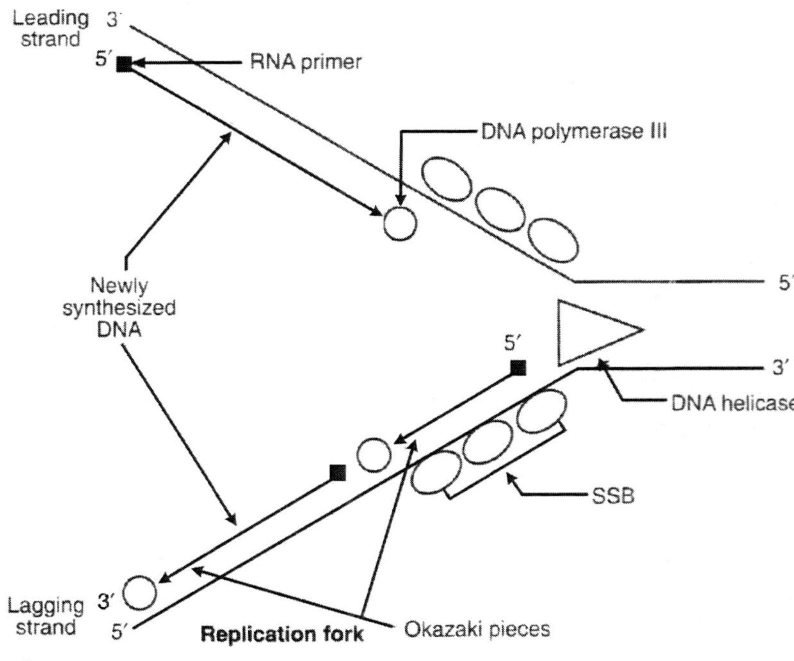


**Fig. 6:** Steps of replication

a. Unwinding of double-stranded DNA
   - DNA helicases binds near fork forcing the strands apart using energy provided by ATP
   - This separation is maintained by helix destabilizing proteins or replication protein A.
b. Relaxation of supercoiled DNA
   - As replication proceeds, DNA becomes positively supercoiled downstream from fork
   - This supercoiling constraints are relieved by DNA topoisomerase which remove superhelicity and produce negative supercoiling and underwinding
   - Topoisomerase I relaxes supercoiling by causing single strand break (nicking of one strand) and resealing it after it winds one turn
   - Topoisomerase II breaks both stands of DNA by using energy provided by ATP
c. Synthesis of small RNA primer
   - Short piece of RNA (5–12 nucleotide long) is synthesized by primase activity of DNA polymerase $\alpha$
   - These are inserted in leading strand (one) and lagging strand (for each Okazaki fragment)
   - This RNA primer enhances efficiency of proofreading at the end of DNA synthesis
d. Synthesis of complementary DNA strands
   - DNA polymerase is responsible for synthesis of DNA synthesis by reading parental strand in 3' - 5' direction and synthesizing new DNA in 5' - 3' direction
   - Therefore, 2 newly synthesized stretches of nucleotide chains grow in opposite direction
   - Strand that is being copied in direction of advancing fork is called leading strand and is synthesized continuously (hence also called continuous strand)
   - Other strand is called lagging strand and is synthesized in fragments (1,000–5,000 base pair long) called Okazaki fragments, which eventually join to become single continuous strand
   - As each deoxyribonucleoside triphosphate is joined, a pyrophosphate is released so that only dAMP, dGTP and dTTP are incorporated
e. Removal and replacement of RNA primer with deoxyribonucleotides
   - RNA primer blocks further synthesis of DNA strand
   - Then, RNA primer is removed by RNAse H1 and FEN-1 protien
   - Gap is filled by synthesis of DNA polymerase $\alpha$ and $\delta$
f. Joining of DNA fragments
   - DNA ligase fills gaps between DNA strand filling RNA primer and leading strand or gaps between Okazaki fragments on lagging strands
   - It catalyzes formation of phosphodiester bond between 3' hydroxyl at the end of one DNA segment and 5' hydroxyl group at the end of another DNA segment by using ATP yielded energy
g. Proofreading and correction of mismatched bases
   - DNA polymerase has proofreading activity by its 3'–5' exonucleases and checks to make sure that bases added are complementary to template (parent DNA) otherwise they are removed and replaced by correct bases
h. Telomerer replication
   - Telomere is a non-informational repeat sequence at the end of a chromosome (sequence in humans—GGGTTA)
   - It is replicated by enzyme telomerase
   - Telomere allows replication of linear DNA to its full length thus preventing shortening of chromosomal DNA, i.e. loss of genetic information.

## Inhibitors of Replication

- Substances interfering of DNA synthesis are mostly used as anticancer or antiviral drugs.

*Examples*

| *Drug* | *Mechanism* |
|---|---|
| • Methotrexate | Competitive inhibition of dihydrofolate reductase<br>Inhibition of synthesis of purine and pyramidine nucleotides |
| • 5-fluorouracil | Suicide inhibition of thymidylate synthetase Inhibition of dTMP synthesis |
| • 6-mercaptopurine | Inhibit synthesis of purine nucleotides |

| | |
|---|---|
| • Acyclovir | Inhibits DNA polymerase (Herpes) |
| • Zidovudine | Inhibits DNA polymerase (HIV) |
| • Cytosine arbinoside | Inhibits replication |
| • Daunorubicin and doxorubicin | Inhibit replication |
| • Actinomycin D | Inhibit replication |
| • Cyclophosphamide, nitrogen mustard | Cross linking of DNA |
| • Cisplatin | Cross linking of DNA |
| • Etoposide | Topoisomerase inhibitor (in eukaryotes) |
| • Nalidixic acid | Topoisomerase inhibitor (in bacteria) |

### Significance

- Replication is a unique process of transfer of genetic information by which new daughter DNA is synthesis while preserving old parent DNA (semiconservative method)
- Any error in replication results in loss of genetic information, mutation and cellular death due nonexpression of genetic information.

## SHORT ESSAYS

### 3. Glycogenolysis.

Refer Question No. 1 June 2007 (RS2).

### 4. Transmethylation reactions.

- Transmethylation reactions are reactions involving transfer of methyl group (-$CH_3$) to an acceptor from a methyl donor.

### Methyl Donor

- Active methionine (SAM/S-adenosylmethionine).

### Reaction

S-adenosylmethionine + Acceptor $\xrightarrow{\text{Methyl transferase}}$ Methylated product + S-adenosylhomocysteine

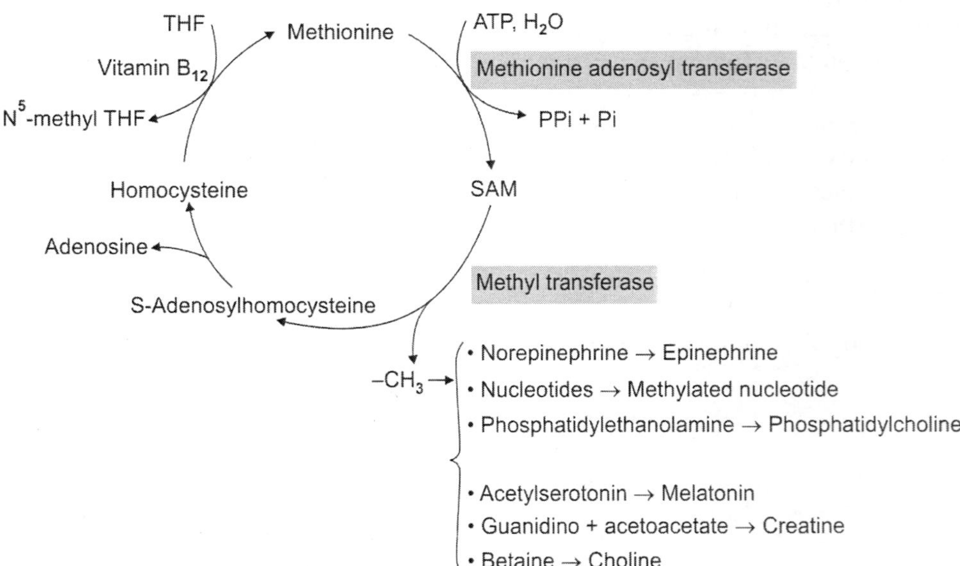


**Fig. 7:** Transmethylation reaction

*Examples*

| *Methyl group acceptor* | *Methylated product* |
|---|---|
| • Norepinephrine | Epinephrine |
| • Guanidoacetate | Creatine |
| • Ethanolamine | Choline |
| • Serine | Choline |
| • Acetyl serotonin | Melatonin |

## Significance

- Many compounds become functionally active only after methylation
- Protects proteins from immediate degradation thus helps to control protein turnover.

## 5. Metabolism of chylomicrons.

Refer Question No. 6 June 2005 (RS2).

## 6. Noncompetitive enzyme inhibition.

Refer Question No. 3 June 2007 (RS2).

## 7. Rappaport Leubering cycle.

- Rappaport Leubering cycle is a supplementary pathway of glucose oxidation operating in erythrocytes to produce 2,3-bisphosphoglycerate
- It occurs in RBCs in a unique fashion as to bypass glycerophosphate kinase reaction, whereas rest of glycolysis proceeds normally
- Also called as 2,3-bisphosphoglycerate pathway.

| *Principle organ* | *Intracellular site* | *Substrate* | *Product* |
|---|---|---|---|
| • Erythrocytes | • Cytosol | • 1,3-bisphosphoglycerate | • 3-phosphoglycerate |

## Pathway

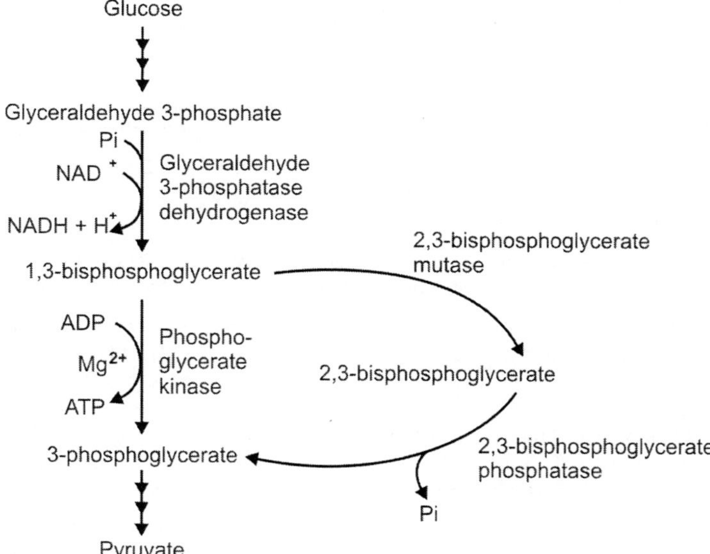


**Fig. 8:** Rapaport Leubering cycle

## Significance

a. Produces 2,3-bisphosphoglycerate
   - This pathway yield 2,3-bisphosphoglycerate which is essential for oxygen carrying function of RBCs
   - 2,3-bisphosphoglycerate when combined with hemoglobin, reduces its oxygen affinity thus helping unloading of oxygen at tissue level
   - The amount of glucose metabolized through this pathway is increased in conditions leading to hypoxia like high altitude to increase production of 2,3-bisphosphoglycerate.

b. Loss of 2 ATPs per glucose
   - As in this step, step 6 of glycolysis is bypassed, ATP produced by substrate level phosphorylation is not produced thus eventually resulting in loss of 2 ATPs per glucose molecule
   - However, only 15–25% of glucose is metabolized through this pathway.

## 8. Deficiency manifestations of vitamin A.

Refer Question No. 2 Dec. 2009 (RS2).

## 9. Protein-energy malnutrition.

- Protein-energy malnutrition is most common nutritional disorder of developing countries.



### Causes

| *Primary* | *Secondary* |
|---|---|
| • An insufficient intake of food causing undernutrition<br>• Insufficient intake of one or more of the essential nutrients, specially proteins | • Inadequate absorption or utilization of essential nutrients<br>• Increase in requirement, destruction or excretion of certain nutrients |

### Types

| | *Marasmus* | *Kwashiorkor* | *Marasmic-kwashiorkor* |
|---|---|---|---|
| • Cause | Severe deficiency of both dietary energy and proteins | Due to diet very low in proteins | |
| • Features | Characterized by muscle wasting with normal serum protein levels | Characterized by edema with decreased serum albumin levels | Features of both marasmus and kwashirokor, i.e. muscle wasting and edema |

### Features

| *Features* | *Marasmus* | *Kwashiorkor* |
|---|---|---|
| a. Definition | • PEM arising due to diet deficient in energy and protein<br>• Most common in tropics—result of starvation in small children | • PEM occurring due to diet very low in proteins |
| b. Mechanism | • Diet may be adequate in qualitative term but insufficient in calories for rapidly growing child | • Diet very low in proteins but provides enough calories to satisfy need of the child |
| c. Causes | • Exclusively breastfed infant of a malnourished mother (milk supply is grossly reduced)<br>• Prolonged breastfeeding with inadequate supplementation of other foods<br>• Artificial feeds (inadequate, less nutritive in proteins and calories)<br>• Fear of diarrhea (less feeding) | • Premature termination of breastfeeding<br>• Use of over diluted milk<br>• Artificially fed and weaned children (occurs weeks or months after weaning)<br>• Feeding of low quality proteins (cereal grains, starchy foods and roots)<br>• No milk, eggs, etc. |
| d. Predisposing factors | • Premature babies<br>• Local diseases<br>• Malformations of mouth and nose (interfere with adequate feeding) | • Infectious diseases like acute diarrhea, respiratory infections, measles (add to deterioration of diet, poorer utilization, and higher requirement) |
| e. Age | • Infants (less than one year) | • Older children (usually 2nd or 3rd year of life) |

*Contd...*

*Contd...*

| *Features* | *Marasmus* | *Kwashiorkor* |
|---|---|---|
| f. Clinical features: | | |
| i. Growth | • Mild retarded growth (child is grossly emaciated, and underweight)<br>• Depleted of subcutaneous fats with muscle | • Server retardation in growth and development<br>• Child is not emaciated rather looks blown up due to edema |
| ii. Muscles | • Muscle wasting (characteristic) | • Weak and atrophic |
| iii. Behavior | • Very hungry and cries continuously | • Apathy and anorexia (early manifestations)<br>• Child is less lively and refuses to eat |
| iv. Diarrhea and vomiting | • Frequent small dark green mucus stools of "hunger diarrhea" (aggravates disease further)<br>• Vomiting more common | • Diarrhea almost always present and becomes chronic and remittent |
| v. Skin and mucous membranes | • Skin is thin, attached to bone, flaccid and wrinkled<br>• Bony prominences are marked<br>• Mucous membranes of mouth are usually reddish | • Skin lesions although not always present are very characteristic, patches of hyperpigmentation exfoliation, desquamation and ulceration are seen in skin of legs, buttocks and perineum<br>• Unlike marasmus, some subcutaneous fats are present |
| vi. Edema | • Absent | • Pitting edema (main clinical characteristic for diagnosis)<br>• Soft and painless, usually first affects legs and then spreads to upper extremities and face |
| vii. Hairs and facies | • Hairs usually thin and lustreless<br>• Typical face of marasmic child compared to "little monkey | • Hairs usually dry and thin<br>• Black hairs become brown or reddish yellow and sometimes even white<br>• Depigmented hairs alternate with more pigmented hairs (Flag sign)<br>• "Moon facies" |
| g. Water and electrolyte balance | • Dehydration and electrolytes imbalance (due excessive diarrhea and vomiting) | • Dehydration and electrolytes imbalance (due excessive diarrhea and vomiting) |
| h. Biochemical findings | • Serum albumin almost normal (2–3 g/dL)<br>• Blood urea level normal<br>• Serum cortisol increased<br>• Fasting glucose reduced<br>• Serum $K^+$ normal | • Serum albumin markedly reduced (0.5–2 g/dL)<br>• Blood urea level reduced<br>• Serum cortisol normal or decreased<br>• Fasting glucose reduced<br>• Serum $K^+$ decreased |



## 10. Extracellular buffers.

Refer Question No. 2 June 2012 (RS2).

## 11. Functions of selenium.

- Selenium is a trace element.

| *Dietary sources* | *Daily requirement* | *Normal serum level* | *Location* |
|---|---|---|---|
| • Meat, sea food, liver, kidney and plants | • 50–100 µg/day | • 50–100 µg/dL | • Liver, testes |

### Functions

a. Antioxidant functions
   - Nonspecific intracellular antioxidant complementary to vitamin E preventing hepatic necrosis and muscular dystrophy
   - Prevents lipid peroxidation and protects cell against free radicals
   - Component of glutathione peroxidase (present in abundance in RBCs) which decomposes organic peroxides and hydrogen peroxides thus suppresses oxidative stress in erythrocytes.

b. Metabolic functions
   - Present in 5 deiodinase which converts thyroxin to $T_3$
   - Present in thioredoxin reductase, an enzyme involved in purine nucleotide metabolism
   - Binds to heavy metals, preventing their toxicity.

c. Others
   - Maintains structural integrity of biological membranes
   - Necessary for normal development of spermatozoa
   - Selenocysteine can be considered 21st amino acid with genetic code UGA (a termination codon) which is inserted into selenium-containing enzymes.

### Significance

| | *Deficiency* | *Toxicity (selenosis)* |
|---|---|---|
| Causes | • Low soil content<br>• Parenteral nutrition<br>• Malnutirition | • Handling of metal polishes, antirust compounds |
| Clinical features | • Hypothyroidism, liver necrosis, cirrhosis, cardiomyopathy and muscular dystrophy | • Hair loss, falling of nail, diarrhea, weight loss and garlicky odor in breath |

## 12. Acute phase proteins.

- Acute phase proteins are certain plasma proteins secreted as a nonspecific response to stimulus of infection, injury, inflammation or cancer.

| *Examples* | *Role* |
|---|---|
| • C-reactive protein<br>• $\alpha_1$ antitrypsin<br>• Ceruloplasmin<br>• $\alpha_2$ macroglobulin<br>• Complement proteins<br>• Mannose binding lectin<br>• Haptoglobin<br>• Fibrinogen | • Acute phase proteins help in modulation of inflammatory response in following ways:<br>– By stimulating complement activity<br>– Opsonization and emacrophagic phagocytosis<br>– Inactivation of proteases released by bacteria |

### Significance

- Estimation of acute phase proteins is important for evaluation of acute phase response
- It also helps to note response of body to treatment or surgery.

Revised Scheme 2

# SHORT ANSWERS

## 13. Nutritional classification of amino acids.

- Amino acids are a group of organic compounds containing two functional groups—amino and carboxyl.

### Classification Based on Nutritional Requirment

- Nutritional classification of amino acids based on their requirement by body into three classes.

| *Essential amino acids* | *Semiessential amino acids* | *Nonessential amino acids* |
|---|---|---|
| Amino acids which cannot be synthesized by body and their need has to fulfilled from food | Amino acids which can be synthesized by adults from nonessential amino acids | Amino acids which can be synthesized in body and hence need not be supplied in diet |
| • Phenylalanine<br>• Tryptophan<br>• Threonine<br>• Lysine<br>• Leucine<br>• Isoleucine<br>• Methionine<br>• Valine | • Arginine<br>• Histidine | • Glycine<br>• Alanine<br>• Serine<br>• Cysteine<br>• Aspartate<br>• Aspargine<br>• Glutamate<br>• Glutamine<br>• Tyrosine<br>• Proline |

## 14. Significance of serum amylase.

- Amylase is a carbohydrate splitting enzyme.

| *Reaction catalyzed* | *Sources* | *Normal serum level* |
|---|---|---|
| • Hydrolysis of α (1–4) glycosidic bond of starch to produce maltose, maltotriose and limit dextrins | • Pancreas, salivary gland | • 50–120 U/L (80–180 somogy units/dL) |

### Significance

- Estimation of serum amylase helps in diagnosis of pancreatic and salivary gland disorders.

| *Serum level >1000 times* | *Serum level <1000 times* |
|---|---|
| • Acute pancreatitis (investigation of choice)—peak value within 8–12 hours | • Mumps<br>• Parotitis<br>• Salivary duct stone<br>• Chronic pancreatitis<br>• Pancreatic carcinoma<br>• Obstruction to pancreatic duct |

## 15. Endoplasmic reticulum.

- Endoplasmic reticulum is network of interconnecting membranes enclosing channels or cisternae extending from outer nuclear membrane to outer plasma membrane.

### Types

| | *Rough endoplasmic reticulum* | *Smooth endoplasmic reticulum* |
|---|---|---|
| Features | • Studded with ribosomes on cytoplasmic side giving it a granular appearance | • Does not contain ribosomes |
| Functions | • Protein biosynthesis by ribosomes located on them<br>• Post-translational modifications of proteins such as glycosylation | • Synthesis of lipids (phospholipids, cholesterol)<br>• Synthesis of steroid hormones (in adrenals, gonads and placenta)<br>• Metabolism of glycogen (in liver and muscles)<br>• Metabolism of drug metabolism by microsomal cytochrome P-450 system (in liver and kidney)<br>• Store house for $Ca^{2+}$ (sarcoplasmic reticulum of skeletal muscles) |

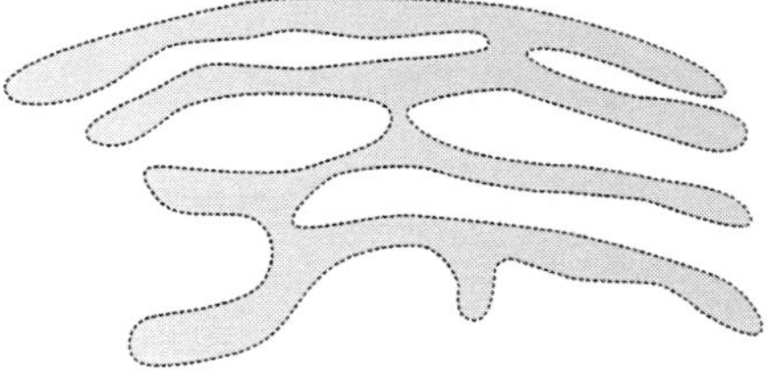

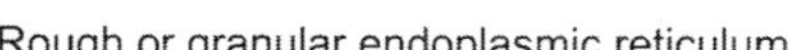

Rough or granular endoplasmic reticulum

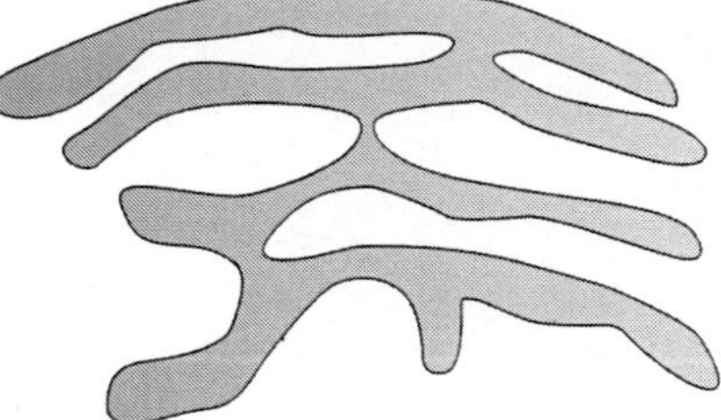

Smooth or agranular endoplasmic reticulum

**Fig. 9:** Types of endoplasmic reticulum

## 16. Niemann-Pick disease.

- Niemann-Pick disease is a lipid storage disorder.

| *Inheritance* | *Deficient enzyme* | *Pathology* |
|---|---|---|
| • Autosomal recessive | • Sphingomyelinase, a lysosomal enzyme | • Accumulation of sphinomyelin in liver, spleen and brain |

### Clinical Features

- Affects children, arises at birth or infancy

- Child presents with hepatosplenomegaly and progressive mental retardation (due to accumulation of sphingomyelins in brain)
- Cherry-red spot in macula
- Usually fatal, most die by age of 2 years.

## 17. Denaturation.

- Denaturation is disorganization of native structure of protein with concomitant loss of biological activity.

| *Causes* | *Features* |
|---|---|
| a. Physical agents<br>– Heat (temperature >60°C)<br>– Violent shaking<br>– X-ray<br>– UV radiation<br>b. Chemical agents<br>– Strong acids and strong bases<br>– Organic solvents (acetone, alcohol)<br>– Urea and guanidium hydrochloride<br>– Detergents<br>– Heavy metals (arsenic, mercury, lead) | • Loss of secondary, tertiary and quaternary structure of a protein (native helical structure)<br>• Primary structure is not lost (peptide bonds not hydrolyzed)<br>• Loss of biological activity<br>• Becomes insoluble<br>• Increased viscosity and decreased surface tension<br>• Increased ionisable and sulfhydral groups of proteins (due to loss of hydrogen and disulfide bonds)<br>• Easily digestable<br>• Usually irreversible but may be reversible (renaturation)<br>• Crystallization is not possible |

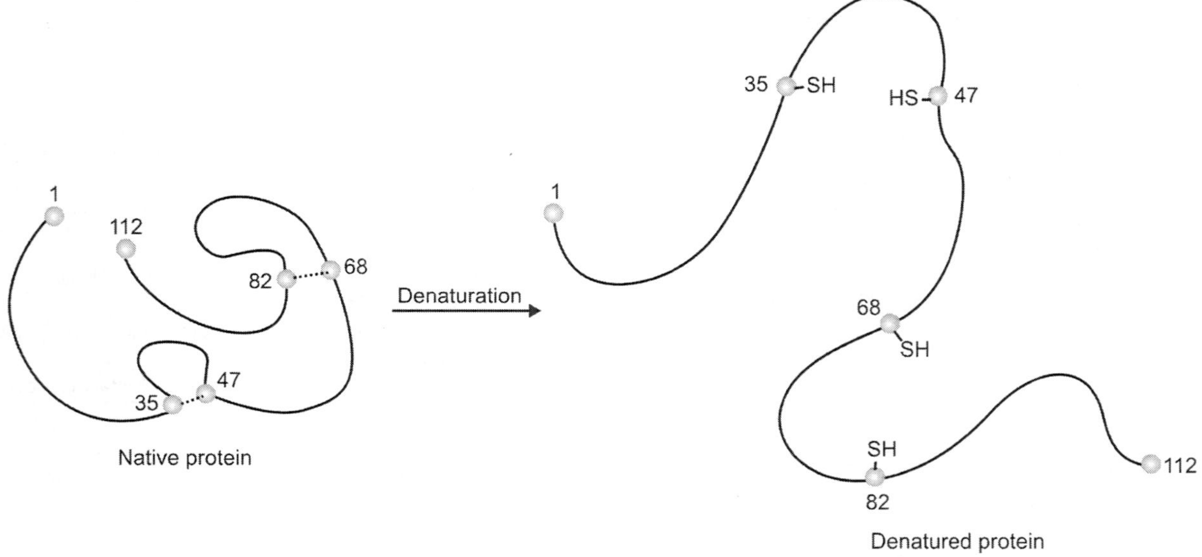


**Fig. 10:** Denaturation



## Significance

- Cooking of proteins renders them denatured thus making them easily digestible and even gastric acid in stomach does same function
- Denaturing can be used for selective isolation of protein of interest.

## 18. Methemoglobin.

Refer Question No. 10 June 2016 (RS2).

## 19. Dietary fiber.

Refer Question No. 21 Dec. 2007 (RS2).

## 20. Respiratory quotient.

- Respiratory quotient is ratio of volume of $CO_2$ produced to volume of $O_2$ consumed

$$\text{Respiratory quotient (RO)} = \frac{\text{Volume of } CO_2 \text{ produced}}{\text{Volume of } CO_2 \text{ consumed}}$$

### Respiratory Quotients of Nutrients

- Carbohydrate : 1
- Lipids : 0.7
- Proteins : 0.8
- Mixed diet : 0.85

### Conditions Lowering Respiratory Quotient

- Respiratory quotient is lowered when rate of utilization of fat increases in relation to carbohydrates as in:
  - Diabetes mellitus
  - Starvation
  - Consumption of ketogenic diet (high in lipid content).

### Significance

- Respiratory quotient is index of metabolic state of an individual and is altered in physiological and pathological states.

## 21. Renal glycosuria.

- Renal glycosuria is condition where glucose is excreted in urine due to decrease in renal threshold of glucose.

| *Causes* | *Mechanism* | *Diagnosis* |
|---|---|---|
| Physiological<br>• Pregnancy<br>Pathological<br>• Hereditary—absent or defective carrier protein<br>• Acquired<br>– Diseases of renal tubules (Fanconi's syndrome)<br>– Heavy metal poisoning ( Pb, Hg, Cd)<br>• Lowering of renal threshold<br>• Experimental renal glycosuria (drugs like phloridzin) | • Quantity of glucose in glomerular filtrate is increases when more glucose is filtered through glomerular membrane due to decreased renal threshold (renal glycosuria) or increased glucose in blood (hyperglycemic glucosuria) and this increased glucose cannot be reabsorbed resulting in excretion of excess glucose in urine<br>• Renal threshold of glucose is 180 mg/dL, above which glucose appears in urine | • By Benedict's qualitative test: Detects reducing sugars (screening test)<br>• Oral glucose tolerance test: Normal response in changes of plasma glucose but presence of glucose in urine samples (confirmatory test) |

## 22. Lesch-Nyhan syndrome.

Refer Question No. 10 June 2005 (RS2).

# MBBS PHASE I EXAMINATION
## DECEMBER 2010
## (Revised Scheme 2)

### LONG ESSAYS

#### 1. Describe the metabolism of phenylalanine and tyrosine. Add a note on tyrosinemia.

Phenylalanine and tyrosine are 2 structurally similar aromatic amino acids.

**Features**

- Phenylalanine is an essential amino acid but tyrosine is synthesized from phenylalanine
- Both are partly glucogenic and partly ketogenic
- They are precursors of biologically important compounds like proteins, catecholamines, thyroid hormones, melanin etc.

A. Synthesis of tyrosine from phenylalanine:
   *Tissue site*
   – Liver
   *Steps*

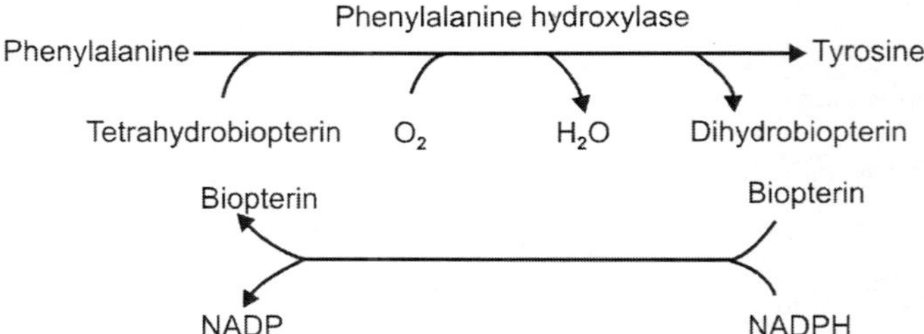


   *Significance*
   – Presence of tyrosine in food proteins spares phenylalanine from being converted to tyrosine thus reducing dietary requirements of phenylalanine.

B. Importance of phenylalanine and tyrosine (products synthesized):
   a. Protein synthesis
      - Phenylalanine and tyrosine as amino acids are building blocks of proteins
   b. Synthesis of catecholamines (nonadrenaline and adrenaline)
      *Tissue site*
      - Adrenals

*Steps*

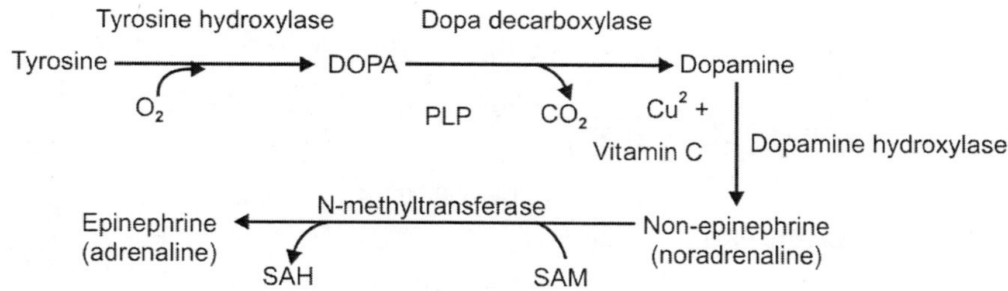


c. Synthesis of thyroid hormones (tri-iodo thyronine and tetra-iodo thyronine)

*Tissue site*

- Thyroid

*Steps*

i. Iodination of tyrosin molecule of thyroglobulin to form mono-iodo tyrosine (MIT) catalyzed by thyroid peroxidase and $H_2O_2$

$$\text{Tyrosin} + I_2 \xrightarrow[H_2O_2]{\text{Thyroid peroxidase}} \text{MIT}$$

ii. Further iodination of some MIT molecules to form di-iodo tyrosine (DIT)

$$\text{MIT} + I_2 \xrightarrow[H_2O_2]{\text{Thyroid peroxidase}} \text{DIT}$$

iii. Coupling of one MIT with one DIT gives $T_3$

$$\text{MIT} + \text{DIT} \longrightarrow T_3$$

iv. Coupling of two DIT gives $T_4$

$$\text{DIT} + \text{DIT} \longrightarrow T_4$$

v. Release of $T_3$ and $T_4$ from thyroglobulin by breakdown of peptide bonds by proteolytic enzymes.

d. Synthesis of melanin (a black pigment of skin, hair, etc.)

*Tissue site*

- Melanoblasts located in skin

*Steps*

Tyrosine —(Tyrosinase; $O_2$, $Cu^{2+}$)→ DOPA —($Cu^{2+}$)→ DOPA quinone → 5,6-dihydroxyindole

Several steps and polymerization ↓

Melanin

C. Catabolism of phenylalanine and tyrosine

– Phenylalanine is first converted to tyrosine and rest of pathway is same for both

*Steps*

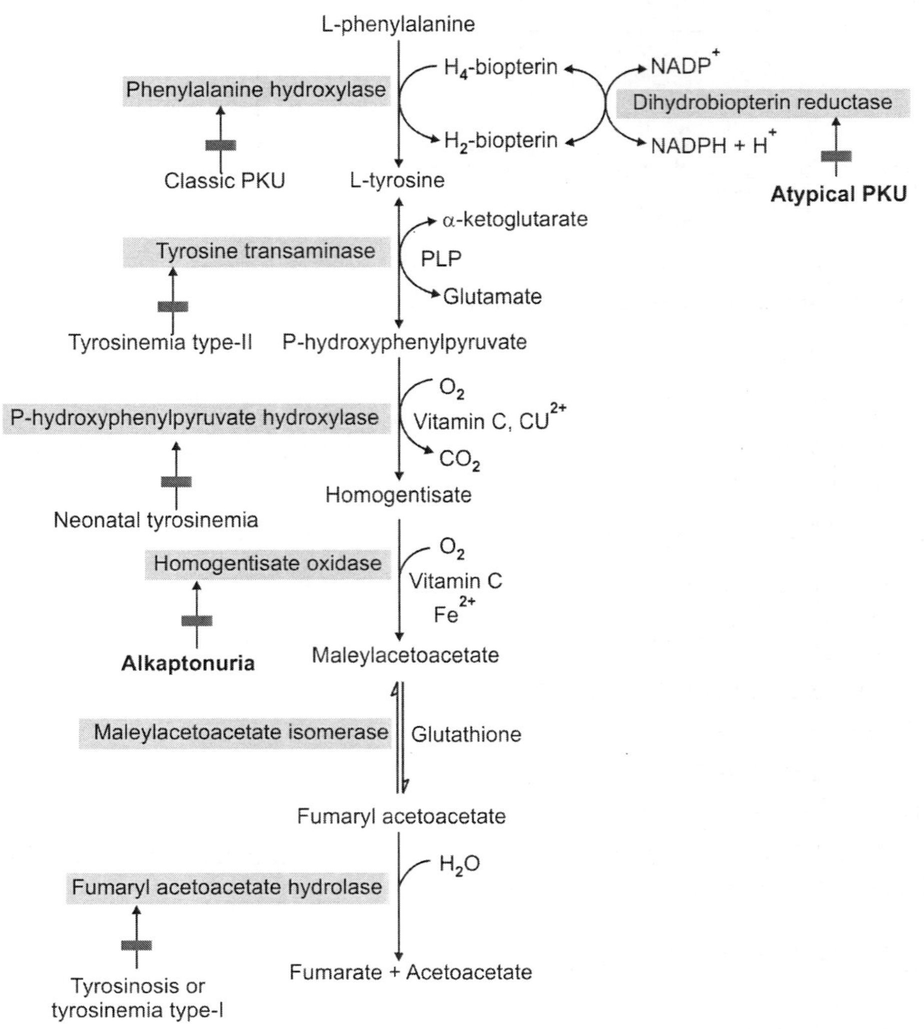


**Fig. 1:** Catabolism of phenylalanine and tyrosine

*End Products and their Fate*

- Fumarate → glucose (by gluconeogenesis)
- Acetoacetate (ketone body).

## Inborn Errors of Metabolism

a. Phenylketonuria (PKU)
   – Most common inborn error of phenylalanine metabolism

| *Inheritance* | *Deficient enzyme* | *Types* | |
|---|---|---|---|
| | | *Classical phenylketonuria* | *Non-classical phenylketonuria* |
| • Autosomal recessive | • Phenylalanine hydroxylase | • Type I<br>Deficiency of phenylalaline hydroxylase<br>• Type II and III<br>Partial deficiency of phenylalaline hydroxylase | • Type IV<br>Deficiency of dihydrobiopterin reductase<br>• Type V<br>Deficiency of enzyme synthesizing coenzyme biopterin |

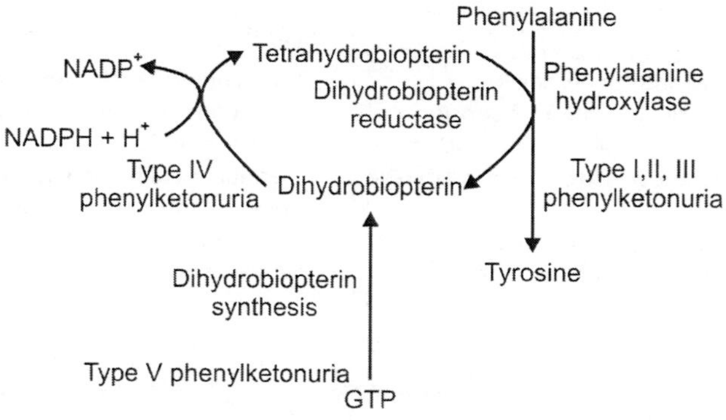


**Fig. 2:** Phenylketonuria—types

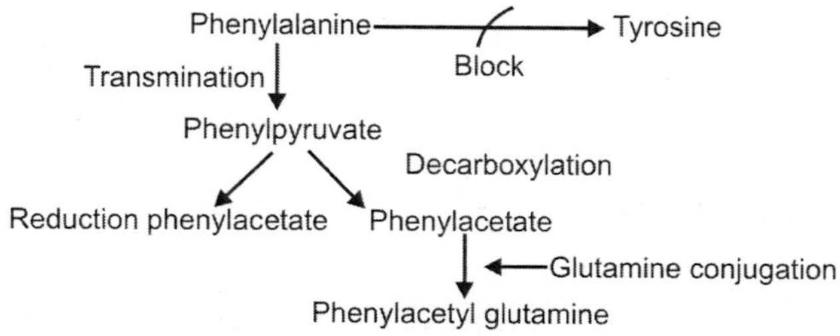


**Fig. 3:** Metabolites accumulated in phenylketonuria

– These end products, i.e. phenyl pyruvate, phenyl lactate, phenyl acetate and phenyl acetyl glutamine are excreted in urine along with phenylalanine.

| *Clinical features* | *Diagnosis* | *Treatment* |
|---|---|---|
| • Mental retardation (due to low serotonin level)<br>• Light skin and hair color (due to inhibition of melanin synthesis)<br>• Seizures, agitations and tremors<br>• Eczema and mousy odor of skin, hair and urine (due to increased phenylketones)<br>• Hypopigmentation of skin (due to defective synthesis of tyrosine) | • Ferric chloride test (screening test) where urine turns blue green on addition of ferric chloride and color change persists for 2–4 minutes<br>• Positive Guthrie's test, i.e. growth of bacillus subtilis on addition of patients blood or urine<br>• Positive dinitrophenylhydrazine test, i.e. yellow or yellow-white precipitates in urine due to the reaction of DNPH with keto acids<br>• Quantitative tests to estimate phenylalanine and phenylketones by mass spectrometry<br>• Prenatal diagnosis by DNA analysis of amniotic or trophoblastic cells<br>• Detection of carrier state by elevated phenylalanine levels after oral dose of phenylalanine | • Dietary restrictions<br>• Tetrahydrobiopterin supplements |

b. Alkaptonuria (Black urine disease)
   – Inborn error of tyrosine metabolism

| *Inheritance* | *Deficient enzyme* | *Biochemical defect* |
|---|---|---|
| • Autosomal recessive | • Homogentisate oxidase | • Accumulation of homogentisic acid in body and its excretion in urine |

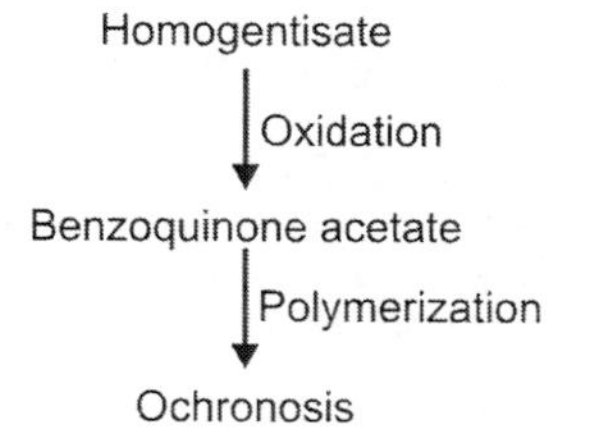


(Black colored alkapton bodies that binds to connective tissue)

**Fig. 4:** Alkaptonuria

| *Clinical features* | *Diagnosis* | *Treatment* |
|---|---|---|
| • Benign condition manifesting by 3rd and 4th decade<br>• Oochronosis (pigmentation of cartilages due to deposition of alkaptone bodies on the cartilages of nose, pinna of ear and sclera)<br>• Arthritis (due to binding of homogentisic acid to collagen in cartilage and intervertebral discs)<br>• Darkening of urine on standing—resembles coke (due to atmospheric oxidation of homogentisic acid to alkaptone bodies) | • Ferric chloride test (screening test) where urine turns green on addition of ferric chloride<br>• Quantitation of homogentisic acid in urine by high pressure liquid chromatography<br>• Identification of homogentisic acid | • Dietary restrictions of phenylalanine and tyrosine<br>• Vitamin C administration |

c. Albinism

| *Inheritance* | *Deficient enzyme* | *Biochemical defect* | *Clinical features* |
|---|---|---|---|
| • Autosomal recessive | • Tyrosinase | • Defective synthesis of melanin due to absence of tyrosinase in melanoblasts | • Light color skin and hairs<br>• Photophobia (due to hypopigmentation of optic fundus)<br>• Nystagmus and low visual acuity<br>• Skin sensitive to UV rays (increasing risk of skin cancer) |

d. Tyrosinemia
– Rare inborn error of tyrosine metabolism

*Types*

| | *Type I* | *Type II (Richner Hanhart syndrome)* | *Transient neonatal tyrosinemia* |
|---|---|---|---|
| Deficient enzyme/ cause | • Fumarylacetoacetate hydrolase and/ or malylacetoacetate isomerase | • Tyrosine transaminase | • Due to liver immaturity |
| Biochemical defect | | • Accumulation and excretion of tyrosine and its metabolites (p-hydroxyphenyl pyruvate, p-hydroxyphenyl lactate, phydroxyphenyl acetate, N-acetyl tyrosine and tyramine) | • Relative deficiency of p-hydroxyphenylpyruvate hydroxylase |
| Clinical features | • Acute hepatic failure in infancy and chronic cirrhosis in adults<br>• Vitamin D resistant rickets, amino aciduria, glycosuria and phosphaturia (due to generalized transport defect in proximal tubules) | • Mental retardation<br>• Photophobia (due to corneal erosions)<br>• Palmoplanter keratosis (lesions of palms and soles) | • Not severe, transient condition |

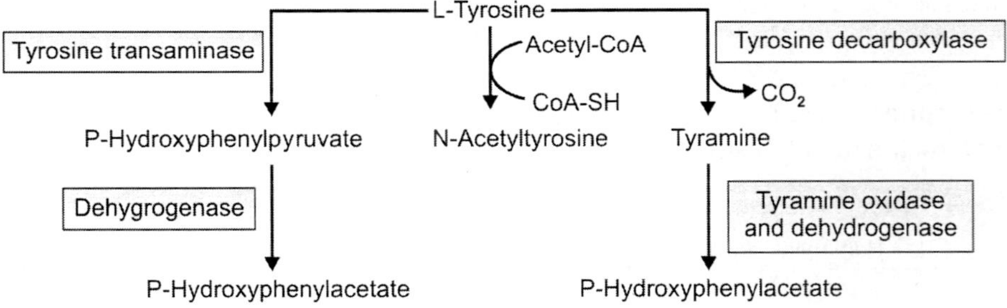


**Fig. 5:** Tyrosinemia

| *Diagnosis* | *Treatment* |
|---|---|
| • High levels of tyrosine and phenylalanine in blood and urine<br>• Increased urinary excretion of DOPA and other tyrosine metabolites | • Dietary restrictions<br>• Ascorbic acid in neonatal tyrosinemia |

## Clinical Significance

- Phenylalanine is an essential amino acid which is required for synthesis of various important compounds in body
- Phenylketonuria is a common inborn error associated with phenylalanine metabolism.

**2. Explain the steps of activation, initiation, elongation and termination of protein biosynthesis.**

Refer Question No. 2 Dec. 2008 (RS2).

## SHORT ESSAYS

### 3. Proto-oncogenes and oncogenes.

- Proto-oncogenes are cellular oncogenes detected on normal animal and human cell and promote normal growth and differentiation of cells
- Oncoqenes are cancer causing genes derived from proto-oncogenes.

#### Products of Oncogene

- Oncogenes encode proteins called oncoproteins which resemble the normal products of protooncogenes.

| Product | Oncogene |
|---|---|
| a. Extracellular growth factor | |
| i. β - chain of PDGF (platelet derived growth factor) | Sis |
| ii. FGF (Fibroblasts growth factor) | hst, k53 |
| b. Transmembrane growth factor receptors | |
| i. EGF receptors (epidermal growth factors) | erb B1, her-2/neu (erb B2) |
| ii. CSF receptor (colony stimulating factor) | Fms |
| c. Intracellular signal transduction proteins | |
| i. GTP binding (guanosine triphosphate) | Ras |
| ii. Nonreceptor tyrosine kinase | Abl |
| d. Nuclear regulatory protein | |
| i. Transcription activators | Myc, n-myc |
| e. Cell cycle regulatory proteins | |
| i. Cyclins | cyclin d |
| ii. Cyclin-dependent kinase | CDK-4 |
| f. Apoptotic inhibitors | |
| i. Anti-apoptotic gene | bcl-2 |

#### Mechanism of Activation of Cellular Oncogenes

- A normal gene or protooncogene is converted or activated in oncogene by:
  - Change in the structure of the gene
  - Change in the regulation of gene expression.

| *Point mutation and deletion* | *Chromosomal translocation* | *Gene amplification* |
|---|---|---|
| • Mutation of viral oncogene sequence increases tumerogenic ability of acute transforming retroviruses<br>*Example*<br>– Rat sarcoma virus oncogen or r–ras is carried in bladder cancer, pancreatic adenocarcinoma, cholangiocarcinoma | • Transfer of a portion of one chromosome to another<br>• Implicated in pathogenesis of leukemias and lymphomas<br>*Example*<br>– Philadelphia chromosome (P. 9,22)<br>- C-abl proto-oncogene is translocated from chromosome 9 to 22<br>- Seen in 95% cases of chronic myeloid leukemia<br>– C-myc proto-oncogene is translocated from chromosome 8 to 14 in 75% cases of Burkitt's lymphoma | • Increase in number of copies of a gene due to chromosomal alteration<br>*Example*<br>– Neuroblastoma having n-myc HSR region<br>– erb-B in breast and ovarian cancer |

## Significance

- Protooncogenes are normal genes located on human chromosomes regulation growth and differentiation of human cells which can genetically transform into oncogenes which produce cancer.

### 4. Explain substrate level phosphorylation.

Refer Question No. 4 Dec. 2014 (RS2).

### 5. Rapoport-Luebering cycle.

Refer Question No. 7 June 2010 (RS2).

### 6. Define $K_m$ (Michaelis constant) value of an enzyme. Write about its importance with a suitable example.

- $K_m$ value is substrate concentration at which velocity of enzyme catalyzed reaction is half of $V_{max}$
- Also called Michaelis-Menten constant or Brig's and Haldane's constant
- K stands for constant and m stands for Michaelis
- It describes relationship between substrate concentration and rate of reaction.

## Features

- $K_m$ value is substrate concentration at half maximal velocity
- Expressed in moles/L
- Denotes that 50% of enzyme molecules are bound with substrate at that particular substrate concentration
- Constant for an enzyme
- Independent of enzyme concentration
- Signature of enzyme, i.e. each substrate has individual $K_m$
- Denotes affinity of enzyme for substrate.

## Significance

- $K_m$ is an index of affinity of enzyme towards substrate, i.e. low $K_m$ means higher affinity for substrate and high $K_m$ means low affinity for substrate.

  *Example*
  - $K_m$ of hexokinase for glucose is 0.05 mmol/L whereas that of glucokinase is 10 mmol/L thus hexokinase acts on glucose at lower concentration (fasting condition) whereas glucokinase acts on glucose at higher concentration (immediately following meals).
- $K_m$ provides measure of substrate concentration required for significant catalysis to occur
- $K_m$ is useful to distinguish type of enzyme inhibition
  - Km is increased in competitive inhibition whereas it is unaltered in non-competitive inhibition.

### 7. Compounds derived from cholesterol.

Refer Question No. 3 June 2009 (RS2).

### 8. Explain the catabolism of purine.

Refer Question No. 2 June 2007 (RS2).

### 9. What is anion gap? Explain normal anion gap acidosis and high anion gap acidosis with examples.

Refer Question No. 9 June 2005 (RS2).

## 10. Radioactive isotopes of iodine and their clinical application.

- Isotopes are different forms of same element having same number of protons (atomic number) but different number of neutrons
- Radioactive isotopes are isotopes that emit radiation due to instability of nucleus (also known as radio nuclides).

### Radioactive Isotopes of Iodine

- Radioactive isotopes of iodine are called radioactive iodine.

### Types

| | $^{131}I$ | $^{125}I$ |
|---|---|---|
| Radiations | Emits beta and gamma radiations | Emits gamma radiations |
| Half life | About 8 days | About 60 days |

### Clinical Applications

| *Diagnostic uses ($^{131}I$ is used to label various substances to assess)* | *Therapeutic uses* |
|---|---|
| • Thyroid function test (↑uptake in hyperthyroidism and ↓ uptake in thyroid cancer)<br>• Fat absorption<br>• Hepatic function<br>• Pulmonary function<br>• Renal functions<br>• Plasma volume<br>• Turnover rate of a substance in body (rate of synthesis and breakdown) | • Thyroid cancers<br>• Primary thyrotoxicosis (hyperthyroidism/toxic nodular goiter)<br>• Cardiac diseases<br>• Controlling ectopic arrythmias |

## 11. What is the normal range of serum potassium and write about hypokalemia.

- Potassium is principle intracellular cation.

### Normal Range

- 3.4–5 mEq/L.

### Hypokalemia

- Hyopokalemia is decreased potassium level below 3 mmol/L.

### Causes

| *Increased renal excretion* | *Shift or redistribution of potassium (entry of $K^+$ into cell in exchange for $H^+$)* | *Gastrointestinal loss* | *IV administration of $K^+$ free fluids* | *Drugs* |
|---|---|---|---|---|
| • Cushing's syndrome<br>• Hyperaldosteronism<br>• Renal tubular acidosis<br>• Adrenogenital syndrome | • Alkalosis<br>• Insulin therapy<br>• Hypokalemia periodic paralysis | • Prolonged diarrhea or vomiting<br>• Defiant dietary intake<br>• Malabsorption<br>• Pyloric obstruction | | • Osmotic diuretics<br>• Corticosteroids |

| *Clinical features* | *ECG changes* | *Laboratory diagnosis* | *Treatment* |
|---|---|---|---|
| • Anorexia, nausea, vomiting<br>• Abdominal distention and ileus<br>• Irritability<br>• Muscular weakness, fatigue and cramps<br>• Decreased reflexes<br>• Hypotension<br>• Tachycardia and palpitations<br>• Cardiomegaly<br>• Cardiac arrhythmias<br>• Cardiac arrest | • Flattening, lowering or inversion of T wave<br>• Prominent U wave<br>• Depression of ST segment | a. Urine potassium level<br>– >25 mmol/day (renal loss of potassium)<br>– <25 mmol/day (extra renal loss of potassium)<br>b. Plasma bicarbonate level<br>– Decreased (renal tubular acidosis)<br>– Increased (Cushing's syndrome) | • Potassium supplementation<br>• Treatment of underlying cause |

## 12. Mention five biochemical functions of pyridoxine in the body with examples.

Refer Question No. 2 June 2006 (RS2).

## SHORT ANSWERS

## 13. Enumerate reactive oxygen species and their characteristics.

Refer Question No. 17 Dec. 2008 (RS2).

## 14. What are xenobiotics? What is the role of glutathione in detoxification?

- Xenobiotics are compounds which may be accidently ingested or taken as drugs or compounds produced in body by bacterial metabolism
  (Gr. Xenos - Strange, foreign)

*Examples*

- Food addictives, food contaminants, drugs, microbial toxins, etc.

### Role of Glutathione in Detoxification

- Glutathione is a tripeptide formed from glutatamate, cysteine and glycine
- It is an active conjugating agent, conjugating cysteine residue with xenobiotics
- Compounds conjugating with glutathione are alkyl or aryl halides, alkanes, nitro-compounds and epoxides.

## 15. List metabolic functions and clinical significance of lysosomes.

- Lysosomes are intracellular cytosolic organelles shaped as spherical vesicles enveloped by a single membrane
- Discovered by Rene de Duve in 1950.

### Metabolic Functions

a. Digestion of cellular substances like protein, lipids, carbohydrates and nucleic acids
   - Also called as digestive tract of cells, lysosomes are actively involved in digestion of cellular substances due acidic pH of lysosomal matrix which facilitates degradation of different compounds like proteins, lipids, carbohydrates and nucleic acids.

b. Maintaining cellular components in dynamic state.

c. Digestion of foreign substances.

### Clinical Significance

- Lysosomes contains numerous hydrolyses (enzymes) like $\alpha$-glucosidase, cathepsins, lipases, ribonucleases and leakage of these into cytoplasm can lead to degradation of functional macromolecules of cells resulting in cell death. Such leakage of lysosomal enzymes is seen in arthritis, muscles diseases, allergic disorders etc.
- Usually degraded compounds leave lysosome by diffusion for reutilization; however in certain instances it may accumulate especially lipids and proteins in form of lipofuscin which is referred to as wear and tear or aging pigment
- In certain genetic diseases, lysosomal enzymes are deficient or absent leading to accumulation of lipids or polysaccharides causing storage disorders. Inclusion cell (I-cell) disease is another rare disorder wherein the lysosomal enzymes are seen in blood but not in lysosomes.

## 16. Role of dietary fiber in health and disease.

Refer Question No. 21 Dec. 2007 (RS2).

## 17. Write any six functions of vitamin C.

Refer Question No. 2 Dec. 2005 (RS2).

## 18. What is genetic code? Explain.

Refer Question No. 2 June 2011 (RS2).

## 19. Renal threshold for glucose and its significance.

- Renal threshold is concentration of glucose in blood below which it is completely reabsorbed by renal tubules.

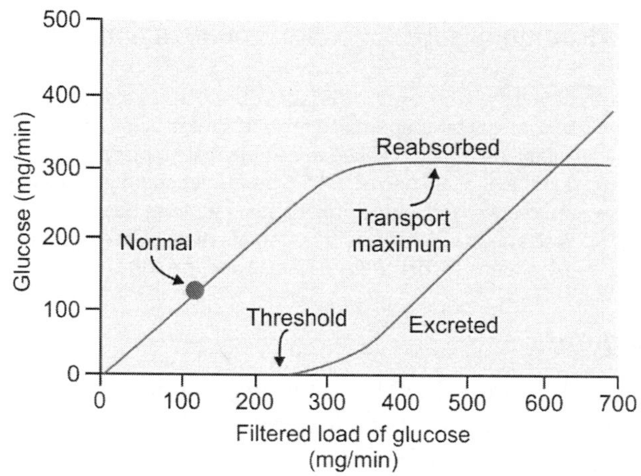


**Fig. 6:** Renal threshold for glucose

### Normal Value

- 175–180 mg/dL.

### Significance

- If glucose level in blood exceeds this level, glucose appears in urine (glycosuria)
- Glucose appears in urine even when renal threshold is reduced (renal glycosuria).

## 20. List biochemical changes in protein–energy malnutrition.

Refer Question No. 9 June 2010 (RS2).

## 21. Absorption of iron in the body.

Refer Question No. 11 June 2007 (RS2).

## 22. Structure of immunoglobulin.

- Immunoglobulins are a heterogeneous group of serum proteins, which either function as antibodies or are chemically related to antibodies.

### Structure of Immunoglobulins

- All immunoglobulins molecules basically consists of two identical heavy (H) chains and two identical light (L) chains held together by disulfide linkages and non-covalent interactions
- Thus, immunoglobulin is a Y-shaped tetramer.

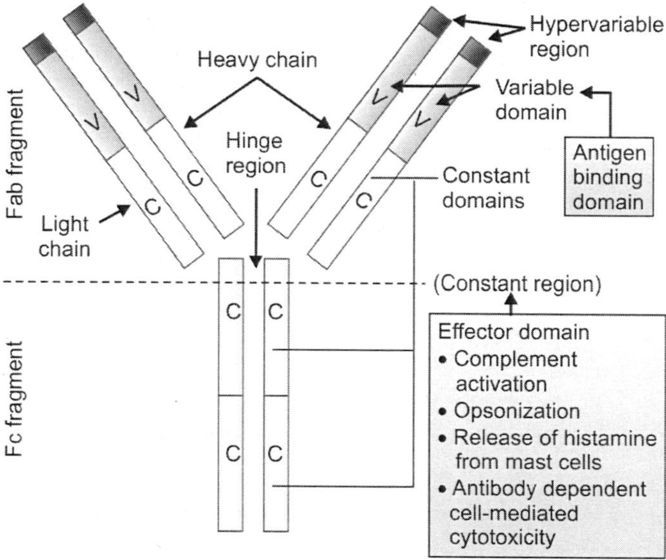


**Fig. 7:** Structure of immunoglobulin

## Chains

- All immunoglobulins consists of two identical heavy (H) chains and two identical light (L) chains.

| *Heavy chains (H)* | *Light chains (L)* |
|---|---|
| • Longer, contains approximately 450 amino acids each and has molecular weight of 55000-70000 and is linked to carbohydrate moiety<br>• 2 H chains are joined by 1-5 S-S bonds depending upon class of immunoglobulins<br>• Structurally and antigenically distinct for each class<br>• Based on structure of constant region, there are 5 types of heavy chains, namely alpha (α), gamma (γ), delta (δ), epsilon (ε) and meu (μ) | • Shorter, have about 212 amino acids each and have molecular weight of about 23000<br>• Similar in all types of human immunoglobulin and are 2 types namely kappa(κ) and lambda (λ) |

## Regions

- Each chain either H or L has two regions namely constant region (C) and variable (V)
- Constant region of a chain is made of homologus sequences whereas variable regions have variable amino acid sequence
- Amino terminal half of L chain is variable region while carboxy terminal half is constant region
- Whereas ¼ of H chain is variable and rest ¾ is constant
- Amino acid sequence of this variable region is responsible for specificity of immunoglobulin to a particular antigen.

## Fractions

- Depending upon solubility of fractions of immunoglobulins, there are two fractions of immunoglobulins, namely Fc and Fab fragments.
- Fc fragment is composed of carboxyterminus of H chains and Fab fragment is composed of aminoterminus of H chains and L chains
- Portion of H chain in Fab fragment is called Fd piece which carries a carbohydrate moiety which is distinct for each class of immunoglobulins
- Fc fragment is concerned with properties of immunoglobulin such as complement fixation, placental transfer, skin fixations and catabolic rate.

## Types and Functions of Immunoglobulins

| *Type (GAMED)* | *H-chain* | *L-chain* | *Serum concentration* | *Functions* |
|---|---|---|---|---|
| a. Immunoglobulin G (IgG) | γ | κ or λ | 800–1500 mg/dL | • Can enter into extravascular space<br>• Only immunoglobulin that can cross placenta and transfer maternal immunity to fetus<br>• Plays an important role in opsonization<br>• Triggers foreign cell destruction mediated by complement system (activates both complement pathways)<br>• Only immunoglobulin that plays a role in antibody dependent cell mediated cytolysis<br>• Predominant antibody in secondary immune response |
| b. Immunoglobulin A (IgA) | α | κ or λ | 150–400 mg/dL | • Found mostly in body secretion on such as saliva, tears, sweat milk and the walls of intestine (secretory antibody)<br>• Predominantly present in colostrum thus helps in immunity building of infants<br>• Responsible for local immunity by inhibiting adherence of micro-organisms to surface of mucosal cells and are effective locally |
| c. Immunoglobulin M (IgM) | μ | κ or λ | 50–200 mg/dL | • Found predominantly in intravascular compartment and on surface of B lymphocytes<br>• Predominant class of antibodies produced in primary responses to an antigen<br>• Natural antibodies because they are produced without any known antigenic stimulation<br>• Most effective against invading parasitic and viral infections |

*Contd...*

*Contd...*

| *Type (GAMED)* | *H-chain* | *L-chain* | *Serum concentration* | *Functions* |
|---|---|---|---|---|
| d. Immunoglobulin E (IgE) | ε | κ or λ | 0.02–0.05 mg/dL | • Mediate hypersensitivity and anaphylaxis reactions<br>• Fixes to mast cells and basophils and on subsequent exposure to allergen release histamine<br>• Binds with other leukocytes and helps in release of mediators of inflammation |
| e. Immunoglobulin D (IgD) | δ | κ or λ | 1–10 mg/dL | • IgD along with IgM is predominant immunoglobulin on surface of human B lymphocytes and may be involved in differentiation of these cells<br>• Has antibody activity towards certain antigens like insulin, diptheria toxoid and certain thyroid antigens |

# MBBS PHASE I EXAMINATION
## JUNE 2011
## (Revised Scheme 2 & 3)

## LONG ESSAYS

### 1. Discuss the formation and fate of ketone bodies.

- Ketone bodies are water soluble and energy yielding compounds produced in excess during excessive breakdown of fatty acids.

### Examples

- Acetone
- Acetoacetate
- β-hydroxybutyrate.

### Ketogenesis (Formation of Ketone Bodies)

| *Principle organ* | *Subcellular site* | *Pathway* |
|---|---|---|
| • Liver | • Mitochondria | • HMG CoA lyase pathway |

*Steps*

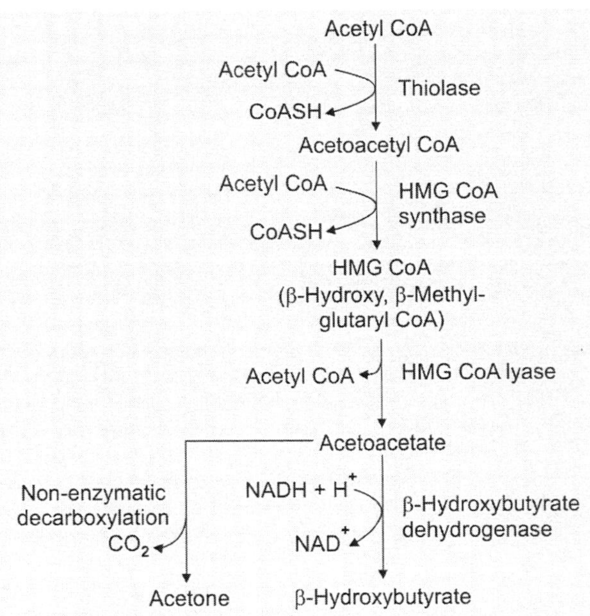


**Fig. 1:** Ketogenesis

*Regulation*

| *Rate limiting enzyme* | *Substrate availability* | *Regulation of β oxidation* | *ATP availability* |
|---|---|---|---|
| • HMG CoA synthase<br>**Inducers**<br>• Fasting, increased fat intake, diabetes mellitus | • Excess availability of fatty acids for oxidation (in starvation and diabetes) → ↑ ketogenesis | • ↑ glucagon and ↓ insulin resulting in inhibition of acetyl CoA carboxylase which decreases malonyl CoA resulting in increased β oxidation of fatty acids (in starvation) | • ↑ β oxidation produces more ATP through TCA cycle resulting in availability of acetyl CoA for ketogenesis |

## Ketolysis (Utilization of Ketone Bodies)

| *Principle organ* | *Fate of individual ketone bodies* | | |
|---|---|---|---|
| | *β-hydroxy butyrate* | *Acetaoacetate* | *Acetone* |
| • Extrahepatic tissues (brain, heart, skeletal muscles, kidney) | • Converted into acetoacetate by β-hydroxybutyrate dehydrogenase | • Activated to form acetoacetyl CoA either by transfer of CoA molecule from succinyl CoA or directly using CoA and ATP<br>• Acetoacetyl CoA is cleaved by enzyme thiolase in presence of CoASH to gives 2 molecules of acetyl CoA which enters TCA cycle to yield energy | • Some is converted back to acetoacetone<br>• Excess is excreted out through lungs giving fruity smell to breath<br>• Some undergoes propanediol pathway which is glycogenic |

*Steps*

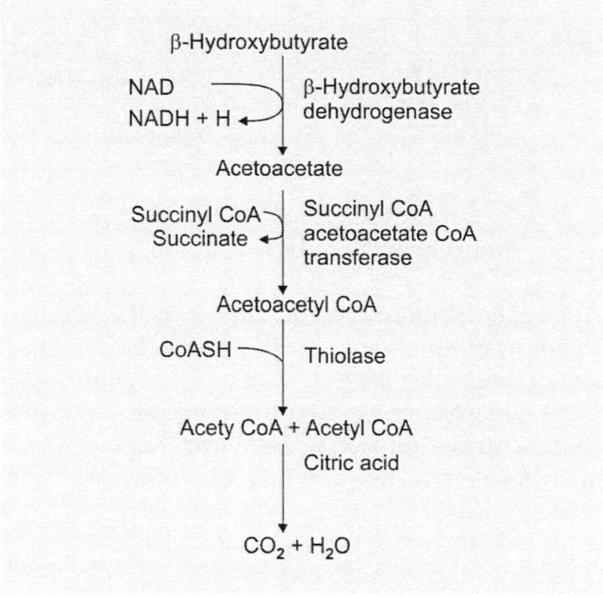


**Fig. 2:** Ketolysis

*Clinical Significance*

***Ketosis***

Ketosis is condition where there is accumulation of abnormal amount of ketone bodies in tissues and body fluids (ketonemia) and urinary excretion of β-hydroxybutyric acid exceeds 200 mg daily (ketonuria) and breath smells of acetone.

***Causes***

- Starvation
- Untreated diabetes
- Alkalosis
- Pregnancy toxemia
- Prolonged either anesthesia

- High fat feeding
- After severe exercises
- Injection of anterior pituitary extracts.

*Metabolic Derangements*

- When dietary supply of glucose is deprived as in starvation, any available oxaloacetate is diverted for gluconeogenesis to meet obligatory glucose requirements of brain
- To provide the alternate source of fuel, lipolysis is increased thus increasing mitochondrial level of acetyl CoA but oxaloacetate is deficient
- Hence citric acid cycle cannot utilize excess acetyl CoA which become substrate for ketogenesis
- When there is deficiency of insulin, like diabetes mellitus, lipolysis is accelerated producing more acetyl CoA
- Similarly in deficiency of insulin which has inhibitory effect on gluconeogenesis is absent thus decreasing the availability of oxaloacetate for citric acid cycle.

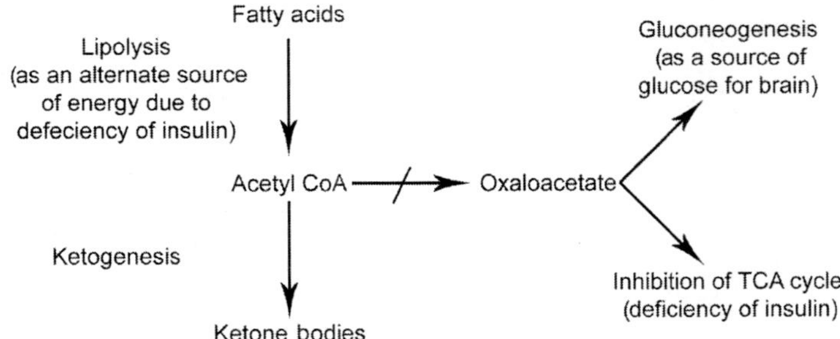


**Fig. 3:** Metabolic derangement of ketolysis

*Consequences*

- Ketone bodies namely acetoacetate and β-hydroxy butyric acid are acids and when they accumulate, metabolic acidosis results
- Plasma bicarbonate is used up for buffering these acids and hence its level falls
- Patients have typical acidotic breathing or Kussmaul's breathing due to compensatory hyperventilation
- Smell of the breath of ketosis patient is acetone like
- There is loss of important electrolytes like $Na^+$ and $K^+$ as they are excreted in urine as salts of ketone bodies
- There is dehydration due to osmotic diuresis induced by ketonuria, $Na^+$ loss in urine and associated vomiting.
- Thus consquences of ketosis are hypokalemia, dehydration and acidosis which are contributory for lethal effects of ketosis.

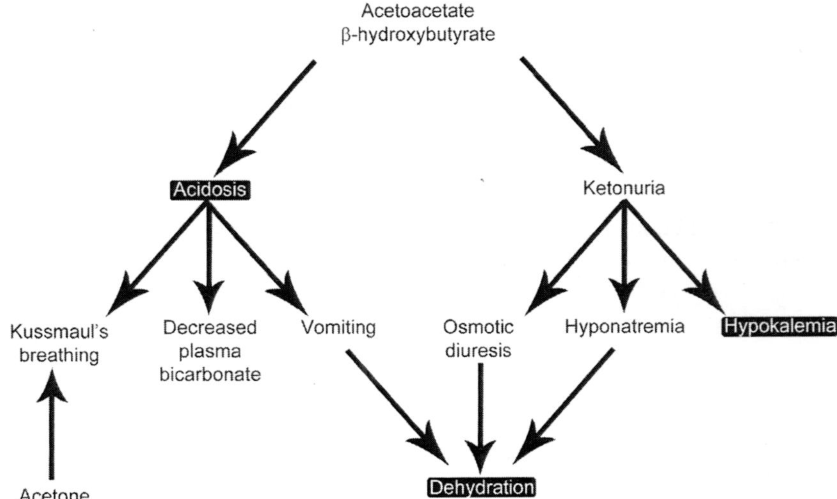


**Fig. 4:** Consequences of ketosis

## Prevention (in Diabetics)

- Regular and prompt treatment with insulin
- Avoiding starvation
- Eating lots of carbohydrates (antiketogenic)
- Minimizing use of ketogenic substances like fatty acids and amino acids.

## 2. What is genetic code? Describe the process of eukaryotic translation.

### Genetic Code

Genetic code is a 3 base sequence in mRNA that codes for a specific amino acid during protein synthesis.

### Features

- A genetic code is constituted by the base sequence in a part of mRNA.
- Each codon is a triplet of bases, i.e. A, U, G and C
- Each codon directs incorporation of a specific amino acid from 5' – 3' direction
- Based on permutations and combinations of purine pyramidine bases, there exist 64 codons.

### Types

| *Specific codons* | *Initiation codon* | *Termination codon* |
|---|---|---|
| • 61 codons, each of which code for a specific amino acid are specific codons | • AUG which codes for methionine is chain initiation codon | • UAA, UAG and UGA codon do not code for any amino acid are chain termination codons<br>• Also called nonsense codon |

### Characteristic of Genetic Code (DUSK)

| **Characteristic of genetic code** *(DUSK)* |
|---|
| ✓ Degeneracy<br>✓ Universality<br>✓ Specificity<br>✓ K(c)ommaless |

| *Specificity* | *Universality* | *Degeneracy* | *Nonoverlapping and commaless* |
|---|---|---|---|
| • A specific codon always codes for a single amino acid | • Same code specifies same amino acid in all organisms<br>• However, exception to this is genetic code of mitochondria which is not universal | • Some amino acids have more than one codon, i.e. 61 codon code for 20 amino acids | • Code is read from AUG continuously without punctuation |

**For Translation**

Refer Question No. 2 Dec. 2008 (RS2).

## SHORT ESSAYS

## 3. Glycogenolysis.

Refer Question No. 1 June 2007 (RS2).

## 4. Decarboxylation of amino acids.

Refer Question No. 2 June 2006 (RS2).

## 5. Diagnostic uses of enzymes.

- Besides catalyzing body reactions, enzymes are also used clinically to diagnose and treat numerous conditions.

## Diagnostic Uses

| *Enzyme* | *Sources* | *Normal level* | *Increased in* | *Decreased in* |
|---|---|---|---|---|
| • Alanine transaminase (ALT/SGPT) | Liver | 5–35 U/L | Viral hepatitis<br>Alcoholic liver disease | — |
| • Aspartate transaminase (AST/SGOT) | Liver, heart, muscle | 5–40 U/L | Viral hepatitis (marked increase)<br>Alcoholic liver disease<br>Myocardial infarction (significant and peak rise in 24–48 hours)<br>Congestive cardiac failure<br>Muscular dystrophy | — |
| • Alkaline phosphatase (ALP) | Bone, liver, intestine, placenta | 30–115 U/L | Obstructive jaundice, rickets, pregnancy, intestinal cancer | — |
| • Amylase | Salivary glands, pancreas | 10–90 U/L | Parotitis, pancreatitis, mumps, pancreatic carcinoma | — |
| • Lipase | Pancreas | | Specific for pancreatitis | — |
| • Creatinine kinase (CK) | Heart, muscle, brain | 20–150 U/L | Myocardial infarction, muscular dystrophy, alcoholic myopathy, muscle trauma | — |
| • Lactate dehydrogenase (LDH) | Heart, muscle, liver, lungs, RBC | 40–240 U/L | Viral hepatitis, alcoholic hepatitis, myocardial infarction, Congestive cardiac failure, muscular dystrophy | — |
| • Acid phosphatase (ACP) | Prostate, RBC | 2–12 U/L | Prostatic cancer, hemolytic states | — |
| • Aldolase | Muscles, liver, erythrocyte and heart | 2–7 U/L | Muscle diseases, viral hepatitis, myocardial infarction, malignancy, hemolytic anemia | — |
| • γ-glutamyl transferase (GGT) | Liver | 10–50 U/L | Hepatitis, obstructive jaundice, chronic alcoholic liver disease | — |
| • 5′ nucleotidase | Liver | 2–10 U/L | Hepatitis, obstructive jaundice | — |
| • Pseudocholinesterase | Liver, heart | 2–5 U/L | Myocardial infarction | Cirrhosis of liver<br>OP poisoning |
| • Ceruloplasmin | Liver | 15–60 mg/dL | Inflammatory states | Wilson's disease |

## 6. Fatty acid synthase complex.

Refer Question No. 1 June 2006 (RS2).

## 7. Detoxification by oxidation.

Refer Question No. 7 Dec. 2005 (RS2).

## 8. Nitrogen balance.

Refer Question No. 12 June 2005 (RS2).

## 9. Function of albumin.

Refer Question No. 8 Dec. 2012 (RS2).

## 10. Biochemical functions and deficiency manifestations of vitamin D.

Refer Question No. 9 June 2007 (RS2).

## 11. Functions of iodine.

- Iodine is an important trace element, essential in diet for normal functioning of thyroid.

| *Sources* | *Daily requirement* | *Distribution* | *Functions* |
|---|---|---|---|
| • Sea foods, eggs, dairy products, iodized salt | • 150 µg | • Total body content: 50 mg<br>• Thyroid gland: 15 mg | • Iodine is essential for synthesis of thyroid hormones in thyroid gland<br>• It is essential for growth and development of fetus, deficiency of which causes cretinism |

### 12. Structure of mRNA.

Refer Question No. 8 June 2013 (RS2).

## SHORT ANSWERS

### 13. Free radicals and disease.

Refer Question No. 16 June 2005 (RS2).

### 14. Active transport.

Refer Question No. 15 Dec. 2015 (RS2).

### 15. Essential amino acids.

Refer Question No. 5 Dec. 2009 (RS2).

### 16. Any three enzymes unique to gluconeogenesis.

Refer Question No. 1 June 2009 (RS2).

### 17. Uncouplers of oxidative phosphorylation.

Refer Question No. 1 June 2010 (RS2).

### 18. Types and causes of beri-beri.

Refer Question No. 8 June 2005 (RS2).

### 19. Causes of sickle cell anemia.

Refer Question No. 20 Dec. 2007 (RS2).

### 20. Immunoglobulin A (IgA) and immunoglobulin M (IgM).

Refer Question No. 22 Dec. 2010 (RS2).

### 21. Describe any three renal function tests.

- Renal functional tests are tests carried out to test the functional capacity of kidneys.

#### Indications

- Detection of renal diseases
- Assessment of prognosis of renal disease
- Monitoring renal function during treatment of diseases
- Monitoring renal damage (such as tubular proteinuria) during transplant rejection.

#### Classification

| *To screen for renal diseases* | *To assess renal function* | | |
|---|---|---|---|
| | *Tests for glomerular function* | *Tests to measure renal plasma flow* | *Tests for tubular function* |
| • Complete urine analysis<br>• Plasma urea and creatinine<br>• Plasma electrolytes<br>• Intravenous pyelography<br>• Ultrasound scanning<br>• Radioactive renogram<br>• Radioactive scanning | • Urea clearance test<br>• Creatinine clearance test<br>• Inulin clearance test<br>• Cr 51 – EDTA clearance test | • Para amino hippurate test<br>• Filtration fraction | • Reabsorption studies<br>• Secretion tests<br>• Concentration and dilution tests<br>• Renal acidification |

a. **For creatinine clearance test**
Refer Question No. 9 Dec. 2005 (RS2).

b. **Urea clearance test**
- Blood urea clearance is an expression of number of mL of blood/plasma which are completely cleared of urea by kidney per minute
- Urea clearance is less than GFR, because urea is partially reabsorbed.

*Procedure*
- After a normal breakfast, at 9 am the patient is given a cup of water and instructed to void the bladder and discard the urine
- At 10 am bladder is completely emptied and urine is measure for volume and urea levels
- At same time, blood urea levels are also estimated from a blood sample taken.

*Calculations*
- Urea clearance = U x V/P
where,
U = urine urea (in mg/dL)
P = plasma urea (in mg/dL)
V = urine excreted (in mL/min)

*Inference*
i. Maximum urea clearance (Cm)
- Clearance which occurs when urinary volume exceeds 2 mL/min
- Normally when 750 mL of plasma passes through the kidney per minute, only about 10% of urea is removed thus urea clearance is 75 mL/min
- This is called maximum urea clearance.

ii. Standard urea clearance (Cs)
- Clearance which occurs when urinary volume decreases to <2 mL/min
- It is calculated as:

$$\text{Standard urea clearance} = \frac{U \times \sqrt{V}}{P}$$

- Normal standard urea clearance is 54 mL/min

**Interpretation of urea clearance value**

| *Values* | *Interpretation* |
|---|---|
| 100–70% | Normal |
| 40–70% | Mild impairment |
| 20–40% | Moderate impairment |
| <20% | Severe impairment |

c. **Concentration and dilution test**
i. Concentration test
- Simple bedside procedures, easy to carry out and extremely important.

*Principle*
- Based on the ability of kidneys to concentrate urine and based on measuring specific gravity of urine.

*Procedure (Fishberg concentration test)*
- Patient is allowed no food or water after a meal at 6 pm
- Next day at 7 am, the bladder is emptied and specimen is discarded and the second specimen is collected at 8 am and its specific gravity is measured.

*Inference*

| | *Specific gravity of urine* | *Volume of urine* |
|---|---|---|
| Normal | >1.022 | Volume of urine in night is half of volume of urine in day |
| Tubular dysfunction | 1.010 (fixed)—isosthenuria | Nocturia (increased excretion of urine at night) |

ii. Dilution tests
- More sensitive and less harmful than concentration test.

*Principle*
- Ability of the kidneys to eliminate water is tested by measuring urinary output after ingesting a large volume of water.

*Procedure*
- Patient is not allowed to drink any water after midnight
- Bladder is emptied at 7 am and a water load is given (1,200 mL over next 30 minutes)
- Hourly urine samples are collected for next 4 hours separately
- Volume, specific gravity and osmolality of each sample are measured.

*Inference*

| | *Volume of urine* | *Specific gravity of urine* | *Osmolality* |
|---|---|---|---|
| Normal | Excrete all volume within 4 hours | Atleast one sample shows <1.003 | Atleast one sample shows <50 milliosmol/kg |
| Tubular dysfunction | <80% of water excreted within 4 hours | 1.010 (fixed) | |

**22. Deficiency features of orotic aciduria. Explain the biochemical basis of manifestations.**

Refer Question No. 10 June 2005 (RS2).

# MBBS PHASE I EXAMINATION
## DECEMBER 2011
## (Revised Scheme 2 & 3)

### LONG ESSAYS

**1. Describe the reactions of urea cycle. Discuss the interrelation of urea cycle and citric acid cycle. What is the reference range for serum urea?**

- Urea cycle is a cyclic pathway converting ammonia to urea
- Also called Kreb's Henseleit cycle.

| *Principle organs* | *Intracellular site* | *Substrate (Ammonia synthesis)* | *Product* |
|---|---|---|---|
| • Liver | • First 2 reactions in mitochondria and remaining in cytoplasm | • Ammonia (formed by following methods in body)<br>i. Transdeamination (transamination followed by oxidative deamintion)<br>- Major source of ammonia<br>- Occurs in cytoplasm of hepatocytes<br>- All amino acids are transaminated to glutamate followed by deaminated by glutamate dehydrogenase<br>ii. Non-oxidative deamination<br>- Hydroxy amino acids like serine and threonine are undergo non-oxidative deamination by enzyme dehydratase to form corresponding keto acids and ammonia<br>iii. Oxidation deamination<br>- 2 enzymes D-amino acid oxides and L-amino acid oxides, oxidize amino acids to corresponding ketoacids and liberates free ammonia. They utilize FAD and FMN respectively | • Urea (Carbon and oxygen derived from $CO_2$ and one $NH_2$ each from free ammonia and aspartate) |

## Pathway

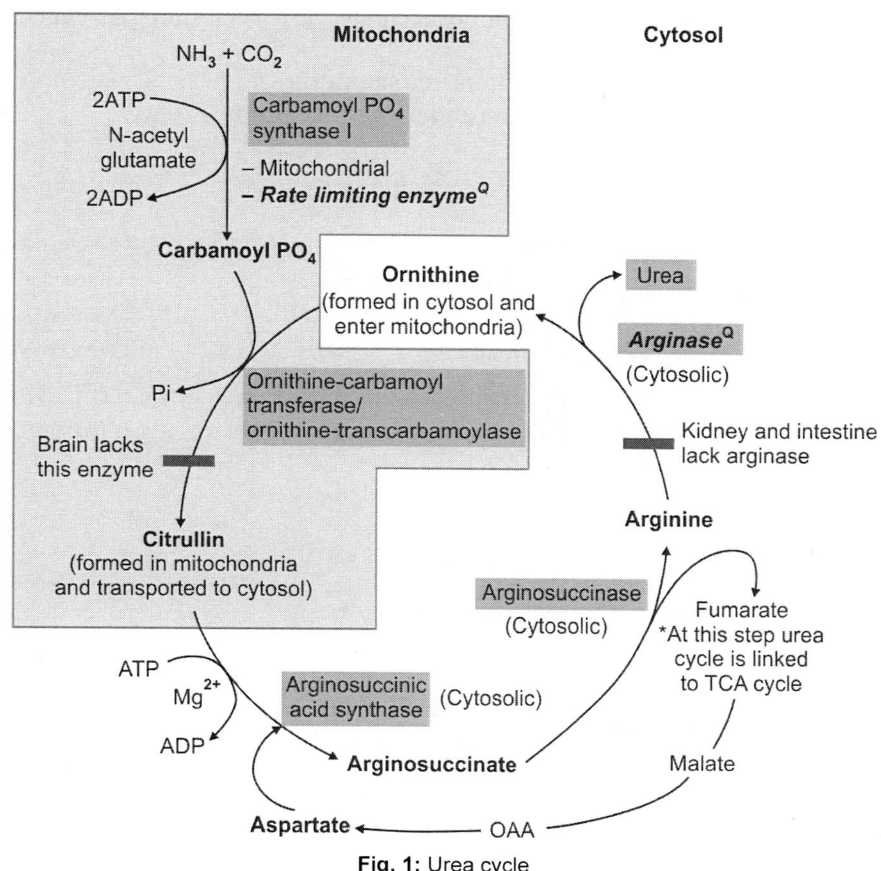


**Fig. 1:** Urea cycle

## Energetics

| *Reaction* | *Enzyme* | *ATP used* |
|---|---|---|
| $NH_3 + CO_2 \rightarrow$ Carbamoyl phosphate | Carbamoyl phosphate synthetase I | - 2 ATPs |
| Citrulline → Argininosuccinate | Argininosuccinate synthase | - 2 ATPs |
| | **Total** | **- 4 ATPs used** |

## Regulation

| *Key enzymes* | *Type of regulation* | *Inhibitor* | *Activator* |
|---|---|---|---|
| • Carbomyl phosphate synthase 1 (Rate limiting enzyme) | Allosteric regulation | Carbomyl phosphate | N-acteyl glutamate |
| • Ornithine transcarbamoylase | Feedback inhibition | Citrulline | — |
| • Arginosuccinate synthase | Feedback inhibition | Arginosuccinate | — |

## Significance

- Urea cycle detoxifies toxic $NH_3$ into urea which is less toxic and water soluble
- It synthesizes Arginine from ornithine which can be used for protein synthesis.

## Relationship between Urea Cycle and TCA Cycle

- Conversion of argininosuccinate to arginine by argininosuccinate lyase yields fumarate which provides link between urea cycle and TCA cycle
- This fumarate is converted to malate which then enters mitochondria
- In mitochondria, malate is converted to oxaloacetate and then to aspartate.

## Inherited Disorders of Urea Cycle

| Inborn error | Deficient enzyme | Inheritance |
|---|---|---|
| Hyperammonemia type I | Carbamoyl phosphate synthase I (CPS-I) | Autosomal |
| Hyperammonemia type II | Ornithine transcarbamoylase (OTC) | X-linked |
| Citrullinemia | Arginosuccinate synthase | Autosomal |
| Arginosuccinic aciduria | Arginosuccinase | Autosomal |
| Hyperargininemia | Arginase | Autosomal |

## Uremia

- Uremia is elevated levels of blood urea level.

Normal blood urea level

- 15–40 mg/dL

## Causes of Uremia

| *Prerenal causes* | *Renal disorders* | *Post renal causes* |
|---|---|---|
| • Dehydration<br>• Diabetic coma<br>• Fever | • Acute glomerulonephritis<br>• Nephrosis<br>• Chronic pyelonephritis<br>• Malignant hypertension | • Renal stones<br>• Stricture of urethra<br>• Enlarge prostate<br>• Urinary bladder tumors |

## Diagnostic Significance

- Normal plasma urea level is 15–40 mg/dL
- Plasma urea level is an indicator of renal and liver functions
- Increased plasma urea levels are seen in renal failure (impaired excretion) and burns (increased protein breakdown)
- Decreased plasma urea levels suggest severe liver diseases (decreased synthesis)

### 2. What is gluconeogenesis? Describe the pathway in detail and add a note on its significance.

Refer Question No. 1 June 2009 (RS2).

## SHORT ESSAYS

### 3. Classify transport mechanisms across cell membranes. Define uniport, symport and antiport. Give an example of each.

- Transport system across cell membrane is classified based on number of solutes transported and direction of their transport.

## Classification

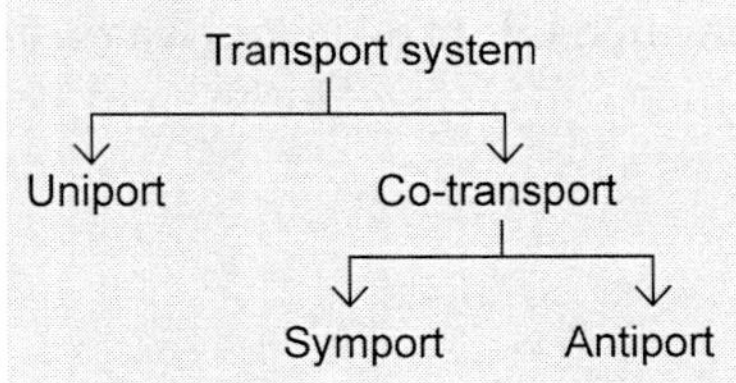

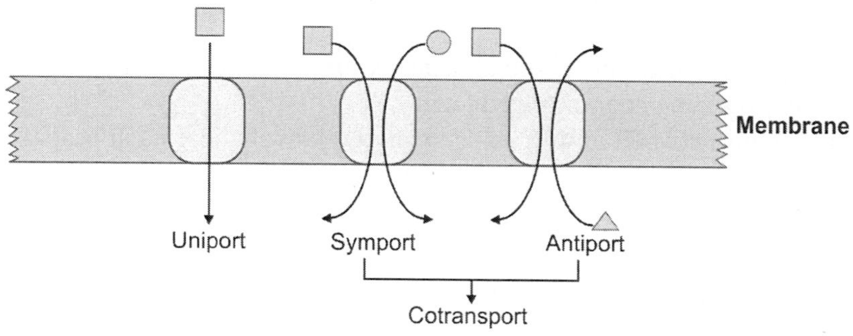


**Fig. 2:** Types of transport mechanisms

| *Types* | *Uniport* | *Co-transport* | |
|---|---|---|---|
| Features | • Transfer of one single molecule in a uni-direction along concentration gradient | • Transfer of molecule depending upon simultaneous or sequential transfer of another molecule<br>• Movement of substance against a concentration gradient is coupled with movement of second substance down concentration gradient by coupling with active energy requiring process | |
| | | *Symport* | *Antiport* |
| Solute molecules/ions transported across cell membrane | • Single solute molecule | • 2 solutes molecules in same direction | • 2 solutes molecules in opposite direction |
| Examples | • Glucose transport in various cells<br>• Calcium pump | • Na dependent glucose transport<br>• Amino acid transport | • Sodium pump<br>• Chloride bicarbonate exchange in RBCs |

## 4. Define primary, secondary, tertiary and quarternary structure of protein. What are the noncovalent forces which preserve the secondary structure?

Proteins are polymers of L-$\alpha$ amino acids structurally organized in a complex through four levels namely:

a. Primary structure
b. Secondary structure
c. Tertiary structure
d. Quaternary structure.

### Primary Structure of Protein

- A linear sequence of amino acids with a unique number and sequence
- Amino acids are held together by covalent peptide bonds linking an amino group of one amino acid to carboxyl group of adjacent amino acid.

#### *Bonds Involved*

- Covalent peptide bonds.

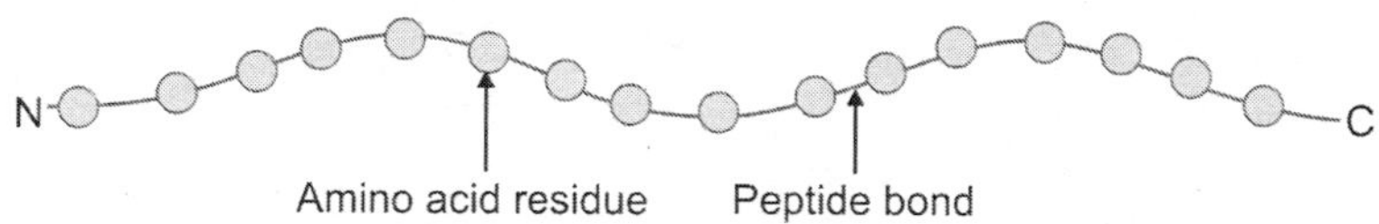


**Fig. 3:** Primary structure of protein

#### *Significance*

- Primary structure of protein is unaltered by denaturation.

## Secondary Structure of Protein

- Spatial arrangement of protein in a three dimensional structure formed by folding or coiling
- Consist of a helically coiled, zig-zig, linear or mixed form
- Results from stoic relationship between amino acids located relatively near each other in peptide chain.

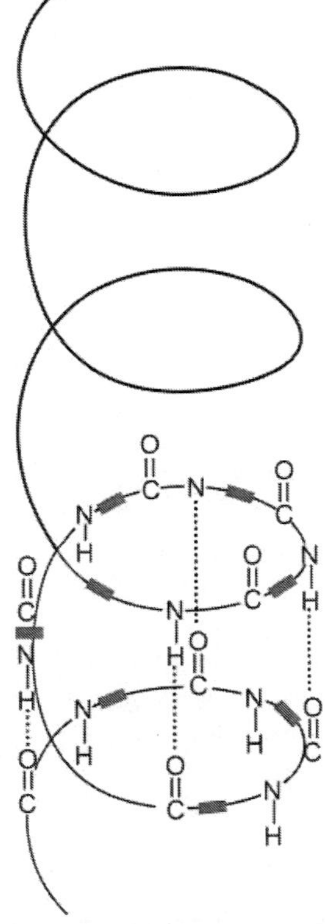
Fig. 4: Secondary structure of proteins—α-helix

### *Bonds Involved*

- Covalent bonds like hydrogen bonds
- Noncovalent bonds like van der Waals forces.

### *Types*

i. α-helix
   - Most common spiral structure of protein
   - Has a rigid arrangement of polypeptide chain.

   *Features*
   - Tightly packed coiled structure with amino acid side chains extending outward from central axis
   - Stabilised by extensive hydrogen bonding
   - All amino acids except 1st and last participate in hydrogen bonding
   - Each turn of α helix contains 3.6 amino acids and travels a distance of 0.54 nm and spacing between each amino acid is 0.15 nm
   - Formed spontaneously with lowest energy
   - Right handed α helix is more stable than left handed α helix
   - Disturbed by certain amino acids (particularly proline) like acidic (Asp, Glu) or basic (Lys, Arg, His) amino acids.

   *Examples*
   - Albumin, keratin

ii. β-pleated sheets
   - Composed of two or more segments of fully extended peptide chains, arranged either in parallel (same) or anti-parallel (opposite) direction
   - Stabilized by hydrogen bonds which may be interchain in case of two or more polypeptide chains or may be intrachain when a single polypeptide chain folds upon itself
   - Core structure of globular proteins

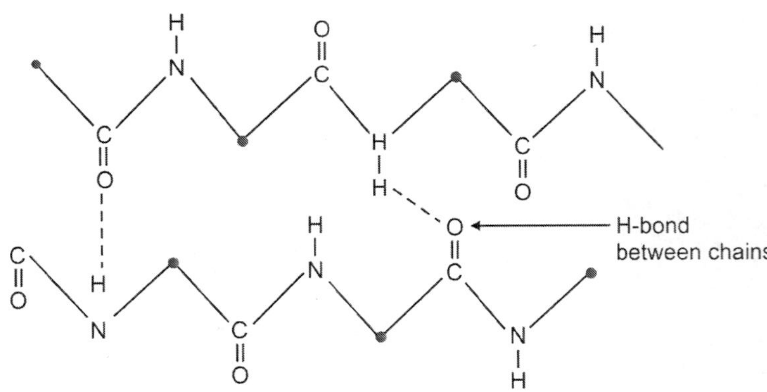

Fig. 5: Secondary structure of proteins—β-pleated sheet

*Example*
- Hemoglobin, silk.

iii. Triple helix
- Arrangement of 3 parallel helical chains wound in triple helix
- Occurs due to abundance of small amino acids like glycine, proline, hydroxyproline, alanine.

*Example*
- Collagen.

## Tertiary Structure of Protein

- Three-dimensional arrangement of protein
- Compact structure where hydrophobic side chains are held inside and hydrophilic groups are on surface of protein
- Offers stability of the molecule.

### *Bonds Involved*

- Covalent bonds like disulfide bond, hydrogen bond
- Noncovalent bonds like electrostatic (ionic), hydrophobic bonds, van der Waals forces.

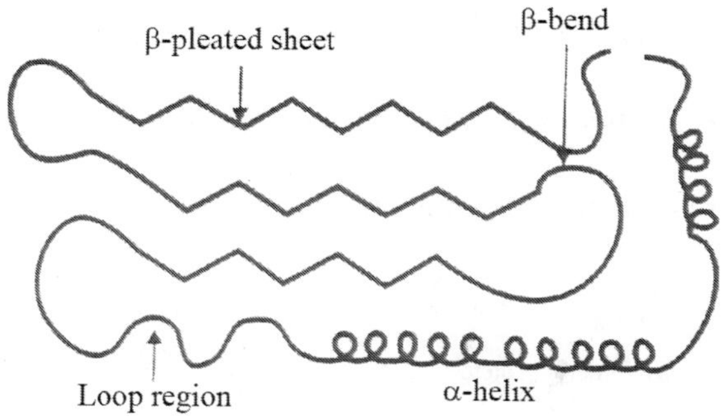

**Fig. 6:** Tertiary structure of protein

*Significance*
- Tertiary structure is very essential for functions of proteins
- It helps in formation of active site of enzymes by bringing 2 or more distant amino acids together by protein folding.

## Quaternary Structure of Protein

- Spatial arrangements 2 or more polypeptide chain subunits to form a functional unit
- Each polypeptide is called monomer, protomer or subunit and protein is called oligomer
- Thus a protein with 2 polypeptide chain is called dimer, 3 polypeptides as trimer and so on.

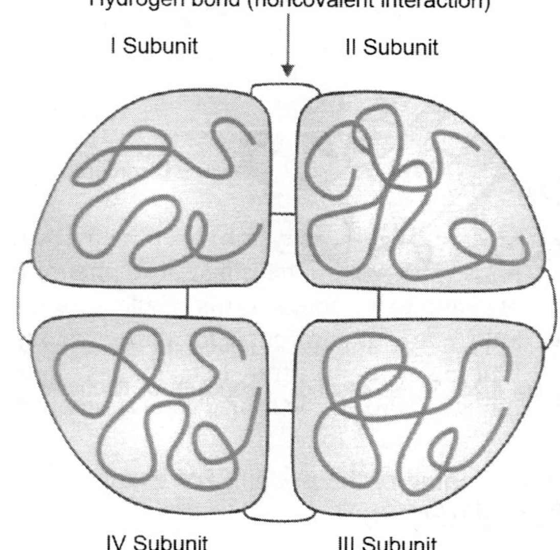

**Fig. 7:** Quaternary structure of protein

### *Bonds Involved*

- Noncovalant bonds namely hydrogen bonds, hydrophobic interactions and ionic bonds.

### *Types*

i. Homomeric proteins
- Proteins with identical subunits
- Example: Lactate dehydrogenase of muscle form (M4)

ii. Heteromeric proteins
   - Proteins with non-identical subunits
   - Example: Hemoglobin with 2α and 2β subunits.

*Significance*
- Quaternary structure of protein is essential for functioning of proteins by interaction between subunits to modify functions of oligomeric protein (cooperativity)
- Subunit interaction of hemoglobin helps in oxygen binding.

## 5. Explain the mechanism of action of allosteric enzymes? Name the allosteric inhibitor and allosteric activator for phosphofructokinase and acetyl CoA-carboxylase.

- Allosteric enzymes are enzymes that possess a distinct region called allosteric site other than active site and whose activity is regulated by allosteric mechanism
- (Gr. allo = other).

### Mechanism of Action

- Allosteric enzymes have complex quaternary structure and possess multiple subunits
- They have one catalytic site where substance binds and another separate allosteric site where modulator (activator, inhibitor) binds
- Binding of regulatory molecule can either enhance activity (allosteric activation) or inhibit activity (allosteric inhibition) of enzyme
- Binding of positive modifier alters configuration of substrate binding site to favor substrate binding and it is called positive cooperativity
- Binding of negative modifier decrease activity of substrate binding site and is said to be negative co-operativity.

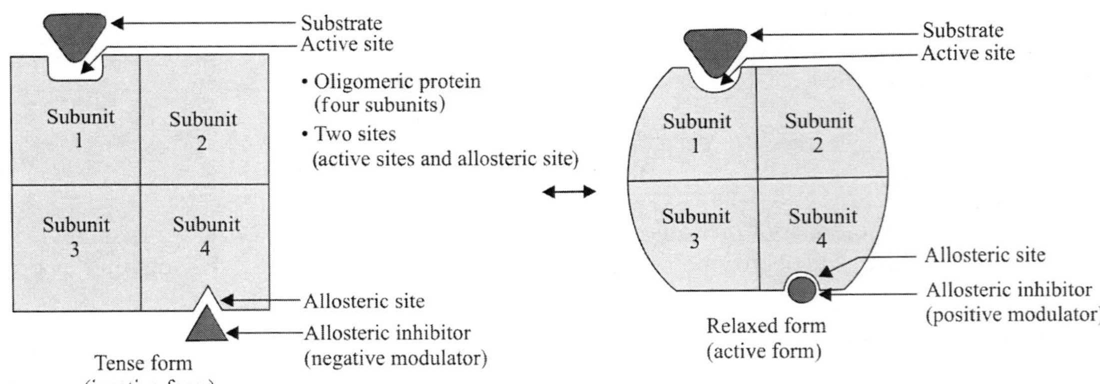


**Fig. 8:** Allosteric enzymes—mechanism of action

### Features

- Most of allosteric enyzmes are oligomeric in nature with identical or different subunits
- Allosteric enzymes demonstrate a phenomenon of cooperativity, i.e. change in activity of one subunit due to binding of ligand to another subunit of allosteric enzyme
- Substrate saturation curve for allosteric enzyme is sigmoid shaped (S-shaped curve) because of cooperativity indicating binding of one substrate to facilitates binding of additional substrate molecules to other active sites
- Allosteric enzyme exhibit 2 states namely, tense state (T form) refers to less active subunit and relaxed state (R form) refers to more active subunit.

### Modulators

- Modulators or effectors are molecules that bind to allosteric sites of allosteric enzyme and change their activity

| | *Positive modulator (activator)* | *Negative modulator (inhibitor)* |
|---|---|---|
| • Site of binding | • Activator site | • Inhibitor site |
| • Effect of biding of binding allosteric enzyme | • Stabilizes enzyme in more active conformational form | • Stabilizes enzyme in inactive conformational state |
| • Effect on velocity curve | • Shifts to left (towards lower substrate concentration) | • Shift to right (towards to higher substrate concentration) |
| • Km Value | • Decreased | • Increased |

*Examples*

| *Enzymes* | *Metabolic pathway* | *Positive Modifier* | *Negative Modifier* |
|---|---|---|---|
| • Phosphofructokinase | Glycolysis | AMP, ADP | ATP, citrate |
| • Acetyl CoA carboxylase | Fatty acid synthesis | Citrate | Palmitic acid |
| • Isocitrate dehydrogenase | TCA cycle | ADP, $NAD^+$ | ATP |
| • Aspartate transcarbomylase | Pyrimidine nucleotide synthesis | ATP | CTP |
| • Fructose 1,6 biphosphatase | Gluconeogenesis | Citrate | AMP |

## Significance

- Allosteric enzymes frequently catalyze early committed and rate limiting step (irreversible) in a metabolic pathways and such regulatory enzymes are called key enzymes or rate limiting enzymes thus allosteric acts as regulatory enzymes of a metabolic pathway.

## 6. Outline the steps for synthesis of cholesterol. Discuss the rate limiting step and regulation of synthesis of cholesterol.

Refer Question No. 1 June 2016 (RS2).

## 7. Describe the reactions of citric acid cycle.

Refer Question No. 1 June 2008 (RS2).

## 8. Briefly outline the steps of de novo synthesis of purine.

Refer Question No. 2 June 2013 (RS2).

## 9. Hormonal regulation of fluid and electrolyte.

- Fluid and electrolyte balance is interrelated evident by fact that concentration of sodium determines total fluid content of body.

## Hormonal Regulation of Fluid and Electrolytes

- Hormones involved in regulation of fluid and electrolytes are:

| *Antidiuretic hormone (vasopressin)* | *Aldosterone* | *Renin-angiotensin system* | *Atrial natriuretic factor* |
|---|---|---|---|
| • Increases permeability of renal collecting ducts to water, leading to water reabsorption<br>*Mechanism of action*<br>• Vasopressin binds to V2 receptors on collecting duct cells and activates adenyl cyclase increasing levels of cyclic AMP resulting in insertion of water channels into luminal membrane | • Enhances reabsorption of sodium in distal renal tubules in exchange for potassium and hydrogen ions | • Regulate water and electrolyte balance by stimulating release of aldosterone | • Inhibits release of antidiuretic hormone and aldosterone<br>• In large doses, it increases excretion of sodium in urine |

Interrelationship of various hormones on water and electrolytes can be represented as follows

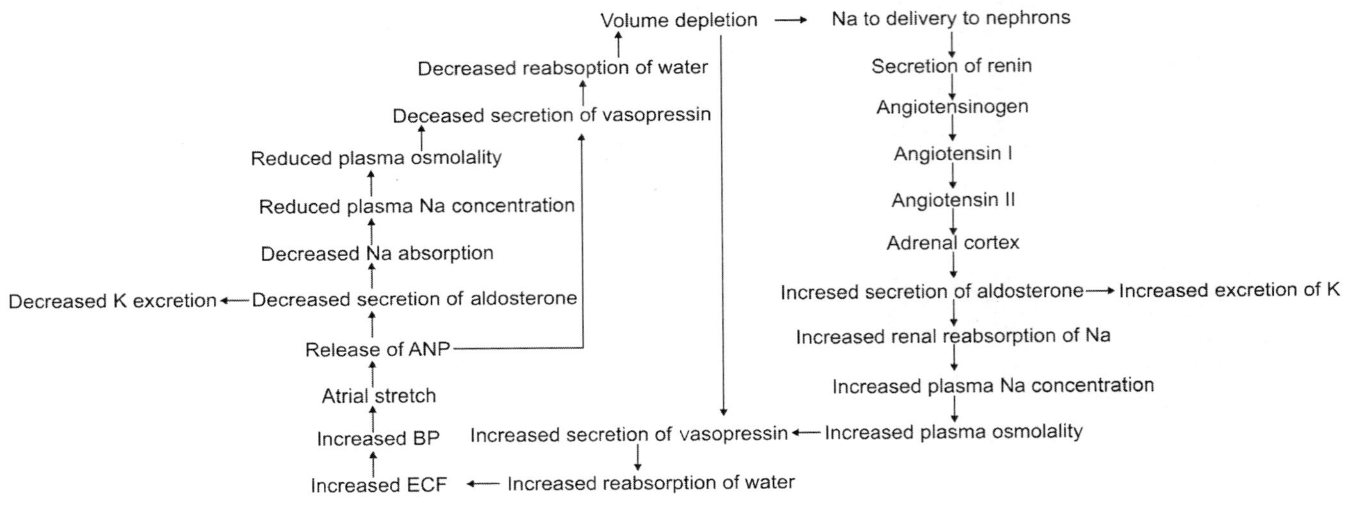


**Fig. 9:** Hormonal regulation of fluid and electrolytes



**Significance**

- A harmony of these hormones is essential to maintain fluid and electrolyte balance in body and any aberration due to hyper- or hypo-secretion of these hormones may lead to edema, dehydration, and electrolyte abnormalities.

### 10. Briefly explain the renal mechanisms involved in maintenance of pH of blood.

Refer Question No. 2 June 2012 (RS2).

### 11. Sources, biochemical role and dietary requirement of vitamin A.

Refer Question No. 2 Dec. 2009 (RS2).

### 12. Protein calorie malnutrition.

Refer Question No. 9 June 2010 (RS2).

## SHORT ANSWERS

### 13. Oncogenes.

Refer Question No. 3 Dec. 2010 (RS2).

### 14. Thyroid function tests—routine and anti-TPO.

- Thyroid function tests comprises biochemical, pathological and radiological investigations carried out to assess thyroid functions and help confirm diagnosis of any thyroid disorder and also its relation to anterior pituitary.

| *Tests* | *Normal range* | *Interpretation* | *Remarks* |
|---|---|---|---|
| a. Hormonal studies | | | |
| i. Serum protein bound iodine | 3.5–8 µg/dL | | Cheap and simple test: Nonspecific and unreliable (i.e. measures non hormonal form of iodine) |
| ii. Free serum thyroxin (F-T4) | 0.7–2 ng/dL | ↓ hypothyroidism<br>↑ hyperthyroidism | Measured by competitive protein binding or radioimmune assay methods:<br>• More sensitive<br>• Excludes interference disease or drugs on TBG |

*Contd...*

*Contd...*

| Tests | Normal range | Interpretation | Remarks |
|---|---|---|---|
| iii. Total serum tri-iodothyronine ($T_3$) | 80–200 ng/dL | • ↑ hyperthyroidism, acute thyroiditis, thyrotoxicosis<br>• ↓ hypothyroidism | • Estimated by radioimmunoassay method<br>• Effective test<br>• But very difficult |
| iv. Total serum thyroxine ($T_4$) | 5.4–11.5 μg/dL | • ↓ hypothyroidism<br>• ↑ hyperthyroidism | Evaluates extent of hormone deficiency or excess |
| v. T3 resin uptake | 0.91–1.21 μg | • ↓ hyperthyroidism<br>• ↑ hypothyroidism | Measures unoccupied $T_3$ binding sites by fixing of radiolabeled $T_3$ to free thyroid binding proteins in blood |
| vi. Free thyroxin index (FTI) | 3.5–8 | | • Calculated as serum $T_4 \times T_3$ uptake%<br>• Accurately reflects thyroid status of an individual (best single test) |
| vii. Serum thyroid stimulating hormone (TSH) | 0.2–5.4 μU/mL | • ↑ hyperpitutirsm, primary hypothyroidism<br>• Undetectable in hyperthyroidism<br>• ↓ primary hyperthyroidism, secondary and tertiary hypothyroidism | Measured by immunoassay |
| viii. TSH stimulation test | 200 μg IV dose of TRH raises TSH level to 10 μU/mL in 20 min and slowly returns to normal by 2 hours | • ↑ hypothyroidism<br>• No response in hyperthyroidism | • Measures response of thyroid stimulating hormone to thyrotrophin releasing hormone<br>• Useful for distinguishing primary from pituitary hypothyroidism |
| ix. $T_3$ or $T_4$ suppression test | | • Suppression of TSH—hyperthyroidism<br>• No response—pituitary disorder | • Measures response of thyroid hormone on TSH secretion<br>• Used to confirm hyperthyroidism |
| x. Thyroid binding globulin (TBG) | 12–28 mg/mL | • ↑ hypothyrodism, drugs (estrogen), pregnancy<br>• ↓ hyperthyroidism, drugs (androgen), chronic liver disease, nephrotic syndrome | Helpful to evaluate availability of free hormone in plasma |
| b. Radioisotope studies | | | |
| i. Thyroid iodine uptake test | 1–3% after 2 hours<br>15–15% after 24 hours | • ↓ hypothyroidism, thyrotoxicosis, subacute thyroidits<br>• ↑ hyperthyroidism | Measures rate and proportion of uptake of iodine or technetium isotopes by thyroid gland |
| ii. Thyroid scan | Functioning (hot) areas take up radioisotopes whereas nonfunctioning (cold) areas do not uptake radioisotopes | | • Following administration of radioisotopes of iodine or technetium, scanning is done after 24 hours and 30 minutes respectively<br>• Also detects ectopic thyroid tissue or retrosternal goiter |
| c. Autoimmunity tests | | | |
| i. Anti-thyroglobulin | <8% | ↑ autoimmune thyroid disease | Not present in remission |
| ii. Anti-TPO (thyroperoxidase) | <100 IU/L | ↑ autoimmune thyroid disease | • More sensitive test<br>• Detectable during remission |
| iii. Anti-thyroid receptor | Negative | — | Confirms Graves' disease including neonatal conditions |
| iv. Thyroglobulin | 5–25 mg/dL | ↑ goiter, inflammation of thyroid | Thyroid cancer marker |

### 15. Cytochromes.

- Cytochromes are heme enzymes helping in cellular oxidation
- They have an iron atom which can oscillate between $Fe^{2+}$ (ferric) and $Fe3^{+}$ (ferrous) state during oxidation and reduction (in contrast to Hb iron which remains in ferrous state).

*Examples*

| *Cytochromes* | *Location* | *Function* |
|---|---|---|
| • Cytochrome aa3 (Cytochrome oxidase)<br>• Cytochrome b<br>• Cytochrome c and c1 | Inner mitochondrial membrane | • Are members of electric transport chain as follows: Flavoproteins → CoQ → Cyt b → Cyt c1 → Cyt c → Cyt $aa_3$<br>• Serve as transfer electron from flavoprotein to cytochrome oxidase<br>• All cytochromes except cytochrome oxidase are anaerobic dehydrogenases |
| • Cytochrome $b_5$<br>• Cytochrome $p_{450}$ | Smooth endoplasmic retinaculum | Xenobiotics (drug metabolism, steroid metabolism) |

### 16. GTT graph for renal glycosuria.

- Renal glycosuria is excretion of glucose in urine

*GTT graph for renal glycosuria*

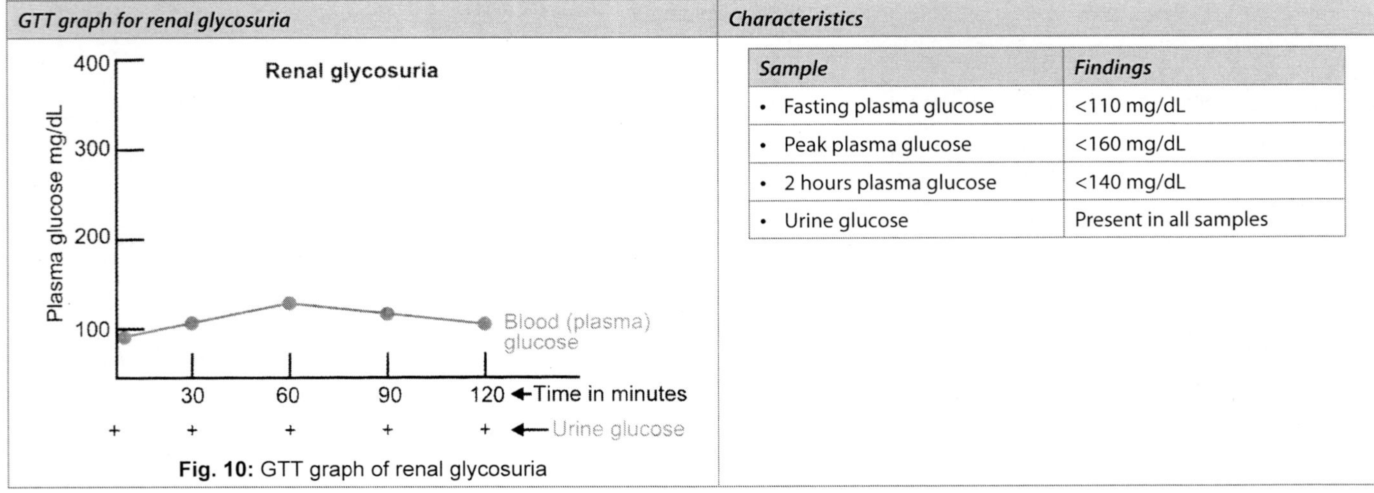


Fig. 10: GTT graph of renal glycosuria

*Characteristics*

| *Sample* | *Findings* |
|---|---|
| • Fasting plasma glucose | <110 mg/dL |
| • Peak plasma glucose | <160 mg/dL |
| • 2 hours plasma glucose | <140 mg/dL |
| • Urine glucose | Present in all samples |

### 17. Antioxidants.

Refer Question No. 6 June 2008 (RS2).

### 18. Operon concept.

Refer Question No. 10 Dec. 2013 (RS2).

### 19. Bence Jones proteins.

Refer Question No. 18 Dec. 2005 (RS2).

### 20. What is porphyria? Mention the defect and signs and symptoms of acute intermittent porphyria.

Refer Question No. 9 June 2015 (RS2).

### 21. Enumerate three functions of the liver and three tests with reference ranges to assess them.

Refer Question No. 11 Dec. 2008 (RS2).

## 22. What is a chimeric DNA molecule? Give the applications of recombinant technology.

- Chimeric DNA is hybrid combination of DNA of interest (foreign DNA) and vector DNA.
- Also called recombinant DNA or hybrid DNA
- (Chimera = Greek; a monster with lion's head, goat's body and serpent's tail).

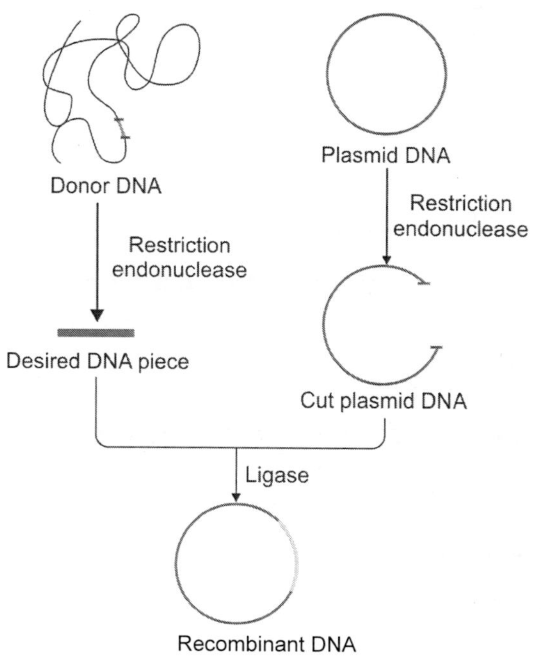


**Fig. 11:** Chimeric DNA

**For application of recombinant technology**

Refer Question No. 2 June 2008 (RS2).

# MBBS PHASE I EXAMINATION

## JUNE 2012

## (Revised Scheme 2 & 3)

## LONG ESSAYS

### 1. Give an account of metabolism of phenylalanine. Add a note on disorders associated with its metabolism.

Refer Question No. 1 Dec. 2010 (RS2).

### 2. What is the normal pH of blood? Explain the mechanism of how it is regulated.

- Normal pH of blood is 7.4 ± 0.5.

### Regulation of Blood pH (Acid-Base Balance)

- pH blood is regulated by following mechanism.

a. Buffer system in body
b. Renal mechanism—regulation of concentration of $H^+$ and $HCO_3^-$ ions in blood by ultimate excretion of excess of acid or base
c. Respiratory mechanism—regulation of excretion of $CO_2$ and hence regulation of $H_2CO_3$ in blood.

*A. Buffer System in Body*

Buffer is a mixture of weak acid and its conjugate base or weak base and its conjugate acid that resists change in pH on addition of a acid or alkali.

*Types*

i. Mixture of a weak acid with their salt with a strong base
   Example: Bicarbonate buffer
ii. Mixture of a weak base with their salt with a strong acid

*Important buffers in body are*

| *Location* | *Buffers present* |
|---|---|
| • Plasma | • Bicarbonate buffer<br>• Phosphate buffer<br>• Protein buffer |
| • Erythrocytes | • Hemoglobin buffer<br>• Protein buffer |
| • Bone | • Phosphate buffer |
| • Urine | • Phosphate buffer<br>• Ammonia buffer |

| Components | Location | Action |
|---|---|---|
| a. Bicarbonate buffer system<br>– Most important plasma buffer<br>– An open buffer system, i.e. its components are present in two separate communicating compartments<br>*Features*<br>– Effective in buffering bases and non-volatile acids<br>– When an acid ($H^+$) is added to the buffer, base of the buffer ($HCO_3^-$) is used up to form the weak acid and the concentration of base falls $HCO_3^+ + H + \rightarrow H_2\,CO_3$<br>– When strong base is added to the buffer, the weak acid of the buffer is used up to form conjugate base and water and concentration of acid falls.<br>– $H_2CO_3 + OH^- \rightarrow HCO_3^- + H_2O$ | | |
| – Bicarbonate and carbonic acid | • Plasma | • Whenever the bicarbonate buffer neutralizes any acid or base the replacement of one of the member of buffer pair by other member changes the buffer ratio and consequently blood pH<br>• But buffer ratio is immediately restored by altering either the respiratory elimination of $H_2\,CO_3$ as $CO_2$ or urinary elimination of $HCO_3^-$ |
| b. Phosphate buffer system<br>– Second most important buffer next to bicarbonate buffer though its concentration is only 8% of that bicarbonate buffer in blood | | |
| – Diphasic phosphate ($HPO_4^{2-}$) as base and mono basic phosphate ($H_2PO^{4-}$) as acid | • Plasma, bone and urine | • Buffer ratio is adjusted by renal elimination not by respiratory elimination<br>• It corrects acidosis in chronic renal failure |
| c. Protein buffer system<br>– Accounts for 1–2% of buffering capacity of blood | | |
| – Acidic proteins and their anion at isoelectric pH as conjugate bases | • Plasma, RBCs | |
| d. Hemoglobin buffer system<br>– Major buffer present intracellularly in erythrocytes | | |
| – Hemoglobin and reduced hemoglobin (HHb) | • RBCs | • Hemoglobin acts as buffer by forming carbaminohemoglobin when $CO_2$ interacts with amino group of hemoglobin |
| e. Ammonia buffer system<br>– Major buffer system in kidney for removal of hydrogen ions | | |
| – Ammonia and ammonium ions | • Urine | • Ammonia formed in distal renal tubular cells traps hydrogen ions to form ammonium ions which cannot be reabsorbed and hence excreted as ammonium chloride<br>• Accounts for renal regulation of acid-base balance |

## *B. Renal Regulation of Blood pH*

- Kidneys acts as second line defence in acid-base imbalance
- This important function of kidneys is usually referred to as acidification of urine
- While excreating hydrogen ions, kidney simultaneously reabsorb bicarbonate from glomurlar filtrate.

*Mechanism of action*

| | |
|---|---|
| a. Excretion of $H^+$ and generation and resorption of $HCO_3^-$ | • Occurs in proximal convulated tubules<br>• $CO_2$ combines with $H_2O$ to form carbonic acid with help of carbonic anhydrase<br>• This carbonic acid then ionizes to give $H^+$ and $HCO_3^-$<br>• Hydrogen ions are secreted in exchange for $Na^+$ which are reabsorbed along with $HCO_3^-$ into blood<br>• This serves to excrete $H^+$ and generate bicarbonate thereby increasing the alkali reserve |

| | |
|---|---|
| b. Reabsorption of bicarbonate | • Bicarbonate in glomerular filtrate in proximal convulated tubules combines with $H^+$ to form carbonic acid<br>• Carbonic anhydrase on brush border dissociates it int o $H_2O^+$ and $CO_2$<br>• $CO_2$ diffuses into cell and combine with $H_2O$ and ionizes to give $H^+$ and $HCO_3^-$<br>• Hydrogen ions are secreted in exchange for $Na^+$ which are reabsorbed along with $HCO_3^-$ into blood<br>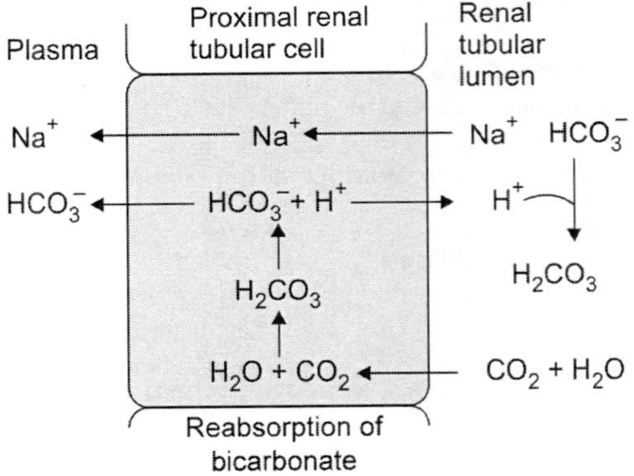<br><br>**Fig. 1:** Reabsorption of bicarbonate<br>• There is no net excreation of $H^+$ or generation of new bicarbonate. So this mechanism helps to maintain a steady state of acid–base balance. |
| c. Excretion of titrable acid | • Major titrable acid present in urine is sodium acid phosphate<br>• Due to $Na^+ - H^+$ exchange, $Na_2HPO_4$ (basic phosphate) is converted to $NaH_2PO_4$ (acid phosphate) which is excreted<br>• Excretion of titrable acid enables constant excretion and elimination of acid from body<br>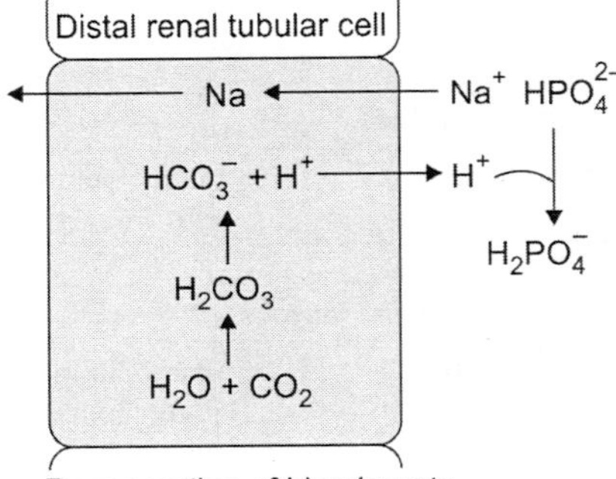<br><br>**Fig. 2:** Excretion of titrable acid |
| d. Excretion of $NH_4^+$ (ammonia buffer mechanism) | • Occurs mainly at distal convulated tubules<br>• Excreted $NH_3$ traps $H^+$ in the urine to become $NH_4^+$ and thus large quantity of acid is excreted<br>• Glutaminase in tubular cells hydrolyze glutamine to $NH_3$ and glutamic acid<br>• $NH_3$ diffuse into lumen and combine with $H^+$<br>• $NH_4^+$ formed cannot diffuse back into cells and therefore excreted as ammonium chloride<br>• Glutaminase activity is increased in acidosis so more $NH_4^+$ is excreted<br>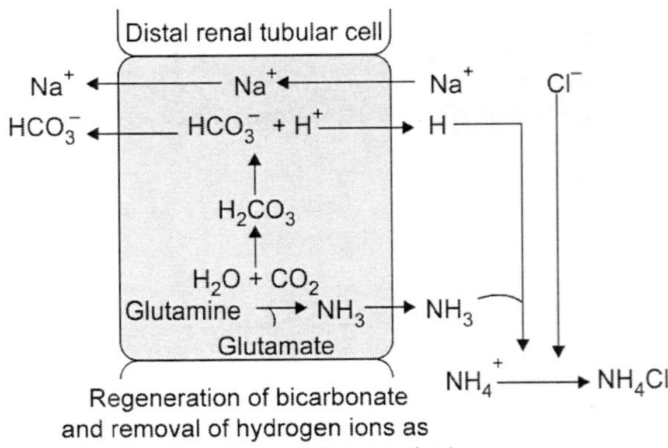<br><br>**Fig. 3:** Excretion of $NH_4^+$ (ammonia buffer mechanism) |

- Thus renal regulation of pH can be summarized as follows:

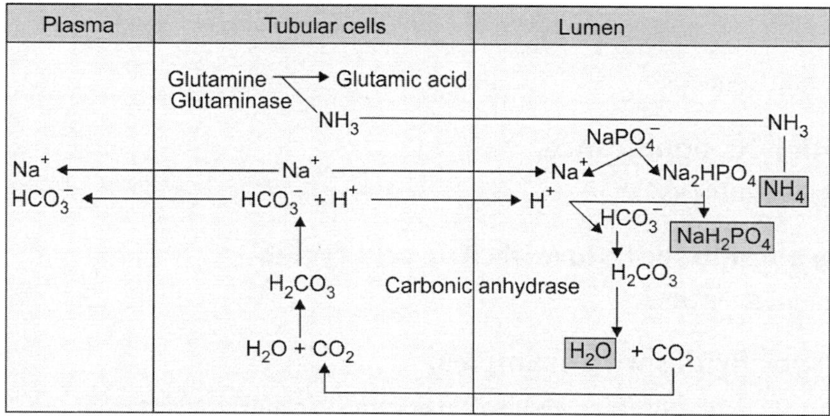


**Fig. 4:** Summary of renal regulation of pH

### *C. Respiratory Regulation of Blood pH*

- Lungs play first line of defence in pH regulation along with body buffers
- It responds to any change in pH immediately but it cannot proceed to completion
- This action is mediated through chemoreceptors in respiratory center.

*Mechanism of action*

| *Regulation of respiratory rate* | *Through hemoglobin buffer* |
|---|---|
| • In acidosis $pCO_2$ (partial pressure of $CO_2$) is increased leading to increased diffusion of $CO_2$ from body (hyperventilation)<br>• Decrease in $H^+$ concentration depresses respiratory center with consequent slow and shallow respiration (hypoventilation) resulting in retention of $CO_2$ | • Lungs also regulate pH through hemoglobin buffer system as follows:<br>i. At tissue<br>– $HbO_2 \rightarrow Hb + O_2$ (to tissue)<br>– $CO_2$ (from tissue) + $H_2O$ (ECF) $\rightarrow H_2CO_3$<br>– $Hb + H_2CO_3 \rightarrow HHb + HCO_3^-$<br>ii. At lungs<br>– $HHb + O_2 \rightarrow HHbO_2 \rightarrow HbO_2 + H^+$<br>– $HCO_3^- + H^+ \rightarrow H_2CO_3 \rightarrow H_2O + CO_2$ (expired) |

## Significance

- Proper and prompt interaction of body buffers, lungs and kidneys is essential for a well-balanced regulation of body pH.

## Importance of Maintaining Acid-Base Balance (Regulation of Body pH)

- pH is based on concentration of hydrogen ion concentration in body
- Acid-base balance, i.e. hydrogen ion concentration has a widespread effect on function of body's enzyme systems
- Hydrogen ion is highly reactive and will combine with bases or negatively charged ions at very low concentrations
- Proteins contain many negatively charged and basic groups within their structure
- Thus, a change in pH will alter the degree ionization of a protein, which may in turn, affect its functioning
- At more extreme hydrogen ion concentrations a protein's structure may be completely disrupted
- Enzymes function optimally over a very narrow range of hydrogen ion concentrations
- For most enzymes this optimum pH is close to the physiological range for plasma (pH= 7.35 to 7.45)
- As enzymes have a huge number of functions around the body, an abnormal pH can result in disturbances in a wide range of body systems
- Thus, disturbances in pH may result in abnormal respiratory and cardiac function, derangements in blood clotting and drug metabolism, to name but a few
- Therefore, it is important to maintain the acid-base balance or hydrogen ion concentration within the normal range in body.

## SHORT ESSAYS

### 3. Cori's cycle.

Refer Question No. 1 June 2009 (RS2).

### 4. What is $K_m$? Mention its significance.

Refer Question No. 6 Dec. 2010 (RS2).

### 5. What is meant by amphibolic nature of citric acid cycle?

Refer Question No. 1 June 2008 (RS2).

### 6. Explain enzyme specificities with examples.

- Specificity is characteristic property of active site of an enzyme to catalyze a particular reaction.

#### Types

- Stereospecificity
- Reaction specificity
- Substrate specificity.

| *Sterospecificity (optical specificity)* | *Reaction specificity* | *Substrate specificity* | | |
|---|---|---|---|---|
| | | *Absolute substrate specificity* | *Relative substrate specificity* | *Broad specificity* |
| • Acts on only one isomer of a substrate due to specific binding of distinct regions of substrate to enzyme active sites<br>• However, isomerase enzymes do not exhibit stereospecificity | • Ability of a substrate to undergo different types of reactions, each catalyzed by different enzymes | • Acts only on specific substrate and not even on other structurally similar substances | • Act on structurally similar or related substrates | • Acts on closely related substrates |
| *Examples* | | | | |
| • Hexokinase acts only on D-hexoses<br>• Glucokinase acts only on D-glucose | • Amino acids can undergo transamination, decarboxylation, oxidative deamination, etc. | • Glucokinase acts only on glucose and not on other monosaccharides | • Group specificity<br>– Trypsin hydrolyzes peptide linkage involving arginine or lysine<br>• Bond specificity<br>– Glycosidases acts on glycosidic bonds of carbohydrates | • Hexokinase acts on glucose, fructose, mannose, etc. |

### 7. Transmethylation.

Refer Question No. 4 June 2010 (RS2).

### 8. Standard urea clearance test.

- When the urinary volume is less than 2 mL/min, the rate of urea elimination is reduced, because relatively more urea is reabsorbed in the tubules, and is proportional to square root of urinary volume.
- Such clearance is termed as standard clearance of urea (Cs)

$$Cs = \frac{u \times \sqrt{v}}{B}$$

*Average normal value*

- 54 mL/min

### Significance

- Provided no prerenal factors are temporarily reducing the clearance of urea, the volume of blood cleared of urea per minute is an index of renal function
- If a larger volume than normal is cleared/mt, renal function is satisfactory
- If a smaller volume is cleared, renal function is impaired.

### 9. Salvage pathway.

Refer Question No. 11 Dec. 2005 (RS2).

### 10. Briefly outline the steps of de novo synthesis of purine.

Refer Question No. 2 June 2013 (RS2).

### 11. Mention the sources, RDA and factors affecting calcium absorption.

Refer Question No. 2 June 2009 (RS2).

### 12. Deficiency manifestation of vitamin A.

Refer Question No. 2 Dec. 2009 (RS2).

## SHORT ANSWERS

### 13. Free radicals.

Refer Question No. 16 June 2005 (RS2).

### 14. Mitochondria.

- Mitochondria are spherical oral or rod like subcellular organelles
- They are called powerhouse of the cell because they are involved in ATP production through electron transport chain and oxidative phosphorylation which are located in the inner mitochondrial membrane
- Mitochondria are absent in erythrocytes.

### Structure

- Mitochondria are elongated organelle surrounded by two concentric layers, outer and inner membrane.

| | *Features* | *Functions* |
|---|---|---|
| Outer membrane | • Consists mostly of phospholipids and contains a considerable amount of cholesterol<br>• Also contains many copies of protein called porin | Porin and other proteins form channels that permit substances with molecular weights of <10,000 to diffuse freely across outer mitochondrial membrane |
| Inner membrane | • Very rich in proteins and contains high proportion of phospholipid, cardiolipin<br>• Highly folded and these tightly packed inward folds are called cristae | • Selective permeability (impermeable to polar and ionic substance)<br>• Cristae contains components of electron transport chain and oxidative phosphorylation thus is involved with production of ATPs |
| Inter membrane space | Space between outer membrane and inner membrane | Contains few enzymes like adenylate kinase |
| Matrix | • Large internal compartment<br>• Contains DNA and ribosomes | • Contains enzymes involved in intermediary metabolism such as enzymes of citric acid cycle and β-oxidation of fatty acids<br>• Site of metabolic reactions and replication of mitochondrial DNA |

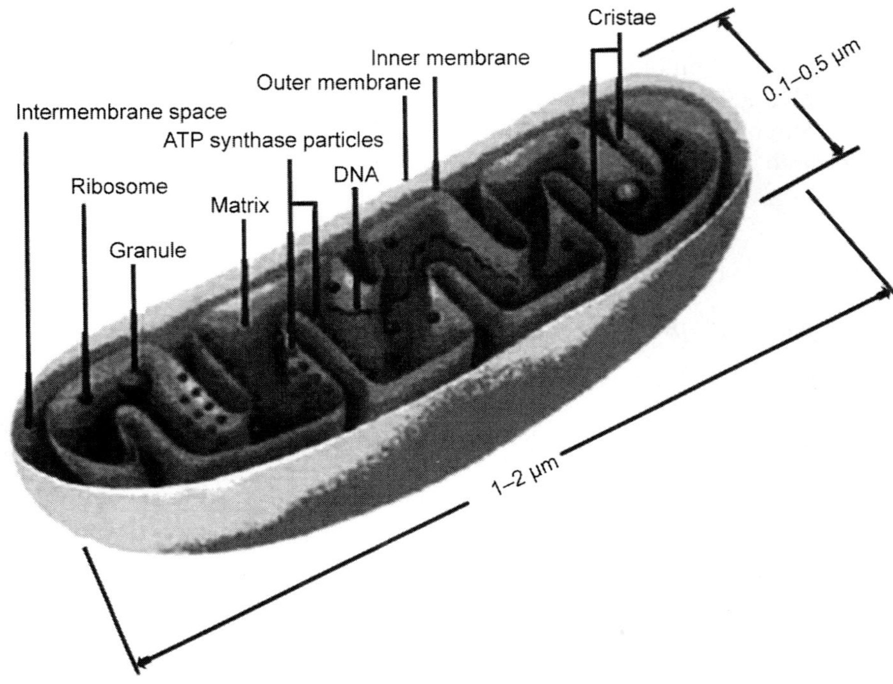


**Fig. 5:** Structure of mitochondria



## Significance

- Inherited disorder of mitochondrial metabolic function
  - Fumarase deficiency (mitochondrial encephalomyelopathy)
  - Multiple acyl CoA dehydrogenase deficiency (organic aciduria or glutaric aciduria type II)
- Inherited disorder of oxidative phosphorylation
  - LEON disease
- Mitochondrial dysfunction is one of the early events in cells undergoing apoptosis (programed cell death)
- Mitochondrial function can be inhibited by cyanide and carbon monoxide which inhibit cytochrome oxidase (component of electron transport chain) thus decreasing ATP synthesis
- Megamitochondria (larger mitochondria) is seen in viral hepatitis and alcoholic liver disease
- Erythrocytes lack mitochondria; therefore, anaerobic glycolysis provides energy requirement of erythrocytes.

## 15. Steattorrhea.

- Steatorrhea or fatty stool is condition characterized by loss of lipid in stool, i.e. when average daily excretion of fat exceeds 6 g/day.

## Causes

| *Defective digestion of fat due to deficiency of pancreatic lipase* | *Defective absorption of fat due to* |
|---|---|
| • Chronic pancreatic disorder<br>• Surgical removal of pancreas | • Deficiency of bile acids and salts due to bile duct obstruction—gallstones, tumors of head of pancreas, enlarged lymph node<br>• Diseases of intestines—celiac disease, sprue, Crohn's disease<br>• Surgical removal of large length of the intestine |

## Significance

- Steatorrhea is commonly seen in disorders associated with pancreas, biliary obstruction, severe liver dysfunction, etc.

## 16. Hartnup's disease.

- Hartnup's disease or neutral amino aciduria is an inherited disorder of tryptophan metabolism.

| *Inheritance* | *Cause* | *Features* | *Biochemical features* |
|---|---|---|---|
| • Autosomal recessive inheritance | • Due to inherited defect in intestinal and renal tubular transport of tryptophan and other neutral amino acids (alanine, serine, threonine, valine and histidine) | • Characterized by pellagra like features due to decreased synthesis of NAD from tryptophan<br>• Skin lesions include erythematous and eczematous skin rash<br>• Neurological manifestations are cerebellar ataxia and emotional disturbances | • Low plasma levels of tryphophan and other neutral amino acids<br>• Neutral aminoaciduria<br>• Increased urinary excretion of indoacetic acid and indolepyruvic acid |

## 17. Derivatives of tryptophan.

- Tryptophan is an aromatic amino acid
- It is an essential amino acid which cannot be synthesized in body and its daily requirement has to be supplied only through diet.

### Derivatives of Tryptophan

a. Protein and peptides
   - Tryptophan is one of the standard amino acid present in proteins and peptides

b. Serotonin
   - Serotonin or 5-hydroxy tryptamine is an important monoamine synthesized from tryptophan.

| *Site of synthesis* | *Biosynthesis* | *Catabolism* |
|---|---|---|
| • GIT mucosa<br>• Brain<br>• Mast cells and platelets | 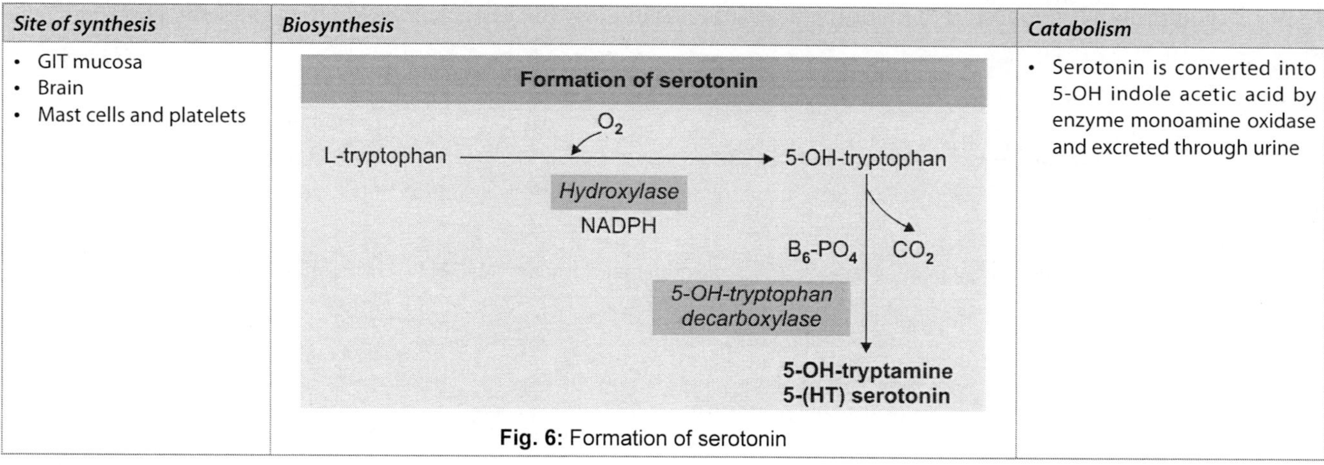<br>**Fig. 6:** Formation of serotonin | • Serotonin is converted into 5-OH indole acetic acid by enzyme monoamine oxidase and excreted through urine |



*Functions (Action)*
- Neurotransmitter in brain
- Regulation of cerebral activity (excitation of brain)
- Reduces sensitivity to pain
- Induces sleep
- Controls behavior pattern
- Potent vasoconstrictor
- Contraction of smooth muscles in bronchioles and arterioles
- Evokes release of peptide hormones from GIT and is necessary for GIT motility
- Stimulates respiratory and circulatory chemoreceptors causing tachycardia, rise in BP and hyperpnea
- Produces melatonin in pineal gland.

*Significance*
- Overproduction of serotonin occurs due to carcinoid tumors causing flushing, sweating, intermittent diarrhea and fluctuating hypertension
- Deficiency of serotonin produces depression, psychosis, etc.

c. Melatonin
   - Melatonin is a pineal gland hormone derived from tryptophan.

*Synthesis of melatonin*

| *Site of synthesis* | *Precursor* | *Biosynthesis* | *Regulation* |
|---|---|---|---|
| Pineal body | Serotonin | Serotonin → (Acetyl CoA → CoASH; Serotonin acetyl transferase) → N-acetyl serotonin ($CH_2-NH-C(=O)-CH_3$) → (S-adenosyl methionine → S-adenosyl homocysteine; Methyl transferase) → Melatonin<br>**Fig. 7:** Synthesis of melatonin | • Rate limiting enzyme—serotonin N-acetyl transferase<br>• Factors influencing—light |

*Functions*
- Modulation of in circardian rhythms or diurnal variations of body (sleep-wake cycle)
- Inhibits production of melanocyte stimulating hormone (MSH) and adrenocorticotropic hormone (ACTH)
- Inhibitory effect on ovarian functions
- Involved in neurotransmission

d. NAD and NADP (coenzymes of niacin)
   - Trypatophan is converted to nicotinic acid (niacin) in body (60 mg is converted to make 1 mg NAD).

*Steps*

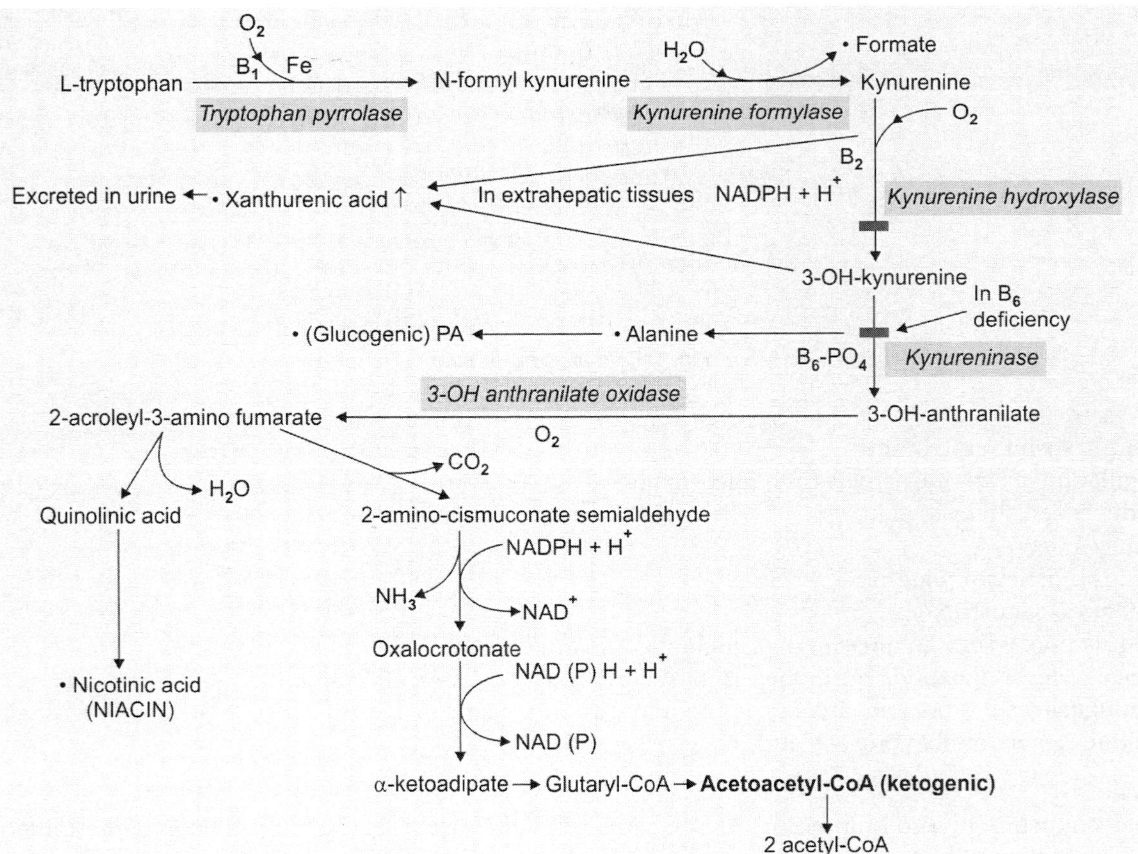


**Fig. 8:** Formation of NAD and NADP

e. Glucose and ketone bodies
   - Tryptophan is both glucogenic and ketogenic amino acid
   - Glucogenic: It yields alanine that forms pyruvate which can be converted to glucose
   - Ketogenic: It is also catabolized to acetyl CoA that forms ketone bodies.

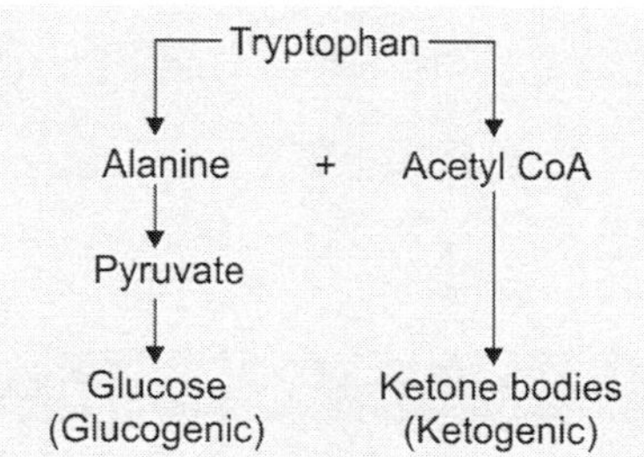


**Fig. 9:** Formation of glucose and ketone bodies

## Significance

- Tryptophan is an essential amino acid whose daily requirement needs to supplied only through diet and omission of tryptophan in diet leads to tissue wasting and negative nitrogen balance
- It is also important because it is as it involved in synthesis of NAD, NADP which are involved in numerous metabolic reactions.

## 18. Menke's disease.

- Menke's disease or Menke's syndrome is a rare inborn error of copper metabolism.

| Inheritance | Cause | Features | Biochemical features |
|---|---|---|---|
| • Sex linked recessive inheritance | • Mutation in gene coding of copper binding P type ATPase in intestinal mucosal cell<br>• This causes defect in transport of copper from intestinal mucosal cell into blood resulting in deficiency of copper in other tissues of body<br>• Copper may be trapped in metallothionein | • Especially affects male infants<br>• Characterized by growth failure, mental retardation and kinky or silky hairs with depigmentation<br>• Death occurs early in infancy | • Low serum copper level<br>• Low serum ceruloplasmin<br>• Low copper stores in liver |

## 19. Specific dynamic action of food stuff.

- Specific dynamic action (SDA) of food is extra heat produced over and above calorific value of food
- The extra heat produced comes from constituents of tissues; thus, ingestion of protein causes high SDA because of several reactions of proteins such as transamination and urea synthesis
- Heat of SDA can be utilized for body temperature regulation but not for muscular or cellular work
- Thus it is also known as calorigenic action or thermogenic action or thermic action (effect) of food.

## SDA of Food

- Proteins—30% (highest)
- Carbohydrates—5%
- Fat—15%.

## Significance

- Balanced diet
   - SDA of food has to be kept in mind while prescribing a balanced diet; SDA of balanced diet is 10%
   - SDA percentage has to be added to required calorie intake to make up for calorie deficit by SDA, i.e. for a person requiring 1,600 cal/day, he should receive extra 160 cal (total 1,760 cal) by a balanced diet

- Temperature regulation
  - Heat of SDA can be utilized for body temperature regulation, hence in cold climates, diet rich in protein is recommended.

## 20. Types and causes of beri-beri.

Refer Question No. 8 June 2005 (RS2).

## 21. Functions of vitamin K.

- Vitamin K is fat-soluble vitamin
- Named K from koagulation (German).

| *Forms* | *Sources* | *RDA* | *Absorption, transport and storage* |
|---|---|---|---|
| • $K_1$ (phylloquinone) found in plants<br>• $K_2$ (menaquinone) found in animals (produced by intestinal flora)<br>• $K_3$ (menadione) is synthetic form | *Dietary*<br>• Cabbage, cauliflower, tomato, spinach<br>• Egg yolk, meat, liver, cheese and dairy products<br>*In vivo*<br>• Synthesized by intestinal bacterial flora | • 50–100 mg/day | • Absorbed along with fat and is dependent on bile salts<br>• Transported along LDL<br>• Stored in liver (mainly) and other tissues |

| *Biochemical functions* | *Deficiency* | |
|---|---|---|
| | *Causes* | *Features* |
| • Vitamin K acts as cofactor for enzyme carboxylase which activates inactive precursors of clotting factors prothrombin, factors VII, IX and X by carboxylation of glutamic acid residue present in them<br>• Helps in post-transcriptional modification of blood coagulation factors<br>• Enhances calcium binding capacity of some proteins of bone, spleen, placenta and kidney<br>• Necessary as cofactor in oxidative phosphorylation | • Faulty absorption (lack of bile salts)<br>• Loss into feces (diarrheal diseases)<br>• Antibiotic administration (killing of bacterial flora) | • Profuse bleeding with minor cuts due to increased clotting time<br>• Bruising tendency, ecchymotic patches, mucosal hemorrhage<br>• Hemorrhagic disease of newborn due to deficient hepatic store of vitamin K in newborns |

## 22. Functions of copper.

Refer Question No. 22 Dec. 2008 (RS2).

# MBBS PHASE I EXAMINATION
## DECEMBER 2012
## (Revised Scheme 2 & 3)

## LONG ESSAYS

### 1. Define lipids. Classify lipids with an example for each. Mention the functions of the lipids.

- Lipids are organic substances relatively insoluble in water, soluble in organic solvents like alcohol, ether; actually or potentially related to the fatty acids and utilized by living cells.

#### Classification of Lipids (Modified from Bloor)

A. Simple lipids
   - Esters of fatty acids with various alcohols
     a. Triacylglycerols: Esters of fatty acids with glycerol
        Example: Tripalmitin, triolein, groundnut oils
     b. Waxes: Esters of fatty acids with monohydroxy aliphatic alcohols other than glycerol
        Example: Esters of acetyl alcohol, bees wax, lanolin

B. Complex lipids
   - Esters of fatty acids with alcohol containing additional groups like phosphate, nitrogenous base, carbohydrates, protein, etc.
     a. Phospholipids: Lipids containing phosphoric acid residue and nitrogenous base
        i. Glycerophospholipids: Glycerol as alcohol
           Example: Lecithin, cephalin
        ii. Sphingophospholipids: Sphingosine as alcohol
           Example: Sphingomyelin
     b. Glycolipids: Lipids containing a fatty acid, carbohydrate, nitrogenous base and alcohol (sphingosine)
        i. Cerebrosides, e.g. Kerasin, Cerebron
        ii. Gangliosides, e.g. GM–1, GM-2
     c. Sulfolipids: Lipids-containing sulfate group
        Example: Sulfatid
     d. Aminolipids: Lipids-containing amino group
     e. Lipoproteins: Macromolecular complexes of lipids with proteins
        Example: Chylomicrons, VLDL, LDL and HDL

C. Derived lipids
   - Derivates obtained by hydrolysis of simple and compound lipids, which still possess general characteristics of lipids
     a. Fatty acids
        i. Saturated: Acetic acid
        ii. Unsaturated: Palmitic acid
        iii. Cyclic: Hydrocarpic acid
     b. Monoglycerides and diglycerides
     c. Alcohols
        i. Straight chain alcohols
        ii. Glycerols

iii. Alcohols containing β-ionone ring—vitamin A
iv. Cholesterol and other steroids

D. Miscellaneous lipids
   - Compounds possessing characteristics of lipids
     a. Aliphatic hydrocarbons: Iso-octadecane
     b. Eicosanoids (Prostaglandins, prostacyclins, thromboxanes, leukotrienes)
     c. Carotenoids
     d. Sequalene
     e. Vitamin E and K.

E. Neutral lipids
   - Lipids which do not posses any charge
   - Example: Triglycerides, cholesterol esters.

**Functions (Biomedical Importance)**

a. Energy reserve
   - Triacylglycerols stored in adipose tissue serves as stored form of energy
   - Oxidation of fatty acids provides about 22% of energy requirement of cells.
b. Insulation
   - Subcuteneous fat is an effective insulating material.
c. Thermogenesis
   - Brown adipose tissue rich in mitochondria is involved in thermogenesis.
d. Protection of internal organs
   - Internal organs are protected against trauma or shock by fat surrounding them.
e. Maintain cell integrity and regulate cell permeability
   - Lipids maintain cell integrity by being integral component of cell membrane
   - As component of cell membrane, they regulate membrane permeability.
f. Regulation of metabolism, growth and reproduction
   - Important lipid compounds regulate various body functions
   - Vitamin A is required for vision in dim light, growth differentiation, reproduction and maintenance of epithelial cell integrity
   - Essential amino acids are required for normal growth, reproduction, prevention of fatty liver and lowering plasma cholesterol
   - Cortisol regulates carbohydrate metabolism and inflammation
   - Aldosterone regulates sodium and water metabolism
   - Testosterone is essential for spermatogenesis
   - Estradiol and progesterone are important for regulation of menstrual cycle and maintenance of pregnancy.
g. Visceral functions
   - Prostaglandins cause inhibition of gastric secretions and constriction of uterine muscles.
h. Chemical mediators
   - Prostaglandins and platelet activating factors acts as mediators of inflammation
   - Leukotrienes function as mediators of anaphylactic and allergic reactions.
i. Blood coagulation and vascular reactivity
   - Prostacyclins cause coronary vasodilatation and inhibition of platelet aggregation
   - Thromboxanes cause vasoconstriction and promote platelet aggregation
   - Phospholipids are required for blood clotting process
   - Vitamin K is required for synthesis of active form of blood clotting factors
   - Platelet activating factor is a potent stimulator of platelet aggregation
j. Digestion, absorption and transport of lipids
   - Bile acids are essential for solubilization of cholesterol in bile, excretion of cholesterol, digestion of triacylglycerols and absorption of fats as well as fat soluble vitamins.

k. Medicinal use
   - Prostaglandins ($PGE_2$) are used in treatment of peptic ulcer and induction of labor
   - Digoxin is used in treatment of cardiac failure and cardiac arrhythmias
   - Cortisol is used as an anti-inflammatory drug.

## 2. Describe the synthesis of pyrimidine and its regulation.

- Pyrimidine are synthesized in body step by step from glutamine and carbon dioxide by de novo synthesis
- It differs from de novo synthesis of purine nucleotides in fact that here ring structure of pyrimidine is formed first and then ribose phosphate is added where in purine synthesis, ring structure is built upon ribose phosphate.

<table>
<tr><th>Sites</th><th>Substrates</th><th>Products</th></tr>
<tr>
<td>Tissue site<br>• Liver<br>Intracellular site<br>• Cytosol (rest of the reactions)<br>• Mitochondria (dihydroorotate → orotic acid)</td>
<td>
<table>
<tr><th>Source</th><th>Atom</th></tr>
<tr><td>• Aspartate</td><td>N-1, C-4, C-5 and C-6</td></tr>
<tr><td>• Glutamine (amino group)</td><td>N-3</td></tr>
<tr><td>• $CO_2$</td><td>C-2</td></tr>
</table>
N–3 from glutamine<br>N–1, C–4, C–5,C–6 from aspartate<br>C–2 from $CO_2$<br>
Fig. 1: Sources of carbon and nitrogen atoms in pyrimidine
</td>
<td>• Uridine triphosphate (UTP)<br>• Cytidine triphosphate (CTP)<br>• 2-deoxythymidine monophosphate (dTMP)</td>
</tr>
</table>

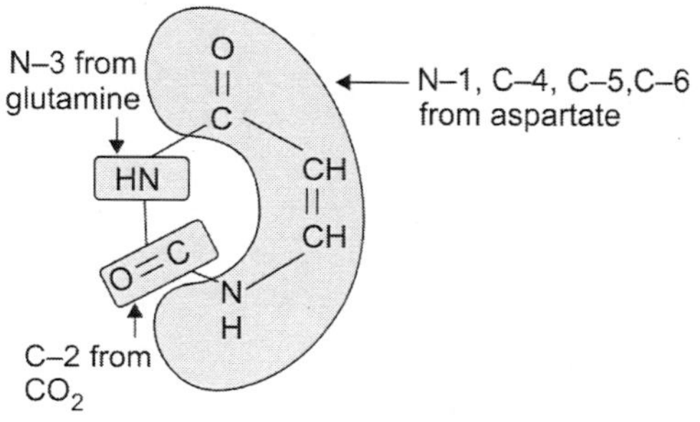

## Pathways

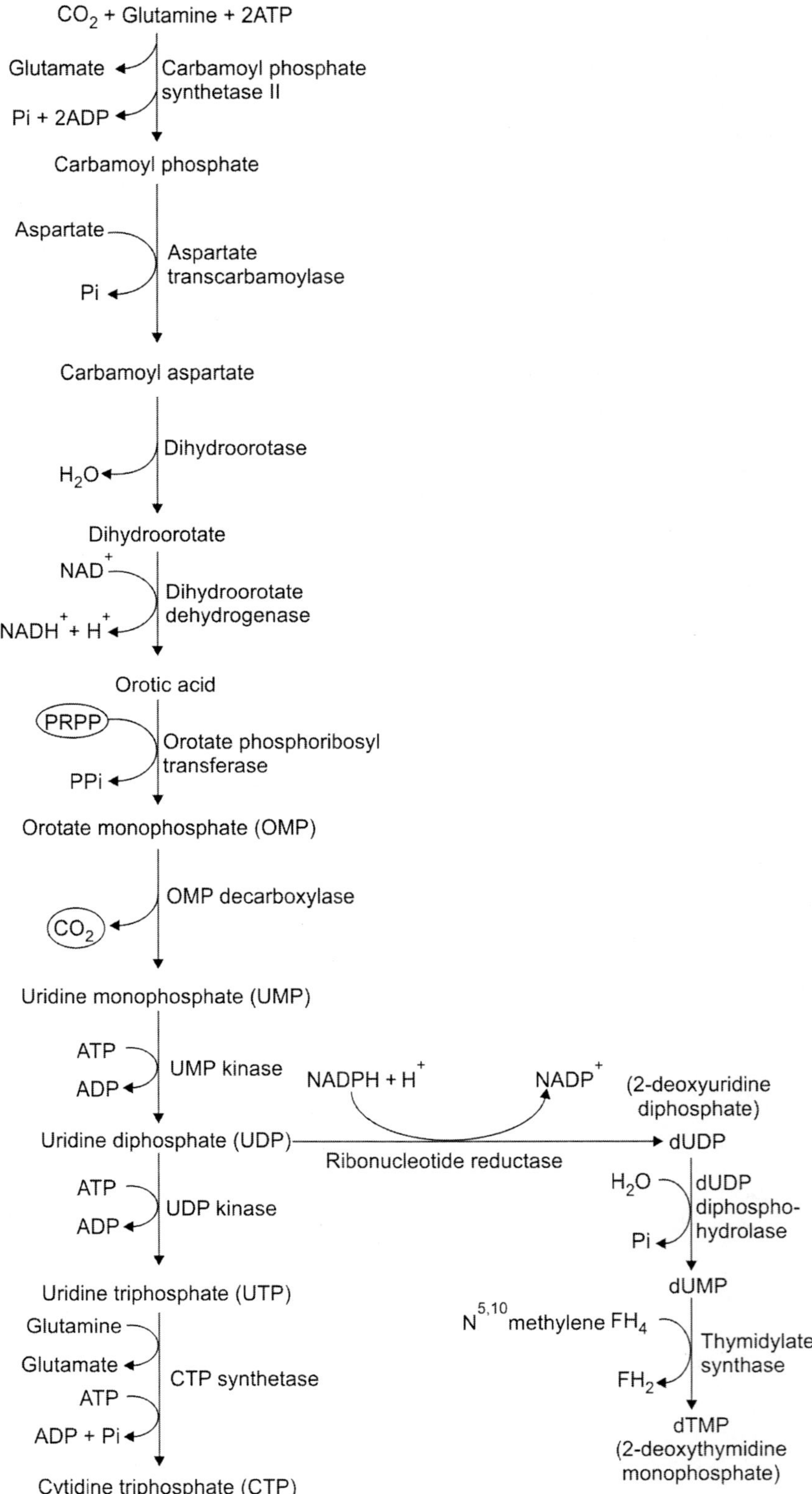


**Fig. 2:** Pyrimidine synthesis

## Regulation

| *Enzyme* | *Type of regulation* | *Inhibitor* | *Stimulator* |
|---|---|---|---|
| • ATCase—Aspartyl transcarbamoylase (Committed and rate limiting enzyme in bacteria) | Allosteric regulation | CTP and UTP | ATP |
| • CPS II—Carbamoyl phosphate synthetase II (key enzyme in animals) | Feedback regulation | UMP and UTP | ATP and PRPP |
| • OMP decaroxylase | Competitive inhibition | UMP and CMP | — |
| • CTP synthetase | Feedback regulation | CTP | GTP |

## Significance

- In eukaryotes first 3 enzymes,viz,CPSII, ATC and DHOase are present as a multienzyme complex and referred to as 'CAD', taking the first letters of the 3 enzymes and also the last 2 enzymes, OPRTase and OMP decarboxylase are also present as a single functional complex. Both complexes are cytosolic
- Because of this clustering of enzymes, the synthesis is well-coordinated.

## SHORT ESSAYS

### 3. Discuss the metabolic changes during diabetes mellitus.

Refer Question No. 5 Dec. 2008 (RS2).

### 4. Absorption and storage of iron.

Refer Question No. 11 June 2007 (RS2).

### 5. Is tyrosine an essential amino acid? Justify. Write the reactions of three important biological products formed from tyrosine.

Refer Question No. 1 Dec. 2010 (RS2).

### 6. Give a diagrammatic representation of mechanism of steroid hormone action.

Refer Question No. 7 June 2008 (RS2).

### 7. Draw a neat diagram of a cell and its organelles. Explain the functions of each.

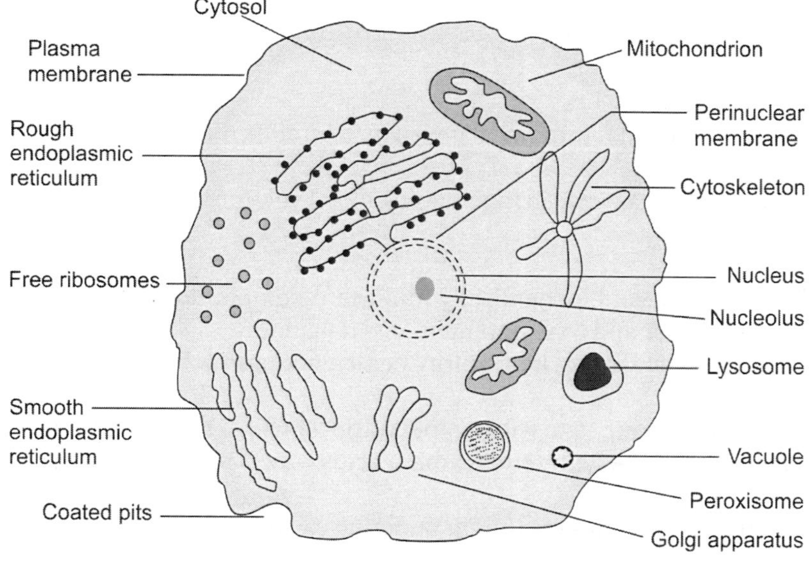


**Fig. 3:** Structure of cell

## Subcellular Organelles

- Subcellular organelles are distinct internal membranous structures present within a eukaryotic cell.

| *Subcellular organelles* | *Functions* |
|---|---|
| a. Nucleus | Replication, transcription, DNA repair, rRNA ribosome synthesis |
| b. Endoplasmic reticulum (smooth and rough) | Protein synthesis, post-translational modifications of proteins, glycogen metabolism, fatty acid synthesis, steroid metabolism, detoxification, synthesis of cholesterol (part) |
| c. Golgi complex | Intracellular sorting of proteins, post-translational modifications of proteins |
| d. Mitochondria | Power house of cell, oxidative phosphorylation (ETC), ATP synthesis, TCA cycle, fatty acid oxidation, mitochondrial DNA metabolism, ketone bodies production, urea synthesis (part), heme synthesis (part), gluconeogenesis (part), pyrimidine synthesis (part) |
| e. Lysosomes | Intracellular digestion of macromolecules (carbohydrates, proteins, lipids, nucleotides), phagocytosis, receptor mediated endocytosis |
| f. Peroxisomes | Oxidation of amino acids, oxidation of long chain fatty acids, $H_2O_2$ metabolism, bile acid synthesis, plasmalogen synthesis |
| g. Cytosol | Supporting subcellular organelles, protein synthesis, glycolysis, glycogen metabolism, HMP shunt pathway, transaminations, fatty acid synthesis, cholesterol synthesis, heme synthesis (part), urea synthesis (part), pyrimidine synthesis (part), purine synthesis |

### 8. What is normal serum protein level? Mention three important functions of albumin. List conditions when albumin/globulin (A/G) ratio is altered.

- Plasma proteins are proteins circulating in blood.

## Composition

| | *Plasma conc.* | *Fraction* |
|---|---|---|
| • Total plasma proteins | 6–8 g/dL | 100% |
| • Albumin | 3.5–5 g/dL | 55–65% |
| • Globulin | 2.5–3.5 g/dL | |
| – $\alpha_1$ globulin | 0.3–0.5 g/dL | 2–4% |
| – $\alpha_2$ globulin | 0.4–0.8 g/dL | 6–12% |
| – $\beta$ globulin | 0.6–1.1 g/dL | 8–12% |
| – $\gamma$ globulin | 0.8–1.8 g/dL | 12–22% |
| • Fibrinogen | 0.2–0.4 g/dL | |

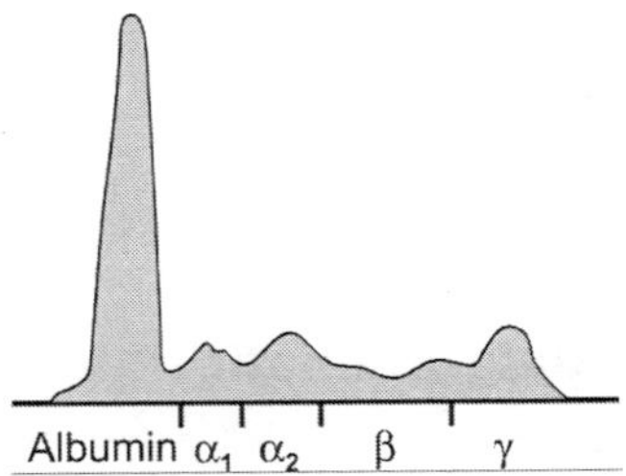


**Fig. 4:** Electrophoresis pattern of serum proteins

## Functions of Albumin

a. Osmotic function
   - Due to its high concentration and low molecular weight, albumin contributes to 75–80% of total plasma osmotic pressure
   - Thus albumin plays a predominant role in maintaining blood volume and exchange of water between tissue fluid and blood.

b. Transport function
   - Plasma albumin binds to several biochemically important compounds like free fatty acids bilirubin, steroid hormones, calcium and copper and transport them in circulation
   - It also helps in transport of many drugs like aspirin, penicillin G and sulfanomides to their target tissues.

c. Nutritive function
   - Albumin in plasma is in a dynamic state with a rapid turnover with a specific half-life
   - It is delivered to cells where it is hydrolyzed for amino acids which are used for synthesis of cellular proteins

d. Buffering function
   - Among plasma proteins, albumin has maximum buffering capacity

e. It exerts low viscosity and helps in blood flow

## Significance

*Hypoalbuminemia*

| *Causes* | *Consequences* |
|---|---|
| • Decreased synthesis: Cirrhosis, chronic liver failure<br>• Decreased amino acid availability: Protein–energy malnutrition, malabsorption syndrome<br>• Loss through urine: Nephrotic syndrome<br>• Loss through skin: Burns<br>• Loss through intestine: Protein losing enteropathy | • Edema is consequence of the hypoalbuminemia when albumin level full below 2.5 g% |

*A/G Ratio*

- A/G ratio is ratio of serum concentration of albumin to globulin.

| *Normal A/G ratio* | *Low (altered) A/G ratio* | |
|---|---|---|
| • 1.2–1.5 : 1 | Decrease in albumin level | Increase in globulin level |
| | • Due to decreased synthesis of albumin by liver<br>– Liver diseases<br>– Severe malnutrition<br>• Due to increased excretion of albumin by kidney<br>– Nephrotic syndrome<br>– Nephritic syndrome<br>– Nephroscleroís | • Due to increased production<br>– Chronic infection<br>– Multiple myeloma |

## 9. Discuss the metabolic function of sodium and potassium.

- Sodium is a major cation of extracellular fluid whereas potassium is a major intracellular cation
- Both are involved in various important physiological processes

| *Sodium ($Na^+$)* | *Potassium ($K^+$)* |
|---|---|
| **Normal serum concentration** | |
| • 135–145 mEq/L | • 3.5–5 mEq/L |
| **Biochemical (metabolic) functions** | |
| a. Regulation of plasma volume<br>– Sodium maintains crystalloid osmotic pressure of extracellular fluid and helps in retaining water in ECF and also regulates distribution of body water in different compartments<br>b. Regulation of acid base balance<br>– In association with chloride and bicarbonate, it regulates the acid base balance<br>– Sodium and hydrogen ion exchange in renal tubule acidify urine<br>c. Maintains blood viscosity of blood<br>– Salts of sodium with globulins are soluble and sodium and potassium both maintain viscosity of blood<br>d. Neuromuscular excitability<br>– Along with other electrolytes, sodium is involved in neuromuscular irritability<br>e. Generation of resting membrane potential<br>– Poor permeability of cell membrane to sodium creates a potential difference of –70 to –95 millivolts across membrane which is called as resting membrane potential<br>f. Component of sodium potassium pump<br>– Sodium potassium pump sends out 3 ions of sodium for every 2 ions of potassium pumped in<br>– This Na-K pump is essential for maintenance of cell volume<br>g. Absorption of nutrients<br>– Sodium is involved in absorption of glucose, galactose and amino acids by secondary active transport in both proximal intestine and renal tubules<br>h. Role in cardiac function<br>– Sodium is required for initiating and maintaining heart beat | a. Regulation of intracellular volume<br>– Potassium maintains intracellular osmotic pressure and water balance in cells<br>b. Regulation of acid base balance<br>– Potassium regulates acid base balance<br>c. Neuromuscular excitability and transmission of nerve impulse<br>– Along with other electrolytes, potassium is involved in neuromuscular irritability<br>– It is also involved in transmission of nerve impulse<br>d. Generation of resting membrane potential<br>– Potassium is an important determinant of resting membrane potential of excitable tissues like nerves and muscles<br>e. Functioning of sodium-potassium ATPase<br>– Sodium potassium pump maintenance high intracellular potassium level by using energy to pump in 2 ions of potassium for 3 molecules of sodium pumped out<br>f. Secretion of gastric acid<br>– In stomach, potassium is exchanged for hydrogen ions which is utilized for secretion of hydrochloric acid (gastric acid)<br>g. Activation of intracellular enzymes<br>– Certain enzymes like pyruvate kinase, glycogen synthase are dependent on potassium for its optimum activity<br>– Adequate intracellular concentration of potassium is required for proper protein biosynthesis by ribosomes<br>h. Role in cardiac action<br>– Extracellular potassium influences activity of cardiac muscles<br>– Excessive potassium is myotoxic |

**10. Clinical importance of alpha-fetoprotein (AFP) and prostate-specific antigen (PSA). Give their normal values.**

- Alpha-fetoprotein and prostate-specific antigen are tumor markers.

| | *Alpha-fetoprotein (AFP)* | *Prostate specific antigen (PSA)* |
|---|---|---|
| Features | • Alpha-fetoprotein (AFP) is a tumor marker for liver cancers<br>• Produced by liver and yolk sac in fetal life<br>• Is a oncofetal glycoprotein | • Prostate-specific antigen (PSA) is a tumor marker for prostatic cancer<br>• Product of prostatic epithelium and secreted in seminal fluid<br>• 32 kD glycoprotein<br>• Demonstrated in tissue biopsy as well as in serum |
| Normal level | • <10 µg/L | • 0–4 ng/mL |
| Significance | • Marked increase in AFP levels (>400 µg/L) is seen in hepatocellular carcinoma and germ cell carcinoma of testis<br>• Moderate increase is seen in benign hepatic disorders like cirrhosis, hepatitis and pregnancy | • Level between 4–10 ng/mL suggestive of high-risk<br>• Levels above 10 ng/mL diagnostic of prostatic carcinoma (generally higher in low grade tumor than in high grade tumor) |
| Applications | • For diagnosis of hepatocellular carcinoma and germ cell carcinoma<br>• For monitoring therapy and determining prognosis of hepatocellular carcinoma and germ cell carcinoma | • Determines prostatic origin of metastasis<br>• Distinguishes high grade prostatic cancer from urothelial carcinoma, colonic carcinoma, lymphoma and prostitis |

**11. Give the key reactions of renal mechanism in acid base balance.**

Refer Question No. 2 June 2012 (RS2).

**12. What is gout? Give its clinical manifestations and line of treatment.**

Refer Question No. 2 June 2007 (RS2).

## SHORT ANSWERS

### 13. Glutathione.

- Glutathione is a tripeptide containing glutamic acid, cysteine and glycine (chemical name is γ-L – glutamyl-cystinyl – glycine)
- Widely distributed in tissues but richly present in erythrocytes.

#### Synthesis

- In cytosol with help of ATP and does not require RNA.

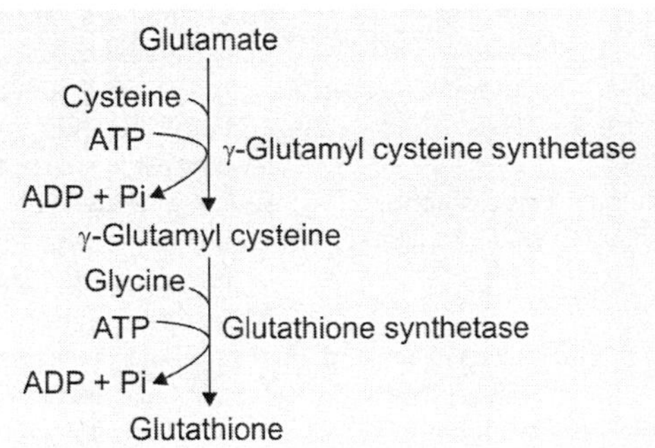


**Fig. 5:** Synthesis of glutathione

## Functions

a. Oxidation-reduction reactions (an important reducing agent in tissues)
   - Suppress oxidative stress in cell (antioxidant function) by donating $H_2$, it converts $H_2O_2$ to water under action of glutathione peroxidase
   - Keeps -SH group containing enzymes in reduced state (active state), e.g. glyceraldehyde 3-P dehydrogenase
   - Maintains red cell membrane stability and protects lens proteins
   - Prevents oxidation of hemoglobin to methemoglobin.

b. Coenzymes for many enzymes
   - Glutathione-insulin transhydrogenase catalyzing catabolism of insulin
   - Formaldehyde dehydrogenase catalyses oxidation of formaldehyde to formic acid
   - Glyoxylase which converts methylglyoxal to lactic acid
   - Maleyl- acetoacetate isomerase helping cis-trans isomerization of maleyl-acetoacetate to fumaryl-acetoacetate.

c. Along with glutathione transhydrogenase, helps to cause reductive cleavage of S-S linkage in thyroglobulin glycoprotein

d. Intestinal absorption of amino acids through γ-glutamyl cycle

e. Reduced (G - SH ) glutathione is required for
   - Conversion of dopa-quinone to glutathione
   - Prostaglandin synthesis by cyclooxygenase pathway as coenzyme
   - Activation of methionine to S-adenosyl methionine

f. Acts as detoxifying agent in by transferring the cysteinyl group catalyzed by glutathione S-transferase
   - Organophosphorus compounds
   - Halogenated compounds
   - Nitrogenous substances (chloro dinitro benzene)
   - Heavy metals
   - Drug metabolism.

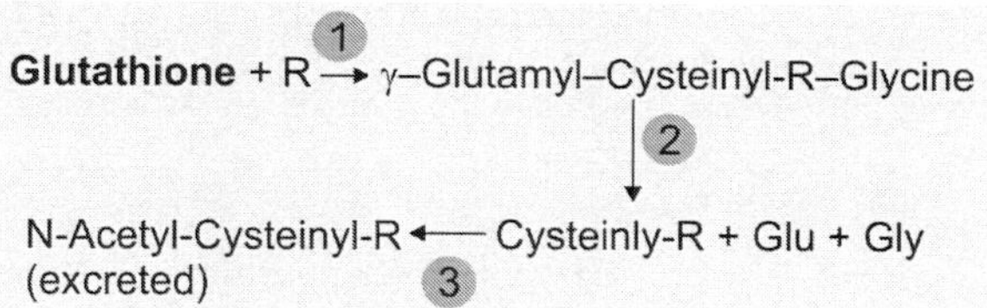


**Fig. 6:** Glutathione as detoxifying agent

## 14. Serotonin.

Refer Question No. 5 June 2008 (RS2).

## 15. Give three enzymes and their therapeutic uses.

Refer Question No. 7 June 2005 (RS2).

## 16. Ionophores.

- Ionophores are compounds transporting small molecular compounds such as ions across cell membranes.

## Types

| | *Carrier ionophores* | *Channel forming ionophores* |
|---|---|---|
| Features | • Carrier ionophores increase the permeability of cell membrane for particular ion<br>• It binds to ion and releases it on other side of membrane | • Channel forming ionophores form a channel in the membrane by creating a space between 2 adjacent phospholipid molecules |
| Examples | • Valinomycin (selective for transport of potassium) | • Gramicidine (facilitates passage of sodium and potassium) |

*Contd...*

Contd...

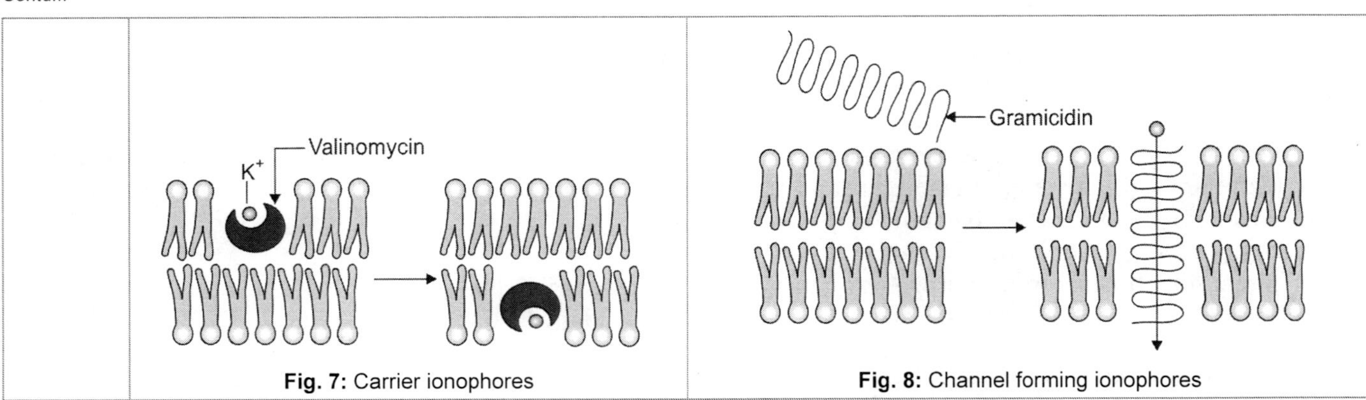


Fig. 7: Carrier ionophores

Fig. 8: Channel forming ionophores

## Significance

- Certain ionophores also act as uncouplers of oxidative phosphorylation.

## 17. Digestion and absorption of disaccharides.

- Disaccharides are product of digestion of limit dextrin and oligosaccharides in intestinal lumen by pancreatic amylase.

### Digestion of Disaccharides

| *Digestion of maltose* | *Digestion of sucrose* | *Digestion of lactose* |
|---|---|---|
| • Intestinal maltase acts on α 1-4 glycosidic linkage to yield 2 glucose molecules<br>Maltose<br>$H_2O$ → Intestinal maltose<br>Glucose + Glucose | • Intestinal sucrase acts on $\alpha_1 - \beta_2$ glycosidic linkage to form a glucose and fructose molecule<br>• Enzyme sucrase is capable of hydrolyzing a large quantity of sucrose | • Intestinal lactase acts on $\beta_1$-4 glycosidic bond to yield a molecule each of glucose and galactose<br>• Enzyme lactase is rate limiting thus utilization of milk sugar (lactose) is limited in humans<br>Lactose<br>$H_2O$ → Intestinal lactase<br>Glucose + Galactose |

### Absorption (of monosaccharides)

- End products of carbohydrate digestion are monosaccharides, namely glucose (>80%), galactose and fructose
- These monosaccharides are absorbed from upper small intestine, i.e. duodenum and proximal jejunum.

| *Absorption of glucose and galactose* | *Absorption of fructose* |
|---|---|
| • Absorption of glucose and galactose is a sodium dependent secondary active transport requiring transporters called sodium dependent glucose transporters (SGLT), namely SGLT1 and SGLT2<br>• Galactose is most efficiently absorbed compared to glucose | • Fructose is absorbed by passive, carrier mediated facilitated diffusion requiring transporter called GLUT 5<br>• It occurs by ping-pong mechanism, i.e. fructose binds to carrier which undergoes conformational change and carries fructose to other side to release it |

Contd...

Contd...

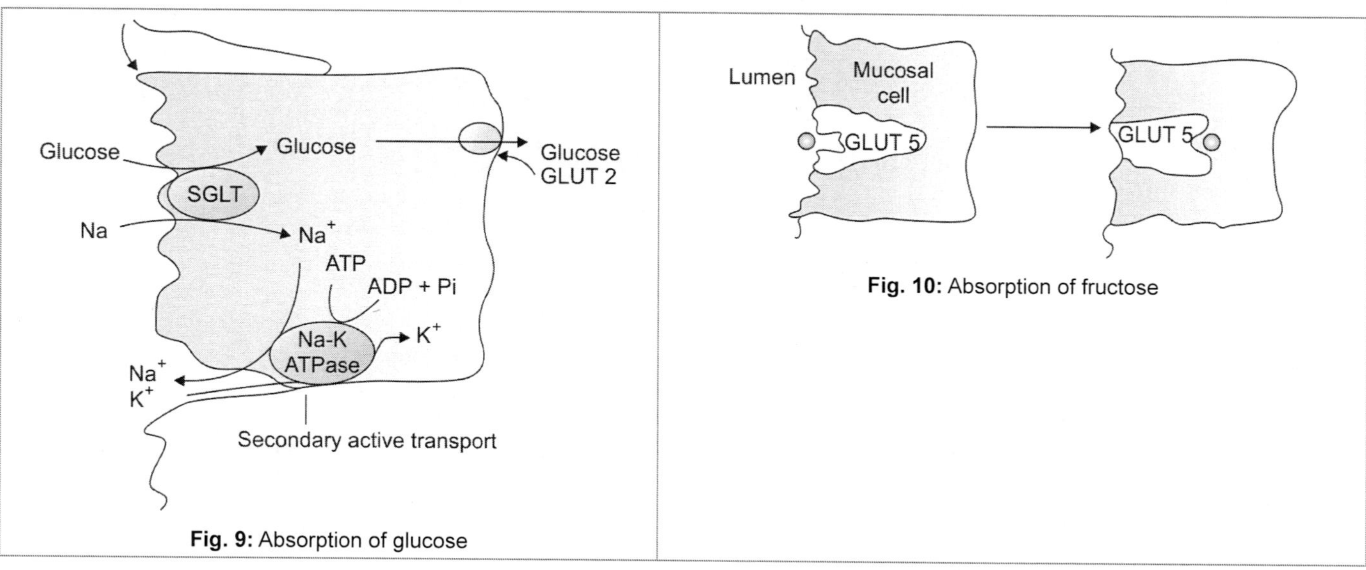


**Fig. 9:** Absorption of glucose

**Fig. 10:** Absorption of fructose

## 18. Antioxidants.

Refer Question No. 6 June 2008 (RS2).

## 19. Four enzymes with copper as integral component.

Refer Question No. 12 June 2017 (RS2).

## 20. Immunoglobulins.

Refer Question No. 22 Dec. 2010 (RS2).

## 21. Causes for xeroderma pigmentosa.

- Xeroderma pigmentosum is a rare skin disorder caused by defect in nucleotide excision repair mechanism of DNA.

| *Cause* | *Pathogenesis* | *Clinical features* |
|---|---|---|
| • Defects in any of several genes that code for XP proteins required for nucleotide excision repair of UV damage in humans<br>• Most common cause is mutation in XPA gene | • Underlying mechanism is defect XP protein needed for thymine (pyrimidine) dimers caused by defective excinuclease | • Characterized by hypersensitivity to sunlight leading to development of skin lesions and skin cancer |

## 22. Specific dynamic action (SDA) and basal metabolic rate (BMR).

**For Specific Dynamic Action**

Refer Question No. 19 June 2012 (RS2).

**For Basal Metabolic Rate**

Refer Question No. 12 June 2006 (RS2).

# MBBS PHASE I EXAMINATION
## JUNE 2013
### (Revised Scheme 2 & 3)

## LONG ESSAYS

**1. What are enzymes? Classify enzymes with one example each. Explain any four factors that affect enzyme activity.**

- Enzymes are biocatalyst synthesized in the living cells which are protein in nature colloidal and thermolabial in character and specific in their action.

### Classification [International Union of Biochemistry (IUB) Classification]

- Enzymes are classified into 6 major classes according to chemical reaction they catalyze and their reaction mechanism
- This functional classification is also called IUB classification as it based on system established by Intenral Union of Biochemistry (IUB)
- According to it, each enzyme is characterized by a code number, known as enzyme which comprises 4 digits separated by dots:
  - 1st digit—indicates major functional class of enzyme
  - 2nd digit—indicates subclass defining specific functional characteristics
  - 3rd digit—indicates sub-subclass indicating nature of reaction
  - 4th digit—indicates specific substrate.

  *Example*
  - Hexokinase is referred to as 2.1.1.1

| *Class* | *Subclass* | *Example* |
|---|---|---|
| A. Class 1: Oxidoreductases (Enzymes that catalyze oxidation-reduction reactions Catalyze addition of oxygen, transfer of hydrogen and transfer of electrons) | a. Oxidases Catalyze transfere of hydrogen or electron from donor, using oxygen as hydrogen acceptor producing either $H_2O$ or $H_2O_2$ | • Cytochrome oxidase Reduced cytochrome C + ½ $O_2$ → oxidized cytochrome C + $H_2O$ |
| | b. Dehydrogenase Catalyze transfer of hydrogen or electrons but hydrogen acceptor is molecule other than oxygen, usually NAD, NADP, FAD or FMN | • Alcohol dehydrogenase Ethyl alcohol + $NAD^+$ → Acetaldehyde + NADH + $H^+$ |
| B. Class 2: Transferses (Enzymes that catalyze transfer of a group from one substrate to another) | a. Aminotransfease Catalyze transfer of an amino group of amino acid to an alpha ketoacid, resulting in formation of a new amino acid and a new ketoacid | • Aspartate aminotransferase Aspartate + α ketoglutarate → Oxaloacetate + glutamate |
| | b. Kinases Catalyze transfer of phosphate from ATP to substrate | • Glucokinase Glucose + ATP → Glucose-6-phosphate + ADP |
| C. Class 3: Hydrolases (Enzymes that catalyze breakage of a bond using water usually involving bonds between C-O, C-N, O-P or C-S) | a. Glycosidases Catalyze hydrolysis of glycosidic bond | • Maltase Maltose + $H_2O$ → Glucose + glucose |
| | b. Phosphatase Catalyze removal of phosphate from substrate | • Glucose-6-phosphatase Glucose-6-phosphate + $H_2O$ → Glucose + Pi |

*Contd...*

*Contd...*

| *Class* | *Subclass* | *Example* |
|---|---|---|
| D. Class 4: Lyases (Enzymes that catalyze zaddition or removal of water, ammonia or carbon dioxide by cleaving C-C, C-S or C-N bonds) | a. Lyases Catalyze cleavage of C-C bonds | • Citrate lyase Citrate + CoASH → Acetyl CoA + Oxaloacetate |
| | b. Decarboxylase Catalyze removal of $CO_2$ from substrate | • Glutamate decarboxylase Glutamate → Gamma amino butyric acid + $CO_2$ |
| E. Class 5: Isomerases (Enzymes that catalyze transfer of groups within same substrate molecule) | a. Isomerases Catalyze interconversion of cis-trans isomers and functional isomers | • Phosphohexose isomerase Glucose-6-phosphate → Fructose-6-phosphate |
| | b. Epimerases Catalyze interconversion of epimers | • Phosphopentose epimerase Ribulose-5-phosphate → Xylulose-5-phosphate |
| F. Class 6: Ligases (Enzymes that catalyze formation of new covalent bonds using high energy from ATP) | a. Carboxylase Catalyze formation of C-C bonds using $CO_2$ as substrate | • Pyruvate carboxylase Pyruvate + $CO_2$ + ATP → Oxaloacetate + ADP + Pi |
| | b. Synthetases Catalyze linking of 2 molecules in ATP dependent reactions | · Glutamine synthetase $NH_3$ + Glutamate + ATP → Glutamine + ADP + Pi |

## Factors AFfecting Enzyme Activity (Velocity of Enzyme)

- Activity or velocity of an enzyme catalyzed reaction is influenced by several factors which are:

a. Concentration of enzyme
   - In beginning, velocity of enzymatic reaction is directly proportional to the enzyme concentration
   - When substrate concentration is in large, excess of exceeding that of $V_{max}$, more enzymes molecules enables conversion of progressively larger number of substrate.

b. Concentration of substrate
   - Increase in substrate concentration gradually increases velocity of enzyme reaction
   - However, this is true up to a certain concentration after which increasing concentration of substrate does not further increase velocity of reaction
   - On plotting a graph taking velocity on Y axis and substrate concentration on X axis, a rectangular hyperbola is obtained showing three different phases.
     i. At low substrate concentration, velocity of reaction is directly proportional to substrate level
     ii. In second phase, substrate concentration is not directly proportional to enzyme activity
     iii. In final phase, velocity is independent of substrate concentration

c. Concentration of product
   - Excess concentration of product may reduce velocity of reaction by occupying active sites of enzymes
   - In some reversible reaction, it is also possible that, high concentration of products may favors reverse reaction forming back substrate.

d. Effect of temperature
   - Velocity of an enzyme reaction increases with rise in temperature up to a maximum and then declines. Thus a bell-shaped curve is usually obtained
   - Temperature at which the maximum enzyme activity is seen is called the optimum temperature of that enzyme. Optimum temperature of most of the enzymes lies between 40–45°C.

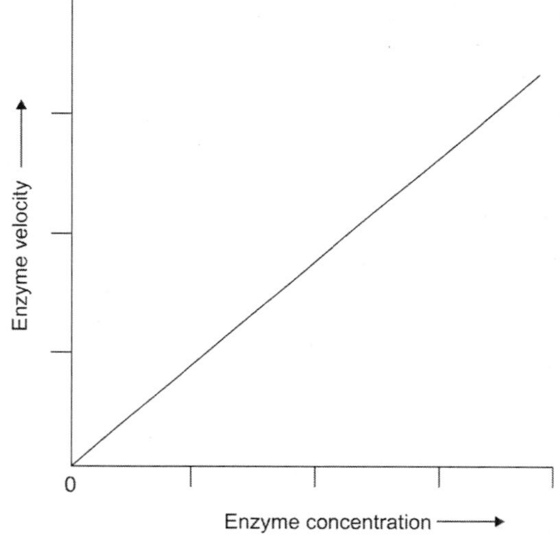


**Fig. 1:** Effect of enzyme concentration on enzyme velocity

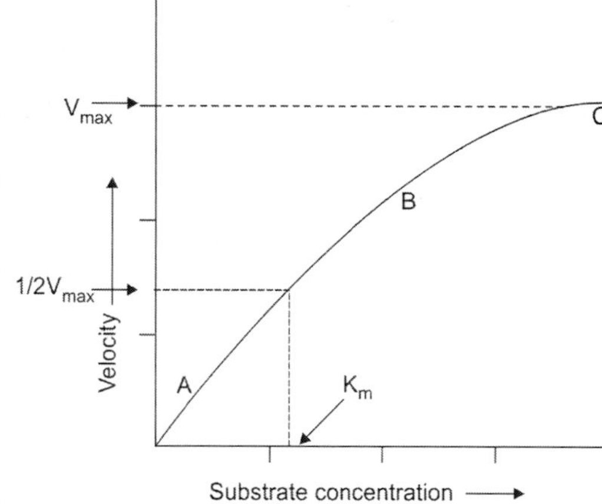


**Fig. 2:** Effect of substrate concentration on enzyme velocity

- A rise in temperature increases total energy of chemical system with result the activation energy is increased
- However, after crossing optimum temperature, enzymes undergoes denaturation thus reducing reaction velocity.

e. Effect of pH
- Increase in $H^+$ concentration considerably influences enzyme activity and gives a bell-shaped curve similar to one obtained on effect of temperature
- Like optimum temperature every enzymes has an optimum pH below and above which activity of the enzyme declines. For most of the enzymes, it lies in range of 6–8.
- Concentration of $H^+$ alters ionization of active sites or substrates
- It also influences separation of coenzymes from holoenzyme complex.

f. Effect of activator and coenzymes
- Activity of certain enzymes is greatly dependent of metal ions activators and co-enzymes.
- These activators and coenzymes enhance velocity by:
  - Maintaining or producing active structural configuration of enzyme
  - Forming substrate enzymes complex
  - Changing structure of substrate
  - Accepting or donating electrons
  - Activating or functioning as nucleophiles
  - Forming ternary complex with enzymes or substrate.

g. Effect of modulators and inhibitors
- Presence of modulators and inhibitors may adversely reduce velocity of reaction.

h. Effect of time
- Time required to completion of an enzyme reaction increases with fall in temperature from its optimum
- However, under ideal and optimum conditions of temperature and pH the time required for enzymatic reaction is less.

i. Effect of light and radiations
- Exposure to UV light, β, γ and X-rays reduces velocity of enzymes reaction by inactivating enzymes.

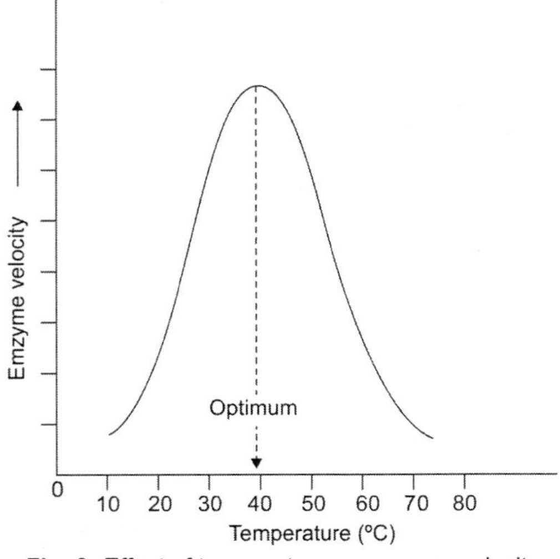

**Fig. 3:** Effect of temperature on enzyme velocity

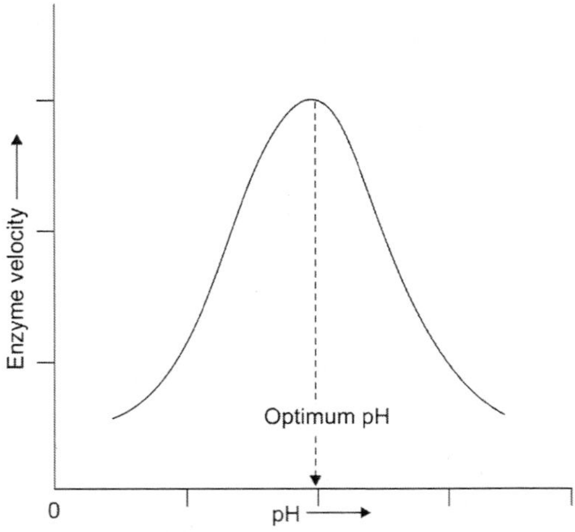

**Fig. 4:** Effect of pH on enzyme velocity



## 2. What are sources of C and N atoms of purine? Describe the biosynthesis of purine and add a note on its regulation.

- Purine nucleotides are synthesized in body step by step from ribose 5-phosphate molecule by de novo synthesis.

<table>
<tr><th>Site</th><th>Substrates</th><th>Products</th></tr>
<tr><td>Tissue site<br>• Liver<br>Intracellular site<br>• Cytosol</td><td><table><tr><th>Source</th><th>Atom</th></tr><tr><td>• Aspartate (amino group)</td><td>• N-1</td></tr><tr><td>• Glutamine (amino group)</td><td>• N-3 and N-9</td></tr><tr><td>• $N^{10}$ formyl tetrahydrofolate</td><td>• C-2 and C-8</td></tr><tr><td>• Glycine</td><td>• C-4, C-5 and N-7</td></tr><tr><td>• $CO_2$</td><td>• C-6</td></tr></table><br>C-6 $CO_2$<br>N-1 Aspartate<br>Glycine C-4, C-5, N-7<br>$N^{10}$-formyl tetrahydrofolate C-8<br>$N^{10}$-formyl tetrahydro-folate C-2<br>Glutamine N-3, N-9<br>Fig. 5: Sources of carbon and nitrogen atoms in purine</td><td>• Inosine monophosphate (IMP)<br>• Adenosine monophosphate (AMP)<br>• Guanosine monophosphate (GMP)</td></tr>
</table>

## Reactions

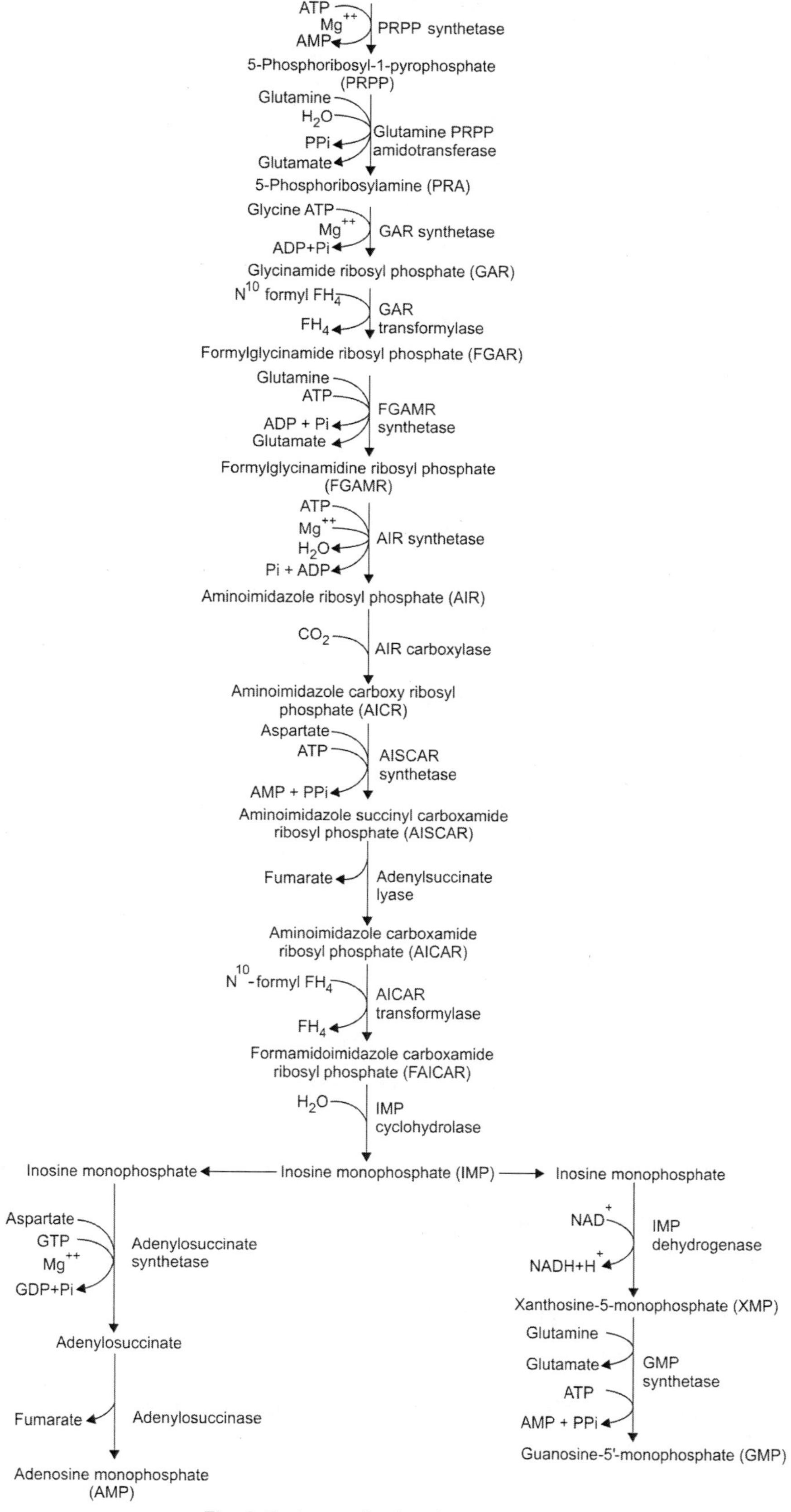


**Fig. 6:** Purine synthesis—de novo synthesis

## Regulation

| *Enzyme* | *Type of regulation* | *Inhibitor* | *Stimulator* |
|---|---|---|---|
| • PRPP synthetase | Feedback regulation | Purine 5-nucleotides (mostly AMP and GMP) | — |
| • Glutamine PRPP amidotransferase (rate limiting enzyme) | Allosteric feedback regulation | AMP and GMP | PRPP |
| • Adenylosuccinate synthetase | Feedback cross regulation | AMP | GTP |
| • GMP synthetase | Feedback cross regulation | ATP | GMP |
| • IMP dehydrogenase | Feedback inhibition | GMP | — |

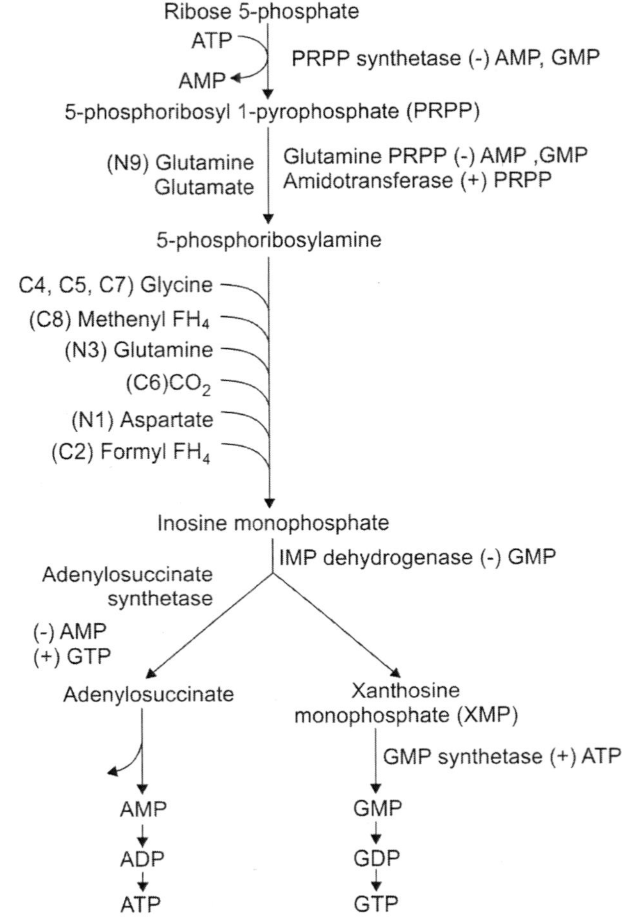


**Fig. 7:** De novo purine synthesis—regulation

## SHORT ESSAYS

### 3. Define gluconeogenesis. How is alanine converted to glucose?

Refer Question No. 1 June 2009 (RS2).

### 4. What is substrate level phosphorylation? Give two examples with complete reaction.

Refer Question No. 4 Dec. 2010 (RS2).

### 5. Classify lipoproteins and write the functions of each lipoprotein.

Refer Question No. 6 June 2005 (RS2).

**6. What are transamination reactions? Giving two examples discuss the importance of these reactions.**

Refer Question No. 2 June 2006 (RS2).

**7. Classify proteins based on their function giving an example for each class.**

- Proteins are polymers of amino acids in which amino acids are linked by peptide bonds.

## Classification

- Proteins are classified in four ways based on their function, composition, shape and nutritive value.

A. Classification based on function (Functional classification of proteins)

| *Class* | *Function* | *Examples* |
|---|---|---|
| a. Enzymes | Catalysis and modulation of metabolism | Glucokinase: Phosphorylation of glucose |
| b. Hormones | Regulation of body function | Insulin: Regulation of blood glucose level<br>Growth hormone: Regulation of growth |
| c. Structural proteins | Structural integrity to body | Collagen in cartilage<br>Keratin in hairs and nails |
| d. Contractile proteins | Contraction of muscles, body motion, cellular movements | Actin and myosin: Muscle contraction<br>Cytoskeletal proteins: Cell movements like phagocytosis |
| e. Transport proteins | Transport of molecules and ions | Hemoglobin: Oxygen transport<br>Albumin: Bilirubin transport |
| f. Storage proteins | Storage of nutrients | Ferritin: Storage of iron<br>Casein: Storage of phosphates in milk |
| g. Protective protein | Defence against injury and infection | Immunoglobulins: Protection against infections<br>Clotting factors: Protection against bleeding |
| h. Proteins in hemostasis | Maintenance of cellular composition and environment | Albumin: Osmotic regulation<br>Hemoglobin: Buffering (acid-base balance) |
| i. Transcription factors | Regulation of gene expression | c-myc: Cell cycle stimulation<br>c-jun: Cell growth, apoptosis |
| j. Receptors | Cellular regulation | Insulin receptors<br>Glucagon receptors |
| k. Genetic proteins | Associated with DNAs, RNAs | Histones |

B. Classification based on composition

a. Simple proteins
- Proteins that contains only amino acids

Example: Albumin, globulins, keratin, lactalbumin

b. Conjugated proteins
- Proteins containing a prosthetic group (non-protein part) in addition to amino acids

Example:

| *Class* | *Prosthetic group* | *Example* |
|---|---|---|
| Hemoprotein | Heme | Hemoglobin, myoglobin |
| Nucleoprotein | Nucleic acids | Histone, ribonucleoprotein |
| Lipoprotein | Lipids | HLD, LDL |
| Glycoprotein | Carbohydrates | Immunoglobulins, $\alpha$-1 antitrypsin |
| Phosphoprotein | Phosphates | Casein |
| Metalloprotein | Metal | Carbonic anhydrase (zinc), tyrosinase (copper), ferritin (iron) |
| Flavoprotein | Riboflavin | NADH dehydrogenase, xanthine oxidase |
| Chromoprotein | 11-cis-retinal | Rhodopsin |

c. Derived proteins
- Proteins formed from high molecular weight proteins by partial hydrolysis

Example: Peptone and gelatin

C. Classification based on shape

| | *Globular proteins* | *Fibrous proteins* |
|---|---|---|
| Shape | Spherical (ovoid) shape | Long and thin, fiber like |
| Structure | Polypeptide chain is completely folded | Pleated structures |
| Function | Functional role | Structural role |
| Example | Albumin, hemoglobin | Keratin of hair, myosin, collagen |

D. Classification based on nutritive value

| | *Complete proteins* | *Incomplete proteins* |
|---|---|---|
| Composition | Rich in essential amino acids | Not rich in essential amino acids |
| Quality | High biological value | Low biological value |
| Example | Egg protein, milk protein | Rice protein, maize protein |

## 8. Name the different types of RNA. Write their salient features. Mention their functions.

- Ribonucleic acid (RNA) is a polymer of ribonucleotides held together by 3' – 5' phosphodiester bridges.

### General Feature of RNA

- Sugar in RNA is ribose
- Bases in RNA are adenine (A), guanine (G), cytosine (C) and uracil (U)
- RNA is usually a single stranded polynucleotide which may fold upon itself to form a specific structure (Clover leaf model of tRNA)—secondary structure
- Due to single stranded nature of RNA, Chargaff's rule is not obeyed
- RNA can be subjected to hydrolysis by alkali due to presence of hydroxyl group.

### Types of RNA

| | *Cellular composition* |
|---|---|
| • Messenger RNA (mRNA) | 5–10% |
| • Transfer RNA (tRNA) | 10–20% |
| • Ribosomal RNA (rRNA) | 50–80% |



a. Messenger RNA
   - mRNA or messenger RNA is so called because it carries genetic information from DNA for protein synthesis.

   **Distribution**
   - 5-10% of total cellular RNA.

   **Size**
   - It is relatively large single stranded RNA molecule
   - Size varies greatly in its molecular weight due variation in its chain length.

   **Structure**
   - mRNA carries adenine, guanine, cytosine and uracil as major bases along with some minor bases as methyl purines and methyl pyrimidines

   **Structural features**
   - Cap—an inverted 7 methyl GTP attached to 5' end
   - Polyadenylate tail (Poly A tail)—consists of 200-300 AMP residues at 3' end
   - 5 UTR (5' untranslated region)—located at 5' end
   - 3' UTR (3' untranslated region)—located at 3' end
   - Coding region—lies between 5' and 3' ends and contains number of codons which are a sequence of 3 bases which stands/codes for an amino acid. Codons are of three types, i.e. initiating codon which is always AUG for methionine, specific codon for different amino acids and terminating codons which are UGA, UAA and UAG.

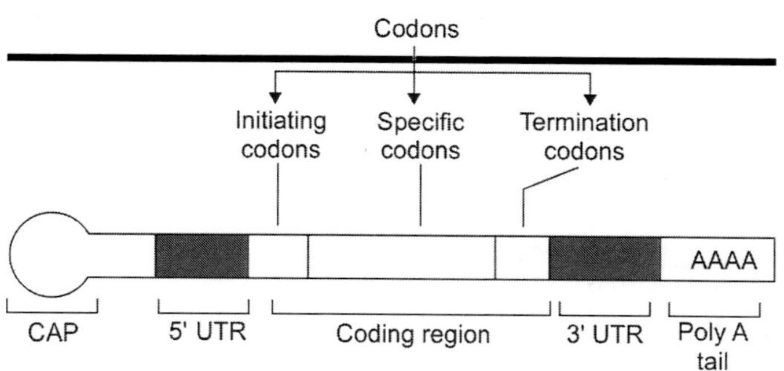


**Fig. 8:** mRNA—structure

**Function**

- mRNA takes an active part in translation, i.e. protein biosynthesis as follows:
  i. Carrier of genetic information
    * It is on this mRNA strand, the genetic information for protein synthesis is present in form of codons
    * This information is copied from DNA in nucleus by transcription and then carried to cytoplasm of cell for translation.
  ii. Serves as template
    * mRNA also functions as template for protein synthesis on which protein synthesis proceeds condon wise.

b. Transfer RNA
- tRNA is so called as it transfers/carries amino acid for protein synthesis
- Each tRNA is specific for a given amino acid and there are at least 20 different tRNA for 20 different amino acids
- Also called adapter tRNA because it carries specific amino acids on its 3' end corresponding to anticodon at its anticodon arm
- All the tRNA molecules as a class have many features in common.

**Distribution**
- 15–30% of total cellular RNA.

**Size**
- tRNA is smaller in size, smallest of all RNAs
- It consists of about 75 nucleotides
- Molecular weight is 25,000.

**Structure (Clover leaf structure)**
- Each tRNA is capable of folding upon itself to form clover leaf structure
- Where folding takes place nucleotides are complementary to each other and they are hydrogen bonded
- Where folding is not possible there are arms.

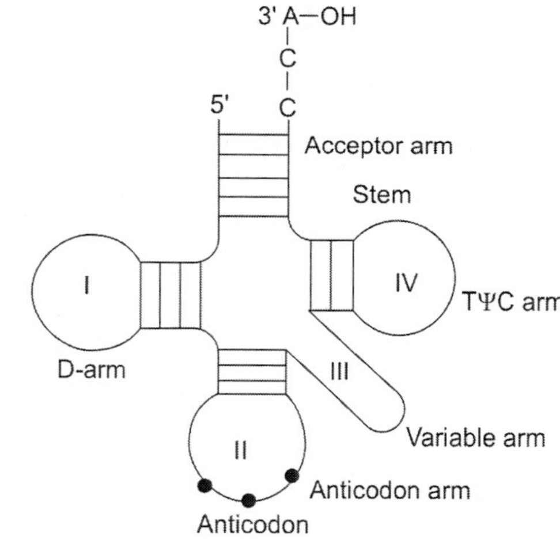


**Fig. 9:** tRNA—structure

**Structural features**
- 5' end starts with a phosphate and guanine
- First arm from 5' end is called D (dihydrouracil arm) arm because it contains a minor base dihydrouracil
- Next to D arm is an anticodon arm which contains a sequence of 3 bases complementary to 3 bases (the codon) on mRNA hence called anticodon
- Some tRNA contain are variable arm (extra arm) which is used to classify tRNA into class I tRNAs (short arm with 3–5 basic pairs) or class II tRNAs (long arm with 13–20 basic pairs)
- Next arm is called Tψ C arm which contains thymine and pseudouracil
- 3' end has sequence of C-C-A-OH. It is here that the ribose is linked to the last base adenine.

**Unusual bases**
- tRNA contain many unusual bases and unusual nucleosides
- Unusual bases include thymine, dihydrouracil, hypoxanthine, 1-methyl adenine and 2-N-dimethyl guanine
- Unusual nucleosides are formed from unusual bases but pseudourindine is an unusual nucleoside present in tRNA formed by unusual glycosidic bond between C-5 of uracil and C-1 of ribose.

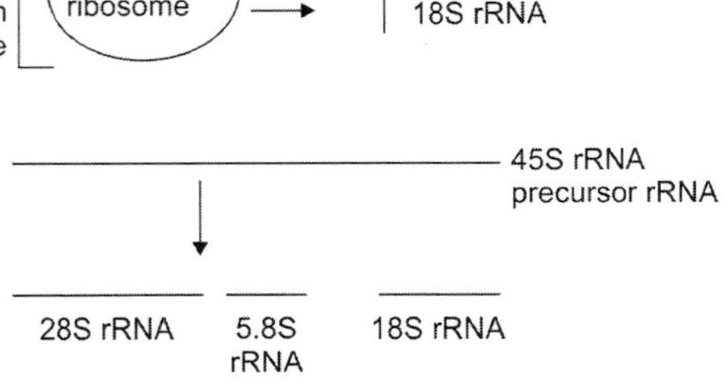


Fig. 10: rRNA—structure

**Function**

tRNA plays an important role in translation, i.e. protein biosynthesis as follows:

- tRNA transfer specific amino acid to site of protein synthesis
- It is also required for incorporating correct amino acid to growing polypeptide chain.

c. Ribosomal RNA
- Ribosomal RNA (rRNA) is factory of protein synthesis
- It is so called because it is found in ribosomes.

**Distribution**
- rRNA accounts for 60–80% of all cellular RNA.

**Size**
- Varies depending upon types of rRNA.

**Structure**
- rRNA composed of 2 major nucleoprotein complexes, namely 60S subunit and 40S subunit
- 60S subunit contains 28S rRNA, 5S rRNA and 5.8S rRNA while 40S subunit contains 18S rRNA.

**Function**
- rRNA takes as a significant role in translation, i.e. protein biosynthesis as follows:
  - They are site of protein synthesis
  - They engage mRNA and tRNA for polypeptide chain synthesis
  - It also serves as a catalyst in formation of peptide bond during polypeptide chain elongation.

## 9. What are buffers? Discuss any two buffer system of the body.

Refer Question No. 2 June 2012 (RS2).

## 10. Give the biochemical functions of niacin with examples and manifestation of its deficiency.

- Niacin or nicotinic acid is a water-soluble vitamin of B complex group
- Also called pellagra preventive factor of Goldberg

| *Chemistry* | *Dietary sources* | *RDA* |
|---|---|---|
| • Pyridine derivative (pyridine 3-carboxylic acid) | • Liver, yeast, whole grains, cereals, pulses (Rich sources)<br>• Milk, fish, egg and vegetables (Moderate sources)<br>• Corn (maize), jowar (Poor sources) | • 15–20 mg for adults<br>• 10–15 mg for children |

### Coenzyme Forms

- Nicotinamide adenine dinucleotide ($NAD^+$)
- Nicotinamide adenine dinucleotide phosphate ($NADP^+$).

### Biochemical (Metabolic) Functions

| *Reaction* | *Enzyme* |
|---|---|
| a. $NAD^+$ dependent | |
| – Carbohydrate metabolism | |
| - Pyruvate → Lactate | Lactate dehydrogenase |
| - Pyruvate → Acetyl CoA | Pyruvate dehydrogenase complex |
| - α-Ketoglutarate → Succinyl CoA | α-Ketoglutarate dehydrogenase complex |

*Contd...*

*Contd...*

| *Reaction* | *Enzyme* |
|---|---|
| – Lipid metabolism | |
| - β-Hydroxy acyl CoA → β-keto acyl CoA | β-Hydroxy acyl CoA dehydrogenase |
| - β-Hydroxybutyrate → Acetoacetate | β-Hydroxybutyrate dehydrogenase |
| - Alcohol → Aldehyde | Alcohol dehydrogenase |
| – Protein metabolism | |
| - α-Keto acids (Leu, Ile, Val) → Acyl CoA thioesters | Branched chain α-keto acid dehydrogenase |
| - Tyramine → ρ-Hydroxyphenyl acetate | Tyramine dehydrogenase |
| b. $NAD^+$ or $NADP^+$ dependent | |
| – Glutamate → α-ketoglutarate + $NH_3$ | Glutamate dehydrogenase |
| – Isocitrate → Oxalosuccinate | Isocitrate dehydrogenase |
| c. $NADP^+$ dependent | |
| – Glucose-6-phosphate → 6 phosphogluconate | Glucose-6-phosphate dehydrogenase |
| – Malate → Pyruvate | Malic enzyme |
| d. NADPH dependent | |
| – HMG CoA → Mevalonate | HMG CoA reductase |
| – Phenylalanine → Tyrosine | Phenylalanine hydroxylase |
| – Folic acid → Tetrahydrofolic acid | Dihydrofoalte reductase |

## Therapeutic Uses

- High doses (3–6 g m/day) to treat hypercholesterolemia and hypertriacylglycerolemia
- Also used to treat elevated plasma HDL levels.

## Deficiency (Pellagra)

- Deficiency of niacin cause pellagra (pelle = skin, agra = rough)

| *Causes* | *Clinical features (3Ds)* |
|---|---|
| • Alcoholism, impaired absorption, leucine rich diet, Hartnup disease | • Dermatitis<br>– Brown, thickened and scaly skin at places exposed to sun, or subjected to pressure or heat (neck, dorsal part of feet, ankle and parts of face)<br>• Diarrhea<br>– Loose stools, often with blood and mucus leading to weight loss<br>– Associated with nausea and vomiting<br>• Dementia (associated with degeneration of nervous tissue)<br>– Anxiety, irritability, poor memory and insomnia, etc.<br>– Ataxia and spasticity also seen<br>• Death (If not treated) |

## 11. What is a restriction endonuclease? Explain their role in recombinant DNA technology.

Refer Question No. 8 Dec. 2015 (RS2).

## 12. Give an account of phosphorus metabolism.

- Phosphorus is an important trace element.

| *Daily requirement* | *Dietary sources* | *Normal plasma level* |
|---|---|---|
| • Children<br>– 1.0 g/day<br>• Adults<br>– 0.8 g/day<br>• Pregnancy and lactation<br>– 1.2 g/day | • Milk, milk products, egg yolk, meat and fish<br>• Vegetables and cereals are also good sources but most of phosphorus is not available for absorption | • Adults<br>– 3–4.5 mg/dL<br>• Children<br>– 5–6 mg/dL |

## Functions

a. Structural role
   - Phosphorus is essential for development of bone and teeth.
b. Component of important compounds
   - Phosphorus is an essential component of compounds like nucleic acids (DNA, RNA), proteins (casein) and phospholipids
   - Phosphorus is component of high energy compounds like ATP, GTP and creatine phosphate
   - Phosphorus is also integral part of many coenzymes like TPP (thiamin pyrophosphate), coeznyme A.
c. Role in respiration
   - Phosphorus as component of 2,3 bisphosphoglycerate, causes release of oxygen from Hb.
d. Role in metabolism
   - Phosphorus is required form phosphrylation of fats and carbohydrates during their metabolism.
e. Role in acid-base balance
   - Phosphate buffer present in blood, urine is involved in acid-base balance.



## Metabolism of Phosphorus

A. Absorption
   - 70% of phosphorus in diet is absorbed as inorganic phosphate from jejunum.

**Factors affecting phosphorus absorption**

| *Factors favoring phosphorus absorption* | *Factors inhibiting phosphorus absorption* |
|---|---|
| • Bile salts<br>• Acidity<br>• Calcium (indirect action): Absorption of phosphorus is optimum when dietary Ca : P ratio is between 1 : 2 and 2 : 1<br>• Cholecalciferol (active vitamin D): Enhances absorption through transcriptional regulation of phosphate absorbing protein<br>• Parathyroid hormone: Stimulates synthesis of active vitamin D | • High calcium-phosphate ratio<br>• Phytates (forms insoluble calcium salts)<br>• Alkalinity<br>• Magnesium and aluminium (forms insoluble salts) |

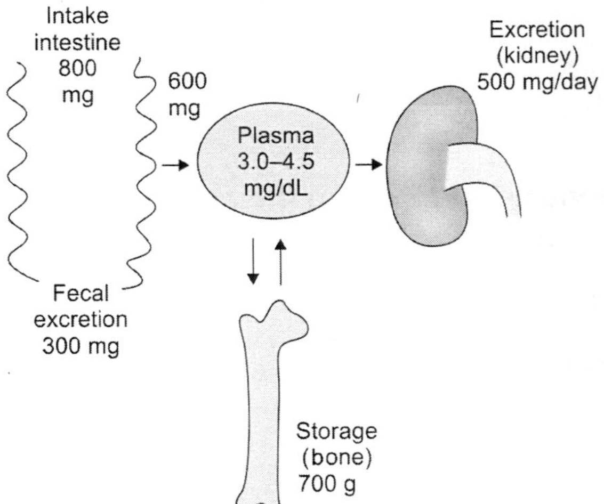


**Fig. 11:** Phosphorus—metabolism

B. Excretion
- Phosphorus in body excreted through urine (2/3rd of ingested phosphorus) and through stool (unabsorbed phosphorus)
- Normally 0.6 g/day is excreted through urine

**Factors affecting renal excretion**

| *Factors decreasing excretion* | *Factors increasing excretion* |
|---|---|
| • Cholecalciferol—increases reabsorption of phosphorus by renal tubules<br>• Growth hormone<br>• Cortisol<br>• Low plasma phosphorus levels | • Parathyroid hormone—decreases renal reabsorption |

## Regulation

- Plasma phosphorus level is maintained by triad of hormones regulating calcium homeostasis as calcium and phosphorus regulation is interlinked.

| *Hormone* | *Cholecalciferol (Active vitamin D)* | *Parathyroid hormone (PTH)* | *Calcitonin* |
|---|---|---|---|
| Effect | • Increases plasma phosphorus level | • Decreases plasma phosphorus levels | • Decreases plasma phosphorus levels |
| Mode of action | • Mediated through transcriptional regulation of gene expression by binding to nuclear receptors | • Mediated through increase in intracellular cAMP levels | • Mediated through increase in intra-cellular cAMP levels |
| Action | • Increases phosphorus absorption from small intestine<br>• Increases renal reabsorption in renal tubules<br>• Increases mobilization of phosphorus from bone into plasma | • Inhibits renal reabsorption of phosphorus | • Inhibits renal reabsorption of phosphorus<br>• Inhibits mobilization of calcium from bone |

# SHORT ANSWERS

## 13. High energy compounds.

- High energy compounds are compounds with high negative free energy change ($\Delta G°$) of -7.0 kcal/mol or more on hydrolysis
- This high free energy is stored in high energy bond which is broken during hydrolysis.

## Factors Contributing to High Energy Bonds

- Increased ionization of charged groups generated by hydrolysis
- Increase in resonance stabilization of products compared to substrate.

## Classification

| *Class* | *Examples* |
|---|---|
| a. Pyrophosphate | ATP, GTP, CTP, UDP-glucose, cyclic AMP, cyclic GMP |
| b. Enol phosphates | Phosphoenolpyruvate |
| c. Acylphosphates | 1,3 bisphosphoglycerate, carbamoyl phosphate |
| d. Acylthioesters | Acetyl CoA, succinyl CoA, s-adenosyl-lmethionine |
| e. Guanidium phosphates | Creatine phosphate |

## Role of High Energy Compounds in Metabolism

| *High energy compounds* | *Energy stored* | *Importance* |
|---|---|---|
| i. ATP | -7.3 | Required for phosphorylation, synthetic reactions and physiological processes (transport, muscle contraction, etc.) |

*Contd...*

*Contd...*

| High energy compounds | Energy stored | Importance |
|---|---|---|
| ii. GTP | -7.3 | Required for protein synthesis, gluconeogenesis |
| iii. CTP | -7.3 | Required for biosynthesis of phospholipids |
| iv. UTP | -7.3 | Required for polysaccharide synthesis |
| v. UDP-glucose | -7.3 | Required for glycogen and lactose synthesis |
| vi. 1,3-bisphosphoglycerate | -11.8 | Used for substrate level phosphorylation |
| vii. Phosphenol pyruvate | -14.8 | Used for substrate level phosphorylation |
| viii. Succinyl CoA | -7.5 | Used for substrate level phosphorylation, heme synthesis |
| ix. Creatine phosphate | -10.5 | Provides energy for muscle contraction |
| x. Carbamoyl phosphate | -12.3 | Intermediate of urea cycle |

## 14. Glycogen storage disorders.

Refer Question No. 4 Dec. 2006 (RS2).

## 15. Enzymes of diagnostic importance.

Refer Question No. 5 June 2011 (RS2).



## 16. FIGLU excretion test.

- FIGLU excretion test is a test to detect deficiency of folic acid
- Also called histidine load test.

| Principle | Procedure | Inference |
|---|---|---|
| • Formiminoglutamate (FIGLU) is an intermediate of histidine metabolism<br>• It is converted into glutamate by transfer of formimino group to $FH_4$ by action of enzyme formiminoglutamate transferase<br>• However, in deficiency of folic acid, this reaction is inhibited thus resulting in accumulation of FIGLU thus increasing it excretion in urine | • Person is given loading dose of 20 g of histidine | • In presence of folic acid deficiency, amount of FIGLU excreted is increased |

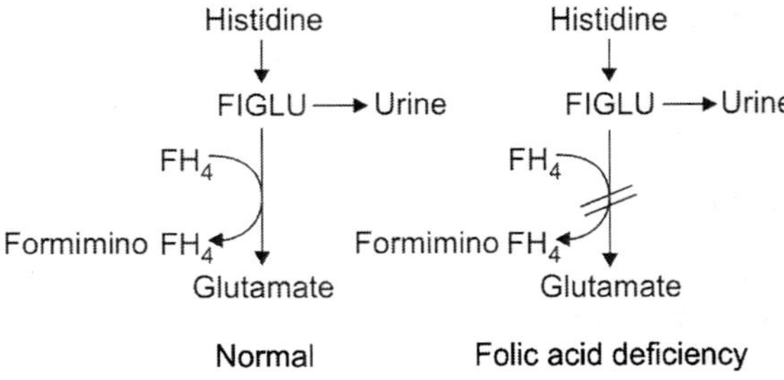


**Fig. 12:** FIGLU excretion test

## 17. Mitochondrial shuttle systems.

Mitochondrial shuttle systems are combination of enzymatic reactions that bypass the impermeability barrier of inner mitochondrial membrane for NADH via substrate pairs linked by suitable dehydrogenases.

*Example:*

| | *Glycerol phosphate shuttle* | *Malate aspartate shuttle (Malate shuttle)* |
|---|---|---|
| Operational in | Brains and skeletal muscles | Liver, heart, kidney |
| Components | α glycerophosphate dihydroxyacetone phosphate redox couple | Malate, oxaloacetate redox couple |
| Mechanism | **Fig. 13A:** Mechanism of glycerol phosphate shuttle | **Fig. 13B:** Mechanism of malate aspartate shuttle |
| Cytoplasm | Dinydroxyacetone phosphate + NADH<br>↓ α - *glycerophosphate dehydrogenase*<br>α - glycerophosphate + $NAD^+$ | Aspartate<br>↓ *Transaminase*<br>Oxaloacetate + NADH<br>↓ *Malate dehydrogenase*<br>Malate + $NAD^+$ |
| Transport into mitochondria | Carrier-mediated transport into mitochondria | Carrier-mediated transport in exchange for α-ketoglutarate (dicarboxylate carrier) |
| Mitochondria | α-glycerophosphate + FAD<br>↓ *α-glycerophosphate dehydrogenease*<br>Dihydroxyacetone phosphate + $FADH_2$ | Malate + $NAD^+$<br>↓ *Malate dehydrogenase*<br>Oxaloacetate + NADH<br>↓ *Transaminase*<br>Aspartate |
| Energetics | - 1ATP (Loss of 1 ATP since $FADH_2$ is formed inside mitochondria instead of NADH) | 0 (Zero loss of ATP) |
| Significance | Unidirectional pathway<br>Not common in humans but is of great importance in insects | Reversible or bidirectional pathway |

## Clinical Significance

NADH produced in cytoplasm during glycolysis, is reoxidized through membrane shuttle systems to generate ATPs.

## 18. Post-translational modifications.

- Post-translational modifications are series of reactions taking place during the protein synthesis or after completion of protein synthesis (most frequent) to make these proteins fully functional.

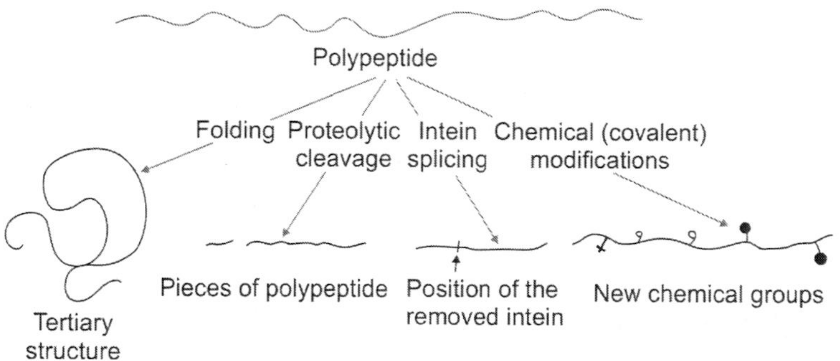


**Fig. 14:** Post-translational modifications

| *Post-translational modification* | *Significance* |
|---|---|
| Protein folding | • Biological function of many proteins is dependent upon their three-dimensional conformation which is achieved through assistance of special heat shock proteins called chaperones<br>• They reversibly bind to hydrophobic regions of unfolded proteins and folding intermediates and favor the interaction on polypeptide surfaces to give specific conformation to a protein<br>• They also stabilize folding intermediates and prevent undesirable interactions of other proteins |
| Proteolysis | |
| a. Removal of initiator amino acid (methionine) | • Formation of functionally active form of protein with unique amino acid sequence |
| b. Proteolysis of proproteins (inactive precursors of proteins)—activated by removal of peptides | *Examples:*<br>• Activation of pancreatic digestive enzymes—protects against autoproteolysis<br>• Activation of blood clotting factors—amplification cascade for clotting process |
| c. Proteolysis of preproproteins (precursor proteins with signal preprotein peptide and proprotein sequence)<br>– Signal peptide of 13–36 amino acids is present on N-terminal end which is recognized by signal recognition particle (SRP) and is removed by signal peptidase | *Examples:* Insulin is secreted as preproinsulin which becomes proinsulin following cleavage of 24 amino acid signal peptide<br>*Significance:*<br>• Signal sequencing is essential for protein targeting and limited proteolysis is essential for secretion of protein and formation of active protein molecule |
| Intein splicing | Inteins are intervening sequences in certain proteins which are removed and exteins are ligated in the appropriate order for the protein to become active |
| Covalent modifications | |
| a. Glycosylation<br>(addition of different carbohydrate residues to asparagine (N-glycosidic bond) or serine and threonine (O-glycosidic bond) in ER and Golgi complex) | *Examples:* Mucoproteins (glycoproteins)<br>*Significance:*<br>• Increased solubility<br>• Functionally active form<br>• Microheterogenecity |
| b. Disulfide bond formation<br>(covalent bonding of cysteine amino acids in same or different peptides by disulfide isomerase) | *Examples:* Disulfide bond in insulin<br>*Significance:*<br>• Functionally active form<br>• Tertiary and quaternary structure<br>• Required for protein function |
| c. Prosthetic (non-protein) group addition | |
| i. Phosphorylation<br>(covalent addition of phosphate by kinase to tyrosine, serine, threonine) | *Examples:* Phosphorylation of serine activates glycogen phosphorylase |
| ii. Hydroxylation<br>[addition of hydroxyl group (vitamin C as co-factor)] | *Examples:* Hydroxylation of proline and lysine—essential for collagen cross linking |
| iii. Gamma carboxylation<br>[addition of carboxyl group to $\gamma$-glutamic acid (vitamin K as co-factor)] | *Examples:* Formation of active forms of clotting factors II, VII, IX, X |
| iv. Prenylation<br>(addition of isoprenyl group to cysteine side chains) | *Examples:* Addition of farnesyl group to p21 ras<br>*Significance:*<br>• Anchoring of proteins to plasma membrane due to its fat solubility |
| v. Acetylation<br>(addition of acetyl group by acetyl transferase) | *Examples:* Acetylation of Histone proteins—regulation of gene expression<br>*Significance:*<br>• Less susceptibility to degradation<br>• Modulation of protein function |

## 19. Base-pairing rule and Wobble hypothesis.

| | *Base-pairing rule* | *Wobble hypothesis* |
|---|---|---|
| Definition | • Base-pairing or Chargaff's rule is a universal rule which states that in body adenine base will pair only with thymine and guanine with cytosine only (A with T and G with C) | • Wobble hypothesis discovered by Frances Crick, states that rules of base pairing are relaxed at the third position, so that a base can pair with more than one complementary base<br>• Some tRNA anticodons have inosine at the third position which can pair with U, C, or A |

*Contd...*

*Contd...*

| | *Base-pairing rule* | *Wobble hypothesis* |
|---|---|---|
| Importance | • Base pairing forms integral part and basis of the Watson-Crick model of double-stranded DNA<br>• It balances number of purines and pyrimidines in any nuclear material<br>• Base-pairing rule has to followed for synthesis of any nuclear material like DNA, RNA and also proteins<br>• It is because of this rule, sequence of bases on DNA can be used to synthesis the proteins, i.e. it helps in phenotypic manifestation of genotype | • Wobble hypothesis explains that for protein synthesis, 61 different tRNA molecules are not required but only half as many |

## 20. Biochemical defect in thalassemia.

- Thalassemias are inherited disorders of hemoglobin synthesis resulting from impaired synthesis of one or more polypeptide chains.

### Biochemical Defect

- Basic biochemical defect in thalassemia is mutation (frameshift mutation or deletion of gene) in respective globin chain synthesis gene resulting in defective transcription, defective post-transcriptional processing of mRNA and defection translation resulting in decreased or defective synthesis of α chain or β chain of globin chain of hemoglobin.

### Types

a. α-thalassemia
b. β-thalassemia
   - Thalassemia major
   - Thalassemia minor
   - Thalassemia intermedia.

### Features

A. α-Thalassemia
   - α-Thalassemia is a disorder of hemoglobin synthesis characterized by defective synthesis of α-globin chain.

   *Causes*
   - By mutation comprising point mutations, insertions and deletions.

   Types [based on number of α globin genes (out of 4) absent]

| *Type* | *Deletion of* | *Clinical features* |
|---|---|---|
| Silent thalassemia | Single globin gene | No clinical effects |
| α thalassemia trait | 2 globin genes | Benign condition, mild anemia |
| α thalassemia minor (Hb H disease) | 3 globin genes | Accumulation of tetramer of chain called hemoglobin H, moderate anemia, splenomegaly |
| α thalassemia major (Hb Bart's) | All 4 globin genes | Accumulation of tetramer of chain called Hb Bart's, hydrops fetalis (fetus survives until birth and then dies) |

B. β-Thalassemia
   - β-thalassemia are disorders of hemoglobin synthesis characterized by defective synthesis of β-globin chain.

   *Causes*
   - Defective transcription due to mutation in the promoter or enhancer region (-88 promoter C → T)
   - Defective RNA processing due to defective splicing caused by mutation in intron-exon region (e.g. IVS - int G → A)
   - Defective translation due to base exchange mutation resulting in formation of non-sense codons with premature termination of polypeptide chain synthesis (e.g. Codon 39, C → T)
   - Frame shift mutation caused by deletion or insertion of bases will also result in defective translation.

*Types*

| | *Thalassemia major* | *Thalassemia minor (β thalassemia trait)* | *Thalassemia intermedia* |
|---|---|---|---|
| Characterized by | Absence of both β-globin genes | Absence of only 1 of globin chain | Intermediate of thalassemia major and minor |
| Genetics | Homozygous state | Heterozygous state | |
| Pathogenesis | Impaired synthesis of one of globin chain → increased synthesis of remaining globin chains → precipitation of unaffected globin chains → hemolysis (inclusion bodies in RBCs) | | |
| Clinical features | • Occurs early in life and affects both sexes equally<br>• Hemolytic anemia, splenomegaly and hepatosplenomegaly | Benign condition manifesting as mild anemia | Moderate degree of anemia<br>Splenomegaly and gallstones |
| Laboratory findings | • ↓ Hb concentration<br>• Reticulocytosis<br>• Hypochromic microcytic anemia<br>• Fragmentation of RBCs<br>• Inclusion bodies in RBCs<br>• Absence of HbA and increased $HbA_2$ and HbF on hemoglobin electrophoresis<br>• ↑ serum iron and ferritin | • Microcytic hypochromic anemia<br>• Presence of HbA and increased $HbA_2$ | ↑ Hb F on hemoglobin electrophoresis |



## 21. Cause of scurvy and beri-beri.

| *Clinical disorder* | *Cause* |
|---|---|
| a. Scurvy | Deficiency of vitamin C |
| b. Beri-beri | Deficiency of thiamine |

## 22. Creatinine clearance test.

Refer Question No. 9 Dec. 2005 (RS2).

# MBBS PHASE I EXAMINATION

## DECEMBER 2013

(Revised Scheme 2 & 3)

### LONG ESSAYS

**1. Describe the citric acid cycle. How is it regulated? Write about its energetic and amphibolic nature.**

Refer Question No. 1 June 2008 (RS2).

**2. Describe the synthesis and breakdown of hemoglobin. Write a note on hemoglobinopathies.**

- Hemoglobin is a chromoprotein responsible for transport of respiratory gases
- It is a conjugated protein containing heme as prosthetic group and 2 pairs of globin chains as apoprotein.

#### Structural Organization (Synthesis) of Hemoglobin

| | |
|---|---|
| Primary | **Globin chain**<br>• α subunit—141 amino acids<br>• β, γ and δ subunit—146 amino acids<br>• All are closely homologous |
| Secondary | • Each globin chain contains several helical segments separated by short non-coiled segments<br>• β, γ and δ chains has 8 helical segments (A, B, C, D, E, F, G and H)<br>• α chain contains 7 segments (it lacks D segment) |
| Tertiary | • Globin chains are highly compact structures<br>• Hydrophilic residues are directed to exterior and hydrophobic residues are directed to interior<br>• Interior hydrophobic residues of globin chain are looped about itself to form a pocket for binding of heme prosthetic group (heme pocket)<br>• One heme associates with each globin chain by non-covalent binding of heme pocket (hydrophobic pocket)<br>**Heme component**<br>• Made of ferrous iron ($Fe^{2+}$) and porphyrin ring (protoporphyrin IX) which contains 4 pyrrole rings<br>• Ferrous iron forms 6 coordinate bonds (ligand bonds); 4 for binding to protoporphyrin IX; 5th bound to proximal<br>• Histidine residue in F helix (β 92 or α 87 histidine) and 6th between oxygen molecule interposed between iron and distal histidine in E helix (β 63 and α 58 histidine) on distal side of porphyrin ring |
| Quaternary | • Each hemoglobin is a tetramer consisting of two pairs of globin chains<br>• HbA is a tetramer of 2 α subunits and 2 β subunits ($\alpha_2\beta_2$) |

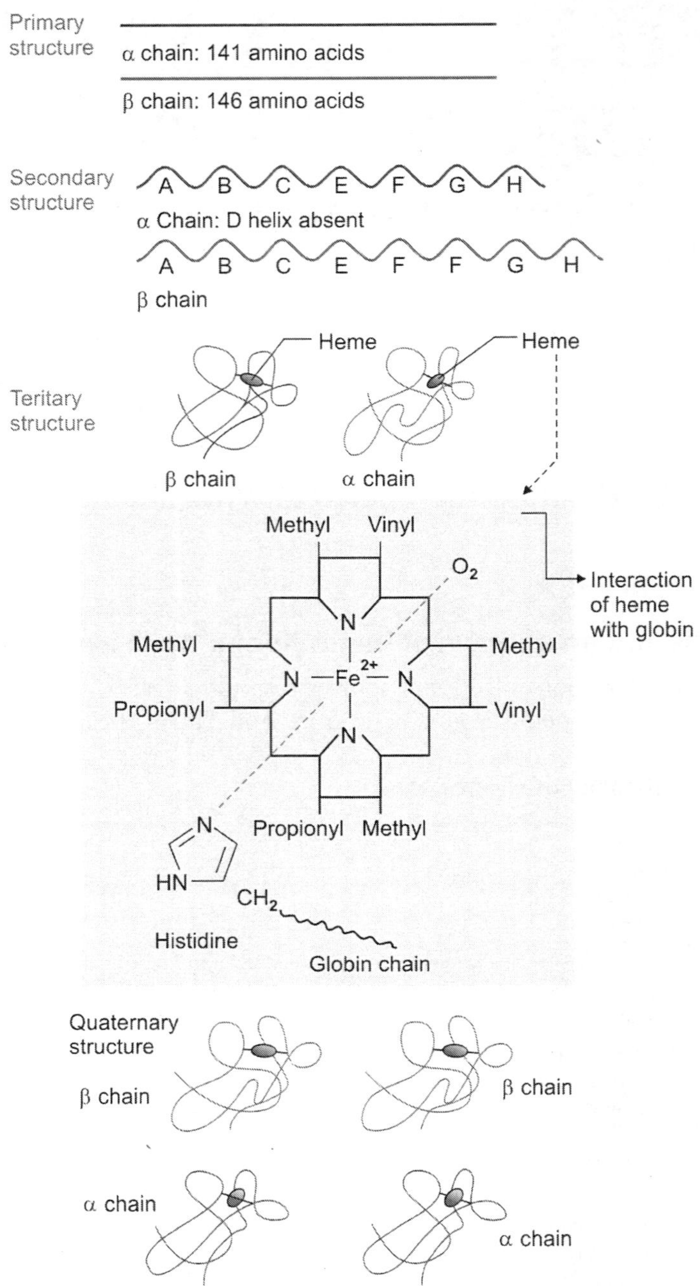


**Fig. 1:** Structural organization of hemoglobin

## Catabolism

- Average life span of an RBC is 120 days
- At end of life span of RBC, they are selectively removed and destroyed by reticulo-endothelial cells of spleen, liver and bone marrow which phagocytose on average about 2.5 - 5 × $10^9$ RBC in 24 hours and catabolize 6–7 g of hemoglobin into more than 200 mg bilirubin
- Heme and globin released are transported in plasma in combination with globulin to hepatocytes and macrophages
- Constituent amino acids are removed from globin chain for reutilization and iron enters iron pool for reuse
- However, iron free porphyrin of heme is degraded in smooth endoplasmic retinaculum of macrophages by heme oxygenase in cooperation with microsomal electron transport system

**For catabolism of hemoglobin**

Refer Question No. 8 June 2007 (RS2).

## Abnormal Hemoglobins

- Abnormal hemoglobins are hemoglobins with defective globin chain
- Clinical disorder thus resulting is called hemoglobinopathies.

*Causes*

- Due to mutation in genes coding for the globin chains
  - Mutations can be genetically transmitted and usually there is a single mutant gene
  - As many as 400 mutations in globin gene are known and 95% of them cause a single amino acid alteration.

*Examples*

| Type | Composition | Chain affected | Alteration |
|---|---|---|---|
| a. HbS | $\alpha_2^A \beta_2^{6\,Val}$ | β | Glutamic acid in 6th position is replaced by valine |
| b. HbC | $\alpha_2^A \beta_2^{6\,Lys}$ | β | Glutamic acid in 6th position is replaced by lysine |
| c. HbD | $\alpha_2^A \beta_2^{121\,Gln}$ | β | Glutamic acid in 121st position is replaced by glutamine |
| d. HbE | $\alpha_2^A \beta_2^{26\,Lys}$ | β | Glutamic acid in 26th position is replaced by lysine |
| e. HbM | $\alpha_2^{87\,Tyr} \beta_2^A$ | α | Histadine in 87th position is replaced by tyrosine |
| f. Hb Sabine | $\alpha_2^A \beta_2^{91\,Proline}$ | β | Leucine in 91st position is replaced by proline |
| g. Hb Chesapeake | $\alpha_2^{92\,Arg} \beta_2^A$ | α | Lycine in 92nd position is replaced by arginine |
| h. Hb Constant spring | $\alpha_2^{172} \beta_2^A$ | α | 172 amino acids in a chain instead of normal 141 |

*Detection of Abnormal Hemoglobins*

i. Finger printing technique
   - Subjecting heat denaturated Hb to action of trypsin which specifically splits protein at site 26 and followed by separation of resulting peptides by electrophoresis in one direction and chromatography at right angle thus detecting abnormal peptides and abnormalities.

ii. Hybridization
   - Detection of abnormal chain by mixing a sample of an abnormal hemoglobin with a mixture of isotopically labeled HbA and subjecting it to low pH and then followed by neutralization.

*Effects of Abnormal Hemoglobins*

- Abnormal hemoglobin gives rise a clinical condition commonly called hemoglobinopathies manifesting as
  - Abnormalities in red cell morphology
  - Definite clinical manifestations like hemolytic anemia/jaundice and other feature in relevance to property of abnormal Hb.

## SHORT ESSAYS

### 3. Describe the fate and functions of methionine.

- Methionine is a sulfur-containing essential amino acid
- It is an aliphatic amino acid and a neutral amino acid
- It is a glucogenic amino acid forming succinyl CoA.

## Metabolic Function of Methionine (Compounds Formed)

a. Proteins and peptides
   - As amino acid, methionine is an important component of proteins and peptides
   - It is the first amino acid to be incorporated during protein biosynthesis (AUG = methionine).

b. Glucose
   - Methionine is a glucogenic amino acid
   - It forms succinyl CoA from propionyl CoA which is formed from homoserine as follows:

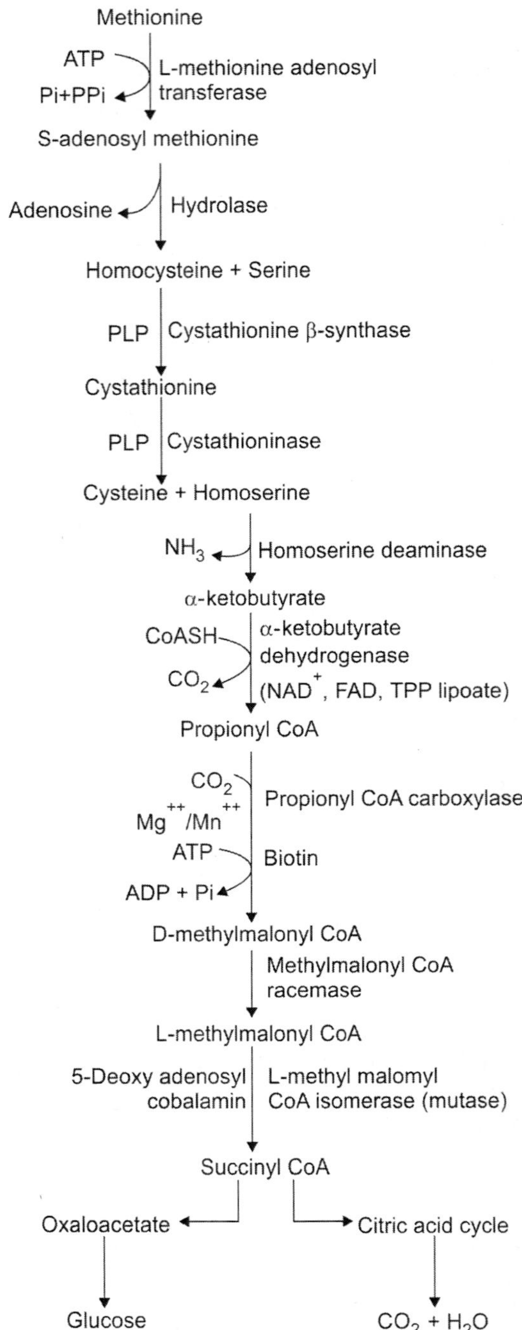


**Fig. 2:** Gluconeogenesis from methionine

- This succinyl CoA can be converted to oxaloacetate to form glucose by gluconeogenesis or it can enter TCA cycle to yield $CO_2$ and water.

Revised Scheme 2 & 3

c. Cysteine
   - Cysteine is another non-essential sulfur-containing amino acid that can be formed from methionine by transulfuration reaction as follows:

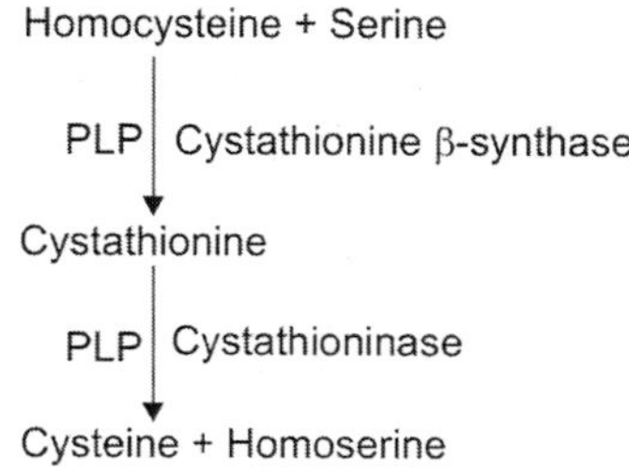


d. Active methionine
   - S-adenosyl methionine (SAM) is active form of methionine
   - It is formed by transfer of adenosyl group from ATP to sulfur group of methionine.

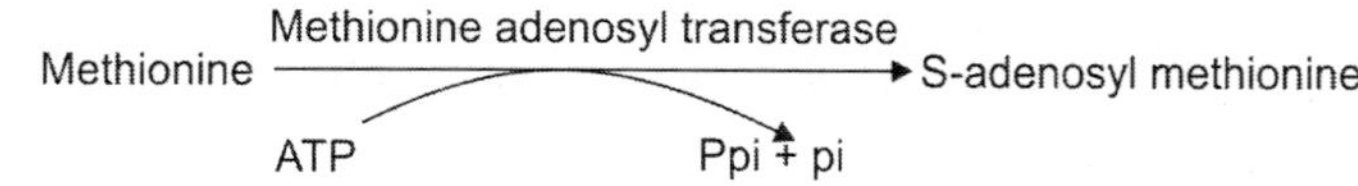


   - Reaction is catalyzed by methionine adenosyl transferase which is also called S-adenosyl methionine synthase

   *Importance*
   - SAM is a major methyl group donor in body
   - It donates it methyl group by transmethylation reactions catalyzed by transmethylase enzyme to be converted into S-adenosyl homocysteine.

*Transmethylase*

SAM → SAH

Acceptor → Methyl acceptor

*Important compounds formed by methylation include:*
   i. Creatinine ← Guanidinoacetate
   ii. Adrenaline ← Noradrenaline
   iii. Melatonin ← N-acetyl serotonin
   iv. A few bases like adenine, guanine of nucleic acids are methylated to methyl adenine and methyl guanine
   v. Detoxification of nicotinic acid or nicotinamide (Nicotinic acid → N-methyl nicotonic acid
   vi. Choline ← Ethnolamine
   vii. Methyl histidine → Histidine
   viii. Anserine ← Carnosine

e. S-adenosyl homocysteine
   - After donating its methyl group SAM is converted S-adenosyl homocysteine (SAH) and then to methionine or homocysteine

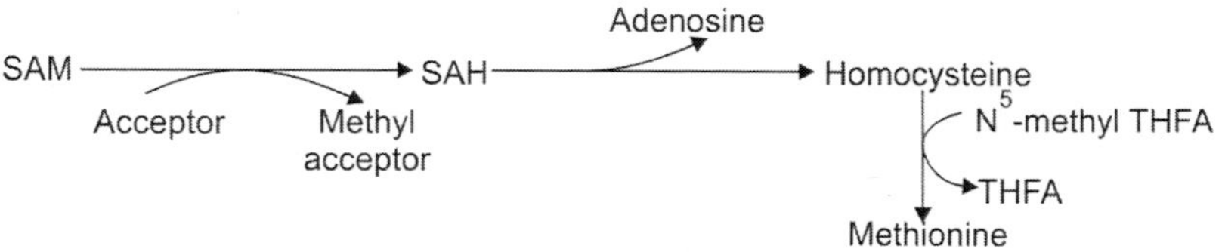

*Catabolism (fate) of methionine*

– Pathway for degradation of methionine is common with that of synthesis of cysteine.

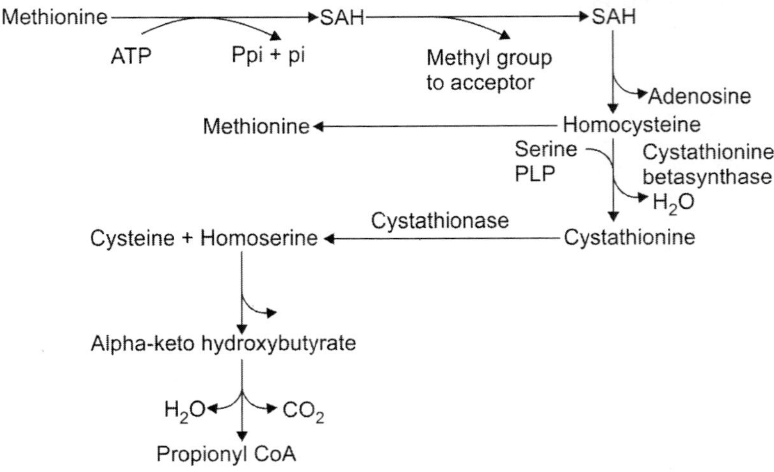


**Fig. 3:** Catabolism of methionine



**For metabolic disorders**

Refer Question No. 7 Dec. 2008 (RS2).

## 4. What are the reactions of HMP pathway? What is the significance of this pathway?

- HMP or hexose monophosphate pathway is an alternate pathway for oxidation of glucose
- It is not involved in energy production but concerned with production of NADPH and pentoses
- Also called pentose phosphate pathway, phosphogluconate pathway or pentose cycle as end products are pentose sugars
- Also referred as HMP shunt as glucose-6-phosphate that enters it, is converted to glyceraldehyde-3-phosphate and fructose 6-phosphate (all intermediates of glycolysis).

| *Tissue site* | *Cellular site* | *Substrate* | *Product* |
|---|---|---|---|
| Erythrocytes, liver, lactating mammary glands, adipose tissue, adrenal cortex, intestines, lens, testes and malignant tissues | Cytosol | Glucose-6-phosphate | NADPH and pentose sugars |

### Reactions

a. Phase 1: Oxidative phase
   – Glucose-6-phosphate is converted to ribulose-5-phosphate with production of 2 NADPH and release of one carbon atom in form of $CO_2$

b. Phase 2: Nonoxidative phase
   – Ribulose-5-phosphate is interconverted to various 3, 5 and and carbon sugars which eventually interact with each other to form fructose-6-phosphate and glyceraldehyde-3-phosphate
   – Thus 3 molecules of glucose-6-phosphate are changed into one ribose-5-phosphate and two xylulose-5-phosphate molecules and finally producing 2 molecules of fructose-6-phosphate and glyceraldehydes-3-phosphate by interaction amongst themselves.

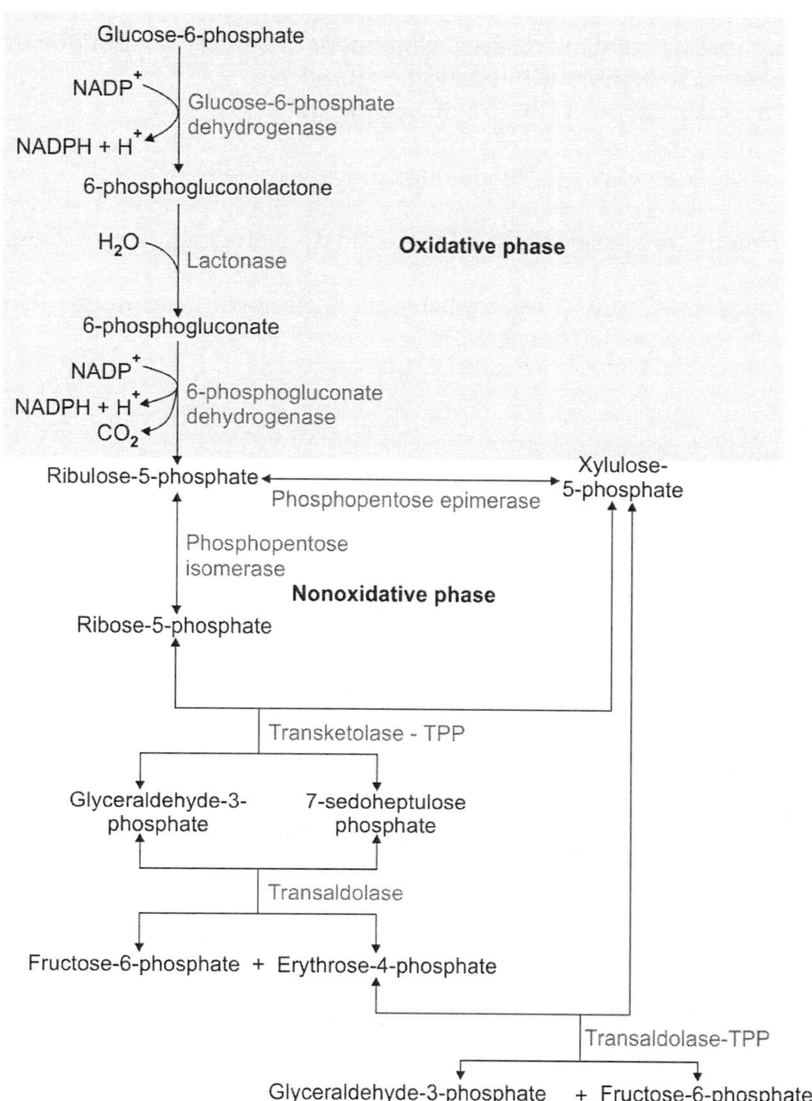


**Fig. 4:** Reaction of hexose monophosphate pathway

## Regulation

| *Key enzyme* | *Modulation* | *Stimulator* | *Inhibitor* |
|---|---|---|---|
| Glucose-6-phosphate dehydrogenase (rate limiting enzyme) | Allosteric regulation | $NADP^+$ | NADPH |
| | Induction (hormonal regulation) | Insulin | — |

## Significance

a. Formation of NADPH
   - NADPH produced in this pathway are used as an electron donor in many reductive synthesis in body like:
     - De novo synthesis of fatty acids
     - Synthesis of cholesterol, steroids, sphingolipids
     - Conversion of oxidized glutathione to reduced glutathione.

b. Provision of pentoses for nucleic acids
   - Ribose-5-phosphate produced during this pathway is used for incorporating ribose into nucleotides and nucleic acids

c. Supply of arbinose-5-phosphate for incorporating arbinose in glycoproteins

d. Role in RBC fragility
   - NADPH formed in this pathway reduces oxidized glutathione to reduced glutathione which in turn remove $H_2O_2$ from RBCs and preserves cell membrane integrity of erythrocytes
   - NADP also reduces rate of oxidation of Hb to methemoglobin.
e. Role in lens metabolism
   - Reduced glutathione is also necessary for maintenance of lens proteins.
f. Role in phagocytosis
   - NADPH generated in this pathway is utilized by NADPH oxidase in producing superoxide anions ($O_2^-$) for destroying phagocytosed material.
g. Fructose-6-phosphate and glyceraldehyde-3-phosphate produced can be used for glycolysis or gluconeogenesis
h. Carbon dioxide produced may be used in $CO_2$ fixation.

## Metabolic Disorders

- Glucose 6-phosphate dehydrogenase deficiency
  - Sex linked inheritance.

  *Pathology*
  - Affects all the cells but more severe in RBCs
  - In RBCs, HMP pathway is the only mean of providing NADPH and thus impaired activity of G6PD impairs synthesis of NADPH in RBCs
  - Erythrocytes require NADPH to keep glutathione in reduced state which is essential for membrane integrity, prevention of methemoglobin formation
  - Thus, GPD dehydrogenease deficiency results in accumulation of methemoglobin and peroxide leading to hemolysis.

## Clinical Features

- Most patients are asymptomatic
- Few develop hemolytic anemia if exposed to oxidant stress by drugs such as primaquine, acetanilide, sulfamethoxazole or infection by production of free radicals.

## Significance

- However, people with G6PD deficiency are resistant to *Plasmodium falciparum* (malaria) infection because the parasite is dependent on HMP pathway and reduced glutathione for growth.

Revised Scheme 2 & 3

## 5. Clinical importance of enzymes in assessment of cardiac disease and liver function.

- Estimation of enzymes has helped diagnose numerous clinical disorders even in absence of significant clinical manifestations.

## Enzyme Profile in Cardiac Disease (Acute Myocardial Infarction)

| | *Normal level* | *Cardiac disorder* | *Significance* |
|---|---|---|---|
| a. Creatinine phosphokinase (CPK-MB) | 4–60 IU/L | After MI the serum value increases after about 6 hours, reaches a peak in 24–30 hours and returns to normal level in 2–4 days | • Serum CPK activity is a sensitive indicator in early stage of myocardial ischemia<br>• It is more useful in subendocardial infarction<br>• There is no increase noted in heart failure and coronary insufficiency |
| b. Aspartate transaminase (AST)/SGOT | 4–17 IU/L | In acute MI, serum activity rises sharply within the first 12 hours with a peak level at 24 hours or over. The level returns to normal within 3–5 days | • Level of the rise of the enzyme activity can be correlated with the prognosis i.e. Levels >350 IU/L are usually fatal, levels >150 IU/L are associated with high mortality and levels <50 IU/L have low mortality<br>• Enzyme level rises even in absence of any detectable ECG change<br>• Rise depends upon the size of the infarct and abnormal level occurs on 2nd day<br>• Extracardiac rise of SGOT seen in muscle and hepatic diseases can be differentiated by simultaneous determination of the SGPT which shows no change in MI<br>• A secondary rise occurs in SGOT in case of reinfarction |

Contd...

*Contd...*

| | *Normal level* | *Cardiac disorder* | *Significance* |
|---|---|---|---|
| c. Lactate dehydrogenase (LDH-1) | 60–250 IU/L | In acute MI, serum activity rises within 12–24 hours attaining a peak at 48 hours at about 1000 IU/L and then returns to normal gradually from 8th–14th days | • The peak rise of the enzyme is roughly proportional to the extent of the myocardial injury<br>• The level remains elevated for a week after other enzyme return to normal<br>• Levels >1500 IU/L are indicators of grave prognosis<br>• Care is taken to avoid hemolysis during estimation as even the RBCs are rich in LDH |
| d. $\gamma$-glutamyl transpeptidase ($\gamma$ - GTP) | Men: 10–47 IU/L<br>Women: 7–30 IU/L | Enzyme rise is quite late, reaching peak between 7th–11th day and lasting as long as a month | • Enzyme rise is due to angioblastic proliferation from vascular endothelium signifying the repair process. Hence it is a useful test in later stages of MI |
| e. Histaminase | 0.12–0.76 PU/mL | Enzyme level above 0.8 PU/mL are suggestive of MI<br>Rise is seen within 6 hours and persists for whole 1 week | • Helps in early diagnosis of MI even when ECG fails to revel any changes<br>• Has more prognostic value as higher the level of rise, worser the prognosis. (Mean value in fatal cases >3.48 PU/mL) |
| f. Pseudo-cholinesterases | 2.17–5.17 IU/mL | Serum enzyme rise is seen within 12 hours and in some case as early as 3 hours also | • Serum enzyme activity is sensitive index for determination of cellular necrosis in myocardium |

## Enzyme Profile in Hepatic Disease

| *Serum enzymes* | *Normal value* | *Rise seen in* | *Fall seen in* |
|---|---|---|---|
| a. Aspartate transaminase (AST)/SGOT | 4–17 IU/L | • Acute liver diseases<br>• Toxic liver cell necrosis | |
| b. Alanine transaminase (ALT)/SGPT | 3–15 IU/L | • Viral hepatitis<br>• Cirrhosis<br>• Toxic liver cell necrosis | |
| c. Lactate dehydrogenase (LDH) | 60–250 IU/L | • Acute hepatitis | |
| d. Alkaline phosphatase (ALP) | 3–13 KA units/dL | • Acute liver disease<br>• Space occupying lesions of liver | |
| e. Aldolase | 2–6 m IU | • Acute liver diseases | |
| f. Amylase | 8–180 somogyi units% | | Acute liver diseases |
| g. Lipase | 9–20 m IU | | Acute liver diseases |
| h. Cholinesterase | 2–5 IU/mL | | Acute liver diseases |
| i. Ceruloplasmin | 3–58 mg% | • Cirrhosis | Hepatolenticular degeneration |
| j. Isocitrate dehydrogenase | 1–4 IU/L | • Viral hepatitis<br>• Sirrhosis | |
| k. Ornithine carbamoyl transferase | 8–20 m IU | • Viral hepatitis<br>• Cirrhosis | |
| l. Leucine amino peptidase | 15–56 m IU | • Superimposed hepatoma in cirrhosis<br>• Liver cell carcinoma<br>• Viral hepatitis<br>• Cirrhosis | |
| m. $\gamma$-Glutamyl transpeptidase | 1–47 IU/L | • Acute hepatobiliary disease<br>• Alcoholic cirrhosis | |
| n. 5′-nucleotidase | 2–17 IU/L | • Acute liver disease | |

## 6. Outline the de novo synthesis of fatty acid. What are the advantages of having a multifunctional enzyme complex?

- De Novo synthesis of fatty acids acid is synthesis of fatty acid from acetyl CoA as source of carbon atom while NADPH providing reducing equivalents utilizing ATP as source energy in a reaction catalyzed by a multienzyme system called fatty acid synthetase.

| Tissue site | Cellular site | Substrate | Product |
|---|---|---|---|
| Liver, adipose tissue and lactating breast | Cytoplasm | Acetyl CoA (source of carbon; derived from citrate)<br>NADPH (Source of reducing equivalents; derived from HMP pathway) | Higher fatty acids (usually palmitic acid) |

*Steps*

a. Reactions of Acetyl CoA carboxylase (Formation of malonyl CoA from acetyl CoA)
   - Acetyl CoA carboxylase carboxylates acetyl CoA to malonyl CoA
   - It requires biotin, $CO_2$, ATP and $Mg^{2+}$ as cofactors
   - It is the rate limiting step.

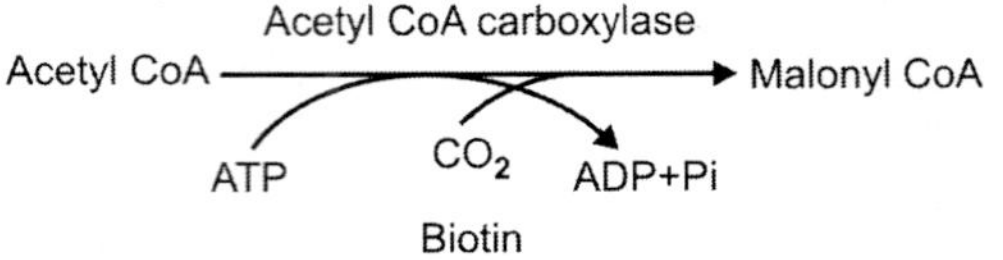


b. Reactions of fatty acid syntheses complex
   - Fatty acid syntheses complex is a multifunctional enzyme

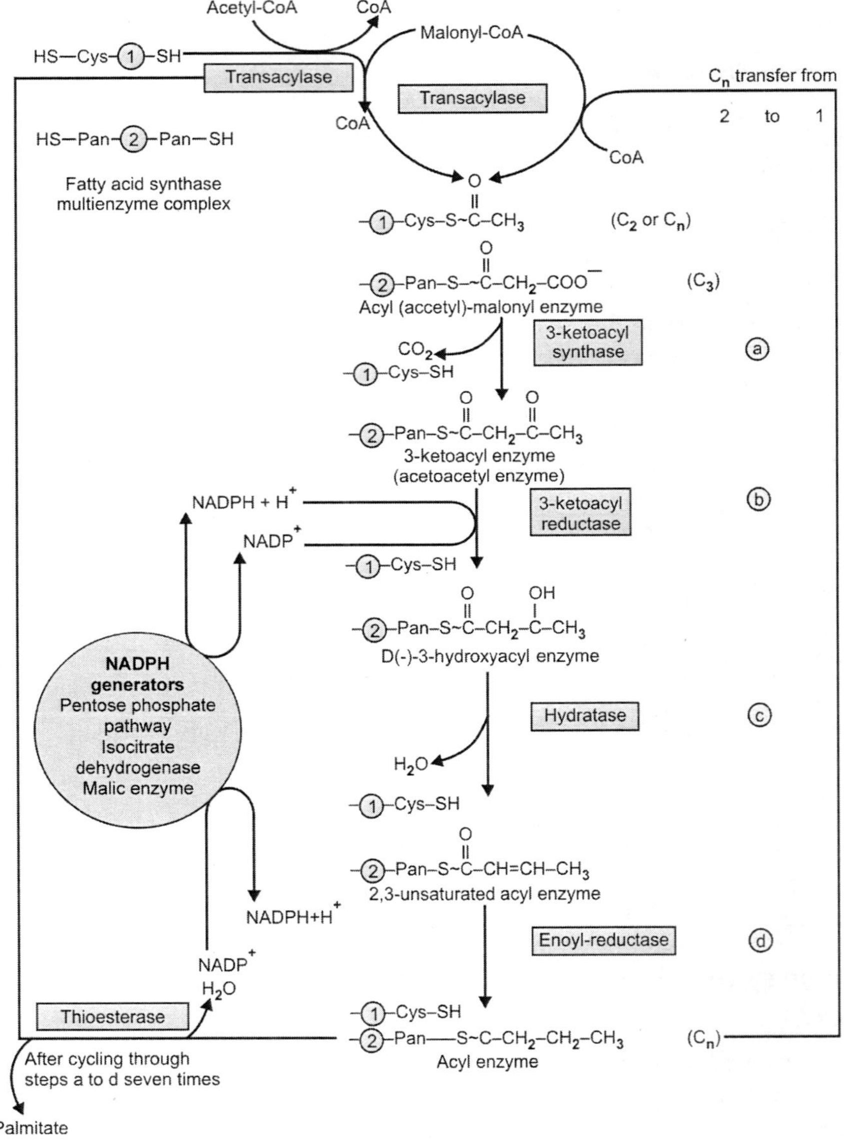


**Fig. 5:** Reaction of fatty acid synthesis complex

- It is a dimer of 2 identical units and each monomer has 7 different enzymes and an acyl carrier protein
- It functions as a single unit catalyzing all the seven reactions.

## Sequence of Reactions (6 Cyclic Reactions)

| Enzyme | Reaction | Remarks |
|---|---|---|
| i. Acetyl CoA – ACP transacylase | Acetyl CoA is transferred to acyl carrier protein (ACP) | Acetyl unit is then transferred from ACP to cystine residue of enzyme making the ACP site vacant |
| ii. Malonyl CoA – ACP transacylase | Transfers calotte from malonyl CoA to ACP | |
| iii. β-ketoacyl ACP syntheses | Transfer to acetyl CoA to malonyl CoA | Decarboxylation reaction with loss of free energy |
| iv. β-ketoacyl ACP reductase | Reduces ketoacyl group to hydroxyacyl group | Requires NADPH |
| v. β-hydrohydroxy ACP dehydratase | Formation of double bond between α and β carbons | Loss of $H_2O$ |
| vi. Enoyl ACP reductase | Reduction of $D^2$ Enoyl ACP to Acyl CoA | Requires NADPH |
| First round of reactions produces 4 carbon compounds (butyrl S-enzyme) and the acyl intermediate is transferred to ACP of fatty acid synthase<br>For synthesis of most abundant fatty acid, i.e. palmitic acid (C-16) the reaction has to the steps mentioned above 6 more times and each time the fatty acid chain is 2 carbon atom more than the previous. Thus at the end of 7 cycles a 16 carbon atom fatty acid, palmitic acid is produced. | | |
| vii. Palmitoyl thioesterase | Separates palmitic acid from enzyme complex | |

- Thus overall reaction can be summarized as follows:
  Acetyl CoA + 7 ATP + 14 (NADPH + $H^+$) → Palmitic acid + 8 CoA + 7 ADP + 7 pi + $6H_2O$.

## Energetics (For Synthesis of Palmitic Acid)

| Reaction | Enzyme | Energy molecule used | No. of cycles | ATPs expenditure |
|---|---|---|---|---|
| Acetyl CoA → Malonyl CoA | Acetyl CoA carboxylase | ATP | 7 | -7 ATP |
| 3-ketoacyl S-enzyme → 3-hydroxyacyl S-enzyme | 3-ketoacyl reductase | NADPH | 7 | -17.5 ATPs |
| 2,3 unsaturated acyl S-enzyme → Acyl S-enzyme | Enoyl reductase | NADPH | 7 | -17.5 ATPs |
| | | | Total | -42 ATPs |

- Thus synthesis of one molecule of palmitic acid requires 42 ATPs.

## Regulation

### *Key Enzyme*

- *Acetyl CoA carboxylase (rate limiting enzyme)*

| Modulation | Stimulator | Inhibitor |
|---|---|---|
| Short-term regulation | | |
| • Allosteric modification | Citrate | Palmitoyl CoA<br>Malonyl CoA |
| • Covalent modification | Insulin (dephosphorylates) | Glucagon<br>Epinephrine<br>Norepinephrine<br>(phosphorylates) |
| Long-term regulation (of enzyme synthesis) | | |
| • Induction | High-carbohydrate diet<br>Insulin | |
| • Repression | Low carbohydrate diet | |

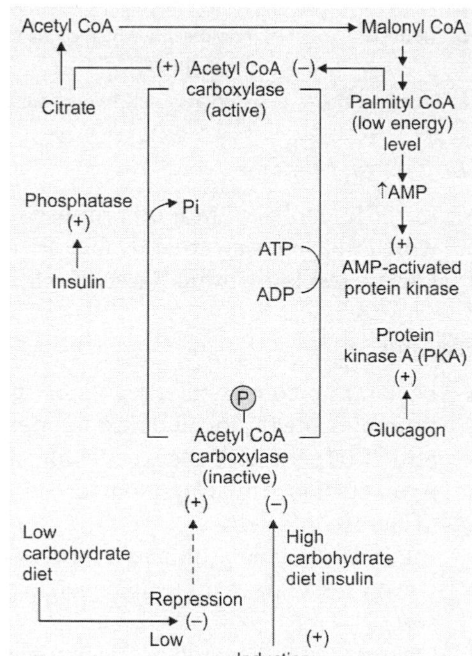

**Fig. 6:** Regulation of lipogenesis

### *Other Enzymes*

- High carbohydrate diet leads to increased synthesis of fatty acid synthase, citrate lyase (provision of acetyl CoA), glucose-6-phosphate dehydrogenase and malic enzyme (provision of NADPH).

**For advantages of multifunctional enzyme complex**

Refer Question No. 1 June 2006 (RS2).

## 7. How is urea synthesized in the body? Give the reactions. What is the significance of urea cycle?

Refer Question No. 1 Dec. 2011 (RS2).

## 8. Explain the structure of tRNA with diagram and mention its function.

Refer Question No. 8 June 2013 (RS2).

## 9. Define BMR. How do you calculate BMR? Discuss four factors that affect BMR.

Refer Question No. 12 June 2006 (RS2).

## 10. Describe with an example regulation of gene expression.

- Genes are parts of DNAs which are responsible for synthesis of certain proteins which is called expression of gene
- All genes of cell are not expressed at all the times because gene expression in regulated to prevent excess protein synthesis.



### Regulation of Gene Expression in Prokaryotes

*Operon Concept*

- Operon is defines as a segment of a DNA strand which is a coordinated unit of gene expression.

*Components*

| | |
|---|---|
| a. Structural gene | • Codes for specific proteins<br>• Present in clusters |
| b. Operator gene | • Controls overall translation process<br>• Located adjacent to structural gene and RNA polymerase has to bind to it first before binding to structural gene |
| c. Regulator gene | • Codes for specific mRNA which translates into a repressor protein which binds to operator gene to stop further movement of RNA polymerase from operator gene to structural gene thus inhibiting (regulating) protein synthesis<br>• Located at a distance from operator gene on same DNA strand |
| d. Inducer | • Molecule which binds to repressor protein, making it unable to bind to operator gene thus promoting (inducing) protein synthesis |
| e. Promoter site | • Binds to RNA polymerase to initiate mRNA synthesis |

*Lac Operon Model*

- In 1961, Jacob and Monod proposed a model for operating of these operon which is called as lac operon model for which they were awarded Nobel prize for medicine in 1965
- Lac operon is an inducible catabolic operon of *E. coil* which regulates lactose metabolism in *E. coli.*

*Features*

- Lac operon consists of a regulatory gene (I), an operator gene (O) and 3 structural genes (Z, Y and A) along with a promoter site (P) located next to operator gene
- Structural genes Z, Y and A codes for enzymes β galactosidase, galactoside permease and galactose acetylase respectively
- β galactosidase hydrolyses lactose into glucose and galactose while galactoside permease is responsible for transport of lactose into cells
- Inhibitor (I) gene produces a repressor molecule, expression of which is constitutive
- Lac repressor has a molecular weight of 150,000 D and has 4 identical subunits which has strong affinity to the operator site
- Operator site is located between promoter and structural genes and has major groove for binding of lac repressor
- For this model, lactose acts as inducer

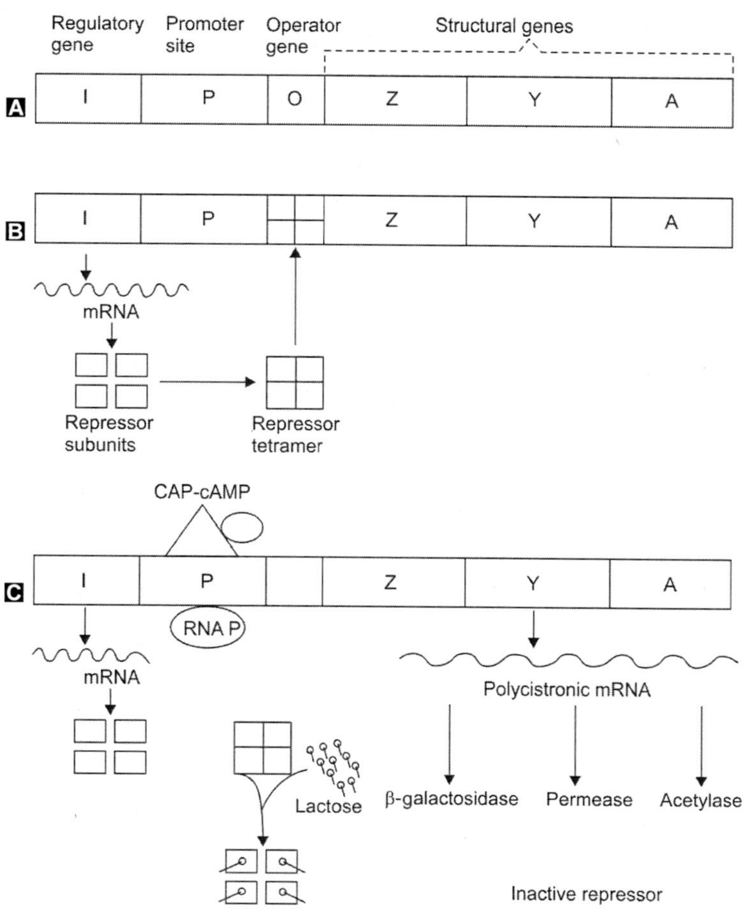


(A) structure of lac operon; (B) Repression of lac operon;
(C) Depression of lac operon (CAP–cAMP–catabolite gene activator protein bound to cAMP; RNAP–RNA polymerase

**Fig. 7:** Lac operon model

*Mechanism of Action*

- Repressor molecule prevents binding of enzyme RNA polymerase to promoter site thereby blocking transcription of structural genes thus when lactose in not available lactose utilizing enzyme are not synthesized
- When lactose in introduced into medium some molecules passively enter into bacterial cell which then binds to repressor molecule and induces a conformational change in repressor
- Repressor gets inactivated and therefore it cannot bind to operator gene thus letting RNA polymerase to act freely
- RNA polymerase then attaches to promoter site and structural genes are transcribed and then translated into 3 enzymes
- Thus lactose induces synthesis of lactose catabolizing enzymes
- When culture medium of bacteria contains both glucose and lactose, bacteria utilize glucose preferentially
- Lactose is catabolized only when glucose is exhausted
- Thus lac operon is induced by lactose only when glucose is not available
- RNA polymerase can attach to promoter site only when catabolite activator protein saturated with cyclic AMP is available
- By an independent mechanism, bacterium accumulates cAMP only when starved
- When glucose is exhausted, cAMP is available in plenty and thus catabolite activator protein (CAP)-cAMP complex is formed
- Then RNA polymerase can identify promoter site
- Thus CAP-cAMP complex acts as a positive regulator for gene expression
- Therefore lac operon is both subjected to positive and negative regulation.

## Regulation of Gene Expression in Eukaryotes

- In eukaryotes, gene expression is regulated as follows:

a. Gene amplification
   - Refers to production of multiple copies of gene by repeated rounds of replication resulting in increased gene expression inturn increased production of protein coded by that gene

   *Significance*
   - Plays significant role in embryonic stages of development
   - It also implicated in development of tumors, development of drug resistance.

**Fig. 8:** Gene amplification

b. Gene rearrangement
   - Refers to mixing of parental DNA from two different sources
   - It could be either homologous recombination, site specific recombination and transposition.

   *Significance*
   - Plays significant role in production of diverse types of antibodies.

c. Post-transcriptional modifications (RNA processing)
   - Primary transcript (product of transcription) undergoes certain covalent modifications to form mature RNA.

d. Alternate mRNA splicing
   - Splicing (removal of introns and joining of exons to produce desired mRNA) can produce different codon combinations resulting in production of different proteins.

e. mRNA editing
   - Refers to enzyme mediated alteration of RNA nucleotide sequence occurring after transcription inform of insertion, deletion or substitution of nucleotides.

f. Degradation of mRNA
   - Adjusting rate of mRNA degradation can regulate gene expression.

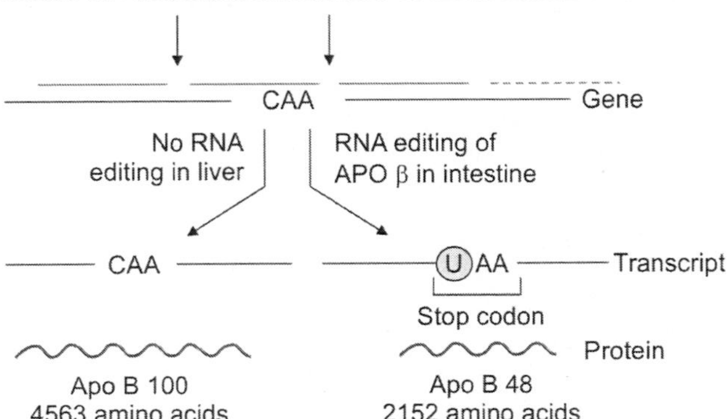


**Fig. 9:** Alternate mRNA splicing

g. Regulator elements
   - Gene expression can also be regulated by regulatory elements like promoters, inducers, hormone responsive elements.

### 11. What do you mean by gene therapy? Discuss its application in medicine.

Refer Question No. 12 Dec. 2007 (RS2).

### 12. Describe the catabolism of purine nucleotide. Add a note on gout.

Refer Question No. 2 June 2007 (RS2).

## SHORT ANSWERS

### 13. Phospholipids.

Refer Question No. 3 Dec. 2009 (RS2).

### 14. Coenzymes.

- Coenzyme is a non protein, organic, low molecular weight and dialyzable substance essential for biological activity of enzyme
- Also known as prosthetic group
- Coenzyme (prosthetic group) + Apoenzyme (inactive enzyme) = Holoenzyme.

### Features

- Take part in reactions involving transfer of hydrogen or any other group
- Either bound tightly to apoenzyme (by covalent linkage) like FMN, FAD and biotin or bound very loosely and transiently like NADP.

### Mechanism

- Coenzymes serve as cosubstrates which often get changed during reaction to lower activation point of enzyme
- But subsequently they are recovered in original form.

*Examples (Types)*

| *Coenzyme* | *Derived from* | *Group transferred* | *Apoenzyme* |
|---|---|---|---|
| **Coenzymes involved in Oxidation – Reduction reactions** | | | |
| • NAD | Niacin | Hydrogen and electron | Lactate dehydrogenase<br>Malate dehydrogenase |
| • NADP | Niacin | Hydrogen and electron | G-6-P dehydrogenase |
| • FMN | Riboflavin | Hydrogen and electron | L-amino acid oxidase<br>NADH dehydrogenase |
| • FAD | Riboflavin | Hydrogen and electron | D-amino acid oxidase<br>Succinate dehydrogenase |
| • Lipoic acid | Lipoic acid | Hydrogen and electron | Pyruvate dehydrogenase complex |
| **Coenzymes involved in group transfer reactions** | | | |
| • TPP | Thiamin | Aldehyde or keto | Transketolase<br>Pyruvate dehydrogenase |
| • PLP | Pyridoxine | Amino or keto | Alanine transaminase<br>Tyrosine transaminase |
| • CoA | Pantothenic acid | Acyl | Thiokinase |
| • $FH_4$ | Folic acid | One carbon moiety | Formyl transferase<br>Thymidylate synthetase |
| • Biocytin | Biotin | $CO_2$ | Pyruvate carboxylase<br>Acetyl CoA carboxylase |
| • Cobalamin | Vitamin $B_{12}$ | Methyl group | Homocysteine methyl transferase<br>L-methyl malonyl CoA mutase |
| • ATP | Adenosine | Phosphate, adenosine, AMP | Kinases |
| • SAM | Methionine | Methyl | Methyltransferase |

### Significance

- Coenzymes play a decisive role in enzyme function.

## 15. Secondary structure of proteins.

Refer Question No. 4 Dec. 2011 (RS2).

## 16. Prostaglandins.

Refer Question No. 15 Dec. 2014 (RS2).

## 17. Transamination.

Refer Question No. 2 June 2006 (RS2).

## 18. Anticancer agents.

- Anticancer agents are drugs which inhibit specific phase of cell cycle.

### Anticancer Agents

| *Cell cycle phase inhibition* | *Drug* | *Mechanism of action* | *Indication* |
|---|---|---|---|
| a. All phases (non-phase specific) | i. Alkylating agents | | |
| | – Cyclophosphamide | Cross linking of bases of DNA, inhibition of strand separation | Lymphomas, myeloid leukemias |
| | – Cisplatin | Forms intrastrand DNA adducts | |
| b. S phase | i. Antimetabolites | | |
| | – 5-fluorouracil | Inhibit thymidylate synthease | Adenocarcinoma of colon and breast |
| | – Methotrexate | Competitive inhibitor of dihydrofolate reductase | Choriocarcinoma, acute leukemia |
| | ii. Purine analogs | | |
| | – 6-mercaptopurine | Inhibits conversion of IMP to AMP | Acute lymphoblastic leukemia |
| | – 6-thioguanine | Inhibits conversion of IMP to AMP | Acute lymphoblastic leukemia |
| c. M phase/$G_1$ phase | i. Microtubule inhibitors | | |
| | – Vincristine and vinblastine | Interferes with assembly of cytoskeleton and inhibits Stathmokinesis (spindle movements) | Leukemias, lymphoma, Wilm's tumor |
| | ii. Anticancer antibiotics | | |
| | – Mitomycin C | Cross bridges are formed between DNA base pairs | Adenocarcinoma of stomach, breast, colon, etc. |
| | – Actinomycin C | Intercalates with guanine bases of DNA, prevents transcription | |
| | – Imatinib | Tyrokinase inhibitor | |
| d. $G_2$ phase | i. Topoisomerase inhibitors | | |
| | – Etoposide | Stabilizes topoisomerase-II-DNA cleavage complexes | Lymphoma<br>Sarcoma |



## 19. Plasmids and oncogenes.

- Plasmids are small, extrachromosomal, independent circular double stranded, self-replicating DNA molecules
- Oncogenes are genes whose products are associated with neoplastic transformation
- Oncogenes are formed from alternation in structure or expression of proto-oncogenes, the normal genes associated with growth and development of body
- cDNA is a synthesized from RNA genome of a virus by reverse transcription is an classical example of plasmids activating oncogene
- cDNA formed from viral RNA is inserted into host genome acts as a promoter of oncogene resulting in transcription.

## 20. Obstructive jaundice and its diagnosis.

- Jaundice is clinical condition characterized by yellow pigmentation of skin and sclera
- Obstructive jaundice or post-hepatic jaundice is caused due to blockage of excretory mechanism of bilirubin.

| *Causes* | *Mechanism* | *Clinical features* |
|---|---|---|
| • Congenital anomalies of the biliary tree<br>• Gall stones<br>• Extrahepatic cholestasis<br>• Biliary atresia<br>• Strictures of bile tree<br>• Tumors (pancreatic or biliary tree) | • Due to obstruction to outflow of bile, all bilirubin conjugated by liver to enters circulation<br>• Thus, it is characterized by excessive presence of only conjugated bilirubin in blood and urine | • Nausea, loss of appetite and gastrointestinal discomfort<br>• Yellow pigmentation of skin and sclera<br>• Dark colored urine due to excessive excretion of bilirubin<br>• Pale, clay colored stool due to absence of stercobilinogen and contains unabsorbed fat<br>• Pruritus (itching) due to deposition of bilirubin in skin |

### Laboratory Diagnosis

| Blood | Urine | Stool | Liver function tests |
|---|---|---|---|
| • Total bilirubin: Elevated<br>• Unconjugated bilirubin: Normal<br>• Conjugated bilirubin: Markedly increased<br>• Alkaline phosphatase: Markedly increased<br>• Gamma glutyl transferase: Markedly increased<br>• AST and ALT: Slightly increase | • Bile pigment: Present<br>• Conjugated bilirubin: Present<br>• Urobilinogen: Absent | • Stercobilinogen: Absent or decreased<br>• Fat: 40–50% increased | • Normal or mildly impaired |

## 21. Abnormal components of urine.

- Pathological constituents of urine are substances which are not usually excreated in urine but appear in urine in some pathological condition.

### Abnormal Components of Urine

| Abnormal constituents | Cause | Test for detection |
|---|---|---|
| a. Proteins | | |
| i. Albumin (if mild injury) or IgG (if severe injury) | Glomerular proteinuria: Nephrotic syndrome, nephritic syndrome, diabetic nephropathy | Heat test, acetic acid test, sulfosalicylic acid test, immunoturbidometry |
| ii. Bence Jones proteins | Overflow proteinuria: Multiple myeloma | Bradshaw test, heat test, immunoelectrophoresis |
| iii. β-2 microglobulin | Tubular proteinuria: Acute tubular necrosis, renal transplant reaction | Nephelometry |
| b. Reducing sugars | | |
| i. Glucose | Diabetic glycosuria: Diabetes mellitus<br>Renal glycosuria: Fanconi syndrome, pregnancy<br>Alimentary glycosuria: Thyrotoxicosis, gastrectomy | Benedict' test, Fehling's test, osazone test |
| ii. Fructose | Hereditary fructose intolerance: Aldolase B deficiency<br>Essential fructosuria: Fructokinase deficiency | |
| iii. Galactose | Galactosemia: Galactose 1 phosphate uridyl transferase deficiency | |
| iv. Xylulose | Essential pentosuria: Xylitol dehydrogenase deficiency | |
| c. Lipids | | |
| i. Cholesterol/TGs | Lipiduria: Nephrotic syndrome | |
| ii. Ketone bodies | Ketosis: Diabetes mellitus, starvation | Rothera's test, Gerhardt's test |
| d. Blood | Glomerulonephritis | Benzidine test, orthotoluidine test |
| e. Bile pigments | Obstructive jaundice: Gallstones, hepatitis, carcinoma of head of pancreas | Fouchet's test |
| f. Bile salts | Obstructive jaundice | Hays test |
| g. Amino acids | Phenylketonuria: Phenylalanine hydroxylase deficiency | Ferric chloride test |

## 22. Radioisotopes.

- Isotopes are different forms of same element having same number of protons (atomic number) but different number of neutrons (atomic weight).

### Radioactive Isotopes

- Isotopes that emit radiation due to instability of nucleus
- Also known as radionuclides.

## Rays

| | *Alpha rays* | *Beta rays* | *Gamma rays* |
|---|---|---|---|
| Emission of | Positively charged electrons | Negatively charged electrons (beta particles) or positively charged positrons | Electromagnetic waves of short wave lengths |
| Features | Low penetrating power<br>Severe damage | | High ionizing capacity<br>Greatest damage |

## Application in Biochemistry

| *In research and studies* | *In diagnosis and treatment* |
|---|---|
| a. To determine metabolic origin of complex molecules such as heme, cholesterol, purines and phospholipids<br>- $^{14}C$ labeled aceto-acetic acid is shown to be incorporated into palmitic acid<br>- $^{14}C$ or $^{15}N$ label in heme is seen following administration of labeled glycine<br>b. To investigate precursor-product relationship in several metabolic pathways like Kreb's cycle, beta-oxidation of fatty acids, urea cycle, fatty acid synthesis, etc.<br>- $^{32}P$ is useful to trace nucleic acid synthesis<br>c. Study of metabolic turnovers<br>- If $^{131}I$ labeled immunoglobulin is injected, quantity of labeled molecules in circulation will be proportional to catabolism of Ig<br>d. Study metabolic pool or total body content of a particular substance<br>- 1 mL of $^{131}I$ labeled albumin is has 1million dps and it is injected in and after attaining equilibrium, i.e. 10–15 minutes, a blood sample of 1 mL is taken and radioactivity is measured which is usually 200 dps. Thus, original count is diluted 5,000 times therefore blood volume is 5,000 mL<br>e. Used in certain endocrine and immunological studies like radioimmunoassay<br>- $^{51}Cr$ is taken up by living cells and label is liberated when cell is lysed and thus it is used to quantitate cell lysis<br>f. In genetic research<br>- $^{3}H$ labeled thyrmidine is incorporated in newly synthesized DNA and therefore used in assessing cell division kinetics<br>g. In elucidating drug metabolism | a. In diagnosis<br>- $^{131}I$ is used in diagnosis of toxic nodular goiter, thyroid carcinoma<br>- $^{90}Sr$ is used for bone carcinoma, osteoporosis<br>- $^{131}I$ Hippuran is used to diagnose renal disorders<br>b. In treatment<br>- In radiotherapy for treatment of radiosensitive carcinomas<br>- Based on principle that radiations produce ionization which damage nucleic acid thus restricting uncontrolled proliferation |

# MBBS PHASE I EXAMINATION
## JUNE 2014
## (Revised Scheme 2 & 3)

## LONG ESSAYS

### 1. Classify amino acid based on their structure giving examples.

- Amino acids are a group of organic compounds containing two functional groups—amino and carboxyl.

### Classification Based on Chemical Structure

- Classification of amino acids based on chemical structure is a comprehensive classification, classifying 20 amino acids into 7 distinct groups based on the presence of side chain (attached to a carbon atom)
- Each amino acid is assigned an abbreviation symbol of 3 letter or 1 letter to represent them in protein structure.

| *Name* | *Symbol* | | *Special group present* |
|---|---|---|---|
| | 3 letters | 1 letter | |
| A. Aliphatic amino acids (amino acids with aliphatic side chains) | | | |
| a. Glycine | Gly | G | |
| b. Alanine | Ala | A | |
| c. Valine | Val | V | Branched chain |
| d. Leucine | Leu | L | Branched chain |
| e. Isoleucine | Ile | I | Branched chain |
| B. Hydroxyl amino acids (amino acid with hydroxyl-OH group) | | | |
| f. Serine | Ser | S | Hydroxyl |
| g. Threonine | Thr | T | Hydroxyl |
| Tyrosine | Tyr | Y (tYrosine) | Hydroxyl |
| C. Sulfur-containing amino acids | | | |
| h. Cysteine | Cys | C | Sulfhydryl |
| Cystine | — | — | Disulfide |
| i. Methionine | Met | M | Thioether linkage |
| D. Acidic amino acid and their amides | | | |
| j. Aspartic acid | Asp | D (asperDic acid) | β-carboxyl |
| k. Asparagine | Asn | N (asparagiNe) | Amide |
| l. Glutamic acid | Glu | E (glutEmic acid) | γ-carboxyl |
| m. Glutamine | Gln | Q (Qtamine) | Amide |
| E. Basic amino acids | | | |
| n. Lysine | Lys | K (letter close to L) | ε-amino |
| o. Arginine (most basic AA) | Arg | R (aRginine) | Guanidinium |
| p. Histidine | His | H | Imidazole |

*Contd...*

*Contd...*

| *Name* | *Symbol* | | *Special group present* |
|---|---|---|---|
| F. Aromatic amino acids | | | |
| q. Phenylalanine | Phe | F (Fenylalanine) | Benzene or phenyl |
| r. Tyrosine | Tyr | Y | Phenol |
| s. Tryptophan | Trp | W (tWiptophan) | Indole |
| G. Imino acid (heterocyclic acid) | | | |
| t. Proline | Pro | P | Pyrrolidine |

**2. Define translation. Describe the steps of translation. Name four inhibitors and their action.**

Refer Question No. 2 June 2005 (RS2).

## SHORT ESSAYS

**3. What is an allosteric enzyme? Describe with two examples.**

Refer Question No. 5 Dec. 2011 (RS2).

**4. Discuss the Embden-Meyerhof pathway that occurs in RBC. Add a note on its energetics.**

- Glycolysis is conversion of glucose into pyruvate or lactate
- Also called Embden-Meyerhof pathway (EM pathway/EMP)
- First pathway in series of glucose metabolism
- It is unique in sense that it can operate under both aerobic and anaerobic conditions.

### Types

| | *Aerobic glycolysis* | *Anerobic glycolysis* |
|---|---|---|
| Tissue site | • All mammalian cells (except RBCs) | • Erythrocytes |
| Intracellular site | • Cytoplasm | • Cytoplasm and mitochondria |
| Substrate | • Glucose | • Glucose |
| Product | • Pyruvate (2 molecules) | • Lactate (2 molecules) |
| ATPs generated | • 7 ATPs | • 2 ATPs |

### Pathway

| *Phase I (preparative phase)* | *Phase II (energy generating phase)* |
|---|---|
| • First 5 steps of glycolysis prepares glucose by phosphorylating it using 2 ATP molecules | • Next 5 steps yield 10 or 4 ATPs (depending upon aerobic or anerobic glycolysis) |

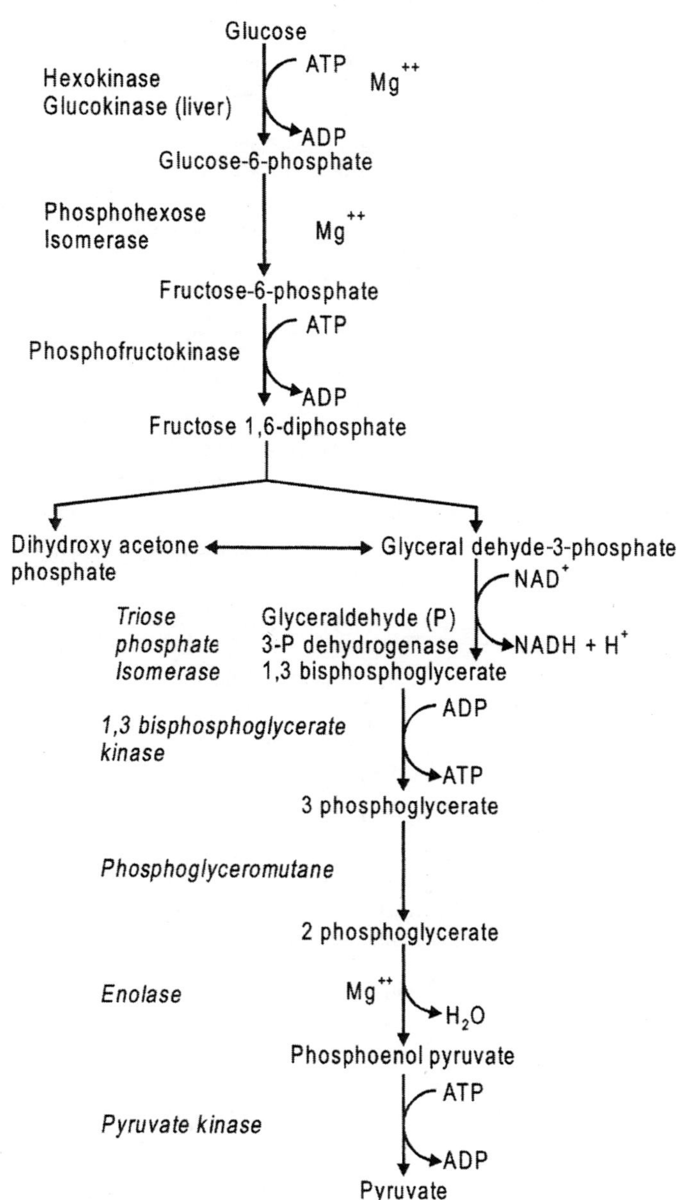


**Fig. 1:** Glycolysis

## Energetics (Per Glucose Molecule)

| *Step* | *Enzyme* | *Type* | *No. of ATP* | |
|---|---|---|---|---|
| | | | *Aerobic glycolysis* | *Anerobic glycolysis* |
| Glucose → Glucose-6-phosphate | Hexokinase/glucokinase | ATP utilized | – 1 | – 1 |
| Fructose-6-phosphate → Fructose 1,6 bisphosphate | Phosphofructokinase-1 | ATP utilized | –1 | – 1 |
| Glyceraldehyde-3-phosphate → 1,3 bisphosphate | Glyceraldehyde 3-phosphate dehydrogenase | Oxidative phosphorylation | + 2.5 × 2 = + 5 | — |
| 1,3 bisphosphoglycerate → 3 phosphoglycerate | 1,3 biphosphoglycerate kinase | Substrate level phosphorylation | + 1 x 2 = + 2 | + 1 × 2 = + 2 |
| Phosphoenol pyruvate → Pyruvate | Pyruvate kinase | Substrate level phosphorylation | + 1 x 2 = + 2 | + 1 × 2 = + 2 |
| | | | 9 –2 = 7 ATPs | 4 – 2 = 2 ATPs |

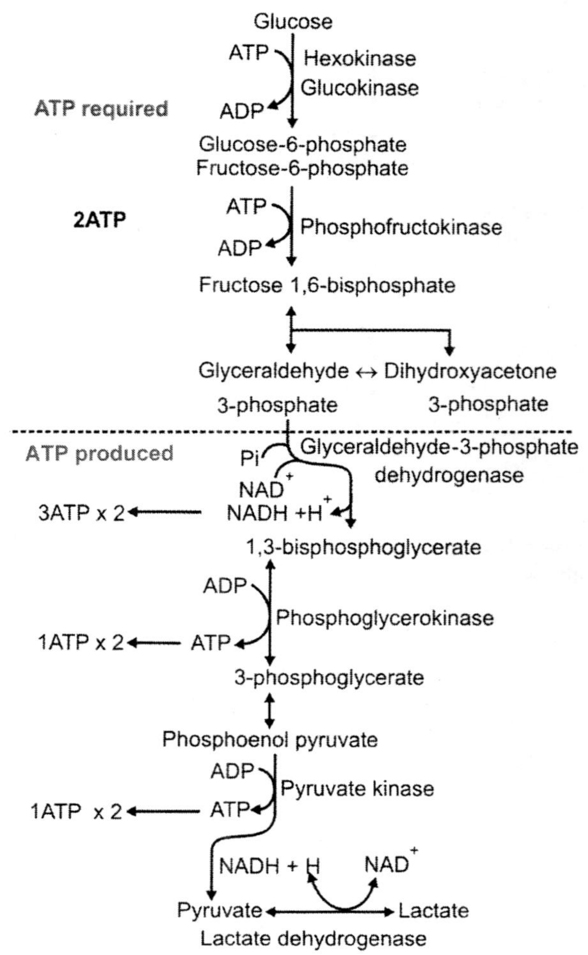


**Fig. 2:** Glycolysis—energetics



## Regulation

| *Key enzymes* | *Type of regulation* | *Inhibitor* | *Activator* |
|---|---|---|---|
| • Phosphofructokinase-1 (Committed step) | Allosteric regulation | ATP, citrate | Fructose 2,6 bisphosphate, AMP |
| • Hexokinase | Feedback regulation | Glucose-6-phosphate | Insulin |
| • Glucokinase | Induction | — | Glucose, insulin |
| • Pyruvate kinase | Allosteric regulation | ATP, NADH, alanine | Fructose 1,6 bisphosphate |
| | Covalent modification | Glucagon (by phosphorylation) | Insulin (by dephosphorylation) |
| | Induction | — | Insulin |
| | Repression | Glucagon | — |

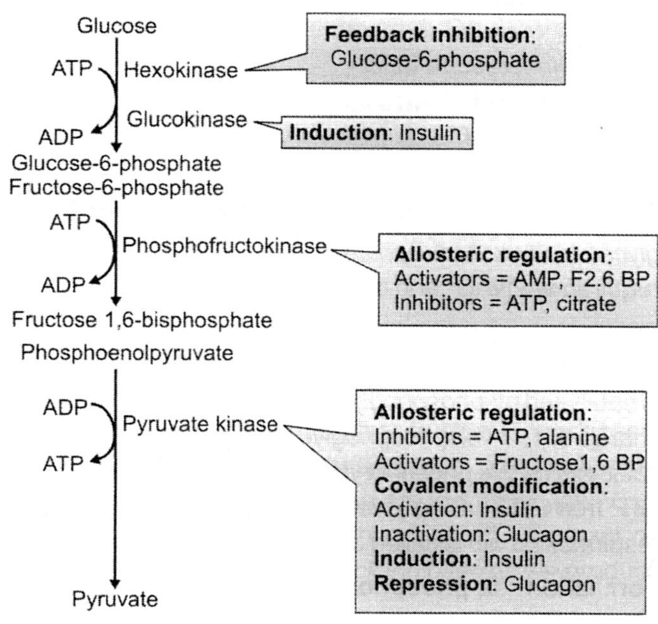


**Fig. 3:** Glycolysis—regulation

## Inhibitor

| *Inhibitor* | *Enzyme* | *Remarks* |
|---|---|---|
| • Iodoacetate | Glyceraldehyde-3-phosphate dehydrogenase | Modifies sulfhydryl group |
| • Arsenate | Glyceraldehyde-3-phosphate dehydrogenase | Competitive inhibition |
| • Flouride | Enolase | Combines with $Mg^{2+}$ required for enolase activation<br>Used as preservative for blood glucose estimation in clinical biochemistry |

## Link to Other Pathways

- Glycolysis provides intermediates to other metabolic pathways

| *Intermediate* | *Pathway* |
|---|---|
| • Glucose-6-phosphate | Pentose phosphate pathway, uronic acid pathway |
| • 1,3-bisphosphoglycerate | Rapaport Leubering pathway |
| • Dihydroxyacetone phosphate | Synthesis of triacylglycerol and phospholipids |
| • Pyruvate | Alanine synthesis |

## Significance

- Glycolysis is first metabolic pathway of glucose metabolism converting $C_6$ compound (glucose) into $C_3$ compound (pyruvate or lactate), however, it is does not cause complete breakdown of glucose
- Anerobic glycolysis is sole source of energy to erythrocytes
- It provides substrates for numerous other pathways like pentose phosphate pathway, uronic acid pathway, lipogenesis, etc.

## 5. What are lipoproteins? Name the lipoproteins and give their functions.

Refer Question No. 6 June 2005 (RS2).

**6. What is biotransformation? Discuss the different phases of biotransformation with an example.**

Refer Question No. 7 Dec. 2005 (RS2).

**7. Components of electron transport chain.**

Refer Question No. 5 June 2007 (RS2).

**8. How is bilirubin formed and excreted? Name the abnormalities associated with bilirubin metabolism.**

Refer Question No. 8 June 2007 (RS2).

**9. Describe the liver function tests based on synthetic and excretory role.**

Refer Question No. 11 Dec. 2008 (RS2).

**10. Write the Henderson-Hasselbach equation and its significance in bicarbonate buffer system.**

- Hasselbach equation is an equation that describes relationship of pH to concentration of acid and base in a buffer system
- It is equation expression of relation between pH, pKa, concentration of acid and conjugate base.

## Expression

$$pH = pKa + \log\frac{[base]}{[acid]} \text{ or } pH = pKa + \log\frac{[salt]}{[acid]}$$

## Derivation

- Dissociation of weak acid, $HA \rightarrow H^+ + A^-$
- Dissociation constant at equilibrium, $K = \frac{[H^+][A^-]}{[HA]}$
- Cross multiplication, $[H^+][A^-] = K[HA]$
- Dividing both sides by $A^-$ : $[H][A^-] = K[HA]$
- Negative logarithm of the equation: $pH = pKa + \frac{\log[A^-]}{[HA]}$ or $pH = pKa + \log\frac{[base]}{[acid]}$

## Significance (Application)

- To calculate pH of blood
- Determine pH of unknown buffer solution
- Determining acid-base status of an individual during disorders of acid-base balance.

## Significance in Bicarbonate Buffer

- Bicarbonate buffer is most important plasma buffer
- It is constituted by:

| *Components* | *Normal concentration* |
|---|---|
| Bicarbonate ($HCO_3^-$) | 24 mmol/L |
| Carbonic acid ($H_2CO_3$) = $pCO_2$ x Sol. constant of $CO_2$ | 1.2 mmol/L = 40 mm Hg × 0.03 |
| pKa of bicarbonate buffer | 6.1 |
| pH of plasma | 7.4 |

- Substituting these in Henderson-Hasselbach equation we have:

$$pH = pKa + \log\frac{[base]}{[acid]}$$

$$7.4 = 6.1 + \log\frac{24}{1.2}$$

$= 6.1 + \log 20$
$= 6.1 + 1.3$
$7.4 = 7.4$

- Thus ratio of $HCO_3^-$ to $H_2CO_3$ at normal plasma pH of 7.4 is 20 under normal healthy condition indicating high alkali reserve in plasma which is essential for maintaining acid-base balance (because body produces acids predominantly).

**For bicarbonate buffer**

Refer Question No. 2 June 2012 (RS2).

## 11. Discuss the biochemical changes during starvation.

- Starvation is a metabolic stress which imposes certain metabolic compulsion on organism and metabolism is reorganized to meet new demands of starvation.

### Causes

- Food scarcity
- Desire for rapid weight loss
- Certain clinical condition.

### Normal Body Metabolism

- Glucose is fuel of choice for brain and muscle but unfortunately body's carbohydrate reserve is very low
- Lipids are predominant reserve of energy in body stored as triacylglycerol in adipose tissues
- Proteins are basically structural constituents but about 1/3 of proteins reserve can be used in starvation for energy needs.

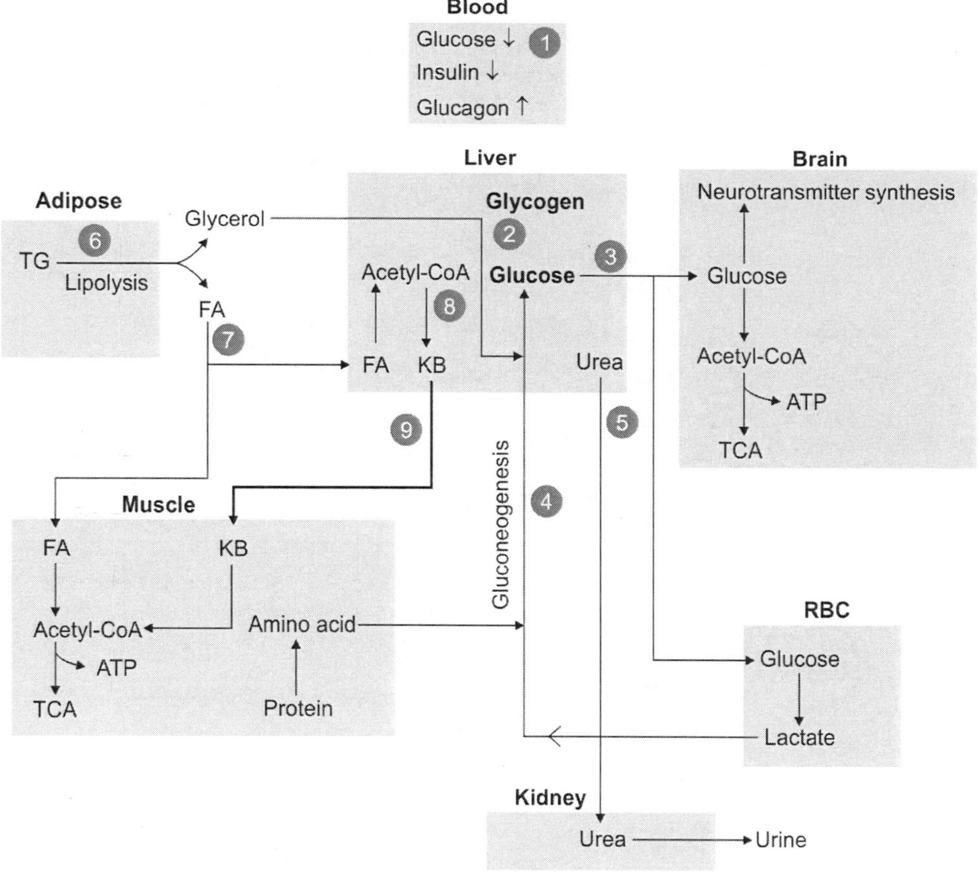


**Fig. 4:** Metabolic changes in short-term starvation

## Biochemical Changes During Starvation (in Reference to Vital Organs)

| | *Liver* | *Adipose tissues* | *Skeletal muscles* | *Brain* |
|---|---|---|---|---|
| Carbohydrate metabolism | Acts a blood glucose buffering organ increasing blood glucose level by:<br>• Increased gluconeogenesis<br>• Elevated glycogenolysis | Reduced uptake and metabolism of glucose | Greatly reduced uptake and metabolism of glucose | Glucose is exclusive source of energy for 2 weeks of starvation courtesy gluconeogenesis from glycerol and amino acids |
| Lipid metabolism | Fatty acid oxidation is increased with an elevated synthesis of ketone bodies from unused acetyl CoA d' to inability of TCA cycle to cope up with excess production of acetyl CoA<br>Ketone bodies slowly and effectively become source of energy for peripheral tissue and brain also adopts itself for ketone body utilization | Increased lipolysis which serves two purposes<br>• Released free fatty acids serve as fuel source for tissues except brain<br>• Glycerol is used as precursor for gluconeogenesis in liver<br>Synthesis of fatty acids and triacylglycerol is totally stopped | Muscles start utilizing free fatty acids and ketone bodies for its energy requirement which after 3 weeks becomes exclusively by free fatty acids and thus there is rise in blood ketone bodies level | Slowly adopts itself to utilize ketone bodies for energy needs beyond 3 weeks |
| Protein metabolism | — | — | Muscle proteins are catabolized to liberate amino acids which are utilized for gluconeogenesis by liver but on prolonged starvation, this protein breakdown is reduced | — |
| Mineral metabolism | • Loss of intracellular $K^+$ thus reducing total body $K^+$<br>• $Na^+$ level maintained in normal range though total mineral content reduced by 10% | | | |
| Water metabolism | • Reduced ECF during first few days d' to stoppage of water intake and continued obligatory losses<br>• ICF volume also falls on prolonged starvation<br>• ECF shows relative expansion d' to shrinkage of cell mass and fluid accumulation<br>• Increase in metabolic water and reduction in GFR reduces need of water intake<br>• Relative expansion of ECF compartment and decreased serum albumin level leads to starvation edema | | | |

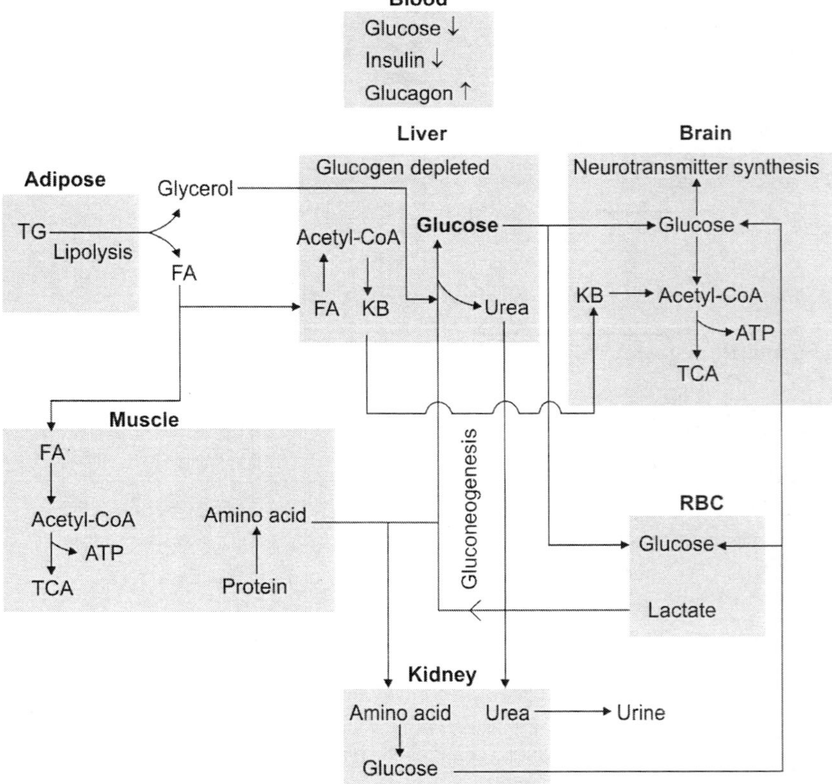


**Fig. 5:** Metabolic changes in long-term starvation

## Clinical Significance

- Biochemical changes occurring during starvation maintain adequate supply of energy sources to various tissues to meet energy demands.

## 12. What are nucleotides? What are the sources of C and N atoms of purine nucleotide? Mention the metabolic disorders associated with purine metabolism.

- Nucleotides are composed of a nitrogenous base, a pentose sugar and a phosphate
- Nucleic acids are polymers of nucleotides.

**Fore sources of C and N atoms**

Refer Question No. 2 June 2013 (RS2).

**Fore metabolic disorders**

Refer Question No. 2 June 2007 (RS2).

## SHORT ANSWERS

## 13. Pyruvate dehydrogenase complex.

Refer Question No. 1 June 2006 (RS2).

## 14. GABA, PUFA and SAM and their importance.

| *GABA (Gamma amino butyric acid)* | *PUFA (Poly unsaturated fatty acid)* | *SAM (S-adenosyl methionine)* |
|---|---|---|
| • Inhibitory neurotransmitter | • Structural components of biological membranes<br>• Participate in cholesterol transport and utilization<br>• Prevent fat accumulation in liver<br>• Essential for prostaglandin synthesis<br>• Maintain proper growth and reproduction | • Methyl group donor to synthesize<br>– Creatine<br>– Epinephrine<br>– Choline<br>– Melatonin<br>• Synthesis of polyamines |

## 15. Importance of iodine.

Refer Question No. 11 June 2011 (RS2).

## 16. FIGLU.

- Formamino glutamic acid (FIGLU) is an intermediate product formed during catabolism of histidine.

## Formation

- From imidazole propionic acid by its hydrolysis by imidazolone propionate acid hydrolase.

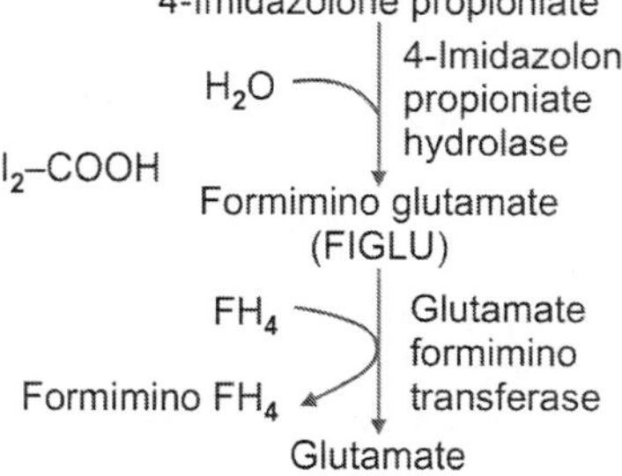


**Fig. 6:** Synthesis and fate of FIGLU

## Fate

- Converted to glutamate and forminino tetrahydrofolate by action of glutamate: Formimino transferase.

## Biomedical Importance

a. Diagnosis of folic acid deficiency (megaloblastic anemia)
   - By detection of FIGLU in urine (sensitive test)—index of folic acid deficiency
   - Folic acid is needed for conversion of FIGLU to glutamate
   - In folic acid deficiency, defect in conversion of FIGLU to formimino $FH_4$ results in increased excretion of FIGLU in urine
   - Best tested by giving 20 g of a loading dose of histidine (histidine load test)
   - Normally <30 mg of FIGLU is excreted per day; value is increased in folate deficiency.

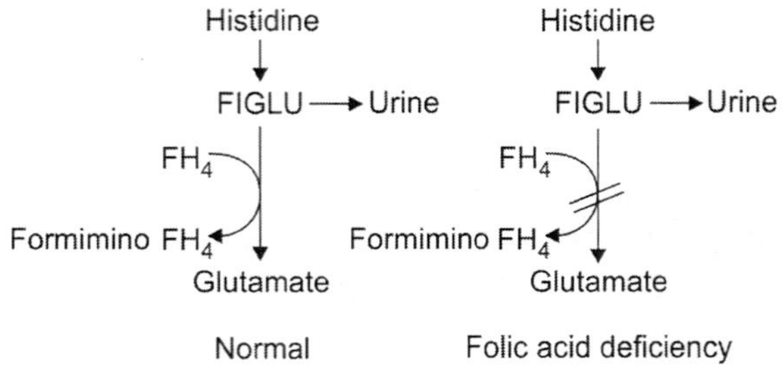

Histidine → FIGLU → Urine; FIGLU → Glutamate ($FH_4$ → Formimino $FH_4$) — Normal

Histidine → FIGLU → Urine; FIGLU ⇸ Glutamate ($FH_4$ → Formimino $FH_4$ blocked) — Folic acid deficiency

**Fig. 7:** FIGLU excretion test

b. One carbon metabolism
   - By contributing to N5-formimino THFA.

## 17. Epimerism and anomerism.

- Epimerism and anomerism are steroisomerism properties of carbohydrates.

| *Epimerization* | *Anomerism* |
|---|---|
| • Epimerization is stereoisomerism in respect of groups of a single asymmetric carbon of a molecule containing more than one asymmetric carbon<br>• Epimers are sugars which differ from each other only in their configuration with regard to a single carbon atom (except anomeric carbon)<br>**Examples**<br>• D-galactose ($C_4$ epimer) and D-mannose ($C_2$ epimer) are epimers of D-glucose<br>• Ribose and xylose are epimers differing in configuration of groups around C-3 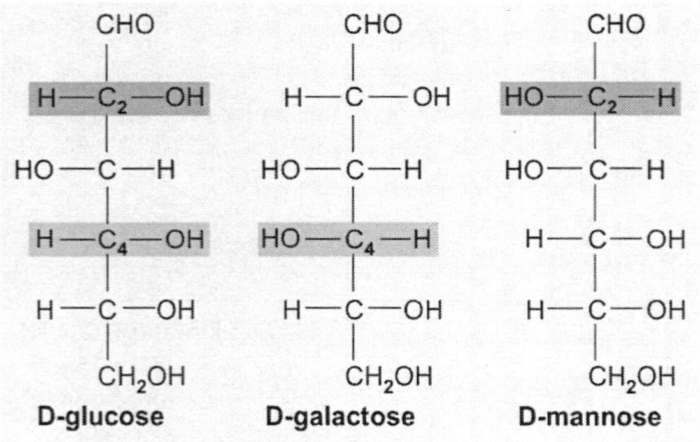<br>D-glucose, D-galactose, D-mannose<br>**Fig. 8A:** Epimerization<br>**Significance**<br>• Interconversion of epimers is catalyzed by epimerases<br>• Example: Phosphopentose epimerase catalyzes conversion of ribulose 5 phosphate and xyluose 5 phosphate | • Anomerism is stereoisomerism in respect 1st carbon atom of a molecule (anomeric carbon)<br>• Anomers are sugars which differ from each other only in their configuration with regard to a anomeric carbon atom<br>**Examples**<br>• α and β cyclic forms of D-glucose<br>– In α - D – glucose, anomeric OH group is to right farthest from CH2OH group and its specific rotation is + 112.2°<br>– In β - D – glucose, anomeric OH group is near to $CH_2OH$ group on to left and its specific rotation of +18.7° 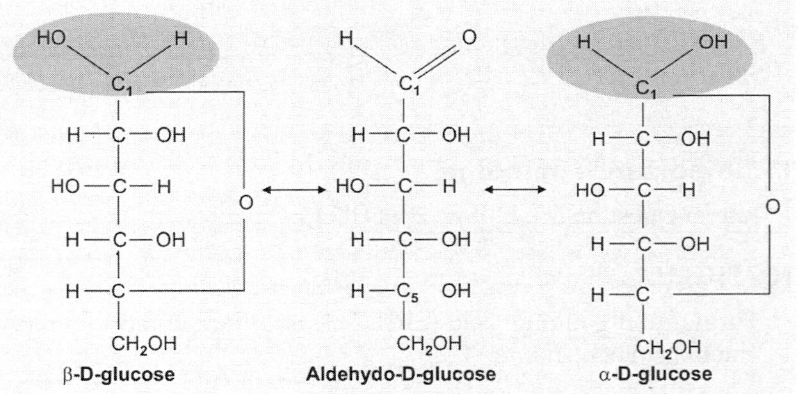<br>β-D-glucose ⟷ Aldehydo-D-glucose ⟷ α-D-glucose<br>**Fig. 8B:** Anomerism<br>**Significance**<br>• Anomerism is responsible for mutarotation of glucose solution |

## 18. Monoclonal antibodies.

- Monoclonal antibodies (McAb) are antibodies produced by a single antibody forming cell or clone directed against a single antigen or antigenic determinant
- Example: Antibodies produced in multiple myeloma.

### Features

- Homogenous and monoclonal
- Produced when a clone of lymphocyte or plasma cell undergoes selective proliferation.

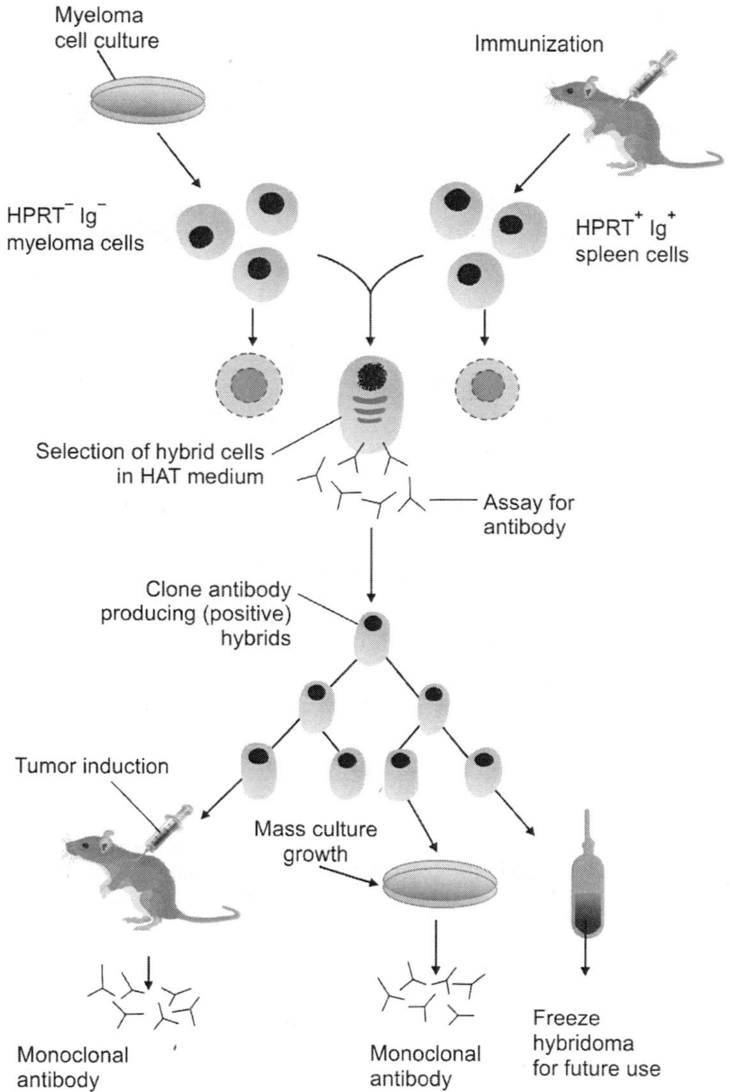


**Fig. 9:** Monoclonal antibodies—production



## Principle

- In laboratory, monoclonal antibodies can be produced from formation of a hybrid cell line (hybridoma) by fusion of a mouse myeloma cell within antibody producing lymphocyte from spleen or lymph node of same inbred stain of mouse
- Such hybrid cells can produce virtually unlimited quantities of monoclonal antibody of any required specificity indefinitely in cell culture conditions.

## Applications

a. Diagnostic use
   - Commercial diagnostic kits for identification of bacterial, viral and other antigens.

b. Test for vaccines
   - Identification and purification of microbial products both for vaccine and for industrial use.

c. Therapeutic use
   - Large and unlimited amount of pure antibody of defined class and subclasses can be prepared for therapeutic purposes.

d. Future use
   - Hybridomas can be frozen and stored for prolonged period, to be revived subsequently if needed.

## 19. PCR and its application.

Refer Question No. 11 June 2006 (RS2).

## 20. Southern blot techniques.

- Southern blotting technique is a technique used for the detection of specific sequences present in DNA
- Blotting refers to process of immobilization of sample nucleic acid on solid support.

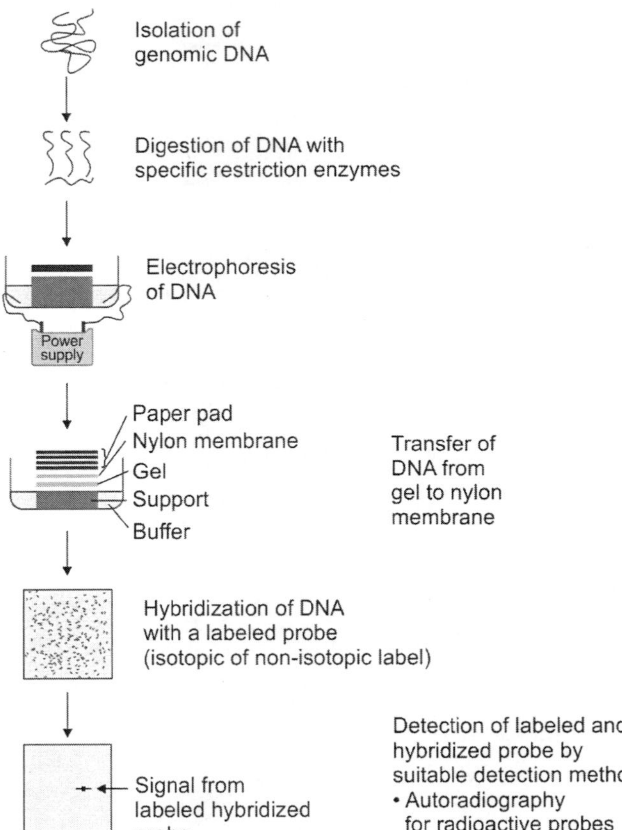


**Fig. 10:** Southern blot technique

### Procedure

a. Isolation of DNA
b. Digestion of DNA with restriction endonuclease
c. Separation of DNA based on size by agarose gel electrophoresis
   - DNA being negatively charged, migrates towards anode
   - Smaller DNA fragments move faster
   - Separated DNA are denatured by exposure to mild alkali
d. Transfer of DNA from the gel to nylon membrane through capillary diffusion or electrophoretic transfer
   - Results in an exact replica of pattern of DNA fragments on gel
e. Fixing of DNA to support by baking (80°C) or using ultraviolet light
f. Hybridization of DNA probe with separated DNA
g. Detection of hybridized DNA with radioisotope or nonisotopic methods.

### Application

- Detection of genes in genome (gene analysis)
- Confirmation of DNA cloning results
- Detection of mutations
- Detect minute quantities of DNA (in forensic medicine)
- Diagnosis of infectious diseases
- Restriction fragment length polymorphism
- DNA finger printing
- To confirm product in polymerase chain reaction.

## 21. Gilbert's syndrome.

- Gilbert's syndrome is an autosomal dominant disorder of bilirubin metabolism characterized by chronic unconjugated hyperbilirubinemia (Bilirubin level <3 mg/dL) and jaundice.

| *Pathology* | *Features* | *Biochemical findings* |
|---|---|---|
| • Defect in uptake of bilirubin by liver cells<br>• Impairment in conjugation due to reduced activity of UDP-glucuronyltransferase<br>• Decreased hepatic clearance of bilirubin | • Seen mostly in males aged 18–25 years<br>• Detected suddenly during examination as mild icterus<br>• Patient usually asymptomatic but can complaints of fatigue, weakness and abdominal pain | • Plasma bilirubin levels—slightly increased but <3 mg/dL (unconjugated fraction) |

## 22. Acute intermittent porphyria.

Refer Question No. 9 June 2015 (RS2).

# MBBS PHASE I EXAMINATION
## DECEMBER 2014
## (Revised Scheme 2 & 3)

### LONG ESSAYS

**1. Describe the mechanisms of blood glucose regulation. What are the causes of hyperglycemia and hypoglycemia?**

Refer Question No. 1 Dec. 2009 (RS2).

**2. Define replication. Describe in detail the process of replication in eukaryotes.**

Refer Question No. 2 June 2010 (RS2).

### SHORT ESSAYS

**3. What are the reactions of β-oxidation of palmitic acid? Give its energetics.**

Refer Question No. 1 Dec. 2008 (RS2).

**4. What is the difference between oxidative and substrate level phosphorylation? Give two examples of substrate level phosphorylation.**

| *Points of comparison* | *Oxidative phosphorylation* | *Substrate level phoshorylation* |
|---|---|---|
| Subcellular site | Mitochondria | Cytosol |
| Mechanism | Electron transferred from oxidation of NADH + $H^+$ and $FADH_2$ to $O_2$ | Direct transfer of phosphate from substrate to ADP |
| Oxygen requirement | Required (done aerobically) | None (done anaerobically) |
| Proton gradient | Required | Not required |
| Enzymes required | ATP synthase | Phosphorylase |

#### Substrate Level Phosphorylation

- Substrate level phosphorylation is coupling of exergenic cleavage of a high energy metabolic intermediate with endergenic phosphorylation of ADP/GDP and a direct utilization of bond energy of metabolic intermediate in synthesizing high energy bond of ATP/GTP
- In other words synthesis of ATP (or GTP) utilizing metabolic intermediates is called substrate level phosphorylation
- Does not require mitochondrial electron transport chain or molecular $O_2$.

#### Mechanism

- Synthesis of ATP from ADP is coupled with hydrolysis of certain high energy compounds generating tremendous free energy which is utilized to bind phosphate to ADP without involvement of electron transport chain and molecular $O_2$.

*Examples*

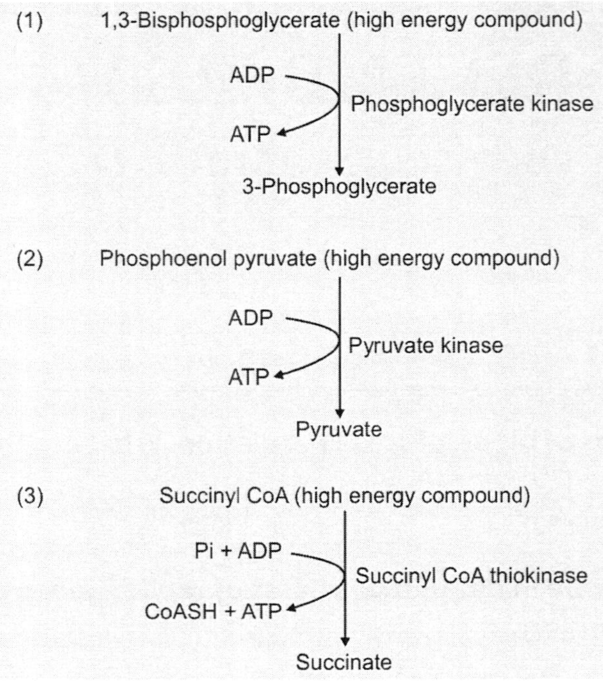




## Significance

- Substrate level phosphorylation occurring during anerobic glycolysis is sole source of energy for erythrocytes (as they lack mitochondria required for oxidative phosphorylation) and vigorously contracting muscles
- In erythrocytes, ATP production by substrate phosphorylation from 1,3-BPG is bypassed by taking Rapoport Lubering pathway.

## 5. Name three enzymes commonly estimated in myocardial infarction. Give its importance and limitations.

- Myocardial infarction (MI) is a form of tissue trauma (oxygen deprivation due to deficient blood supply to heart muscles)
- This anoxic trauma causes necrosis of heart muscles causing release of certain enzymes and proteins into circulation
- Estimation of these enzymes helps to diagnose MI and assess its prognosis.

## Enzyme Profile in Myocardial Infarction

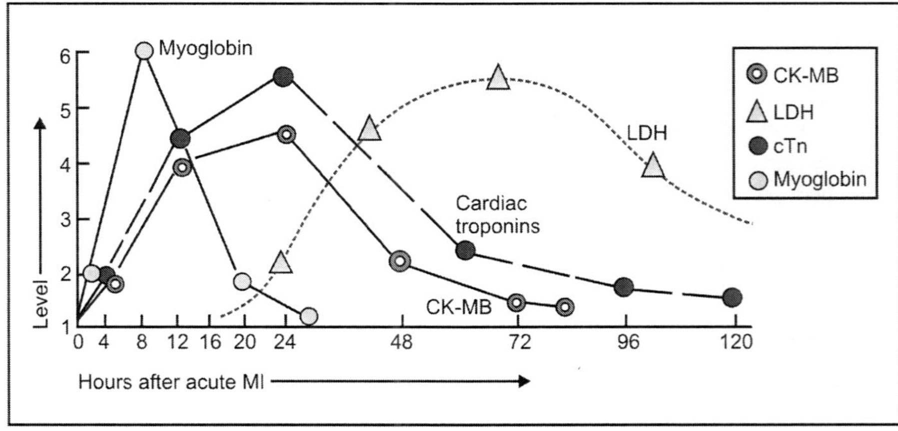


**Fig. 1:** Enzyme profile in myocardial infarction

| | *Creatinine phosphokinase (CK)* | *Lactic dehydrogenase (LDH)* | *Cardiac-specific troponins (cTn)* | *Myoglobin* |
|---|---|---|---|---|
| Feature | Total CK level estimation is not specific but elevation of its CK–MB isoenzymes (myocardium predominant) is specific for myocardial damage<br>*Forms*<br>• CK-MB1: Extracardiac form<br>• CK-MB2: Cardiac form | Total LDH level estimation lacks specificity but estimation of LDH isoenzyme is specific for diagnosis of MI<br>*Forms*<br>• LDH1<br>• LDH2 | Contractile muscle proteins present in human cardiac muscles<br>*Forms*<br>• Cardiac troponin T (cTnT)<br>• Cardiac troponin I (cTnI) | Lacks cardiac specificity and excreted rapidly in urine |
| Significance | CK-MB2: CK-MB1 ratio >1.5 is highly sensitive for diagnosis of acute MI after 4–6 hours of onset of MI and disappears from blood by 48 hours | LDH1: LDH2 ratio >1 is helps in diagnosing MI<br>LDH levels begin to rise after 24 hours and reaches peak in 3–6 days and returns to normal in 2 weeks | Not usually found in blood but their level rise after MI around same time as CK-MB<br>Level remains higher for longer duration, i.e. cTnI for 7–10 days and cTnT for 10–14 days | First cardiac maker to elevate and returns to normal within 24 hours after an attack of MI |

## Significance

- Measurement of levels of these enzymes and proteins help in diagnosing and planning management of a MI patient.

## 6. Define fatty liver. What are the causes of fatty liver? Name the lipotropic factors.

Refer Question No. 6 Dec. 2006 (RS2).

## 7. Describe the digestion and absorption of proteins.

- Proteins in diet are derived from animal or vegetable sources
  - Animal sources: Milk and its products, meat, fish, liver and eggs
  - Vegetable sources: Cereals, pulses, peas, beans and nuts
- All the dietary proteins are denatured while cooking and therefore more easily digested and absorbed.

## Digestion of Proteins

A. Digestion in mouth
   - Proteins are not digested in mouth due to absence of a proteolytic enzyme.

B. Digestion in stomach
   - Gastric juice contains proteolytic enzymes and actual digestion of proteins begins in the stomach.

| *Gastric proteolytic enzymes* | *Action* |
|---|---|
| *Pepsin*<br>• An acid-stable endopeptidase optimally active at pH of 2<br>• Released as pepsinogen which is activated by action of HCl to pepsin which further self-activates pepsinogen | • Acts on peptide bonds to produce proteoses and peptones<br>• Specificity—tryptophan, tyrosine, phenylalanine, glutamate, aspartate |
| *Renin*<br>• Protease found only in infancy and childhood | • Converts casein (a milk protein) to calcium paracaseinate → curdling of milk<br>Casein —Renin→ Paracasein —Spontaneous, $Ca^{++}$→ Calcium paracaseinate<br>(Casein → Proteoses) |
| Gastriscin and gelatinase | |
| *HCl*<br>• An acid present in gastric juice | • Denatures many native proteins to acid metaproteins by clearing electrostatic and hydrogen bonds and enhances action of pepsin on unfolded peptide chain<br>• Lowers gastric pH causing activation of pepsinogen and maintains it for optimum action of pepsin on protein digestion |

C. Digestion in duodenum
– Digested and undigested proteins from stomach are subjected to proteolytic enzymes of pancreatic juice.

| *Pancreatic proteolytic enzymes* | *Action* |
|---|---|
| *Trypsin*<br>• An endopeptidase active at high pH (8–9)<br>• Released as trypsinogen which is activated by enteropeptidase to trypsin which further self-activates trypsinogen | Acts on peptide bonds formed by arginine and lysine |
| *Chymotrypsin*<br>• An endopeptidase<br>• Released as chymotrypsinogen which is activated by trypsin | Acts on peptide bonds formed by tyrosine, tryptophan, phenylalanine, leucine and methionine |
| *Elastase*<br>• An endopeptidase<br>• Released as proelastase which is activated by trypsin | Acts on peptide bonds formed by alanine, glycine and serine |
| *Carboxypeptidase*<br>• An exopeptidase requiring Zn for its action (metalloenzyme)<br>• Released as procarboxypeptidase which is activated by trypsin<br>• 2 types—carboxypeptidase A and carboxypeptidase B | Acts on peptide bond from carboxyterminal end<br>Specificity<br>• Carboxypeptidase A: Alanine, isoleucine, leucine and valine<br>• Carboxypeptidase B: Arginine and lysine |
| Collagenase | Acts on proteins present in collagen |

- Thus protein digestion by pancreatic juice in the duodenum can be summarised as:

| Proteins | |
|---|---|
| ↓ | Trypsin/chymotrypsin/elastase |
| Proteoses and peptones | |
| ↓ | Trypsin/chymotrypsin/elastase |
| Amino acids and polypeptides | |
| ↓ | Carboxypeptidase A and B |
| Amino acids and oligopeptides | |

D. Digestion in small intestine
– Proteins are further digested by proteases present in succus entericus

| *Intestinal proteolytic enzymes* | *Action* |
|---|---|
| *Aminopeptidase*<br>• Nonspecific exopeptidase | Repeatedly cleaves N-terminal amino acids one by one to produce free amino acids and smaller peptides |
| Tri- and dipeptidases | Act on tripeptides and dipeptides respectively |

– The protein digestion in the small intestine by the succus entericus is summarised as:

Oligopeptides —(Aminopeptidase)→ Tri-, di-peptides and amino acids

Tripeptides —(Tripeptidase)→ Dipeptides and amino acids

Dipeptides —(Dipeptidase)→ Amino acids

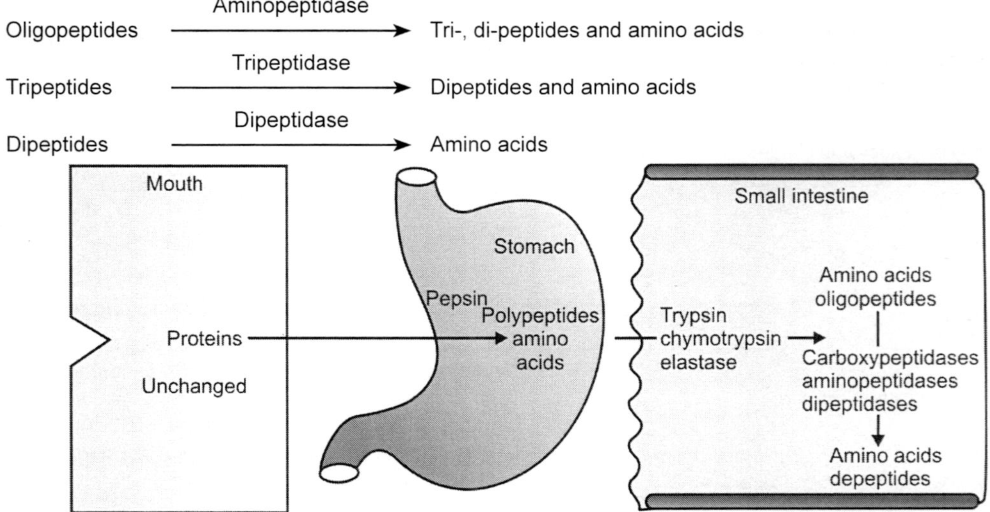


**Fig. 2:** Digestion of proteins

Revised Scheme 2 & 3

## Absorption of Proteins

- End products of protein digestion are peptides, di- and tripeptides and amino acids.

*Site of Absorption*

- Upper small intestine (duodenum and proximal jejunum).

A. Peptides
   - Only very small amounts are absorbed by endocytosis (pinocytosis)
   - Characterized by internalization of small vesicles of plasma membrane containing oligopeptides or small molecular weight proteins

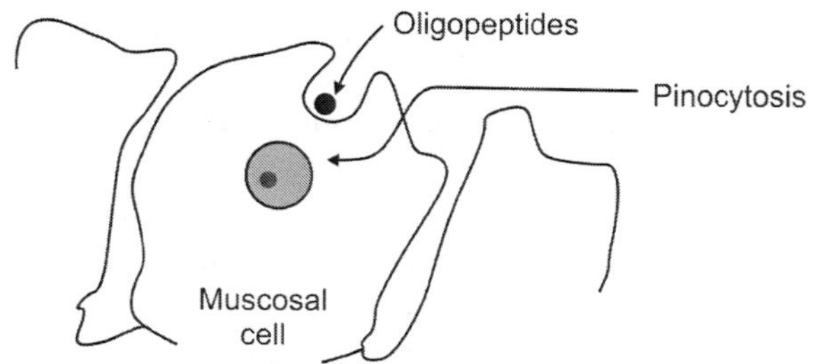

**Fig. 3:** Absorption oligopeptides

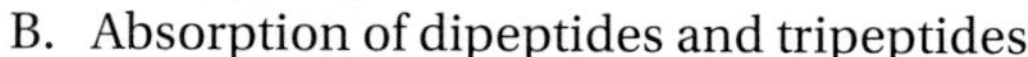

B. Absorption of dipeptides and tripeptides
   - Absorbed by secondary active transport (membrane transport system)
   - Absorbed peptides are hydrolyzed to free amino acids in musosal cell cytosol by dipeptidases and tripeptidases releasing free amino acids which reach liver through the portal circulation

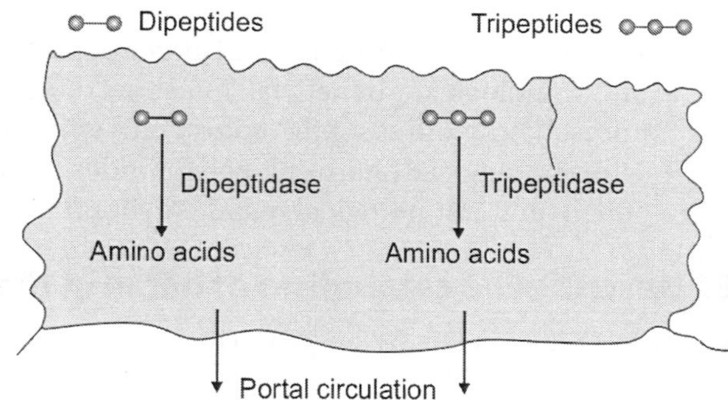

**Fig. 4:** Absorption of dipeptides and tripeptides

C. Absorption of amino acids
   - Transport systems for amino acids are stereospecific for L-amino acids.

*Transport systems for amino acids*

a. Sodium dependent secondary active transport
   - Amino acid and $Na^+$ combines with a common carrier protein located on mucosal surface to form a "carrier-amino acid-$Na^+$ complex"
   - This complex passes into cytoplasmic surface where it dissociates to liberate free amino acid and $Na^+$
   - $Na^+$ is actively pumped out by ATP dependent sodium pump with help of ATPase
   - Amino acid then diffuses out of muscosal cell into portal blood and is transported to the liver.

   *Examples*

   i. Neutral amino acids (glycine, cystine, tryptophan, alanine)
   ii. Dibasic amino acids (arginine, ornithine and lysine)
      - However, cystine (neutral amino acid) also shares this transport mechanism
   iii. Dicarboxylic (acidic) amino acids (glutamate and aspartate)
   iv. Imino acids (proline and hydroxyproline)
      - Glycine (neutral amino acid) also shares this system

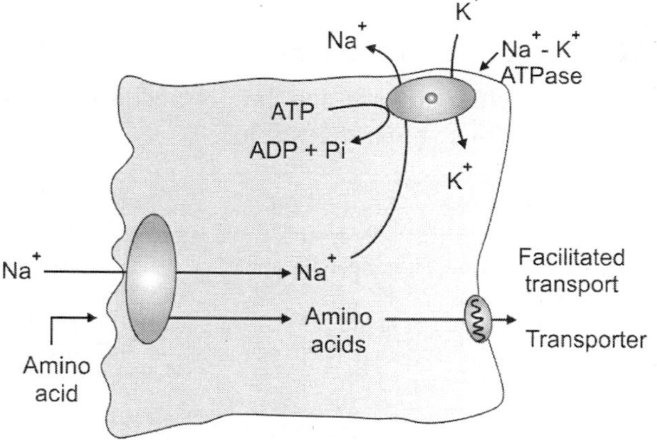

**Fig. 5:** Absorption of amino acids

b. Sodium independent facilitated transport system
   i. Neutral and hydrophobic amino acids (phenylalanine, leucine)
   ii. Basic amino acids (lysine and arginine)

c. γ-glutamyl cycle (Meister cycle)
   - Involved in transport of amino acids at small intestine and renal tubules
   - Requires glutathione (γ-glutamyl cysteinyl glycine)

   *Steps*

   - Glutathione (γ-glutamyl eysteinyl glycine) reacts with amino acid to form γ-glutamyl amino acid in reaction catalyzed by γ-glutamyl transferase
   - This is then translocated into the cell

- In the cytosol, amino acid is released and γ-glutamyl residue is converted to 5-oxyproline
- 5-oxyproline is converted to glutamate in an ATP dependent reaction
- Glutamate is then utilized in reaction forming glutathione
- Cysteinylglycine is hydrolyzed to form cysteine and glycine
- γ-glutamyl cysteine is formed in an ATP dependent reaction into which glycine is incorporated to form glutathione (γ-glutamyl cysteinylglycine)
- Thus the cycle repeats (γ-glutamyl cycle).

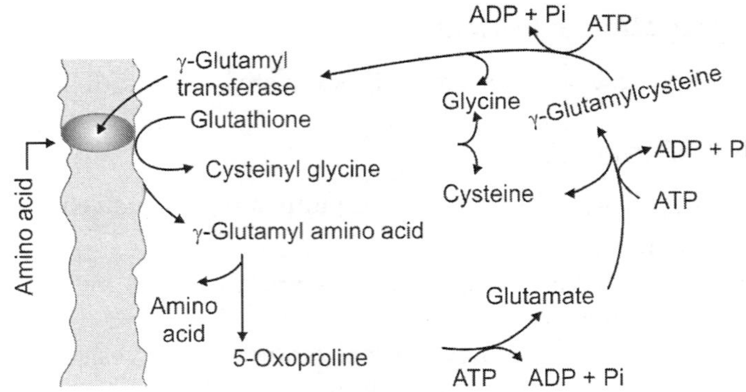


**Fig. 6:** Gamma-glutamyl cycle

## Significance

- Absorption of intact proteins and larger peptides are immunologically significant
  - Immunologically beneficial: Intestinal mucosal cells in neonates are capable of absorbing intact immunoglobulins present in mother's milk (colostrum) which offers protection against infection in newborn
  - Immunologically harmful: Polypeptides derived from gluten (a form of protein present in wheat) if absorbed, may elicit an immunological response (nontropical sprue).

## 8. Describe the catabolism of heme in the body adding a note on clinical significance.

Refer Question No. 2 Dec. 2013 (RS2).

## 9. List the requirements, steps of polymerase chain reaction.

Refer Question No. 11 June 2006 (RS2).

## 10. What is meant by dietary fiber? List the role of dietary fibers.

- Dietary fiber are non-starch polysaccharides which are inert components of carbohydrates with little nutritive value
- Dietary fibers are indigestible.

| *Sources* | *Examples* | *Recommended intake* |
|---|---|---|
| • Vegetables especially green leafy vegetables<br>• Fibrous fruits like pineapple, apple<br>• Brans<br>• Whole grains as lining<br>• Cereals and pulses (>10 g/100 g) | • Cellulose—polymer of glucose<br>• Hemicelluloses—pentoses, hexoses and uronic acid<br>• Lignin—aromatic alcohols<br>• Pectins—partially esterified rhamnogalacturonan | • Daily intake of 40 g is desirable<br>• Indian diet provides about 50–100 g of fiber per day |

## Activities along Gastrointestinal Tract

| *Site* | *Action* |
|---|---|
| Mouth | Stimulates saliva secretion |
| Stomach | Delays gastric emptying |
| Small intestine | Delays absorption |
| Large intestine | Traps water, binds cations |
| Stool | Soften, enlarges, prevents straining |

## Adverse Effects

- Mineral deficiency due to binding of some minerals preventing their proper absorption.

## Role of Dietary Fibers

| *Functions* | *Beneficial effects* |
|---|---|
| • Maintain normal motility of GIT<br>• Adsorption of organic molecules like bile acids, neutral sterols, carcinogens and toxic compounds and facilitating its excretion<br>• Retains water during passage of foods along gut and thereby producing larger, softer stool<br>• Forms bulk of stool, induces peristalasis and reduces tendency of constipation (Roughage action)<br>• Reduces blood glucose levels (delays starch hydrolysis and glucose absorption and improves glucose utilization and insulin sensitivity in target tissues)<br>• Reduces blood cholesterol levels (by binding bile acids and binding dietary cholesterol thus preventing its absorption)<br>• Binds certain minerals and interfere with their absorption | • By reducing intestinal transit time of stool, it reduces toxicity<br>• Inhibits fecal mutagen synthesis<br>• Reduces incidence of colonic polyps, invasive colon cancer<br>• Reduces incidence of stomach, breast and prostate cancer<br>• Reduces incidence of coronary heart diseases<br>• Used in management of irritable bowel syndrome and recurrent diverticulitis<br>• Beneficial in diabetes (slows gastric emptying and attenuate postprandial rise in blood glucose with consequent reduction in insulin secretion)<br>• Reduces body weight since it provides a feeling of fullness without consumption of excess calories |

## 11. What are the causes of respiratory acidosis? List the primary abnormalities of respiratory acidosis.

- Respiratory acidosis is consequent fall in pH after fall in $HCO_3^-/H_2CO_3^-$ ratio by $CO_2$ excess
- Also called primary carbonic acid excess
- Can be either acute (from bronchopneumonia or status asthmaticus) or chronic (from COPD).

$$\frac{HCO_3}{\uparrow H_2CO_3} = pH\downarrow$$

### Causes

| *Obstruction to respiration* | *Depression of respiratory centers* |
|---|---|
| • Bronchopneumonia or lobar pneumonia<br>• Emphysema<br>• Asthma<br>• Respiratory paralysis | • Morphine or barbiturate overdose<br>• Alcohol ingestion |

### Clinical Features

- Decreased respiratory rate, hypotension and coma
- Peripheral vasodilation, tachycardia and tremors (d' to hypercapnia).

### Laboratory Findings (Primary Abnormalities)

| *Blood* | | | *Urine* |
|---|---|---|---|
| | *Acute* | *Chronic* | pH: Acidic<br>↑ excretion of $NH_4Cl$ and $NaH_2PO_4$<br>↑ titrable acidity |
| pH | ↓↓ | ↓ | |
| $pCO_2$ | ↑↑ | ↑ | |
| $HCO_3^-$ | N or ↑ | ↑↑ | |

### Compensatory Mechanism

| *Renal mechanism—primary* | *Respiratory mechanism—secondary* |
|---|---|
| ↑ $pCO_2$ → absorption of more HCO – from tubules → ↑ levels of $HCO_3^-$ and $H_2CO_3$ → restoration of $[HCO_3^-]/[H_2CO_3]$ | ↑ $pCO_2$ → respiratory stimulation → ↑ depth and rate of respiration → ↑ ventilation |

## Summary

| | *Uncompensated* | *Partially compensated* | *Fully compensated* |
|---|---|---|---|
| pH | ↓↓ | ↓ | Normal |
| $pCO_2$ | ↑↑ | ↑ | ↑ |
| $HCO_3^-$ | N | ↑ | ↑ |
| $H_2CO_3$ | ↑ | | ↑ |
| $HCO_3^-/H_2CO_3$ | ↓ | ↓ | Normal |

## 12. Name and explain the functions of plasma proteins with clinical significance.

- Plasma proteins are proteins circulating in blood.

### Composition (Major Proteins)

| | *Plasma concentration* | *Fraction* |
|---|---|---|
| • Albumin | 3.5–5 g/dL | 55–65% |
| • Glubulin | 2.5–3.5 g/dL | |
| – α-1 globulin | 0.3–0.5 g/dL | 2–4% |
| – α-2 globulin | 0.4–0.8 g/dL | 6–12% |
| – β globulin | 0.6–1.1 g/dL | 8–12% |
| – γ globulin | 0.8–1.8 g/dL | 12–22% |
| • Fibrinogen | 0.2–0.4 g/dL | |
| Total plasma proteins | 6–8 g/dL | 100% |

### Functions of Plasma Proteins

a. Transport of substances
   - Plasma proteins combine with various substances and help in their transport in body
   - Albumin, α globulin and β globulin help in transport of enzymes, hormones and respiratory gases
   - Albumin binds and transports free fatty acids and uncojugated bilirubin
   - Specific binding globulins transport vitamins and hormones
   - Transport proteins like transferrin and ceruloplasmin transport metals like iron and copper respectively.

b. Blood coagulation
   - Fibrinogen and prothrombin are essential for blood coagulation as follows:

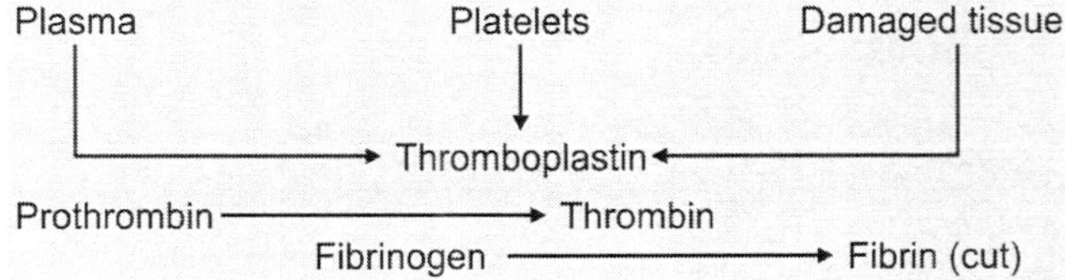


**Fig. 7:** Blood coagulation mechanism

   - Deficiency of fibrinogen or prothrombin results in coagulopathies.

c. Body defense
   - Gamma (α) globulins secreted by plasma cells are called as immunoglobulins or antibodies and are responsible for protection of body from antigens of various microorganisms
   - Complement proteins are involved in immunity against infections
   - Acute phase proteins are plasma proteins that are increased during tissue injury and infection and they are involved in modulation of infection and inflammatory response

d. Maintenance of colloidal osmotic pressure
   - Large molecule of plasma proteins exert an colloidal osmotic pressure as they cannot pass through capillary membrane

- Pressure exerted is directly proportional to concentration of plasma proteins hence its primary function of albumin > globulin > fibrinogen
- Total colloidal osmotic pressure exerted is about 25 mm Hg and by this colloidal osmotic pressure, plasma proteins regulate distribution of fluid between blood and tissue
- Hypoalbuminemia results in edema.

e. Buffering action
  - Albumin maintains acid-base balance in blood by its buffering action.

f. Maintenance of blood viscosity
  - Plasma proteins by virtue of their large size and structural asymmetry are responsible for blood viscosity.

g. Maintenance of blood pressure
  - Plasma proteins by maintaining blood viscosity indirectly maintain blood pressure.

h. Erythrocyte sedimentation rate (ESR)
  - Plasma proteins exert a great influence upon suspension stability of blood
  - Mainly dependent on fibrinogen > globulin > albumin
  - Increase in fibrinogen level enhances Rouleaux formation by RBCs and thus increasing ESR.

i. Production of trephone substance
  - Trephones are substances produced by leukocytes from plasma proteins which are necessary for nourishment of tissue cells in culture.

j. Reserve proteins
  - Plasma proteins serve as store house of proteins to be utilized during period of starvation or protein deficit diet intake.

k. Enzymatic reactions
  - Plasma contains several enzymes which are essential for enzymatic reactions in plasma
  - Example: Lipoprotein lipase, hepatic lipase, renin, and lecithin acyl chloesterol transferase.

l. Miscellaneous
  - Other least important proteins play their necessary role like angiotensinogen's role in release of ADH, aldosterone, etc.



## SHORT ANSWERS

### 13. Mechanism of action of steroid hormones.

Refer Question No. 7 June 2008 (RS2).

### 14. Alkaptonuria.

Refer Question No. 1 Dec. 2010 (RS2).

### 15. Eicosanoids—functions.

- Eicosanoids are group of compounds derived from "Eicosa (20-C) polyenoic fatty acid".

#### Classification

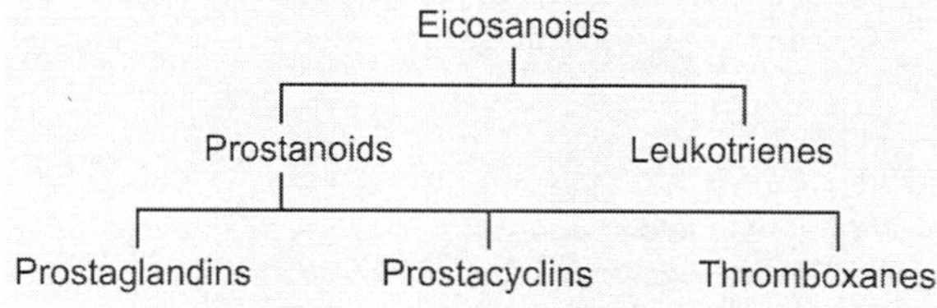


**Fig. 8:** Classification of eicosanoids

## Biosynthesis

- Prostanoids are synthesized by cyclooxygenase pathway and leukotrienes by lipooxygenase pathway.

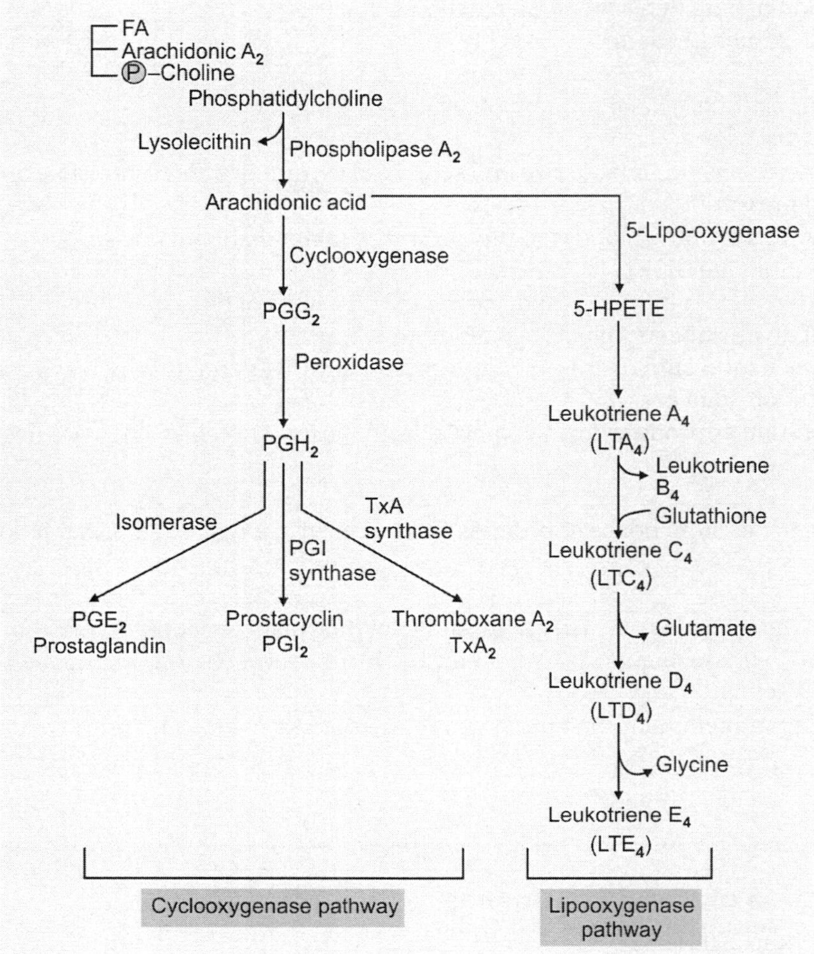


**Fig. 9:** Biosynthesis of eicosanoids

| | *Features* | *Functions* |
|---|---|---|
| Prostaglandins | • Hormone like substances found in almost every mammalian cell<br>• Most potent biologically active substances<br>• Formed from essential fatty acids and each EFA give rise to different series of prostaglandins<br>• Arachidonic acid released from membrane lipids serves as a precursor for series 2 prostaglandin (PGE2, PGF2 and TxA2)<br>• Other eicosapolyenotes released are dihomo γ-linolenate and itimnodnate give rise to series 1 ( PGE1, PGF1 and TxA1) and series 3 (PGE3, PGF3, and TXA3) respectively<br>*Biological action*<br>• Differ on different tissues<br>• General effects are:<br>– Contraction of smooth muscles<br>– Modulating effect on target tissues responding to adinohypophyseal hormones and β adrenergic receptor | • Antihypertensive (lowers blood pressure)<br>• Inhibits platelet aggregation<br>• Inhibits gastric secretion<br>• Stimulates GI musculature<br>• Bronchodilation<br>• Metabolic effect<br>• Increase uterine contraction<br>• Renal action—increase RBF, GFR, diuresis, natriuresis, kaliuresis<br>• Stimulates renin secretion |

*Contd...*

Contd...

| | *Features* | *Functions* |
|---|---|---|
| Prostacyclins | • Synthesized in cyclooxygenase pathway by prostacycline synthase<br>• Principally formed in vascular endothelium and also continually being formed in heart<br>• Also produced in kidneys | • Inhibits platelet aggregation by ↑cAMP level in platelets through activation of adenyl cyclase<br>• Antihypertensive (lowers BP by vasodilation)<br>• Inhibits gastric secretion<br>• Renal action—increases renal blood flow and GFR<br>• Stimulates renin production<br>• Mild inflammatory effects<br>• Counteracts constrictor action of PGs on smooth muscles |
| Thrombaxanes | • Synthesized by thrombaxane synthase mainly in platelets and also in polymorphs, lungs, brain, kidney and spleen via cyclooxygenase pathway | • Enhances platelet aggregation by ↓ cAMP level in platelets through inhibition of adenyl cyclase<br>• Raises BP (potent vasoconstrictor)<br>• Contracts smooth muscles<br>• Induces release of serotonin, $Ca^{++}$ and ADP from platelet |
| Leukotrines | • Produced from arachidonic acid by lipoxygenase pathway in mast cells, basophills, macrophages, neutrophils, platelets and lungs<br>• $LTB_4$ is most potent | • Mainly involved in chemotaxis, inflammation and allergic reactions<br>• Capillary dilatation and vascular permeability<br>• Smooth muscle contraction and constriction of bronchioles<br>• SRS-A (slow reacting substance of anaphylaxis) it is a mixture of $LTC_4$, $D_4$ and $E_4$<br>• Chemotaxis and chemokinetic action—$LTB_4$ in inflammation |

**16. Detoxification reaction—phase I.**

Refer Question No. 7 Dec. 2005 (RS2).

**17. Tertiary and quaternary structure of proteins.**

Refer Question No. 4 Dec. 2011 (RS2).

**18. Discuss the features of Lesch-Nyhan syndrome.**

Refer Question No. 10 June 2005 (RS2).

**19. Draw a neat labeled diagram of tRNA.**

Refer Question No. 8 June 2013 (RS2).

**20. Tumor markers.**

Refer Question No. 6 June 2007 (RS2).

**21. What is meant by renal clearance? How is creatinine clearance calculated?**

Refer Question No. 9 Dec. 2005 (RS2).

**22. What are restriction enzymes? List three features of restriction enzymes.**

Refer Question No. 8 Dec. 2015 (RS2).

# MBBS PHASE I EXAMINATION
## JUNE 2015
## (Revised Scheme 2 & 3)

## LONG ESSAYS

**1. Describe the β-oxidation of fatty acids. Give its energetics and explain the regulation of acetyl CoA in our body.**

**For beta oxidation of fatty acids**

Refer Question No. 1 Dec. 2008 (RS2).

### Regulation of Acetyl CoA

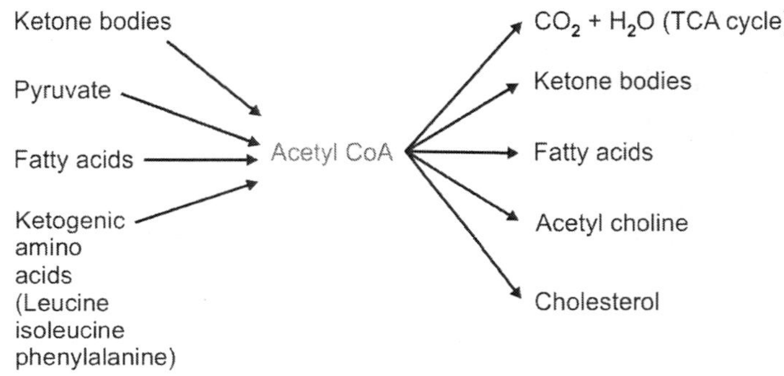


**Fig. 1:** Sources and utilization of acetyl CoA

- Acetyl CoA is an important intermediate of metabolism which generated from carbohydrates, proteins and lipids
- However, major utilization of acetyl CoA is for energy production through TCA cycle
- However excess acetyl CoA is diverted towards synthesis of fatty acids
- The enzyme regulating body acetyl CoA is acetyl CoA carboxylase.

| | *Mechanism* | *Stimulant* | *Inhibitor* |
|---|---|---|---|
| Short-term regulation | Allosteric regulation<br>(Intercoversion between inactive dimeric form to polymeric active form) | Citrate | Long chain acyl CoA |
| | Covalent modification<br>[Phosphorylation (inactive form) and dephosphorylation—active form)] | Insulin | Glucagon<br>AMP |
| Long-term regulation | Induction (increased synthesis) | Excess glucose<br>Insulin | — |
| | Repression (decreased transcription) | — | Low glucose |

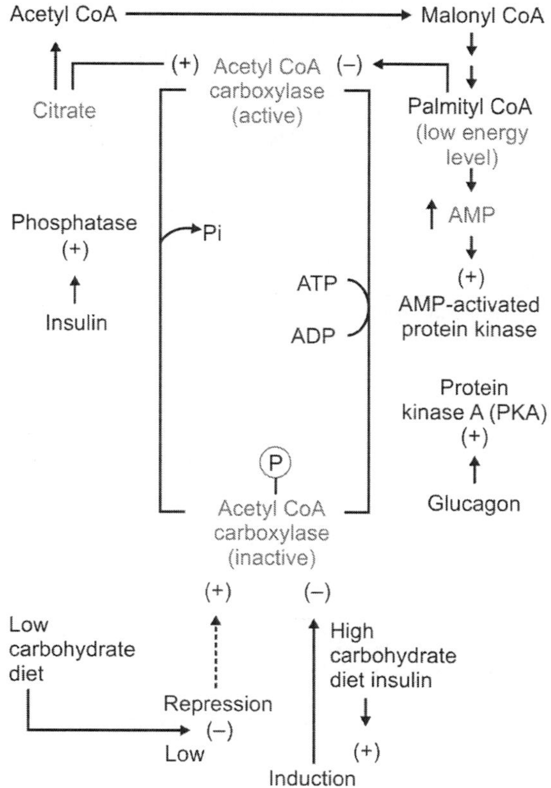


**Fig. 2:** Regulation of acetyl CoA carboxylase

## 2. Draw neat diagram of Watson-Crick model of DNA. Explain its characteristics and the bonds that play a role in the stability of DNA structure.

Refer Question No. 2 June 2010 (RS2).

## SHORT ESSAYS

## 3. How is glycogen digested and absorbed? Describe glycogenolysis in the liver.

- Glycogen a homopolysaccharide present in animals as storage form of carbohydrate
- Carbohydrate consists of many constituents and main bulk of human diet.

### Sources of Carbohydrate in Diet

| *Carbohydrate* | *Food product* |
|---|---|
| • Starch | Cereals |
| • Glycogen | Animal liver and muscles |
| • Cellulose, hemicelluloses and pectins | Cereals, fruits and leafy vegetables |
| • Lactose | Milk and milk products |
| • Sucrose | Sugar and sweets |
| • Fructose | Fruits and honey |
| • Glucose | Fruits and honey |

### Enzymes of Carbohydrate Digestion

- Digestion of carbohydrates is brought about by amyloytic enzymes which convert all complex carbohydrates into simple monosaccharides, absorptive form of carbohydrates.

| *Location* | *Secreted by* | *Enzyme* | *Site of action* |
|---|---|---|---|
| In mouth | Salivary glands | • Salivary amylase | 1-4 glycosidic linkages |
| In intestines | Pancreas | • Pancreatic amylase | a 1-4 glycosidic bonds |
| | Intestinal mucosal cells | • Isomaltase<br>• Maltase<br>• Lactase<br>• Sucrase | 1-4 and 1-6 glycosidic linkages |

## Sites of Digestion

| | |
|---|---|
| • Starch and glycogen | Starts in mouth and completes in small intestine |
| • Cellulose and hemicelluloses | Colon |

## Digestion of Carbohydrates

| | |
|---|---|
| a. In mouth | • Chewed food in mouth is mixed with salivary amylase or ptylin (only amylase in saliva) which breaks down 1-4 glycosidic linkages<br>$\text{Starch} \xrightarrow[\text{4-11pH Cl}]{\text{Ptylin}} \alpha\text{-limit dextrins + maltose + maltotrioses}$ |
| b. In stomach | • Ptylin mixed with food continues its action in stomach till pH of stomach reaches 4, after which it is inactivated<br>• However, no further changes occur in stomach as gastric juice contains only a weak amylase |
| c. In small intestine | • In upper part of intestine, starch, glycogen, limit dextrins are acted upon by pancreatic amylase which is similar to ptylin<br>• It cleaves a 1-4 glycosidic bonds<br>• End products of this digestion are limit dextrins, di- and trisaccharides<br>$\text{Starch or glycogen} \xrightarrow[\text{4–11 pH}]{\text{Pancreatic amylase}} \alpha \text{ limit dextrins} \longrightarrow \text{di- and trisaccharides.}$<br>• Di- and trisaccharides are subjected to action of enzymes on epithelial brush border is maltase, isomaltase, lactase and sucrase<br>• End products of this enzymatic action are monosaccharides which are produced by breaking down both 1–4 and 1–6 linkages<br>$\text{Maltose} \xrightarrow{\text{Maltase}} \text{Glucose + Glucose}$<br>$\text{Isomaltose} \xrightarrow{\text{Isomaltase}} \text{Glucose + Glucose}$<br>$\text{Lactose} \xrightarrow{\text{Lactase}} \text{Glucose + Galactose}$<br>$\text{Sucrose} \xrightarrow{\text{Sucrase}} \text{Glucose + Fructose}$<br>• Monosaccharides are final end product of carbohydrate digestion which are absorbed in small intestine<br>• Glucose forms 80% of this end product and rest 20% is formed by galactose and fructose |

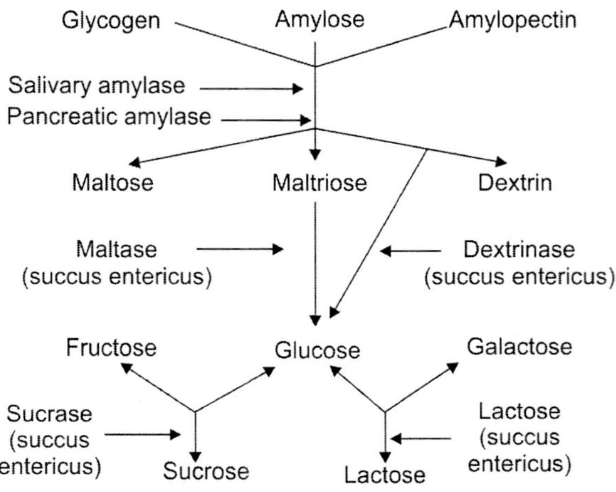


**Fig. 3:** Digestion of carbohydrates

## Carbohydrate Absorption

- Glucose is main form of carbohydrate absorbed
- Mainly absorbed from duodenum and jejunum in form of D-glucose; by an active carrier mediated process involving $Na^+$ monosaccharide symport
- Galactose is also absorbed in similar way by active process (glucose and galactose share same chemical properties)

| Chemical properties necessary for active transport of monosaccharide |
|---|
| ✓ Pyranose ring<br>✓ OH at 2nd carbon atom should project below the ring<br>✓ 6th carbon atom can be $CH_2$ OH or $CH_3$ |

- Intestinal epithelium contains a carrier protein which has 2 binding sites, one for $Na^+$ and other for glucose which transfers both $Na^+$ and glucose from intestinal lumen into mucosal cell cytoplasm
- $Na^+$ then dissociates from carrier to enter cytoplasm down its own concentration gradient, thus reducing affinity of glucose to carrier protein which releases glucose into mucosal cell cytoplasm in-spite of higher sugar concentration there
- Intracytoplasmic $Na^+$ is pumped out by ATP dependent sodium pump ($NA^+$-$K^+$-ATPase) which hydrolyzes ATP and utilise energy for simultaneously transferring 3 $Na^+$ ions outwards and 2 $K^+$ inside mucosal cell.

**For Glycogenolysis**

Refer Question No. 1 June 2007 (RS2).

## 4. How are bile acid synthesized? Mention two functions of bile acids.

- Bile acids are C-24 steroids containing 24 carbon atoms, 2 or 3 hydroxyl groups in steroid nucleus and a side chain ending in carboxyl group
- Bile salts are sodium and potassium salts of conjugated bile acids.

### Types

| *Primary bile acids* | *Secondary bile acids (formed in intestine by deconjugation and decarboxylation by bacteria)* |
|---|---|
| • Cholic acid<br>• Chenodeoxycholic acid | • Deoxycholic acid from cholic acid<br>• Lithocholic acid from chenodeoxycholic acid |

### Properties

- Amphipathic in nature and serve as emulsifying agents in intestine.

### Synthesis

| *Tissue site* | *Subcellular site* | *Substrate* | *Products* |
|---|---|---|---|
| Liver | Peroxisomes | Cholesterol (80% of cholesterol is converted into bile acids) | Glycocholate, taurocholate, glycochenodeoxycholate and taurochenodeoxycholate |

### Reactions

Refer Figure 4 on next page.

### Regulation

| *Reaction* | *Enzyme* | *Mechanism* | *Stimulators* | *Inhibitors* |
|---|---|---|---|---|
| Cholesterol → 7 α-hydroxycholesterol | Cholesterol 7 α-hydroxylase | Covalent modification (phosphorylation) | High cholesterol level | Cholic acid |

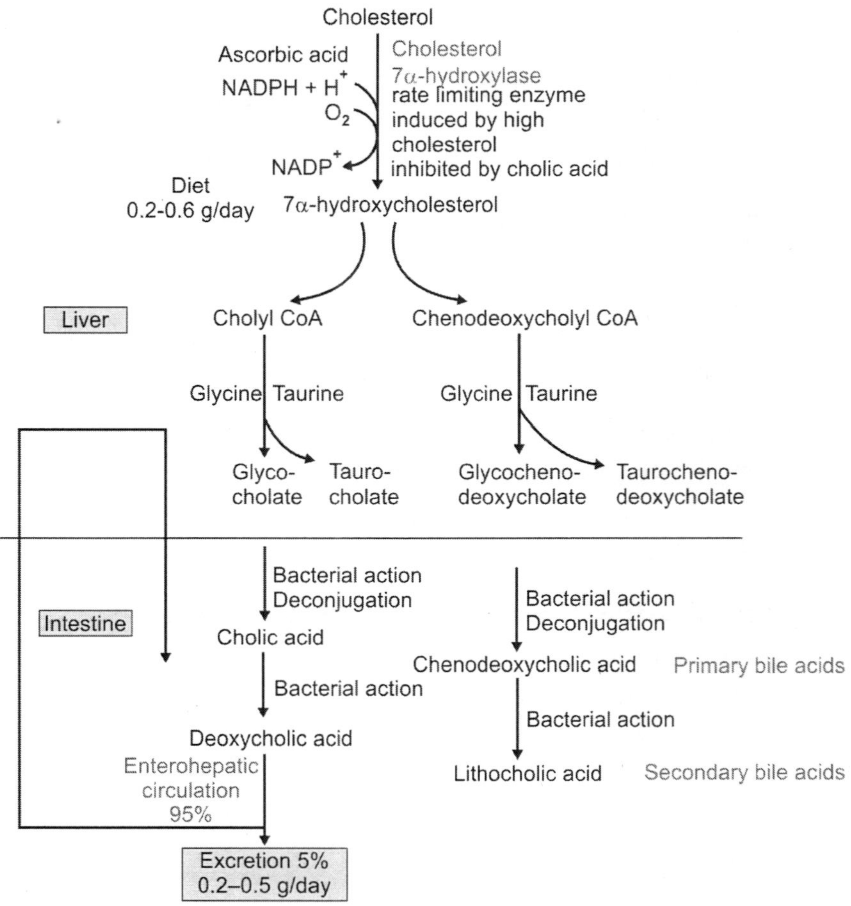


**Fig. 4:** Bile acid synthesis



## Functions (Bile Acids and Bile Salts)

a. Excretion of cholesterol
   - Bile acids (salts) are end product of cholesterol metabolism and they represent the only important pathway for excretion of cholesterol from body.

b. Solubilization of cholesterol
   - Bile acids solubilize cholesterol in bile and prevents precipitation of cholesterol in the bile
   - Hence, they prevent cholesterol stone formation.

c. Digestion and absorption of triacylglycerol
   - Bile salts are required for digestion and absorption of triacylglycerol by virtue of their property of emulsifying agents
   - They function in absorption of triacylglycerols by forming mixed micelles.

d. Absorption of fat-soluble vitamins and cholesterol
   - Fat-soluble vitamins A, D, E, and K require presence of bile salts for their absorption which interact with bile salts to form mixed micelles
   - Cholesterol absorption also requires presence of bile salts.

## Clinical Significance

- Deficiency of bile acids leads to steatorrhea (fatty stool) as lipids are not absorbed from intestine
- It also causes deficiency of fat-soluble vitamins
- Bile acid deficiency predisposes to formation of cholesterol stones.

## 5. Describe the conversion of methionine to cysteine. Add a note on homocystinuria.

**For biosynthesis from cysteine from methionine**

Refer Question No. 4 June 2005 (RS2).

## Homocystinuria

- Group of metabolic disorder characterized by accumulation and increased urinary excretion of homocystine and SAM.

## Inheritance

- Autosomal recessive.

## Types

| *Type* | *Deficient enzyme* | *Remarks* |
|---|---|---|
| • Type I | Cystathionine synthase | Leads to accumulation of homocysteine |
| • Type II | $N^5$–$N^{10}$ methylene THF reductase | |
| • Type III | $N^5$–$N^{10}$ methylene THF homocyteine methyltransferase | Due to impairment in synthesis of methyl cobalamin |
| • Type IV | $N^5$ methyl THF homocyteine methyltransferase | Due to defect in intestinal absorption of vitamin $B_{12}$ |

## Clinical Features (Type I)

- Damage to endothelial cells leading to atherosclerosis (due to deficiency of cystathionine)
- Thrombosis, osteoporosis and mental retardation (due to accumulation of homocysteine)
- Ectopia lentis (juvenile and adult form)
- Death due to myocardial infarction, stroke or pulmonary embolism.

## Laboratory Diagnosis

- Cyanide nitroprusside test to detect homocystinuria.

## Treatment

- Vitamin $B_6$ supplementation (beneficial in $B_6$ responsive type)
- Consumption of diet low in methionine and high in cystine.

### 6. Outline the synthesis of epinephrine and give its functions.

Refer Question No. 7 Dec. 2016 (RS2).

### 7. Give the coenzyme role of pantothenic acid and its importance.

- Pantothenic acid is a water-soluble vitamin.

| *Chemistry* | *Dietary sources* | *Recommended dietary allowance* |
|---|---|---|
| • Pantoic acid joined to β-alanine by a peptide bond<br>• Heat stable but destroyed by acid and alkali | • Yeast, eggs, liver and meat (rich sources)<br>• Vegetables and grains (good sources) | • Adult—10 mg/day<br>• Children—7 mg/day<br>• Pregnancy and lactation slightly higher than adults |

## Metabolism

- Present in food either in free form or coenzyme form (coenzyme form hydrolyzed to free form by action of intestinal pyrophosphatase)
- Free pantothenic is absorbed from upper small intestine by a specific sodium dependent transport system
- Absorbed free pantothenic enters portal circulation and transported to various tissues
- In tissues, vitamin is converted to coenzyme form and stored in liver, heart, brain, kidney and adrenals
- Excreted in urine mainly as free vitamin.

## Biomedical Function (Coenzymes)/Importance

a. Coenzyme A
   - Coenzyme A as a cofactor

- Pyruvate dehydrogenase complex
- α-ketoglutarate dehydrogenase complex
- Fatty acyl dehydrogenase complex
- Thiolase
- Acetoacetyl CoA synthase
- HMG CoA synthase

– Formation of active high energy acyl molecules in body metabolism.

| | *Formation* | *Utilisation* |
|---|---|---|
| Acetyl CoA | From oxidation of pyruvate (derived from carbohydrates and amino acids), amino acids, fatty acids and ketone bodies | • Oxidation through citric acid cycle to provide energy<br>• Converted to acetylcholine (neurotransmitter)<br>• Substrate for synthesis of fatty acids, cholesterol, amino acids and ketone bodies |
| Succinyl CoA | From propionyl CoA (which is formed from oxidation of odd chain fatty acids, valine, isoleucine, methionine) and α-ketoglutarate | • Oxidized through citric acid cycle to provide energy<br>• For metabolism of ketone bodies<br>• For biosynthesis of heme |
| Propionyl CoA | From oxidation of odd chain fatty acids, isoleucine, methionine and valine | Converted to succinyl CoA |

b. 4-phosphopantetheine
- Carrier of acyl groups for de novo synthesis of fatty acids
  - 4-phosphopantetheine is attached to an *acyl carrier protein of fatty acid synthase complex*
  - 4-phosphopantetheine contributes *to peripheral SH* group of fatty acid synthase complex. Acyl intermediates are attached to peripheral SH group during fatty acid synthesis.

## Deficiency

- Deficiency is rare due to wide distribution in diet (induced experimentally by metabolic antagonist such as ω-methyl pantothenic acid).

## Features (Burning Feet Syndrome)

- Numbness and tingling of toes, burning pain in feet, sleep disturbances and depression.

## 8. Describe salvage pathway of purine synthesis and its significance.

Refer Question No. 11 Dec. 2005 (RS2).

## 9. What are porphyrias? Mention four porphyrias with the defective enzyme.

- Porphyrias is metabolic disorder of heme synthesis pathway characterized by increased excretion of porphyrins and porphyrin precursors.

## Classification

| Porphyria | | |
|---|---|---|
| ⇓ | | ⇓ |
| Inherited | | Acquired |
| ⇓ | ⇓ | |
| Erythropoietic porphyria (Enzyme deficiency in RBCs) | Hepatic porphyria (Enzyme deficiency in liver) | |
| Example: Congenital erythropoietic porphyria, erythropoietic protoporphyria | Example: Intermittent acute porphyria (IAP), porphyria cutanea tarda, hereditary caproporphyria, variegate porphyria | |

*Note:* Pattern of excretion of porphyria and its precursors is characteristic for each type.

Revised Scheme 2 & 3

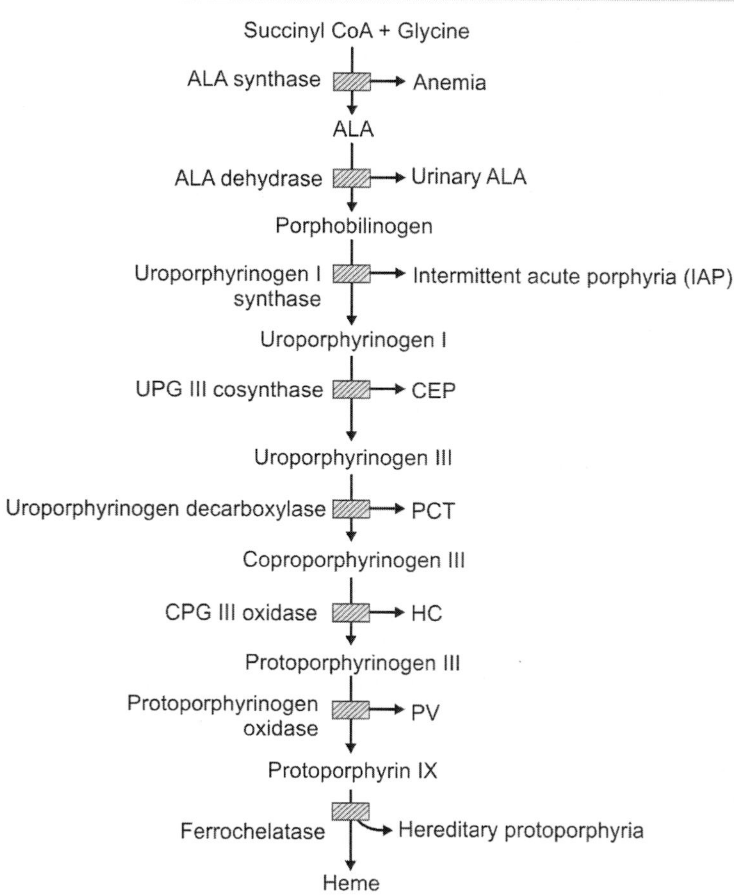


**Fig. 5:** Porphyrias—types

***Prophyrias: AAP Has V(w)asted Capital (Delhi) Election***

- ✓ ALA dehydratase deficiency prophyria
- ✓ Acute intermittent porphyria
- ✓ Porphyria cutanea tarda
- ✓ Hereditary coproporphyria
- ✓ Variegate porphyria
- ✓ Congenital erythropoietic porphyria
- ✓ Erythropoietic protoporphyria

| *Defective enzyme* | *Principal symptoms* | *Laboratory findings* |
|---|---|---|
| **Inherited porphyrias** | | |
| a. 5-ALA dehydratase deficient porphyria (ADP)—autosomal recessive | | |
| – ALA dehydratase | – Neurovisceral | – Zn protoporphyrin in erythrocytes |
| b. Acute intermittent porphyria (AIP)—autosomal dominant<br>– Most common acute porphyria<br>– Not expressed before puberty<br>– Abdominal pain (MC symptom), vomiting, constipation, tachycardia (MC sign), etc.<br>– No abnormal sensitivity to light unlike other hepatic porphyria patients because these do not accumulate porphyrins and protophyrinogen<br>– Aggravated by drugs and steroids metabolized through cytoplasm P450<br>– Relived by hematin, which inhibits enzyme ALA synthase and accumulation of porphobilinogen<br>– Treated with human recombinant erythrocyte PBGD | | |
| – HMB synthase or uroporphyrinogen I synthase | – Neurovisceral | – Urinary ALA and porphobilinogen increased<br>– These colorless compounds upon exposure to light and air form colored compounds causing darkening of urine upon standing |

AIP symptoms (5 P's)

- ✓ Pain in abdomen
- ✓ Polyneuropathy
- ✓ Psychological abnormalities
- ✓ Pink urine
- ✓ Precipitated by drugs (e.g. barbiturates, oral contraceptives and sulfa drugs)

*Contd...*

Contd...

| *Defective enzyme* | *Principal symptoms* | *Laboratory findings* |
|---|---|---|
| c. Porphyria cutanea tarda (PCT)—autosomal dominant<br>– Most common porphyria<br>– Most readily treated porphyria<br>– Caused due to enzyme inhibitors—iron, Cyp1A2, derivatives of uroporphyrinogen<br>– Associated with hemochromatosis<br>– Blistering skin lesions<br>– Exogeneous estrogen is an aggravating factor | | |
| – Urophorphyrinogen decarboxylase | – Cutaneous photosensitivity | – Urinary uroporphyrins I increased<br>– Urine may be pink and upon acidification it fluorescence under UV light |
| d. Hereditary coprophorphyria (HC)—autosomal dominant | | |
| – Coproporphyrinogen oxidase | – Neurovisceral and cutaneous photosensitivity | – Urinary ALA, porphobilinogen and coproporphyrin III and fecal coproporphyrin III increased |
| e. Variegate porphyria (VP)—autosomal dominant | | |
| – Protoporphyrinogen oxidase | – Neurovisceral and cuteneous photosensitivity | – Urinary ALA, porphobilinogen and coproporphyrin III and fecal protoporphyrin IX increased |
| f. Congenital erythropoietic porphyria (CEP)—autosomal recessive<br>– Presents shortly after birth or in-utero as nonimmune hydrops<br>– Predominantly affects erythroid cells in bone marrow<br>– Metabolites accumulated in skin, erythroid cells and erythrocytes<br>– Imbalance between uroporphyrinogen I synthase and cosynthase action causing increased production of type I porphyrins, i.e. uroporphyrinogen I and coproporphyrinogen I<br>– Extreme cutaneous photosensitivity<br>– Repeated attacks of dermatitis and scarring lead to monkey facies<br>– Repeated ulceration and scarring cause mutilation of nose, ear and cartilage<br>– Deposition of porphyrins in teeth making them fluorescent (erythrodontia)<br>– Treated with beta carotene to protect from sunlight and gene therapy using human cDNA UROS retroviral vectors | | |
| – Uroporphyrinogen III cosynthase | – Cutaneous photosensitivity | – Urinary, fecal and red cell uroporphyrinogen I increased<br>– Urine is dark red in color (Pot-wine appearance)<br>– Porphyrine I, porphobilinogen and δ-ALA level in blood |
| g. Erythropoietic protoporphyria (EPP)—autosomal recessive<br>– Due to defect in ferrochelatase (FECH mutation)<br>– Nonblistering photosensivity<br>– Characterized by skin swelling and pain | | |
| – Ferrochelatase | – Cutaneous photosensitivity | – Fecal and red cell protoporphyrin IX increased |
| h. X-linked protoporphyria (XLP)—X-linked<br>– Due to increased activity of ALA synthase 2 due to gain of function mutation | | |
| – ALA synthase 2 | – Cutaneous photosensitivity | – Protoporphyrin in erythrocytes and stool |
| Acquired (toxic) porphyria<br>Exposure to toxic compounds such as hexachlorobenzene, lead, heavy metals causing inhibition of several enzymes in heme synthesis like ALA dehydratase, uroporphyrinogen I synthase and ferrochelatase | | |

| *Diagnosis* | *Clinical features* |
|---|---|
| • Watson and Swartz test by UV fluorescence method<br>– Urine on exposure to UV light emits red fluorescence indicating presence of porphyrins | • Mainly due to accumulation of ALA, PBG and other compounds which have toxic effects<br>*Enzyme deficiency early in pathway*<br>• ALA and PBG accumulates<br>• Abdominal pain and neuropsychiatric symptoms called neurovisceral (NV)<br>*Enzyme deficiency later in pathways*<br>• Porphyrins accumulates<br>• Cutaneous photosensitivity [CP] (redness, urticaria and hyperpigmentation on exposure to sunlight) |

## 10. Explain the role of kidneys in acid-base regulation.

Refer Question No. 2 June 2012 (RS2).

## 11. What is a balanced diet? Discuss the components of a balanced diet.

- A balanced diet (prudent diet) is defined as one which contains a variety of foods in such quantities and proportions that need for energy amino acids, vitamins minerals, fats carbohydrates and other nutrients is adequately met for maintaining health, vitality and general well-being and also makes a small provision for extranutrients to withstand short duration of leanness.

### Prescribing a Balanced Diet (Guidelines)

- Protein requirement calculated to 15–20% of daily energy intake
- Fat requirement limited to 20–30% of daily energy intake
- Carbohydrates rich in natural fibers constitute remaining food energy
- Micronutrient requirements should also be met
- Pattern of food production climatic conditions of the region, economic capacity, religion, customs, taboos, tastes and habits of person should also be borne in mind while prescribing a balanced diet.

### Components (For an Adult Male Weighing 60 kg and Involved in Moderate Work)

| ICMR 1989 recommendation | Vegetarian | Non-vegetarian |
|---|---|---|
| • Cereals | 475 g | 475 g |
| • Pulses | 80 g | 65 g |
| • Leafy vegetable | 125 g | 125 g |
| • Other vegetable | 75 g | 75 g |
| • Roots and tubes | 100 g | 100 g |
| • Fruits | 30 g | 30 g |
| • Milk | 200 g | 100 g |
| • Oil and fat | 40 g | 40 g |
| • Sugar and jaggery | 40 g | 40 g |
| • Meat and fish | — | 30 g |
| • Eggs | — | 30 g |

## 12. What are the sources of dietary fibers? Discuss the importance of it in nutrition. Outline the functions of proteins.

**For dietary fiber**

Refer Question No. 10 Dec. 2014 (RS2).

### Function of Protein

| | |
|---|---|
| a. Growth | • Proteins are involved in tissue formation thus are essential for growth |
| b. Energy | • Proteins are not main source of energy (amino acids oxidation provides only 8% of total energy requirement of cell)<br>• During starvation, proteins are catabolized into amino acids which are then used for gluconeogenesis |
| c. Regulation of body functions | • All enzymes and most of hormones are proteins<br>• Hormones regulate of cell metabolism and control enzyme activity through covalent modification and by regulation of gene expression<br>• Hormone receptors are proteins and they interact with hormone ligands to execute hormone action |
| d. Muscular activity | • Contractile proteins (actin and myosin) bring about muscular contraction |
| e. Protective function | • Immune defence (Immunoglobulins, complement function, $\alpha 2$ microglobulin)<br>• Inflammatory response by acute phase response proteins (C-reactive proteins, $\alpha 1$ acid glycoprotein)<br>• Hemostasis (clotting factors, fibrinogen) |

| | |
|---|---|
| f. Transport function | • Albumin: Bilirubin, free fatty acids, steroids, ions, metals, hormones, drugs, etc.<br>• Hb: Respiratory gases<br>• Ceruloplasmin: Copper<br>• Transcortin: Cortisol<br>• Transferrin: Iron<br>• Lipoproteins: Plasma lipids |
| g. Structural role | • Proteins are components of plasma membrane<br>• Collagen and elastin are structural proteins |
| h. Regulation of acid-base balance and plasma volume | • Plasma proteins (albumin) and Hb acts as buffers and are essential for regulation of acid balance<br>• Albumin exerts osmotic pressure to maintain plasma volume |
| i. Tumor markers | • $\alpha$1 fetoprotein acts as tumor marker |

## SHORT ANSWERS

### 13. Denaturation of proteins.

Refer Question No. 17 June 2010 (RS2).

### 14. Uncouplers of oxidative phosphorylation.

Refer Question No. 1 June 2010 (RS2).

### 15. Reverse cholesterol transport.

- Reverse cholesterol transport is transport of cholesterol esters from peripheral tissue back to liver and steroidogenic tissues for metabolism and excretion through bile.

| *Done by* | *Enzyme responsible* | *Receptors responsible (present in extrahepatic tissues to facilitate cholesterol uptake)* |
|---|---|---|
| HDL | Lecithin cholesterol acyl transferase (LCAT) activated by apo A1 | Class B Scavenger receptors B1 (SR-B1)<br>ATP binding cassette transporters A1 and G1 (ABCA1 and ABGA1) |

#### Mechanism

- High density lipoprotein (HDL) with help of apo-A1, strips off cellular cholesterol from peripheral cells and smooth muscle cells of arteries and apo-A1, activates enzyme "LCAT", which esterifies cholesterol
- Cholesterol esters formed at surface, being hydrophobic, moves into interior and makes discoid HDL to spherical
- Then the mature HDL (good cholesterol) moves to liver where cholesterol is catabolized.

#### Biomedical Importance

- Reverse cholesterol transport is an important function of HDL (Scavenging action of HDL) which helps reduce blood cholesterol level, hence HDL is considered a good cholesterol.

### 16. Bonds stabilizing protein structure.

Refer Question No. 4 Dec. 2011 (RS2).

### 17. UDP-glucuronic acid.

- Uridine diphosphate (UDP) glucoronic acid is the active form of glucoronic acid which is essential for detoxification reactions.

#### Biosynthesis

- Formed through oxidation of UDP glucose in uronic acid pathway.

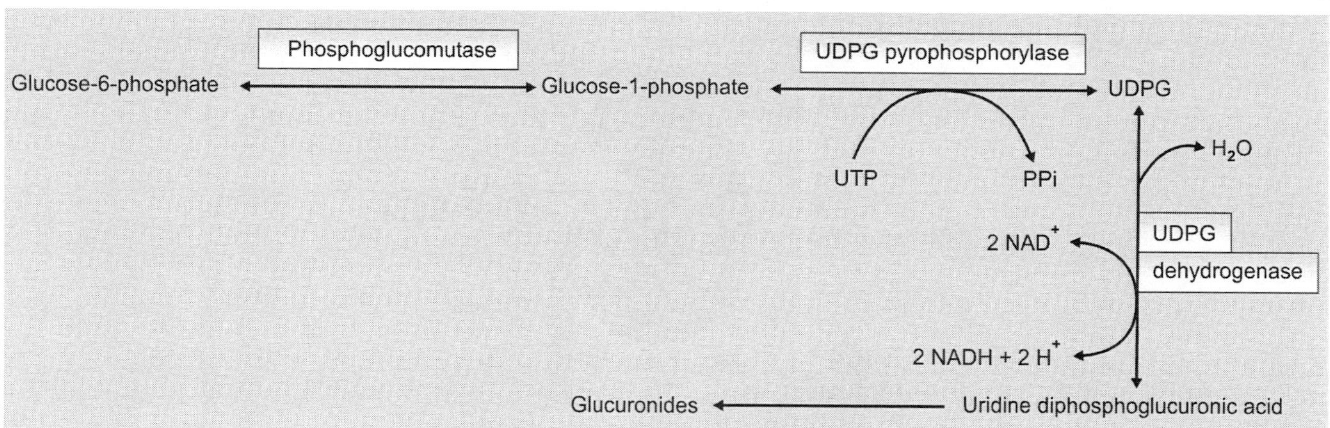


**Fig. 6:** Biosynthesis of UDP-glucuronic acid

## Functions

a. Detoxication reactions (formation of bilirubin diglucuronide)
   - Used for conjugation reactions involved in detoxification of either endogenous substances such as bilirubin or exogenous compounds such as drugs
   - UDP glucuronic acid is a donor of glucuronic acid group, conjugation with which makes a compound highly water soluble for excretion in urine.

   *Examples*
   - Bilirubin to bilirubin diglucoronide
   - Conjugation of benzoic acid to benzoylglucuronic acid.

b. Biosynthesis of glycosaminoglycans
   - UDP glucoronic acid is used in formation hyaluronic acid and heparin.

c. Biosynthesis of L-iduronic acid (an epimer of glucuronic acid)
   - L-iduronic acid is a component of glycosaminoglycans such as heparan sulfate and dermatan sulfate.

## 18. Point mutation.

Refer Question No. 11 June 2005 (RS2).

## 19. Hormones that regulate water balance.

- Major hormones involved in regulating water balance in body at level of kidney are:

| *Hormone* | *Source* | *Site of action* | *Action* |
|---|---|---|---|
| a. ADH (antidiuretic hormone) | Posterior pituitary | Distal tubule and collecting ducts | Increases permeability of distal tubules and collecting duct to increase water reabsorption, thus preventing its loss in urine |
| b. Aldosterone | Adrenal cortex | Distal tubule and collecting duct | Increase $Na^+$ reabsorption and $Cl^-$ reabsortion forming NaCl<br>As NaCl reabsorption increases, osmotic gradient increases and more water moves out of nephron thus preventing its loss in urine |

## Biomedical Significance

- Water is essential component of body and any imbalance leads to dehydration or edema
- Water balance is also important for regulation of blood pressure.

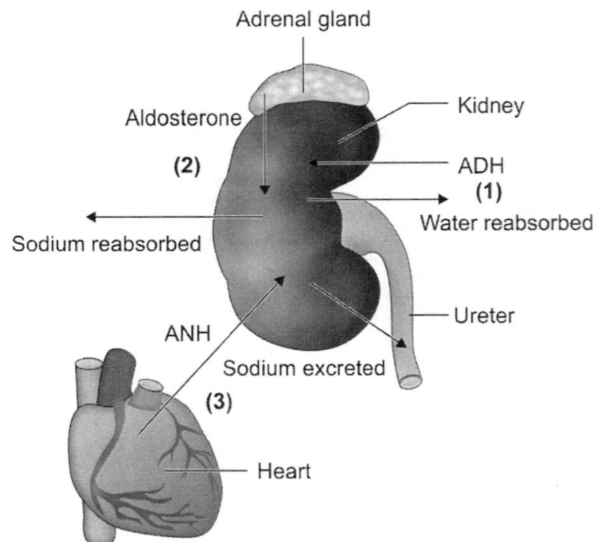


**Fig. 7:** Hormones regulating water balance



## 20. Specific dynamic action (SDA).

Refer Question No. 19 June 2012 (RS2).

## 21. Ribosomal RNA.

Refer Question No. 8 June 2013 (RS2).

## 22. Define antioxidants and give two examples.

Refer Question No. 6 June 2008 (RS2).

# MBBS PHASE I EXAMINATION
## DECEMBER 2015
### (Revised Scheme 2 & 3)

## LONG ESSAYS

**1. Classify enzymes giving an example with the reaction catalyzed.**

Refer Question No. 1 June 2013 (RS2).

**2. Describe the synthesis of DNA. Write a note on replication of DNA.**

Refer Question No. 2 June 2010 (RS2).

## SHORT ESSAYS

**3. Describe the digestion and absorption of lipids.**

- Lipids is an important and essential nutrient
- Triacylglycerols forms major bulk of dietary lipids along with cholesterol and phospholipids.

### Digestion

| *In mouth* | *In stomach* | *In intestine* |
|---|---|---|
| *Enzymes*<br>• Lingual lipase (low optimum pH)<br>*Digestion*<br>• Fat does not undergo major change in mouth and lingual lipase enters stomach along with food | *Enzymes*<br>• Lingual lipase<br>*Digestion*<br>• Acts mainly on short chain and medium chain triglycerides<br>• 30% of triglycerides are digested by 2–4 hours of retention in stomach | *Enzymes*<br>• Pancreatic lipase<br>• Cholesterol esterase<br>• Phospholipase A<br>*Digestion*<br>• Dietary fats are emulsified by bile salts and then hydrolyzed by pancreatic lipase forming diglyceride and then 2-monoglyceride by removing fatty acid from position C1 and C3 (Co-lipase assists lipase in its action) |

### Absorption

- End product of digestion of dietary fat is 2-monoglycerides (because fatty acid at 2nd position cannot be removed by lipase)
- 2-monoglyceride is major absorption form of dietary lipids (72%)
- Unabsorbed 2-monoglyceride is converted to 1-monoglyceride by an isomerase and is absorbed in small quantity (6%)
- 1-monoglyceride is also acted upon by lipase to form glycerol which is too absorbed (22%)
- Fatty acids released are absorbed depending upon their chain length
- Short chain fatty acids are water soluble and are carried directly to liver via portal vein
- Monoglycerides and long chain fatty acids are water insoluble and are rendered water soluble by formation of micelles with the help of bile salts and absorbed by intestinal mucosa.

## Transport

- Inside mucosal cells, fats are again synthesized from 2-monoglyceride, 1-monoglyceride and acyl-CoAs (fatty acids are activated to acyl-CoAs)
- Triglycerides formed in mucosal cells are converted into chylomicrons and transported via lymphatics
- Short chain fatty acids and glycerol being water soluble enter systemic circulation directly (via portal vein).

## Biomedical Significance

- Defective digestion or defective absorption of fat leads to fatty stool/steatorrhea (average daily excretion of fat >6 g/day).

## Causes

| *Defective digestion* | *Defective absorption* |
|---|---|
| • Chronic pancreatic disorder | • Bile duct obstruction—gallstones, tumors of head of pancreas, enlarged lymph node |
| • Surgical removal of pancreas | • Diseases of intestines—celiac disease, sprue, Crohn's disease<br>• Surgical removal of large length of intestine |

## 4. Discuss phenylketonuria under: (i) Enzyme defect; (ii) Manifestation; (iii) Diagnostic test.

Refer Question No. 1 Dec. 2010 (RS2).

## 5. What are mucopolysaccharides. Give their importance with examples.

- Mucopolysaccharides are unbranched hereropolysaccharides made up of disaccharide repeating units composed of an amino sugar (glucosamine/galactosamine) and an acid sugar (D-glucuronic acid/L-iduronic acid)
- Also called as glycosaminoglycans.

## Classification

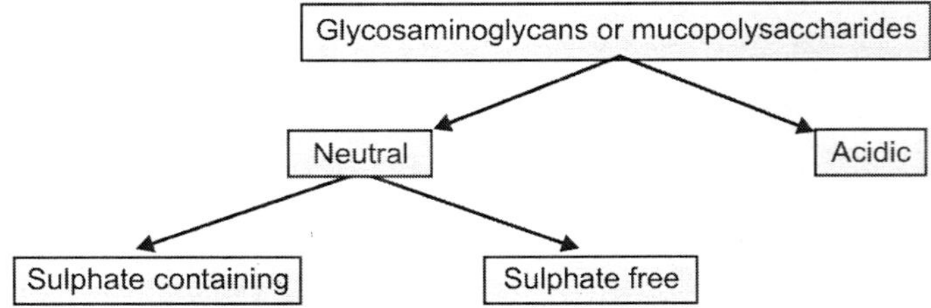


**Fig. 1:** Classification of mucopolysaccharides

## Properties

- Carry large number of negative charges, these chains tend to repel each other
- When water squeezed out, they occupy small volume, when compression is released, they spring back to original hydrated volume because of repulsion of negative charges
- Hence slippery consistency and resilient nature of synovial fluid and vitreous humor
- Special ability to bind to large amount of water, hence forms major component of extracellular matrix.

| | *Disaccharide repeat units* | *Location* |
|---|---|---|
| Neutral mucopolysaccharides | | |
| | | • Various nitrogenous polysaccharides in capsule of pneumococci bacteria<br>• Blood group substances |

*Contd...*

*Contd...*

| | *Disaccharide repeat units* | *Location* |
|---|---|---|
| Acidic mucopolysacharides | | |
| a. Sulphate free | | |
| – Hyalouronic acid | N-acetyl glucosamine, + Glucuronic acid | Connective tissues, tendons, synovial fluids, vitreous humor and umbilical cord |
| – Chondroitin | N-acetyl galactosamine + Glucoronic acid | Cornea and cranial cartilages |
| b. Sulphate containing | | |
| – Keratan sulphate I (does not contain uronic acid) | Galactose + N-acetyl glucosamine | Cornea |
| – Keratan sulphate II | Galactose + N-acetyl glucosamine | Loose connective tissue |
| – Chondroitin sulphate (principle mucopolysaccharide in ground substance) | Glucoronic acid + Sulfated N-acetyl galactosamine | Bones, cartilages, cornea |
| – Heparin [important natural anticoagulant acting both 'in vivo' and 'in vitro, acts as activator for enzyme lipoprotein lipase (clearing factor) and only intracellular mucopolysaccharide] | Glucosamine + L-iduronic acid | Mast cells |
| – Heparan sulphate | Glucosamine + Glucuronic acid | Skin fibroblasts, aortic wall |
| – Dermatan sulphate | N-acetyl galactosamine, iduronic acid/ glucuronic acid | Wide distribution |

## Biomedical Importance

- Mucopolysaccharides are major component of extracellular matrix
- They are present in body fluids such as synovial fluid, vitreous humor
- They offer elasticity and volume to cartilages, cornea, etc.
- Heparin, a mucopolysaccharide is an important natural anticoagulant
- Defect in enzymes degrading mucopolysacharides results in mucopolysaccharidoses resulting in their intralysosomal accumulation.

## 6. Coenzyme form of vitamin $B_{12}$ and its biochemical functions.

- Vitamin $B_{12}$, (anti-pernicious anemia vitamin, cobalamin, extrinsic factor of Castle) is a water-soluble vitamin.

| *Dietary sources* | *Recommended dietary allowance* |
|---|---|
| • Synthesized by only microorganisms (anerobic bacteria) | • Children—0.5–1.5 μg/day |
| • Foods of animal origin are only sources | • Adults—3 μg/day |
| • Liver, kidney, milk, curd, eggs, fish, pork and chicken are rich sources | • Pregnancy and lactation—4 μg/day |

## Biochemical Role

| *Coenzyme forms* | *Functions* |
|---|---|
| • 5′ Deoxyadenosyl cobalamin<br>• Methylcobalamin | • In humans, vitamin $B_{12}$ is present in following enzymes:<br>i. Methyl malonyl CoA isomerase/mutase<br>Methyl malonyl CoA —Isomerase→ Succinyl CoA<br>ii. Homocystine methyl transferase or methionine synthase<br>Homocystine → Methionine (N5 Methyl THFA → THFA) |

## Deficiency Manifestations

- Deficiency of vitamin $B_{12}$ causes pernicious anemia characterized by low hemoglobin level, erythrocytopenia and neurological manifestations.

## Causes

- Autoimmune destruction of gastric parietal cells secreting intrinsic factor thus hampering absorption of vitamin $B_{12}$
- Hereditary malabsoprtion of vitamin $B_{12}$
- Partial or total gastrectomy
- Insufficient production of IF and/or gastric HCl
- Dietary deficiency of $B_{12}$ (seen in strict vegetarians or low socioeconomic strata).

## Clinical Features

| *Hematological features* | | *Neurological features* | *Other features* |
|---|---|---|---|
| *Peripheral blood* | *Bone marrow* | | |
| • Macrocytic type of anemia with megaloblasts, erythroblasts and normoblasts<br>• Granulocytopenia with occasional myelocytes.<br>• Thrombocytopenia<br>• ↓ erythrocyte count and Hb level | • Arrested development of all erythroid, myeloid elements and thrombocytes<br>• Accumulation of megaloblasts and myeloblasts<br>• ↓ megakaryocytes | Due to neuronal degeneration with demyelination and also due to accumulation of methylmalonyl CoA that interferes in myelination:<br>• Paresthesia of fingers and toes<br>• Confusion<br>• Loss of memory<br>• Psychosis in advanced stages | • ↓ DNA synthesis<br>• ↓ serum and urinary $B_{12}$ level<br>• ↑ in fecal $B_{12}$ excretion<br>• ↑ excretion of methyl malonic autoantibodies to intrinsic factor and parietal cells |

## Biomedical Importance

- Through its part in methoinine synthesis reaction, vitamin $B_{12}$ helps converts circulating methyl $FH_4$ to $FH_4$ which is either used for storage as folylpolyglutamate form or is utilized for other reactions such as formation of methylene $FH_4$.

## 7. Describe one carbon metabolism. What is its significance?

- One carbon groups play a pivotal role in donating carbon atoms for synthesis of different types of compounds
- These one carbon compounds are mostly carried by $N^5$ and $N^{10}$ atoms of tetrahydrofolic acid (THFA) derived from folic acid.

## One Carbon Compounds (One Carbon Pool)

| *Group* | *Structure* | *Carrier* |
|---|---|---|
| Formyl | -CHO | $N^5$-formyl-THFA<br>$N^{10}$-formyl-THFA |
| Formimino | -CH=NH | $N^5$-formimino-THFA |
| Methenyl | =CH- | $N^5$, $N^{10}$-methenyl-THFA |
| Hydroxymethyl | $-CH_2OH$ | $N^{10}$-hydroxymethyl-THFA |
| Methylene | $-CH_2-$ | $N^5$, $N^{10}$-methylene-THFA |
| Methyl | $-CH_3-$ | $N^5$-methyl-THFA<br>Methyl cobalamin |

## One Carbon Metabolism

| *Generation (sources)* | *Interconversion* | *Utilization* |
|---|---|---|
| • Conversion of serine to glycine also produces $N^5$, $N^{10}$-methylene THFA (most predominant source)<br>• Formate released from glycine and tryptophan metabolism combines with THF to form $N^{10}$-formyl-THFA<br>• Histidine contributes formimino fragment to produce $N^5$-formimino-THFA<br>• Choline and betain contributes to formation of $N^5$-methyl-THFA | • Different one carbon groups are interconvertible but all one carbon groups are ultimately siphoned into methyl-THFA because reductase reaction is an irreversible reaction | • In formation of one carbon units<br>– $C_2$ of purine<br>– Formylation of methionyl tRNA<br>– $C_8$ of purine<br>– Glycine<br>– Serine<br>– Choline<br>– Deoxy TMP<br>– Transmethylation reactions<br>– Excretion as $CO_2$ |

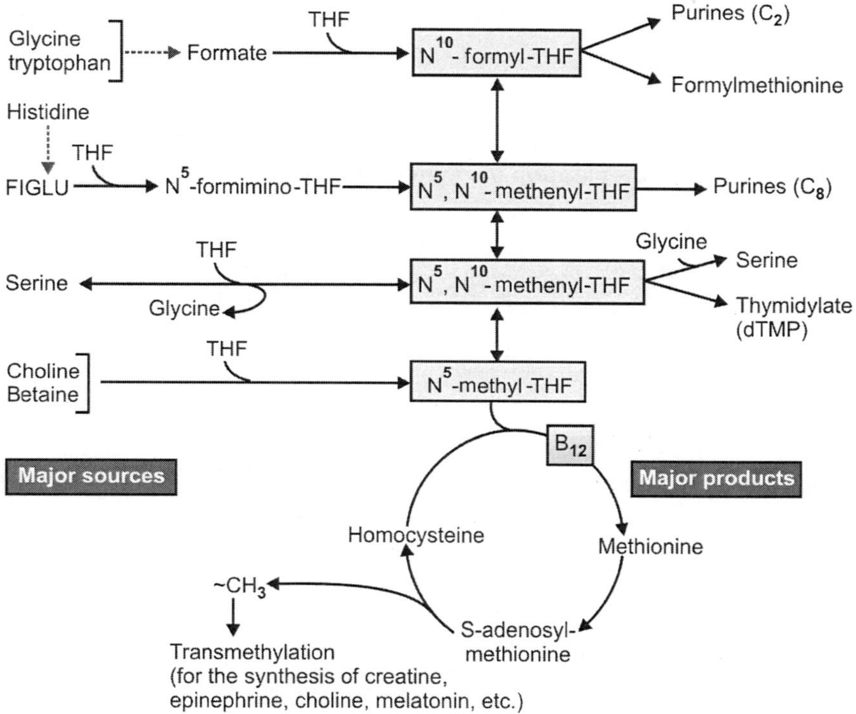


**Fig. 2:** One carbon compound—metabolism

### 8. What is the difference between endonuclease and restriction endonuclease? Give two examples for endonuclease.

| *Point of difference* | *Endonuclease* | *Restriction endonuclease* |
|---|---|---|
| Site of action | Nonspecific | Specific |
| Source | Eukaryotes | Prokaryotes (bacteria) |

## Restriction Endonuclease

- Restriction endonucleases are bacterial enzymes that can split DNA at specific sites
- So named because they can restrict viral replication

*Examples* (They are named for bacteria from which they are isolated)

| *Enzyme* | *Source* | *Recognition sequence* |
|---|---|---|
| a. EcoRI | *Escherichia coli* | 5'....G-/-A-A-T-T-C.....3' |
| b. BamHI | *Bacillus amyloliquefaciens* | 5'....G-/-G-A-T-C-C....3' |
| c. HaeIII | *Haemophilus aegypticus* | 5'....G-G-/-C-G....3' |
| d. HindIII | *Haemophilus influenzae* | 5'....A-/-A-G-C-T-T....3' |
| e. NotI | *Nocardia otitidis* | 5'....G-C-/-G-G-C-C-G-C....3' |

## Actions (Features)

- Restriction endonucleases are endonucleases that cleave DNA at a highly specific sequence
- Most restriction endonucleases make staggered cuts but a few also make straight cuts
- Each restriction endonuclease enzyme recognizes and cleaves a specific double-stranded DNA sequence that is 4 to 7 bp long.
- These DNA cuts result in:
  - Blunt ends (by HpaI)
  - Sticky ends (also called staggered or cohesive ends) by BamHI or EcoRI
- Sticky ends are particularly useful in preparation of chimeric or hybrid DNA molecule.

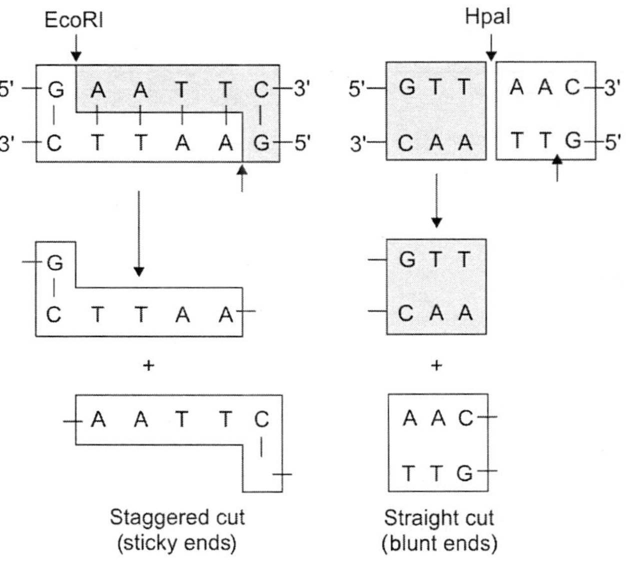


**Fig. 3:** Endonucleases—mechanism of action

## Applications

a. To prepare recombinant DNA (chimeric DNA)
   - Target DNA used in recombinant DNA technique is generated from cellular DNA by action of restriction endonucleases.

   *Procedure*
   - A circular plasmid vector DNA is first cut with a specific restriction endonuclease
   - Human DNA (foreign or insert DNA) is also cut with the same restriction endonuclease, so that same sequences are produced on sticky ends of cut piece.

b. In molecular diagnostics
   - Restriction endonucleases are used in RFLP technique of molecular diagnostics
   - By using different restriction endonucleases for the digestion of a particular DNA, a restriction map with characteristic sites of action can be prepared.

## 9. What are oncogenes? Discuss two tumor markers and their clinical application.

**For oncogenes**

Refer Question No. 3 Dec. 2010 (RS2).

**For tumor markers**

Refer Question No. 6 June 2007 (RS2).

## 10. Diagnostic enzymes used in the assessment of different liver functions.

Refer Question No. 5 Dec. 2013 (RS2).

## 11. Respiratory alkalosis.

- Respiratory alkalosis is increased pH due to decreased $CO_2$
- Also called primary $H_2CO_3$ deficit
- Bicarbonate-carbonic acid ratio is >20.

| *Causes* | *Underlying mechanism* | *Clinical manifestation* | *Compensatory mechanism (renal)* |
|---|---|---|---|
| • High altitude<br>• Hysteria<br>• Hypoxia<br>• Raised intracranial pressure<br>• Brainstem injury<br>• Excessive artificial respiration<br>• Drugs (salicylates)<br>• Lung diseases (pneumonia, pulmonary embolism)<br>• Congestive cardiac failure<br>• Fever, septicemia | Hyperventilation<br>⇓<br>Increased exhalation of $CO_2$<br>⇓<br>Decreased $pCO_2$ | • Hyperventilation<br>• Muscle cramps<br>• Tingling and paresthesia | • Reduction in plasma bicarbonate by:<br>– Increased urinary excretion of $HCO_3^-$<br>– Decreased urinary reabsorption of $HCO_3^-$<br>• Reduction of urinary ammonia formation |

### Biochemical Findings

| *Parameter* | *Uncompensated* | *Compensated* |
|---|---|---|
| • pH | Markedly increased | Slightly increased |
| • $pCO_2$ | Markedly decreased | Decreased |
| • $HCO_3^-$ | Normal | Slightly decreased |
| • Ammonia in urine | Normal | Decreased |

## 12. How is uric acid formed in the body? What is gout? What is the treatment? Explain the basis for the treatment.

Refer Question No. 2 June 2007 (RS2).

## SHORT ANSWERS

## 13. Compare and contrast starch and glycogen.

| | *Starch* | *Glycogen* |
|---|---|---|
| Polymer of | Homopolysaccharide of glucose | Homopolysaccharide of glucose |
| Structure | • Made up of amylose and amylopectin amylose: Linear, helical, α1-4 linkage<br>• Amylopectin branched, α1-6 linkage | • Highly branched<br>• α1-4 linkage linear chain<br>• α1-6 linkage, branched chain |
| Reserve carbohydrate | In plants (potato, cereals, tubers) | In animals (liver and muscle) |
| Color reaction to iodine | Blue color (because of increased absorption of iodine by helical structure of amylase) | Red brown or brown–violet color (because of lack of helical conformation) |
| Role | Major source of glucose in diet | • Liver glycogen: Blood glucose regulation<br>• Muscle glycogen: Energy for muscle contraction |

## 14. Essential fatty acids.

Refer Question No. 4 Dec. 2016 (RS2).

## 15. Transport across cell membrane.

- Transport across cell membrane occurs by two types of mechanisms:
  - Active transport
  - Passive transport.

| **Active transport** | • Movement of a substance against a gradient with utilization of energy |
|---|---|
| Primary active transport | • Energy generated from breakdown of ATP or any other energy compound<br>• Substance to be transported forms a complex with carrier protein which then develops ATPase activity due to conformational change in protein and substance moves across cell membrane |
| Secondary active transport | • Energy generated by transport of one substance across cell membrane is utilized for transport of other substance<br>• Hence also called co-transport<br>*Types*<br>i. Symport: Both molecules move in same direction<br>– Example: $Na^+$ and glucose transport in intestine<br>ii. Antiport: Transport is in different directions.<br>– Example: $Na^+$ – $K^+$ pump in parietal cells of gastric mucosa 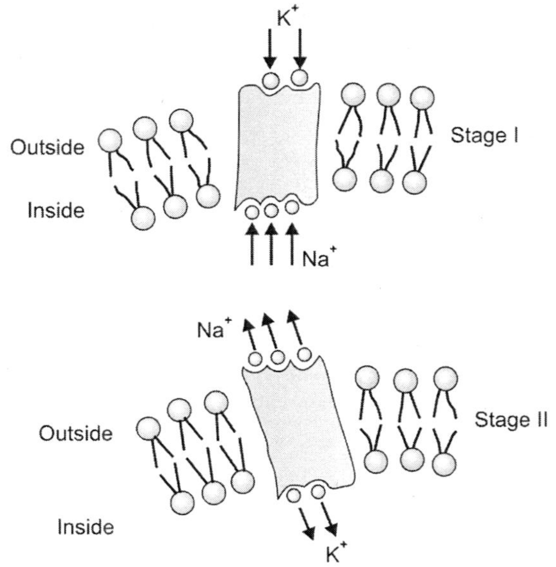<br>$K^+$ Outside Inside $Na^+$ Stage I<br>$Na^+$ Outside Inside $K^+$ Stage II<br>**Fig. 4:** Secondary active transport |
| Endocytosis | • Active transport process for macromolecules like proteins, lipids and small amount of fluid into cell by formation of vesicles<br>• Also called vesicular transport<br>*Mechanism*<br>Contact of macromolecule with cell membrane or membrane receptors (calthrin)<br>⇓<br>Invagination of cell membrane<br>⇓<br>Formation of endocytic vesicle<br>⇓<br>Fusion of noncytoplasmic side of cell membrane<br>⇓<br>Release of vesicle from cell membrane into cytoplasm<br>*Types*<br>• Phagocytosis (cell eating)<br>– Process of ingestion of large particle or microorganisms by specialized cells called phagocytes (e.g. macrophages, neutrophils, monocytes) followed by their digestion<br>– Example: Phagocytosis of bacteria by neutrophills and macrophages |

*Contd...*

*Contd...*

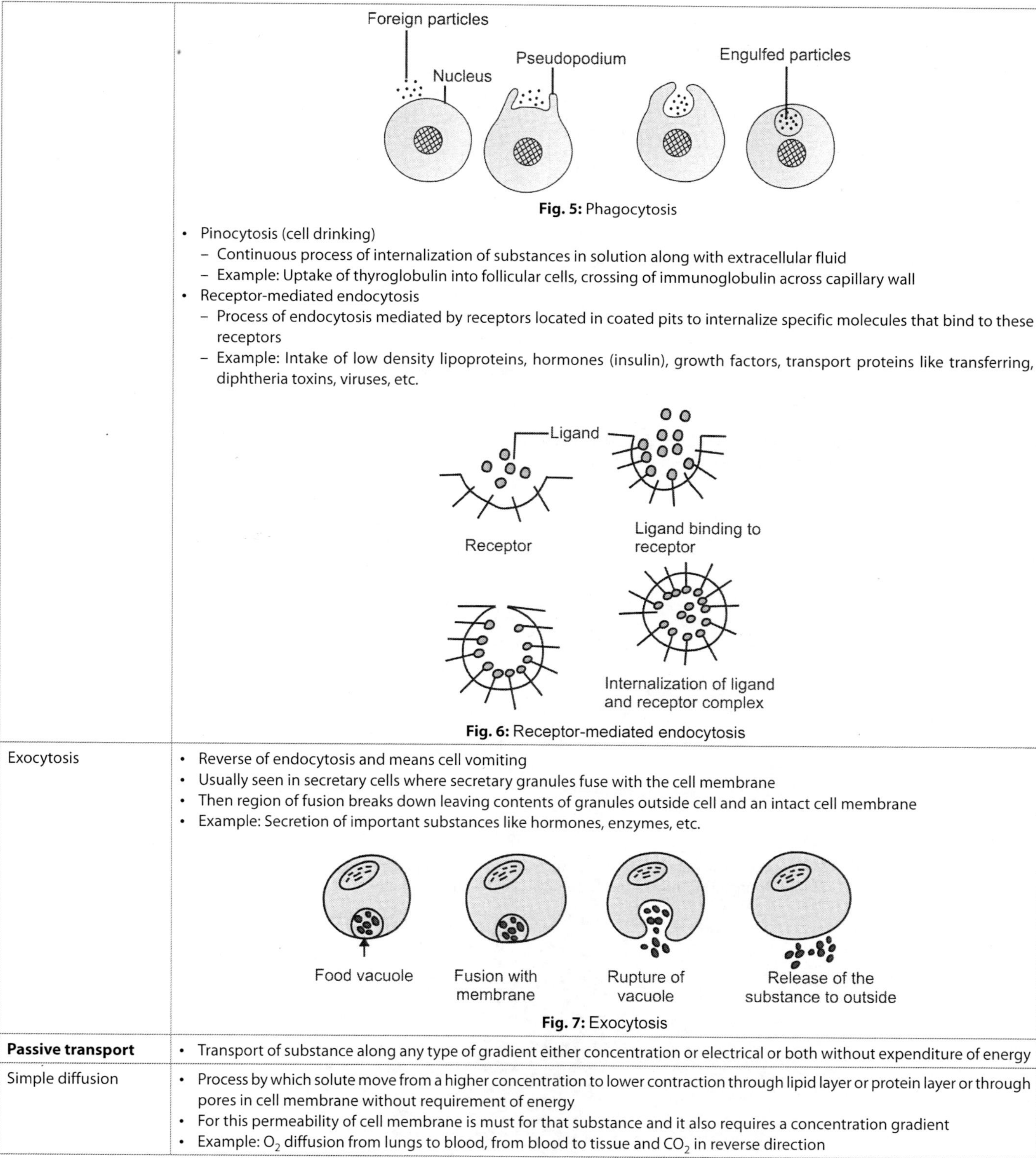


| | |
|---|---|
| | **Fig. 5:** Phagocytosis<br>• Pinocytosis (cell drinking)<br>– Continuous process of internalization of substances in solution along with extracellular fluid<br>– Example: Uptake of thyroglobulin into follicular cells, crossing of immunoglobulin across capillary wall<br>• Receptor-mediated endocytosis<br>– Process of endocytosis mediated by receptors located in coated pits to internalize specific molecules that bind to these receptors<br>– Example: Intake of low density lipoproteins, hormones (insulin), growth factors, transport proteins like transferring, diphtheria toxins, viruses, etc.<br>**Fig. 6:** Receptor-mediated endocytosis |
| Exocytosis | • Reverse of endocytosis and means cell vomiting<br>• Usually seen in secretary cells where secretary granules fuse with the cell membrane<br>• Then region of fusion breaks down leaving contents of granules outside cell and an intact cell membrane<br>• Example: Secretion of important substances like hormones, enzymes, etc.<br>**Fig. 7:** Exocytosis |
| **Passive transport** | • Transport of substance along any type of gradient either concentration or electrical or both without expenditure of energy |
| Simple diffusion | • Process by which solute move from a higher concentration to lower contraction through lipid layer or protein layer or through pores in cell membrane without requirement of energy<br>• For this permeability of cell membrane is must for that substance and it also requires a concentration gradient<br>• Example: $O_2$ diffusion from lungs to blood, from blood to tissue and $CO_2$ in reverse direction |

*Contd...*

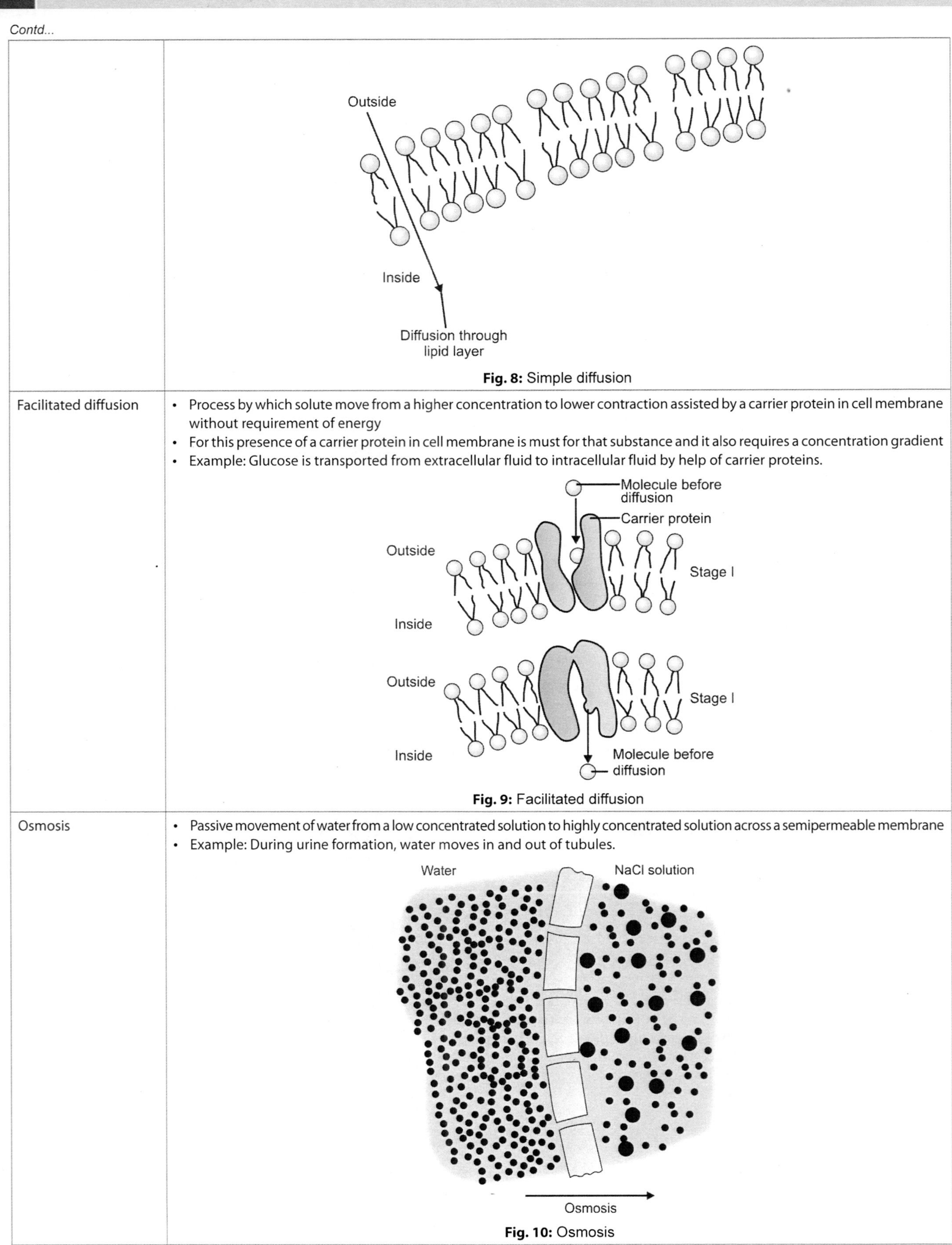


| | |
|---|---|
| | **Fig. 8:** Simple diffusion |
| Facilitated diffusion | • Process by which solute move from a higher concentration to lower contraction assisted by a carrier protein in cell membrane without requirement of energy<br>• For this presence of a carrier protein in cell membrane is must for that substance and it also requires a concentration gradient<br>• Example: Glucose is transported from extracellular fluid to intracellular fluid by help of carrier proteins.<br>**Fig. 9:** Facilitated diffusion |
| Osmosis | • Passive movement of water from a low concentrated solution to highly concentrated solution across a semipermeable membrane<br>• Example: During urine formation, water moves in and out of tubules.<br>**Fig. 10:** Osmosis |

*Contd...*

*Contd...*

| | |
|---|---|
| Filtration | • Process by which a fluid is forced through a membrane due to difference in hydrostatic pressure<br>• Example: Filtration occurs in glomerulus forming glomerular filtrate |
| Through channel or pores | • Channels are pores in cell membrane made up of large protein molecules 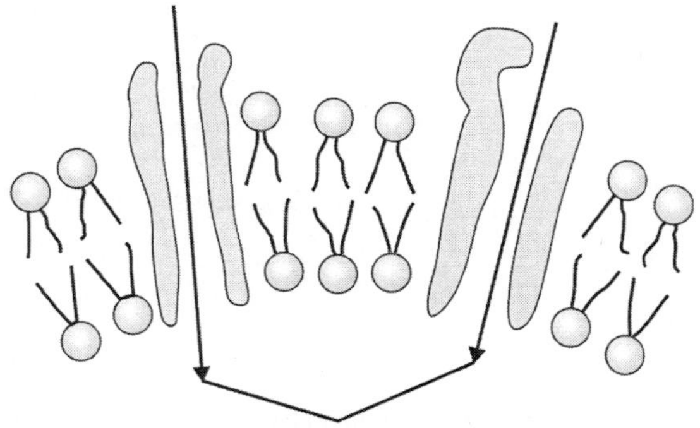<br>Voltage gated channel<br>Ligand gated channel<br>Diffusion through channel proteins<br>**Fig. 11:** Movements across channels<br>*Types*<br>i. Leakage channels<br>– Movements taking place at resting conditions<br>ii. Voltage gated channels<br>– Channels open when there is change in electrical potential across membrane<br>– Example: Calcium channels of sarcotubular system in a muscle<br>iii. Ligands or chemical gated channels<br>– Channel open on combining with a ligand (hormone) or a chemical substance<br>– Example: Sodium channels on neuromuscular junction open on combining with acetylcholine<br>iv. Mechanically gated channels<br>– Channels open by some mechanical factors<br>– Example: Sodium channels in a pacinian corpuscles open on pressure |

## Significance

- Transport of a substance along gradient is passive whereas transport of a substance against gradient requires energy and helps to maintain a balance between extracellular and intracellular fluids.

## 16. Melatonin.

Refer Question No. 17 June 2012 (RS2).

## 17. Polyamines.

- Polyamines are biologically important compounds synthesized from amino acids and contain multiple amino groups (Gr: Poly - Many).

*Examples*

- Putrescine, spermidine and spermine.

## Biosynthesis

- Putrescine is synthesized by decarboxylation of ornithine and later addition of propylamine derived from s-adenosyl methionine produces spermidine and spermine
- Rate limiting enzyme—ornithine decarboxylase (**Shortest half life—10 min**[Q]).

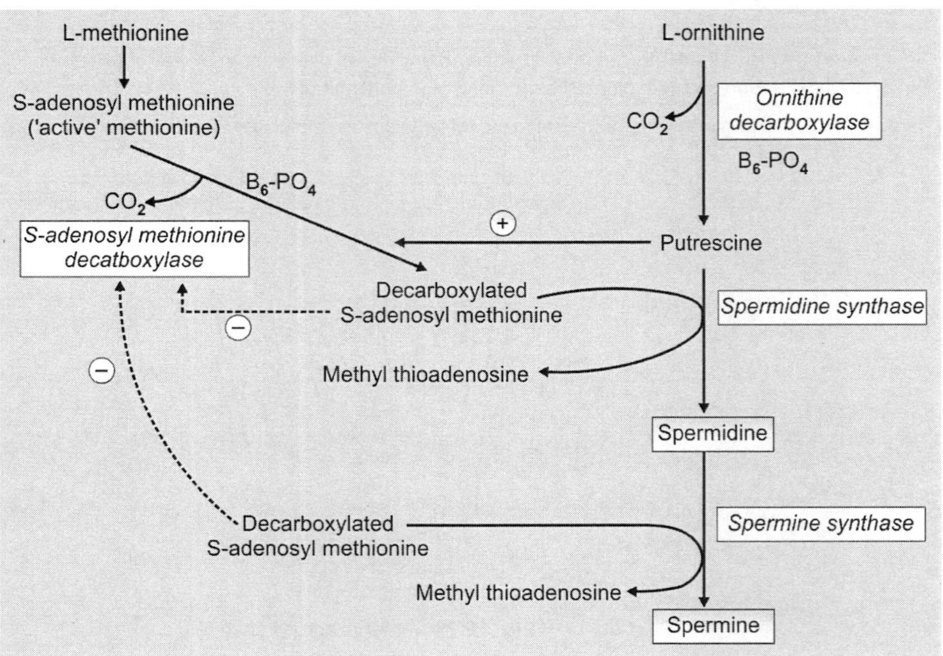


**Fig. 12:** Biosynthesis of polyamines



## Catabolism

- Polyamines are degraded by polyamine oxidase of liver peroxisomes
- Spermine is oxidized to spermidine and then to putrescine.

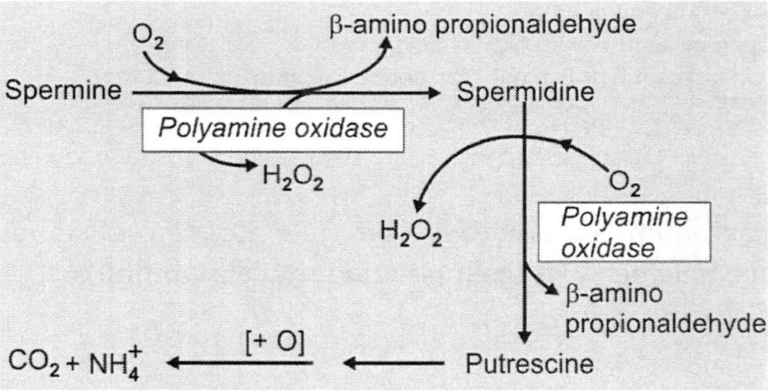


**Fig. 13:** Catabolism of polyamines

## Functions

- Polyamines are basic in nature and possess multiple positive charges; hence they are readily associated with nucleic acids
- Involved in synthesis of DNA, RNA and proteins
- Essential for cell growth and proliferation
- Inhibits some enzymes (protein kinase)
- Involved in stabilization of membrane structure (cell and cellular organelles).

## Biomedical Importance

| *Increased polyamine synthesis in cancer* | *Inhibitors of polyamine synthesis* |
|---|---|
| • In cancer, ornithine decarboxylase activity is increased and increased quantities of polyamines are excreted in urine<br>• Urinary excretion is increased 5–10 times but excretion fluctuates with clinical state and response to treatment and a good correlation has been found between urinary excretion and clinical course<br>• Diagnostically, putrescine is an ideal marker for cell proliferation whereas spermidine is used for assessment of cell destruction | • Drugs such as DFMO (difluoromethyl ornithine) which is a suicide inhibitor of ornithine decarboxylase are used in treatment of infections such as pneumonia caused by *Pneumocystis carinii*, kala azar and sleeping sickness caused by trypanosomes |

## 18. Serum electrophoresis.

- Electrophoresis is a simple, rapid, sensitive and a versatile analytical tool used to study and purify charged molecules.

| *Principle* | *Factors affecting* | *Techniques* |
|---|---|---|
| • Velocity of migration of each molecule in an electric field is dependent upon net charge on the molecule, strength of electric field and is inversely proportional to molecular weight | • Net charge on particles<br>• Mass and shape of particles<br>• pH of medium<br>• Strength of electrical field<br>• Properties of supporting medium | • Zone electrophoresis<br>– Paper electrophoresis (most common)<br>– Gel electrophoresis<br>• Isoelectric focusing<br>• Capillary electrophoresis<br>• SDS-PAGE (sodium dodecyl sulfate polyacryl amide gel electrophoresis)<br>• Immunoelectrophoresis<br>• Radioimmunoelectrophoresis |

## Applications (Diagnostic Importance of Electrophoresis)

- Separation of plasma proteins (simple technique) for detecting changes in proteins fractions and any abnormal proteins
  - In liver diseases: ↓ albumin and ↑$\beta$ and $\gamma$ globulins
  - In multiple myeloma: Extra band called M band separates $\beta$ and $\gamma$ globulin
  - In agammaglobulinemia: Faint v globulin band
- Separation of different types of hemoglobins for detecting hemoglobinopathies
- Separation of isoenzymes and lipoproteins
- Used in Southern blot, Northern blot and Western blot techniques.

## Serum Electrophoresis

- Serum electrophoresis is carried out separate plasma proteins
- A very small amount of serum is applied to a filter paper strip at one place
- Filter paper is placed in a buffer solution (pH 8.6 is chosen as it is greater than isoelectric pH of all plasma proteins thus they have negative charges and migrate towards anode)
- Current is applied for 1 hour through electrode dipped in each buffer compartments
- This causes separation of serum proteins into fractions which is visualized only after staining with a dye (Amido Black)
- After washing off excess stain, 5 characteristic blue bands corresponding to 5 different proteins are seen
- Width and intensity of each band is a measure of relative quantity of that plasma protein
- Results are used for converting bands into peaks
- Thus we obtain a picture like:

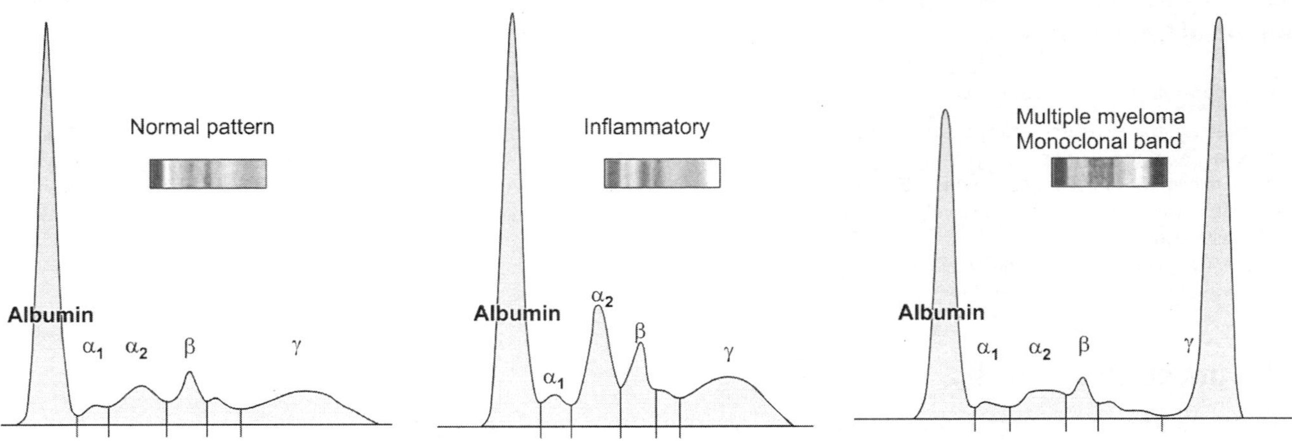


**Fig. 14:** Serum electrophoresis

## 19. Tumor markers.

Refer Question No. 6 June 2007 (RS2).



## 20. Hb as buffering agent.

- Hemoglobin is an important buffer system present in body.

### Location

- Erythrocytes.

### Mechanism of Action (Role of Hemoglobin as Buffer)

- Imidazole nitrogen of histidine present in globin component can act as acid or base to donate H ions or accept H ions
- Deoxygenated hemoglobin has more affinity for H ions
- At tissue levels, deoxygenated hemoglobin accepts H ions to form HHb which is later converted by back to hemoglobin by releasing H ions in lungs
- Also acts buffer system by forming carbamino-hemoglobin by interacting with $CO_2$
- This transport occurs with minimum change in pH (isohydric transport)
- Also serves to generate bicarbonate or alkali reserve by activity of carbonic anhydrase.

**Fig. 15:** Hemoglobin as buffer

## 21. Vitamin K—functions and requirement.

Refer Question No. 21 June 2012 (RS2).

## 22. Point mutation with two examples.

Refer Question No. 11 June 2005 (RS2).

# MBBS PHASE I EXAMINATION

## JUNE 2016

## (Revised Scheme 2 & 3)

## LONG ESSAYS

### 1. Give an account of cholesterol biosynthesis with its regulation. Add a note on atherosclerosis.

- Cholesterol is a sterol present in cell membranes, brain and in lipoproteins.

### Structure

- 27 carbon atom (derived from acetyl CoA) structure in form of a 4 ring structure with an –OH group at C3, a double bond between C5 and C6, methyl carbon at C10 and C13 and a side chain at C17.
- The ring present in cholesterol is a cyclopentanoperhydrophenanthrene(steroid) ring.

### Biosynthesis

| *Tissue sites* | *Subcellular site* | *Substrate* | *Product* |
|---|---|---|---|
| • Liver (major site), intestine, adrenal cortex, testis and ovaries<br>• Adipose tissue, muscle, aorta and neural tissues (low order of synthesis)<br>• Brain of newborn can synthesize cholesterol while adult brain cannot | • Microsomes and cytoplasm | • All 27 carbon atoms in cholesterol are derived from acetyl CoA<br>• Synthesis of cholesterol requires 18 acetyl CoA and after loss of 9 carbon atoms, it gives cholesterol<br>• NADPH | • Cholesterol |

*Steps*

| **Stage I: Synthesis of isopentyl pyrophosphate (source of Isoprenoid unit, the building blocks of cholesterol)** | |
|---|---|
| a. Formation of mevalonate from 3 acetyl CoAs | Acetyl CoA + Acetyl CoA<br>↓ Thiolase (→ CoASH)<br>Acetoacetyl CoA<br>↓ HMG CoA synthase (Acetyl CoA → CoASH)<br>HMG CoA<br>(β-hydroxy, β-methyl glutaryl CoA)<br>↓ HMG CoA reductase ($2NADPH + 2H^+$ → $2NADP^+$, CoASH)<br>Mevalonate (C-6) |

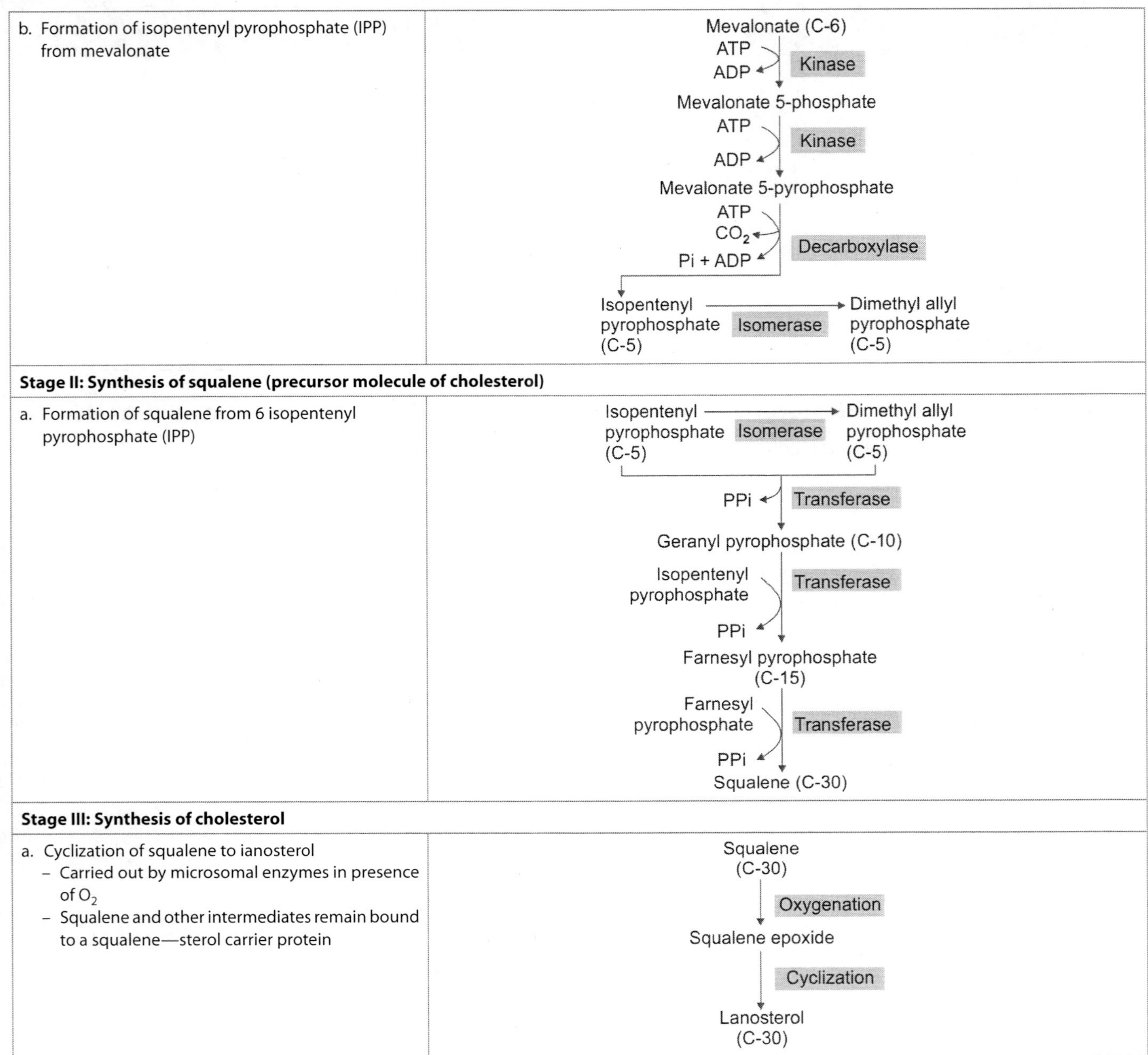

| | |
|---|---|
| b. Formation of isopentenyl pyrophosphate (IPP) from mevalonate | Mevalonate (C-6)<br>ATP → ADP (Kinase)<br>Mevalonate 5-phosphate<br>ATP → ADP (Kinase)<br>Mevalonate 5-pyrophosphate<br>ATP → $CO_2$, Pi + ADP (Decarboxylase)<br>Isopentenyl pyrophosphate (C-5) → (Isomerase) → Dimethyl allyl pyrophosphate (C-5) |
| **Stage II: Synthesis of squalene (precursor molecule of cholesterol)** | |
| a. Formation of squalene from 6 isopentenyl pyrophosphate (IPP) | Isopentenyl pyrophosphate (C-5) → (Isomerase) → Dimethyl allyl pyrophosphate (C-5)<br>→ PPi (Transferase)<br>Geranyl pyrophosphate (C-10)<br>Isopentenyl pyrophosphate → PPi (Transferase)<br>Farnesyl pyrophosphate (C-15)<br>Farnesyl pyrophosphate → PPi (Transferase)<br>Squalene (C-30) |
| **Stage III: Synthesis of cholesterol** | |
| a. Cyclization of squalene to ianosterol<br>- Carried out by microsomal enzymes in presence of $O_2$<br>- Squalene and other intermediates remain bound to a squalene—sterol carrier protein | Squalene (C-30)<br>↓ Oxygenation<br>Squalene epoxide<br>↓ Cyclization<br>Lanosterol (C-30) |

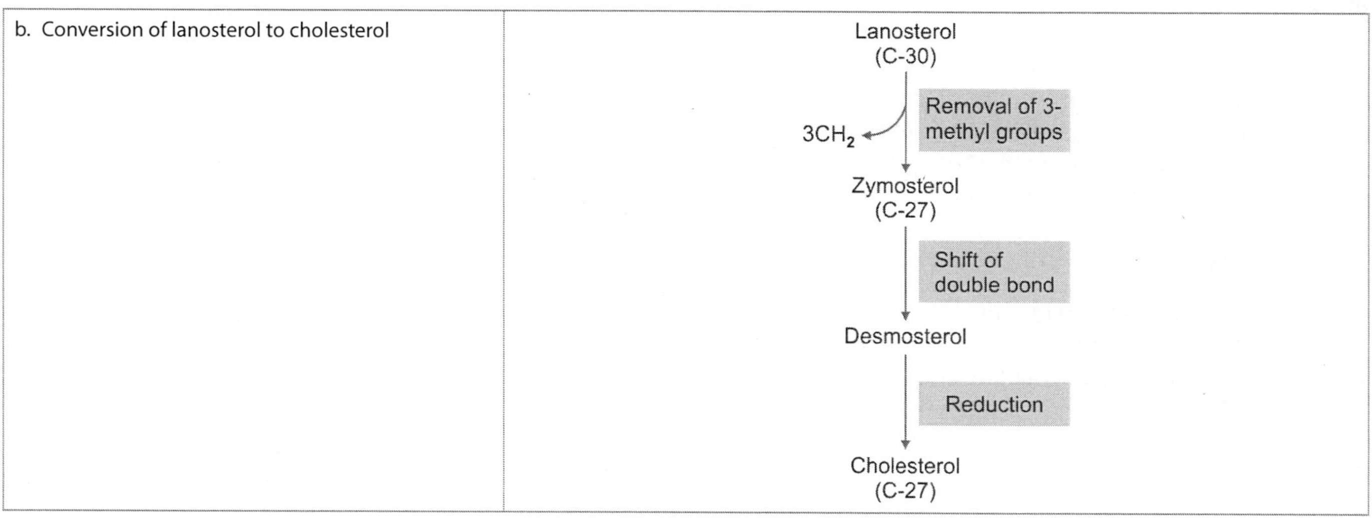


## Energetics

Cholesterol synthesis requires energy only for synthesis IPP, i.e. in stage I

| *Step* | *Enzyme* | *Mechanism* | *ATPs used* |
|---|---|---|---|
| Mevalonate → 5-Phosphomevalonate | Mevalonate kinase | Oxidative phosphorylation | – 1 ATP |
| 5-Phosphomevalonate → 5-Pyrophospho-mevalonate | Phosphomevalonate kinase | Oxidative phosphorylation | – 1 ATP |
| 5-Pyrophosphomevalonate → Isopentenyl pyrophosphate | Pyrophosphomevalonate decarboxylase | Oxidative phosphorylation | – 1 ATP |
| | | Total | – 3 ATP |
| | Total for Cholesterol synthesis | | – 3 x 6 = –18 ATPs |

## Regulation of Synthesis of Cholesterol

Committed/rate limiting step: HMG CoA → Mevalonate

| *Enzyme* | *Regulation method* | *Activator* | *Inhibitor* |
|---|---|---|---|
| HMG CoA reductase (rate limiting enzyme) | Allosteric modulation | | |
| | Reversible covalent modification | Glucagon<br>Cortisol<br>(by phosphorylation) | Insulin<br>Triidothyronine<br>(by dephosphorylation) |
| | Competitive inhibition | | HMG |
| | Induction of synthesis | ↓ Serum LDL-cholesterol | ↑ Serum LDL-cholesterol |
| | Degradation of enzyme by enhancing of activity of HMG CoA hydroxylase | Cholesterol (feedback inhibition)<br>Fasting/starvation | — |

## Biological Significance

- Normal serum cholesterol level—150–225 mg/dL.

## Functions

- Cholesterol is a component of membranes and has modulating effect on fluid state of membranes
- Cholesterol is a poor conductor of electricity and helps to insulate nerve fibers
- Bile acids and bile salts which are important for digestion of fat are derived from cholesterol
- Cholesterol is precursor for synthesis of steroid hormones like glucocorticoids, andrognes, estrogens
- Vitamin $D_3$ is formed from cholesterol.

## Atherosclerosis

- A disease characterized by thickening or hardening of arteries due to formation of atheroma in inner wall of arteries (usually aorta, coronary and cerebral vessels)
- Atheroma, is a collection of lipid, cholesterol (both free and esterified), collagen, fibrous tissue, proteoglycans, calcium, etc.

*Causes*

| *Major constitutional risk factors* | *Major acquired risk factors* | *Minor risk factors* |
|---|---|---|
| • Age: Risk rises with age<br>• Sex: Men are more prone<br>• Genetic predisposition<br>• Familial and racial factors | • Hyperlipidemia<br>• Hypertension<br>• Smoking<br>• Diabetes mellitus | • Environmental influence<br>• Obesity<br>• Oral contraceptive use<br>• Lazy life style<br>• Type A personality |

| *Pathological changes* | *Prevention (lowering plasma lipid level by)* |
|---|---|
| • Slow luminal narrowing causing ischemia and atrophy<br>• Sudden luminal occlusion causing infarction necrosis<br>• Propagation of plague by formation of thrombi and emboli<br>• Formation of aneurysmal dilation and eventual rupture | • Dietary restriction on lipids<br>• Replacement of fat with PUFA<br>• Increased intake of dietary fibers<br>• Exercise<br>• Identification of risk factors and controlling them |

### 2. Describe the replication of DNA in eukaryotes. Mention its inhibitors.

Refer Question No. 2 June 2010 (RS2).

## SHORT ESSAYS

### 3. What are uncouplers? Mention the uncouplers of oxidative phosphorylation.

Refer Question No. 1 June 2010 (RS2).

### 4. Describe tryptophan metabolism.

- Tryptophan is an aromatic amino acid
- It is an essential amino acid which cannot be synthesized in body and its daily requirement has to be supplied only through diet.

## Metabolism

- Kynurenine (Kynurenine-anthranilate) pathway
  - Main pathway for metabolism of tryptophan

| *Principle organs* | *Substrate* | *Product* |
|---|---|---|
| Liver | Tryptophan | 2 molecules of acetyl CoA |

*Steps*

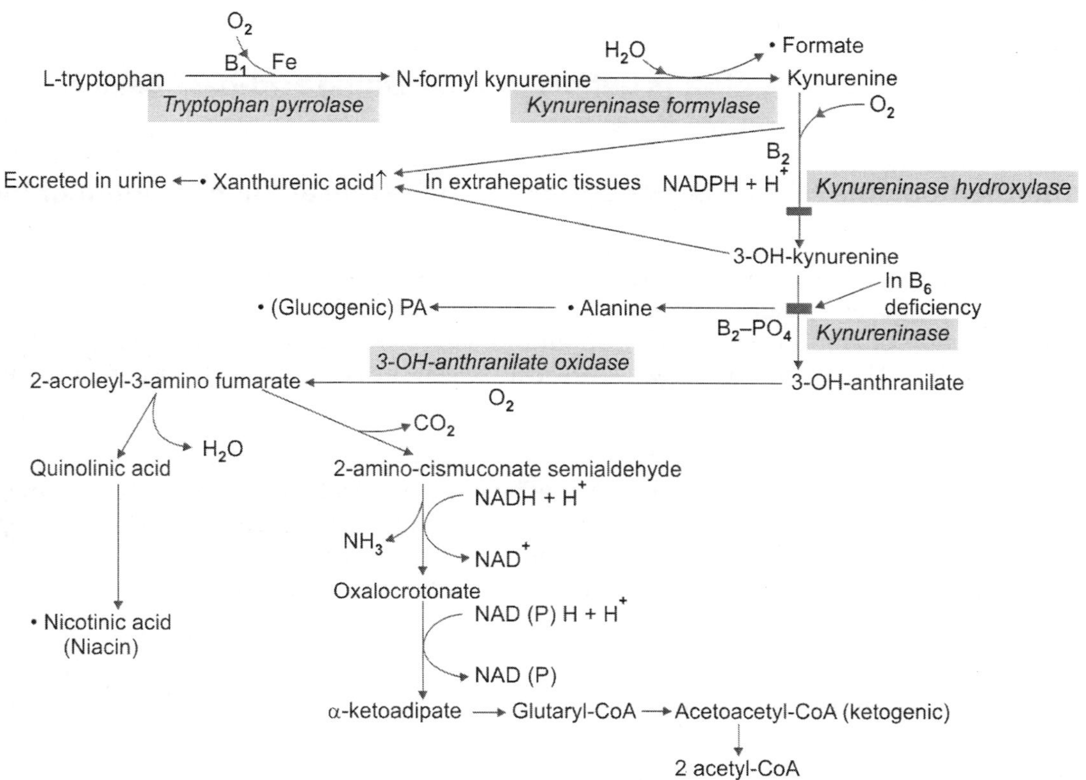


**Fig. 1:** Tryptophan metabolism

*Regulation*

| *Enzyme* | *Stimulant* | *Inhibitor* |
|---|---|---|
| Tryptophan pyrrolase (tryptophan oxygenase)—<br>A Fe-porphyrin metalloprotein | • Cortisol<br>• Trypatophan<br>(by induction of its synthesis) | • NADPH<br>(feedback inhibition) |
| Kynurenine hydroxylase | — | • Estrogen |

## Significance

- Kynureninase, an intermediate enzyme of tryptophan metabolism is a PLP dependent enzyme and is very sensitive to vitamin $B_6$ deficiency
- Lack of PLP blocks, kynureninase reactions thus leading to formation of xanthurenate, increased excretion of which serves as indicator of $B_6$ deficiency.

### 5. Define glycosaminoglycans. Describe its biomedical importance.

Refer Question No. 5 Dec. 2015 (RS2).

### 6. Isoenzymes.

Refer Question No. 1 Dec. 2007 (RS2).

### 7. Describe glycogenolysis. How it is regulated?

Refer Question No. 1 June 2007 (RS2).

**8. Recombinant DNA technology and its applications.**

Refer Question No. 2 June 2008 (RS2).

**9. What are buffers? Explain the plasma buffers in maintaining acid-base balance.**

Refer Question No. 2 June 2012 (RS2).

**10. What is methemoglobin? How it is formed? Mention the causes for methemoglobinemia. How it is detected?**

- Methemoglobin is a hemoglobin derivatives which contains Fe in ferric state (instead of ferrous state)
- It is a true oxidation product of Hb and is also called as oxidized hemoglobin
- For biological function of Hb to carry $O_2$, iron should remain in ferrous ($Fe^{2+}$) state which when oxidized to methemoglobin (with $Fe^{3+}$) is unable to bind to $O_2$ because oxygen site is occupied by a water molecule.

## Formation

- Normally in living system, Hb is spontaneously converted meth-Hb by hydrogen peroxide ($H_2O_2$), free radicals and drugs/poisons (e.g. chlorates, acetanilide, nitrites, nitrobenzene, antipyrin, phenacetin, sulfonals and sulphonamides) but is reconverted to Hb by enzyme methamoglobin reductase using NADPH
- Normally a small amount of methemoglobin is present in body (0.3 g/dL or <1% of Hb).



## Prevention

- Erythrocyte have 2 mechanisms for keeping methemoglobin level <1%

a. By reducing oxidant compounds such as $H_2O_2$ or superoxide before they react with Hb to form methemoglobin
   - Enzyme catalase, glutathione peroxidase with reduced glutathione are important reducing agents for reduction of $H_2O_2$

b. NADH cytochrome b5 methemoglobin reductase system
   - Consists of NADH, a flavoprotein named cytochrome $b_5$ reductase (known as methemoglobin reductase) and cytocbrome $b_5$
   - Reduces heme ferric ($Fe^{3+}$) back to ferrous ($Fe^{2+}$) state.

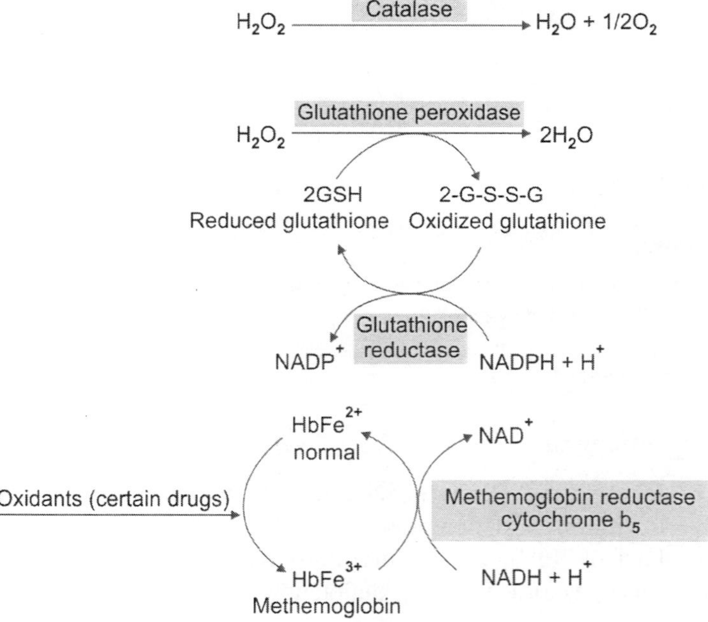


**Fig. 2:** Formation of methemoglobin

## Methemoglobinemia

- Methemoglobinemia is a disorder due to increased concentration of methemoglobin in blood
- Methemoglobin is a derivative of hemoglobin which contain iron in ferric form ($Fe^{3+}$) rather than ferrous form ($Fe^{2+}$)
- In this oxidized state, hemoglobin can neither bind nor transport oxygen
- Normal concentration of methemoglobin in blood is <1%.

*Causes*

| *Congenital (inherited)* | *Acquired (toxic)* |
|---|---|
| a. Famililal methemoglobinemia<br>– Autosomal recessive disorder due to absence (due to mutation) or deficient function of enzyme methemoglobin reductase (enzyme normally reduces $Fe^{3+}$ to $Fe^{2+}$)<br>b. Due to inherited defect (Hb-M)<br>– An abnormal type of hemoglobin formed due to replacement of histidine F8 by tyrosine<br>– Phenolate ion of tyrosine stabilizes iron of hemoglobin M in $Fe^{3+}$ form by forming tight ionic complex<br>c. Glucose-6-phosphate dehydrogenase deficiency<br>– Due to deficiency of NADPH in RBC required for conversion of methemoglobin to hemoglobin | a. Ingestion of certain drugs or chemicals<br>– Drugs like sulfonamides, acetaminophen, phenacetin, amyl nitrate, sodium nitroprusside and chemicals like aniline favor oxidation of $Fe^{2+}$ to $Fe^{3+}$<br>b. Environmental exposure<br>– Exposure to chemicals like nitrobenzene, nitrous oxide in industries<br>– Drinking of water containing nitrates |

*Clinical Features (Become Evident when Methemoglobin Level >10%)*

| *Concentration in blood* | *Clinical feature* |
|---|---|
| • 10–20% | Mild cyanosis |
| • 20–40% | Visible cyanosis, fatigue, dyspnea with activity |
| • 40–60% | Severe cyanosis, severe cardiopulmonary symptoms, tachycardia, tachypnea and depression |
| • >60% | Severe cyanosis, ataxia, dyspnea, loss of consciousness and death |

| *Diagnosis* | *Treatment* |
|---|---|
| a. Spectroscopic analysis of blood<br>– Demonstrates characteristic absorption pattern of methemoglobin<br>- Broad band at 490 mμ in green part near F line<br>- Narrow band at 540 mμ in green part<br>- Narrow band at 575 mμ in yellow part<br>- Band at 634 mμ in red part (most characteristic)<br>b. Electrophoresis<br>– Detects abnormal hemoglobin | a. Methylene blue<br>– 100–300 mg/day orally in mild cases or 2 mg/kg IV in severe cases<br>– Acts by activating NADH or NADPH dependent methemoglobin reductase<br>b. Ascorbic acid<br>– 200–500 mg/day<br>– Can also be used as reducing agent |

**11. What are restriction endonucleases? Give any two examples with their biomedical importance.**

Refer Question No. 8 Dec. 2015 (RS2).

**12. Describe how bilirubin is metabolized in the body. Write the normal values of serum bilirubin.**

Refer Question No. 8 June 2007 (RS2).

## SHORT ANSWERS

**13. Biochemical changes in starvation.**

Refer Question No. 11 June 2014 (RS2).

**14. Competitive inhibition of enzyme activity.**

Refer Question No. 3 June 2007 (RS2).

**15. Rappaport-Leubering cycle.**

Refer Question No. 7 June 2010 (RS2).

## 16. Laboratory diagnosis for hypothyroidism.

- Hypothyroidism is clinical disorder due to decreased circulatory levels of thyroid hormones ($T_3$ and $T_4$)
- Hypothyroidism is termed cretinism in children (associated with physical and mental retardation) and myxedema in adults (characterized by bagginess under eyes, puffiness of face, slowness in physical and mental activities)
- Characterized by reduced BMR, slow heart rate, weight gain, sluggish behavior, constipation, sensitivity to cold, dry skin, etc.

### Laboratory Diagnosis

| | *Primary hypothyroidism* | *Secondary hypothyroidism* |
|---|---|---|
| • Plasma thyroid hormone ($T_3$ and $T_4$) levels | Reduced | Reduced |
| • Free $T_3$ and $T_4$ levels (more sensitive) | Reduced | Reduced |
| • TSH levels | High | Low |
| • Response to TSH | Exaggerated | No response |

## 17. Nonenzymatic antioxidants.

Refer Question No. 6 June 2008 (RS2).

## 18. Balanced diet.

Refer Question No. 11 June 2015 (RS2).

## 19. Reference values.

Refer Question No. 22 Dec. 2007 (RS2).

## 20. Plasma proteins.

Refer Question No. 12 Dec. 2014 (RS2).

## 21. Tests of renal distal tubular function.

Refer Question No. 22 June 2017 (RS2).

## 22. Specific dynamic action.

Refer Question No. 19 June 2012 (RS2).

# MBBS PHASE I EXAMINATION
## DECEMBER 2016
## (Revised Scheme 2 & 3)

### LONG ESSAYS

**1. Explain the effect of different factors on the rate of enzyme catalyzed reactions.**

Refer Question No. 1 June 2013 (RS2).

**2. Discuss RDA, functions and deficiency manifestations of folic acid. How is it interlinked to vitamin $B_{12}$?**

- Folic acid is a water soluble, B complex group of vitamin
- Chemically known as pteroylglutamic acid.

| *Chemistry (composed of 3 constituents)* | *Source* | *RDA* |
|---|---|---|
| • Pteroic acid (pteridine group linked with PABA) linked to glutamic acid<br>• Forms yellow spear-shaped crystals slightly soluble in water and can form metallic salts | • Yeast and green leafy vegetable—spinach, lettuce and cauliflower (rich sources)<br>• Liver, kidney, milk, fruits (poor sources) | • Adults: 200 μg<br>• Pregnancy: 400 μg<br>• Lactation: 300 μg |

#### Biochemical Functions

*Coenzyme forms*

- Folic acid is not biologically active
- Active coenzyme forms of folic acid are:
  - Tetrahydrofolic acid (THFA/$FH_4$)
  - $N^5$ methyl tetrahydrofolic acid ($N^5$ $FH_4$)
  - $N^{5,10}$ methylene tetrahydrofolic acid ($N^{5,10}$ methylene $FH_4$)
  - $N^{10}$ formyl tetrahydrofolate ($N^{10}$ formyl $FH_4$)
  - $N^5$ formimino tetrahydrofolate ($N^5$ formimino $FH_4$)
  - $N^5$ formyl tetrahydrofolate ($N^5$ formyl $FH_4$)
  - $N^{5,10}$ methenyltetrahydrofolate ($N^{5,10}$ methenyl $FH_4$).

*Function*

a. Role in one carbon metabolism
   - Folic acid helps in transfer and metabolism of one carbon compounds
   - Coenzymes of folic acid are involved in transfer of one carbon groups like formate and methyl in reactions involving purine nucleotide, pyrimidine nucleotide and amino acid metabolism

| *Source* | *Carrier* | *Reaction* |
|---|---|---|
| Formyl | $N^{10}$-formyl THFA<br>$N^5$-formyl THFA | $C_8$ of purine |
| Formimino | $N^5$-formimino THFA | FIGLU → Glutamate<br>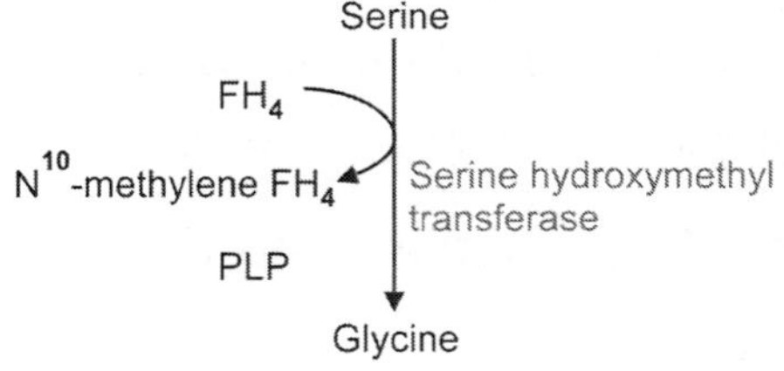 |
| Methenyl | $N^5$, $N^{10}$-methenyl THFA | $C_2$ of purine |
| Methylene | $N^5$, $N^{10}$-methylene THFA | Serine → Glycine<br>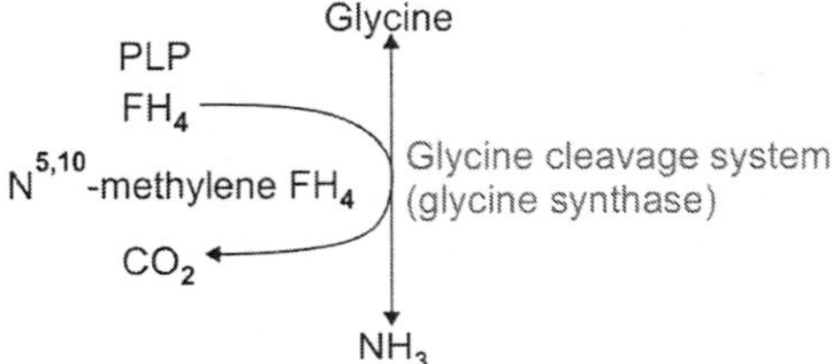<br>Glycine → $NH_3$<br>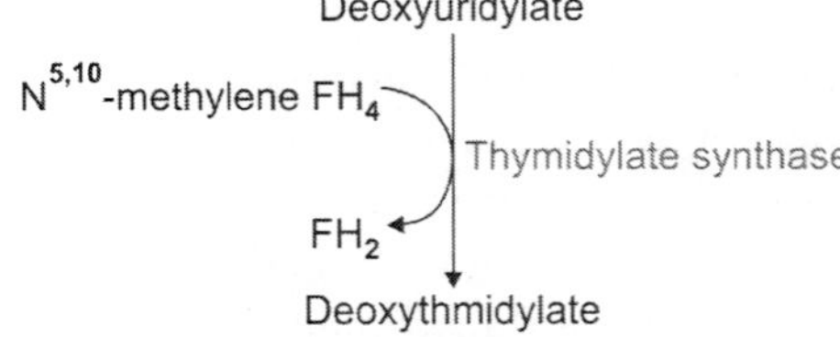<br>dUMP → dTMP |
| Methyl | $N^5$,-methyl THFA | Homocysteine → Methionine<br>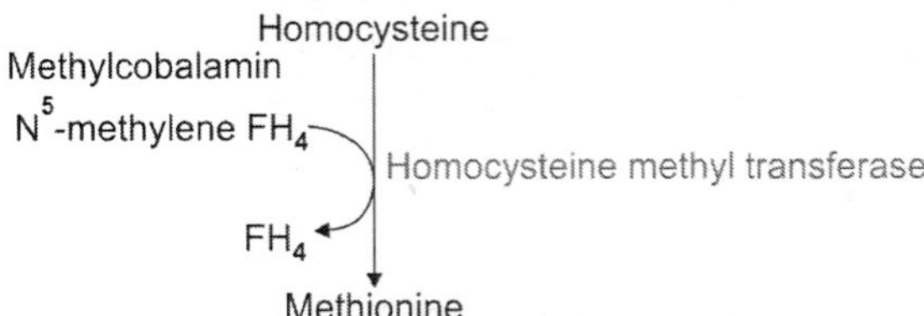 |

Hydroxymethyl $N^{10}$-hydroxymethyl THFA

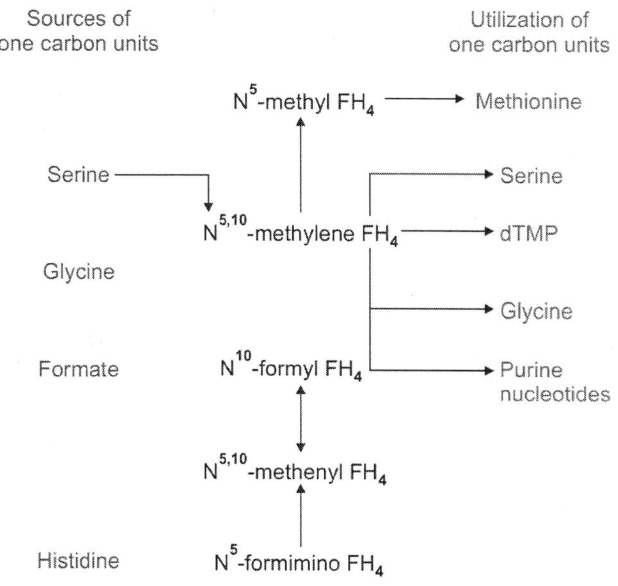


**Fig. 1:** Sources and utilization of one carbon atoms

b. Role in DNA synthesis
   – Folic acid is essential for synthesis of DNA because of its role in synthesis of purines and deoxythymidylate.

## Deficiency Manifestations

*Causes*

| *Dietary deficiency (MC)* | *Impaired absorption* | *Increased demand* | *Others* |
|---|---|---|---|
| • Inadequate intake in alcoholics, anorexia nervosa<br>• Overcooking of food | • Tropial sprue, celiac disease<br>• Drugs (phenytoin, co-trimoxazole) | • Pregnancy<br>• Hemolytic anemia | • Dialysis<br>• Folate antagonist (methotrexate) |

## Clinical Features

a. Megaloblastic anemia
   i. Hyperchromic macrocytic anemia
      - Occurs due to lag in nuclear maturation than cytoplasmic maturation thus nucleus does not disappear
      - RBCs are large, highly basophilic, nucleated and contain little or no hemoglobin
      - These abnormal RBCs are readily trapped in spleen and destroyed and this hemolysis leads to reduction in RBCs life span
      - Thus there is reduced generation and increased destruction RBCs leading to anemia
      - Also associated with leukopenia and thrombocytopenia.
   ii. Glossitis
      - Megablastic changes in mucosa of tongue produces glossitis.
   iii. Paresthesia
b. Neural tube defects
   – Deficiency of folic acid during pregnancy may cause neural tube defects (birth defects involving brain and spinal cord) due to impaired and aberrant neural development.
c. Homocysteinemia
   – Folic acid deficiency increases homocysteine levels in blood which increases risk of coronary artery diseases.
d. Cancer
   – Folate deficiency contributes to etiology of bronchial carcinoma and cervical carcinoma.

## Interlinking of Folic Acid with Vitamin $B_{12}$

- Vitamin $B_{12}$ (methyl cobalamin) is essential for conversion of homocysteine to methionine and formation of $FH_4$ from methyl $FH_4$; in a reaction catalyzed by homocysteine methyl transferase
- In this reaction, circulating methyl $FH_4$ is converted to $FH_4$ which is either used for storage as folylpolyglutamate form or it is utilized for other reactions such as formation of methylene $FH_4$
- In vitamin $B_{12}$ deficiency, impaired conversion of methyl $FH_4$ to $FH_4$ results in accumulation of methyl $FH_4$. This is called methyl folate trap
- Methyl folate trap results in decreased availability of $FH_4$ and $FH_4$ derivatives that are needed for purine nucleotide and thymidylate synthesis
- Thus, vitamin $B_{12}$ results in secondary folate deficiency.

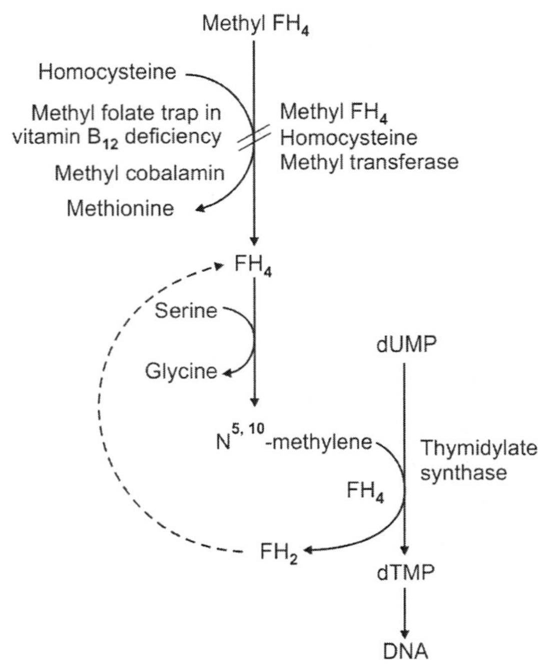


**Fig. 2:** Interlinking of folic acid with vitamin $B_{12}$



## SHORT ESSAYS

### 3. Define gluconeogenesis. Explain the key reactions of gluconeogenesis.

Refer Question No. 1 June 2009 (RS2).

### 4. What are essential fatty acids? What are the functions of essential fatty acids?

- Essential fatty acids are polyunsaturated fatty acids (fatty acids containing >1 double bond) which cannot be synthesized endogenously in the body because body enzymes cannot add a double bond on an existing double bond and at methyl end of molecule
- Thus they have to be supplemented in diet failing which may lead to growth retardation and other deficiency manifestations.

*Examples*

| | |
|---|---|
| a. Linoleic acid (2 double bonds) ($C18:2\ \Delta^{9,12}$) | • 18 carbon molecule with 2 double bonds between 9th and 10th and 12th and 13th carbon<br>• Also called 10-6 series as first double bond from methyl end is at 6th carbon<br>13 12 10 9<br>$CH_3 - (CH_2)_4 - CH = CH - CH_2 - CH = CH - (CH_2)_7 - COOH$ |
| b. Linolenic acid (3 double bonds) ($C18:3\ \Delta^{9,12,15}$) | • 18 carbon molecule of 10-3 series having 3 double bonds between 9th and 10th, 12th and 13th, and 15th and 16th carbon<br>• Most important essential fatty acid<br>16 15 13 12 10 9<br>$CH_3 - CH_2 - CH = CH - CH_2 - CH = CH - CH_2 - CH = CH - (CH_2)_7 - COOH$ |
| c. Arachidonic acid (4 double bonds) ($C20:4\ \Delta^{5,8,11,14}$) | • 20 carbon molecule of 10-6 series having 4 double bonds between 5th and 6th, 8th and 9th, 11th and 12th, and 14th and 15th carbon<br>• Can also be synthesized from linoleic acid by addition of acetyl CoA in presence of PLP<br>• Biologically most important fatty acid<br>15 14 12 11 9 8 6 5<br>$CH_3 - (CH_2)_4 - CH = CH - CH_2 - CH = CH - CH_2 - CH = CH - CH_2 - CH = CH - (CH_2)_3 - COOH$ |

| *Source* | *Daily requirement* |
|---|---|
| • Sunflower oil, safflower oil, cottonseed oil, groundnut oil and peanut oil | • 5–10 g/day |

## Functions

- Growth and reproduction
- Structural elements of tissues, gonads and mitochondrial membrane
- Lower serum cholesterol level by its esterification
- Prevent fatty changes in liver by incorporating into phospholipids
- Prolong clotting time and increase fibrinolytic activity
- Role in vision (docosahexaenoic acid (22:6n-3) present in retinal photoreceptor membranes is formed from linolenic acid and it enhances electrical response of photoreceptors to illumination)
- Components of phospholipids
- Precursor for synthesis of eicosonoids (prostaglandins are synthesized from arachidonic acid by cyclooxygenase enzyme system and leucotrienes are conjugated trienes formed from arachidonic acid in leukocytes by lipoxygenase pathway).

## 5. Briefly discuss the transamination reactions with examples.

Refer Question No. 2 June 2006 (RS2).

## 6. β-oxidation of palmitic acid.

Refer Question No. 1 Dec. 2008 (RS2).

## 7. Explain the synthesis of catecholamines.

- Catecholamines (epinephrine and norepinephrine) are biological amines synthesized from adrenal medulla and brain and so called since they contain catechol ring.

| *Source* | *Principle organs* | *Product (examples)* |
|---|---|---|
| Tyrosine | Adrenal medulla, brain | Ephinephrine, norephinephrine |

## Steps

a. Formation of dihydroxyphenylalanine
   - Reaction is catalyzed by tyrosine hydroxylase

b. Formation of dopamine
   - From dihydroxyphenylalanine by enzyme dopamine decarboxylase and PLP as cofactor

c. Formation of norepinephrine
   - From dopamine by reaction is catalyzed by dopamine β oxidase (dopamine hydroxylase); a copper-containing enzyme and requires vitamin C as a cofactor

d. Formation of epinephrine
   - From norepinephrine by transmethylation reaction catalyzed by phenylethanolamine N-methyl transferase (PMT) and S-adenosylmethionine is methyl donor

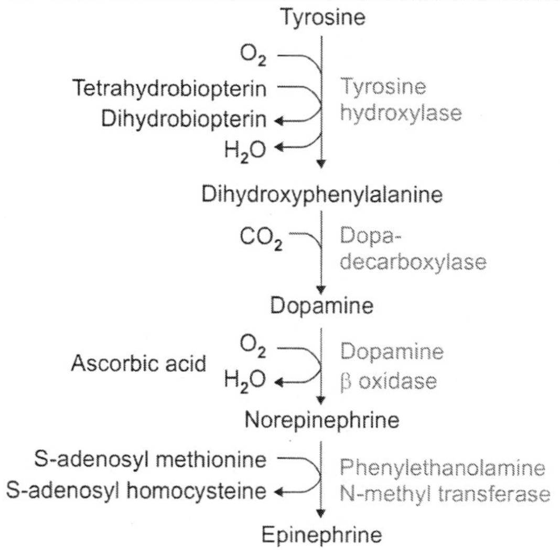

**Fig. 3:** Catecholamine synthesis

## Functions

| | *Epinephrine (adrenaline)* | *Norepinephrine (noradrenaline)* |
|---|---|---|
| a. CVS | | |
| i. Heart rate | Increased | Decreased |
| ii. Force of contraction | Increased | Decreased |
| iii. Excitability of heart muscle | Increased | No change |
| iv. Cardiac output | Raised | Reduced |
| v. Blood pressure | | |
| - Systolic | Increased | Increased |
| - Diastolic | Decreased | Increased |
| - Mean | Increased | Increased |
| vi. Total peripheral resistance | Decreased | Increased |
| vii. Blood vessels | Constriction of some but dilatation of blood vessels in muscles liver and heart | Vasoconstrictor |
| b. Respiration | Stimulated and bronchodilatation | Stimulated |
| c. Smooth muscle | | |
| i. Eye | Dilatation of pupil | Dilatation of pupil |
| ii. Gastrointerdiral tract | Contraction of sphincters, splenic capsule and gallbladder | Contraction of sphincters, splenic capsule and gallbladder |
| | Relaxation of general musculature | Relaxation of general musculature |
| iii. Bladder | Relaxes detrusor | Relaxes detrusor |
| | Contracts internal sphineter and trigone | — |
| iv. Uterus (in vivo) | Inhibits in late pregnancy and during labor and puerperium | Stimulates contractions |
| v. Bronchial smooth muscle | Relaxes | Relaxes |
| vi. Skin | Contraction of arrector pilli and increase secretion of sweat | Contraction of arrector pilli and increase secretion of sweat |
| d. Skeletal muscles | Severe contraction and quick fatigue | — |
| e. Metabolism | | |
| i. General | Increased $O_2$ consumption | Increased $O_2$ consumption |
| ii. Blood sugar | Increased | Increased |
| iii. Blood lactate | Increased | Increased |
| iv. Calorigenesis | Increased | Increased |
| v. Free fatty acids | Increased | Increased |
| vi. Plasma $K^+$ level | Initial rise followed by fall | Initial rise followed by fall |
| f. Blood | RBC count and Hb level increased | RBC count and Hb level increased |
| | Reduced coagulation time | Reduced coagulation time |
| | Increased eosinophil count | No change |
| g. Central nervous system | Stimulated | Stimulated |
| h. Hormones | | |
| i. ACTH | Increased release | Increased release |
| ii. Renin | Increased release | Increased release |
| iii. Glucagon | Increased release | Increased release |
| iv. Insulin | Decreased release | Decreased release |
| i. Secretions | | |
| i. Salivary | Increased | Increased |
| ii. Lacrimal | Increased | Increased |

## 8. Post-translational modifications.

Refer Question No. 10 Dec. 2009 (RS2).

## 9. Biochemical basis of gout and its features.

Refer Question No. 2 June 2007 (RS2).

## 10. Recombinant DNA technology.

Refer Question No. 2 June 2008 (RS2).

## 11. Iron absorption and transport.

Refer Question No. 11 June 2007 (RS2).

## 12. Causes and general features of porphyrias.

Refer Question No. 9 June 2014 (RS2).

# SHORT ANSWERS

## 13. Explain the relationship between $K_m$ and affinity.

- $K_m$ or Michaelis-Menten constant is the substrate concentration (moles/L) to produce half-maximum velocity in an enzyme catalyzed reaction
- It indicates that half of the enzyme molecules are bound with the substrate molecules when the substrate concentration equals the $K_m$ value.

### Relationship between $K_m$ and Affinity

- $K_m$ value is a constant and a characteristic feature of a given enzyme and represents affinity of substrate to the enzyme.

| *$K_m$ value* | *Affinity between enzyme and substrate* |
|---|---|
| • Low $K_m$ value | Strong affinity |
| • High $K_m$ value | Weak affinity |

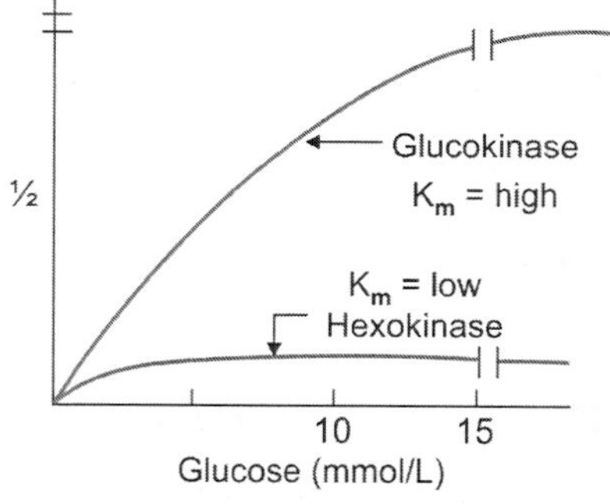


**Fig. 4:** Relationship between $K_m$ and affinity

### Significance

- $K_m$ is an index of affinity of enzyme towards the substrate and is characteristic for each enzyme.

## 14. What is meant by denaturation of proteins? What are the causes of denaturation of proteins?

Refer Question No. 17 June 2010 (RS2).

## 15. Galactosemia.

- Inherited disorder of galactose metabolism seen especially in infants.

| *Inheritance* | *Enzyme deficiency* | *Pathogenesis* |
|---|---|---|
| Autosomal recessive | • Galactose 1-P-uridyl transferase (most common and severe form)<br>• Galactokinase (less common and mild form) | • Inability to metabolize galactose 1-phosphate → its accumulation in liver → Inhibition of galactokinase and glycogen phosphorylase → accumulation of free galactose → galactosemia and galactosuria<br>• Excess galactose converted to galactitol by enzyme aldose reductase |

## Clinical Features

| *At birth (appear normal but later develops)* | *After 2 – 3 months* |
|---|---|
| • Failure to thrive<br>• Lethargy<br>• Vomiting and diarrhea (on ingestion of milk)<br>• Hypoglycemia due to:<br>  – Inability of conversion of galactose to glucose<br>  – Increased insulin secretion<br>  – Inhibition of phosphoglucomutase enzyme<br>• Hepatomegaly and jaundice in neonatal period | • Fatty liver leading to cirrhosis<br>• Mental retardation due to accumulation of galactose and galactose 4-phosphate in cerebral cortex<br>• Cataract due to:<br>  – Osmotic effect of galactitol and dulcitol produced by reduction of galactose in lens by enzyme aldose reductase<br>  – Decreased level of reduced glutathione |

## Laboratory Findings

| *Blood* | *Urine* |
|---|---|
| • Elevated level of galactose<br>• Hypoglycemia<br>• Decreased level of inorganic phosphate (due to its utilization for galactose-1-phosphate) | • Galactosuria—detected by paper chromatography, osazone test, mucic acid test<br>• Albuminuria<br>• Amino aciduria usually serine, alanine and glycine |

| *Treatment* | *Prognosis* |
|---|---|
| • Galactose free diet (removal of milk) improves most symptoms except mental retardation | • Non-fatal and most infant live up to puberty and adulthood as an alternate pathway for galactose utilization is developed |



### 16. Discuss the role of glutathione.

Refer Question No. 13 Dec. 2012 (RS2).

### 17. List the site inhibitors of electron transport chain.

Refer Question No. 5 June 2007 (RS2).

### 18. Protein-energy malnutrition.

Refer Question No. 9 June 2010 (RS2).

### 19. Marker enzymes of liver function test.

Refer Question No. 11 Dec. 2008 (RS2).

### 20. Alkalosis.

| *Sl. No.* | *Metabolic alkalosis* | *Respiratory alkalosis* |
|---|---|---|
| 1. | Primary $HCO_3^-$ excess (absolute or relative) | Primary $H_2CO_3$ deficit |
| 2. | $\frac{HCO_3^-}{H_2CO_3} = pH\uparrow$ | $\frac{HCO_3^-}{H_2CO_3\downarrow} = pH$ |
| 3. | Causes | |
| | • Excessive loss of HCl<br>  – Protracted gastric leavage<br>  – Pyloric obstruction<br>  – High intestinal obstruction<br>  – Pylorospasm<br>• Alkali ingestion and alkali administration<br>• Excessive loss of K leading to 'K' deficiency<br>• X-ray therapy, UV radiation and radiation therapy | • Stimulation of respiratory center:<br>  – CNS disease: Meningitis, encephalities<br>  – Salicylate poisoning<br>  – Hyperpyrexia<br>• Other causes:<br>  – Hysteria<br>  – Apprehensive blood donors<br>  – High altitude ascending<br>  – Injudicious use of respirators<br>  – Some cases of hepatic coma |

Contd...

Contd...

| Sl. No. | Metabolic alkalosis | Respiratory alkalosis |
|---|---|---|
| 4. | Biochemical findings | |
| a. | In uncompensated phase | |
| | Disproportionate increase<br>• ($HCO_3^-$): increased<br>• ($H_2CO_3$): increased or normal<br>• $pCO_2$: increased or normal<br>• Ratio: increased<br>• Total $CO_2$: increased<br>• pH: increased | Disproportionate decrease<br>• ($H_2CO_3$): decreased<br>• ($HCO_3^-$): decreased or normal<br>• $pCO_2$: decreased or normal<br>• Ratio: increased<br>• Total $CO_2$: decreased<br>• pH: increased |
| b. | In fully compensated phase | |
| | • Total $CO_2$ is high but increase in ($HCO_3^-$) and ($H_2CO_3$) proportionate thus pH maintained | • Total $CO_2$ is low but decrease in ($HCO_3^-$) and ($H_2CO_3$) is proportionate thus pH maintained |
| 5. | Compensatory mechanisms | |
| a. | Primary: Respiratory<br>• Depression of respiratory center and hypoventilation leading to retention of $CO_2$ | Primary: Renal<br>• Decreased $H^+$-$Na^+$ exchange<br>• Decreased excretion of acid<br>• Decreased excretion of $HCO_3$<br>• Decreased excretion of $NH_3$<br>• Increased $K^+$ excretion<br>• $Cl^-$ retention |
| b. | Secondary: Renal<br>• Decreased $H^+$-$Na^+$ exchange<br>• Decreased $NH_3$ formation<br>• Decreased bicarbonate reabsorption<br>• Increased $K^+$ excretion<br>• $Cl^-$ retention | Secondary: Respiratory<br>• High pH and low $pCO_2$ produces hypoventilation and increases in $H_2CO_3$ |
| c. | Urinary findings<br>• pH of urine – Alkaline<br>• Decreased $NH_3$<br>• Decreased titratable acidity | Urinary findings<br>• pH of urine—alkaline<br>• Decreased $NH_3$<br>• Decreased titratable acidity |
| 6. | Other findings | |
| | • Low ionic $Ca^{2+}$ leading of tetany<br>• Ketosis and ketonuria<br>• $K^+$ depletion: Hypokalemia<br>• Kidney damage degenerative changes in tubules leading to $N_2$ retention and oliguria | • Low ionic $Ca^{2+}$ leading of tetany<br>• Ketosis and ketonuria<br>• $K^+$ depletion: Hypokalemia<br>• Kidney damage degenerative changes in tubules leading to $N_2$ retention and oliguria |

## 21. Diagnosis importance of serum protein electrophoresis.

Refer Question No. 18 Dec. 2015 (RS2).

## 22. RNA polymerases.

- RNA polymerases are key enzymes of transcription (biosynthesis of RNAs)
- It is a metalloenzyme containing zinc
- It does not possess endo- or exonuclease activity thus it has no ability to repair mistakes in RNA synthesized.

### Types (in Eukaryotes)

| | RNA polymerase I | RNA polymerase II | RNA polymerase III |
|---|---|---|---|
| • Location | Nucleolus | Nucleoplasm | Nucleoplasm |
| • RNA synthesized | rRNA (28S, 18S, 5-8S) | mRNA, small nuclear RNAs | tRNA, rRNA, snRNA, 7S RNA |
| • Inhibitors | | | |
| Actinomycin D | Yes | Yes | Yes |
| α-amanitin<br>(poison obtained from mushroom amanita phylloids) | No | Yes | Less sensitive |

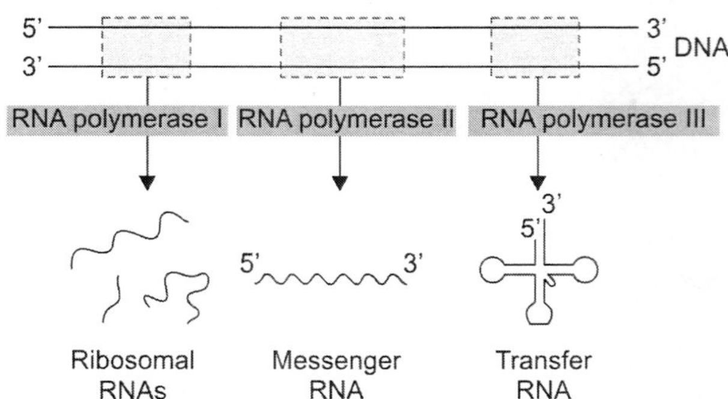


**Fig. 5:** Types of RNA polymerase

## Functions

- RNA polymerase enzyme initiating transcription, i.e. it is required for site specific sequence and it does not require primer to begin transcription
- It is also involved in unwinding of DNA
- It is a component of transcription bubble
- Helps in transcription coupled DNA repair.

# MBBS PHASE I EXAMINATION

## JUNE 2017

(Revised Scheme 2 & 3)

### LONG ESSAYS

**1. Describe the metabolism of phenylalanine. Add a note on its inborn errors.**

Refer Question No. 1 Dec. 2010 (RS2).

**2. Discuss the process of protein biosynthesis. Name three inhibitors of protein biosynthesis.**

Refer Question No. 2 June 2005 (RS2).

### SHORT ESSAYS

**3. Glycogen storage disorders.**

Refer Question No. 4 Dec. 2006 (RS2).

**4. Define isoenzymes. Describe its biomedical importance citing any three examples.**

Refer Question No. 1 Dec. 2007 (RS2).

**5. Describe the decarboxylation reactions of amino acids with four examples. Give its significance.**

Refer Question No. 2 June 2006 (RS2).

**6. Define detoxification. Give any four reactions of phase II detoxification.**

Refer Question No. 7 Dec. 2005 (RS2).

**7. What is HMP shunt? Give it significance.**

Refer Question No. 4 Dec. 2013 (RS2).

**8. Describe heme synthesis and add a note on its regulation.**

Refer Question No. 8 Dec. 2008 (RS2).

**9. Describe recombinant DNA technology. Mention its applications.**

Refer Question No. 2 June 2008 (RS2).

**10. Define biological value of protein. What do you mean by complementary proteins? Give examples. What is the requirement of protein in diet?**

#### Biological Value of Protein

- Biological value is defined as the percentage of absorbed nitrogen retained in the body

$$\text{Biological value of protein} = \frac{\textit{Nitrogen retained}}{\textit{Nitrogen absorbed}} \times 100$$

| *Calculations* | *Biological value of food proteins* |
|---|---|
| • To determine biological value, group of albino rats (21 days old) are fed with protein-free diet for 10 days, followed by feeding diet containing 10% protein for a period of 4 weeks<br>• The nitrogen content in urine and feces are determined and from these the biological value is obtained using the formula | • Egg proteins—94<br>• Milk proteins—84<br>• Meat proteins—75<br>• Rice proteins—68<br>• Wheat proteins—58<br>• Bengal gram—58 |

*Significance*

- Biological value is index of nutritive quality of a protein
- High biological values indicates high quality of proteins and the protein is rich in essential amino acids.

*Disadvantages*

- Does not take into account loss of nitrogen during digestion.

## Complementary Proteins

- Complementary proteins are mixture of 2 or more incomplete proteins to provide biological value of a complete protein
- This is called supplementary action of proteins.

| *Principle* | *Examples* |
|---|---|
| • Nutritional value of a mixture of 2 or more proteins is usually more than the arithmetic mean of the individual values because of the mutual supplementary action of individual amino acids | • Biological value of proteins in cereals can be improved by the addition of pulses and leafy vegetable<br>• Biological value of wheat is 65 (deficient in lysine and threonine) and biological value of Bengal gram is 68 (deficient in methionine); however, the biological value of a mixture of wheat and Bengal gram together is 78 because of the supplementary action of foods |

*Significance*

- Supplementary action of foods allows to enhance the nutritive value of proteins of vegetable origin by appropriate combinations of foods
- Due to the consumption of mixed diets, dietary deficiency of essential amino acids is most uncommon.



## Proteins in Diet (Daily Requirement)

- Adult males 55 g
- Adult females 45 g
- Pregnant woman 55 g
- Lactating woman 65 g
- Children 2 g/kg

## 11. Define codon. What are the salient features of a genetic code?

Refer Question No. 2 June 2011 (RS2).

## 12. List any three trace elements with their biological function.

- Trace elements or micronutrients are nutrients (mineral) which are required in quantity <100 mg/day.

## Classification (Examples)

| *Essential* | *Possibly essential* | *Nonessential* |
|---|---|---|
| Iron, copper, iodine, manganese, zinc, molybdenum, cobalt, fluorine, selenium and chromium | Nickel, vanadium, cadmium and barium | Aluminum, lead, mercury, boron, silver, bismuth, etc. |

| Biochemical role of magnesium | Biochemical role of copper | Biochemical role of flourine |
|---|---|---|
| • Required for formation of bones and teeth<br>• Serves as a cofactor for several enzymes requiring ATP<br>• Necessary for proper neuromuscular function by maintaining neuromuscular irritability and directly acting on myoneural junction | • Essential constituent of several enzymes like *"MACinTACS (sounds like Macintosh)"*<br>– Monoamine oxidase<br>– Ascorbic acid oxidase<br>– Cytochrome oxidase<br>– Tyrosinase<br>– ALA synthase<br>– Catalase<br>– Superoxide dismutase<br>• Necessary for iron absorption and incorporation of iron into hemoglobin<br>• Lysyl oxidase (copper-containing enzyme) is required for conversion of lysine residues of collagen and elastin to allysine which are necessary for cross linking structural proteins<br>• Ceruloplasmin serves as ferroxidase and involved in conversion of $Fe^{2+}$ to $Fe^{3+}$ (transport form of iron)<br>• Necessary for synthesis of melanin and phospholipids<br>• Required for development of bone and nervous system<br>• Increases HDL, thus protects heart | • Necessary for proper development of bones<br>• Prevents development of dental caries by<br>– Forming a protective layer of acid resistant fluoroapatitie with hydroxyapatitie of the enamel and prevents tooth decay by bacterial acids<br>– Inhibiting bacterial enzymes and reducing acid production<br>• Inhibits activities of certain enzymes like sodium fluoride inhibits enolase of glycolytic pathway and fluoroacetate inhibits aconitase of TCA cycle |

## SHORT ANSWERS

### 13. Pellagra.

Refer Question No. 10 June 2013 (RS2).

### 14. Ketosis.

Refer Question No. 1 June 2011 (RS2).

### 15. Components of electron transport chain.

Refer Question No. 5 June 2007 (RS2).

### 16. Hartnup's disease.

Refer Question No. 16 June 2012 (RS2).

### 17. Lipoproteins.

Refer Question No. 6 June 2005 (RS2).

### 18. Mutagens.

- Mutagens are chemical compounds that induce changes in the DNA sequence
- If these changes in DNA are not repaired, it leads to mutations.

#### Examples

- Hydrazine (in edible mushrooms)
- Allyl isothiocyanates
- Aflatoxin (fungus growing on grains and peanuts)
- Alkylating agents—cause alkylation of nitrogen or oxygen residue in DNA bases
- Intercalating agent—gets incorporated between bases causing frame shift mutations
- Deaminating agents—cause deamination of DNA bases.

## 19. Okazaki fragments.

- Okazaki fragments are short, fragmented newly formed DNA located on the lagging strand during the DNA replication
- Discovered by the couple, Reiji and Tsuneko Okazaki.

### Principle

- DNA replication occurs in 5'-3' direction (i.e. as a continuous piece on the leading strand) thus on the lagging strand (3'5' direction), DNA is replicated in fragments.

**Fig. 1:** Okazaki fragments

### Features

- Located on lagging strand (3'-5' direction)
- Synthesized in fragments (100–200 base pair long in eukaryotes) (1–5 kb)
- Separated by ~120 nucleotide RNA primers and are unligated until RNA primers are removed
- Joined together by DNA ligase.

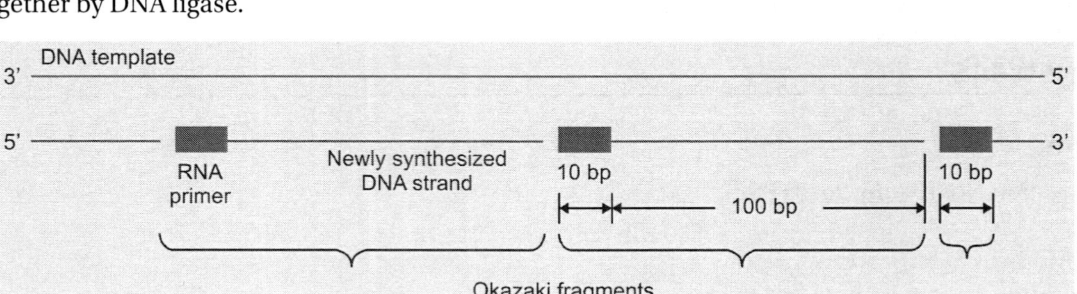


**Fig. 2:** Features of Okazaki fragments

### Significance

- Okazaki fragments eventually join to become single continuous strand
- They are responsible for maintaining our evolutionary development.



## 20. Provitamins.

- Provitamins are precursors of vitamins which are converted into vitamins in the body
- They are substance with little or no vitamin activity, but which can be converted to an active form by normal metabolic processes.

### Examples

| *Provitamin* | *Vitamin* |
|---|---|
| a. β-carotene | Vitamin A |
| b. Erogosterol | Vitamin $D_2$ (Ergocalciferol) |
| c. 7-dehydrocholesterol | Vitamin $D_3$ (Cholecalciferol) |

## 21. Cell cycle.

- Cell cycle is a process in which single parent cell produces two identical daughter cells with accurate duplication of the genetic material and cytoplasm
- The mechanism of cell division is almost same in all dividing cells and has been conserved during evolution.

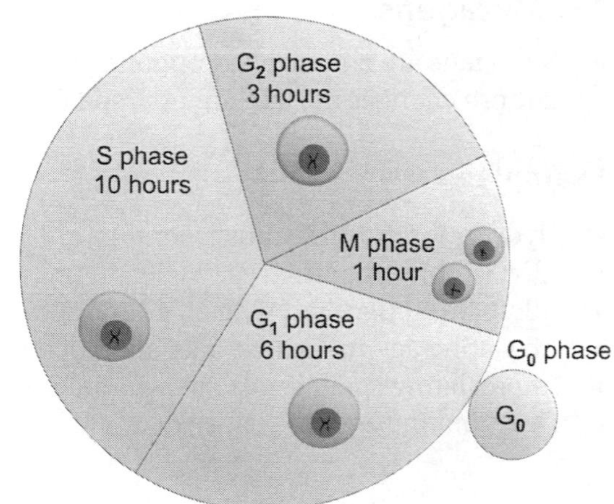


**Fig. 3:** Cell cycle

## Phases

| Phase | Description | Event | Duration |
|---|---|---|---|
| $G_1$ phase (G for gap) | • Gap between M phase and start of S phase<br>• Phase where cell determines its readiness to commit to DNA synthesis | Synthesis of RNA, proteins, lipids and carbohydrates required for S phase occurs during this period | 6 hours |
| S phase (S for stimulation of DNA synthesis) | Phase of DNA replication | • DNA replication<br>• Duplication of centrosome | 10 hours |
| $G_2$ phase | Phase that prepares cells for mitosis | • Determination of fidelity of DNA replication and corrections of any errors<br>• Synthesis of histones | 3 hours |
| M phase (M for mitosis) | Phase where nucleus and then rest of cell divides | • Replicated chromosomes are separated and packaged into 2 nuclei and cytoplasm is divided between the 2 daughter cells by cytokinesis<br>*Stages of mitosis*<br>a. *Prophase*: Chromatin condenses to form well-defined chromosomes and centrosome splits into 2 halves<br>b. *Prometaphase*: Nuclear envelope gets disrupted and nucleolus disappears<br>c. *Metaphase:* Chromosomes align at metaphase plate<br>Significance:<br>– Mitotic inhibitors (colchicines) can arrest cell cycle at this stage<br>– Karyotype analysis is done cells in mitotic stage<br>e. *Anaphase*: Sister chromatids separate and cytokinesis (separation of cytoplasm) is initiated<br>f. *Telophase*: Chromosomes decondense to form chromatin, nuclear envelope gets reformed, nucleolus reappears and cytokinesis (through process of cleavage) is completed | 1 hour |
| $G_0$ phase | Quiescent state where cell are not dividing | • Cells in $G_0$ may be recruited into cell cycle<br>• Progression on appropriate stimulation | -- |

## Regulation

| | | |
|---|---|---|
| Control proteins (regulate the cell cycle progression) | Cyclins | Cyclin A, cyclin B, cyclin C, cyclin E |
| | Cyclin dependent protein kinase | Cdk1, cdk2, cdk4, cdk6 |
| Check points | $G_1$ (restriction point or start point)—progression from $G_1$ to S phase | Cyclin D-cdk4 and cyclin D-cdk6 complexes |
| | S check point—initiation of DNA synthesis | Cyclin E-cdk2 and cyclin A-cdk2 complexes |
| | G2 check point—progression from $G_2$ to M phase | Cyclin A-cdk1 and cyclin B-cdk1 complexes |
| Mechanism | Regulation of protein phosphorylation | Phosphorylation of retinoblastoma protein and activation of E2 transcription factor by Cyclin-Cdk complexes |
| Regulators of Cyclin-Cdk complexes | Growth factor—stimulate cell proliferation (mitogens) or inhibit cell proliferation | • Epidermal growth factor (EGF)<br>• Transforming growth factor α (TGFα)<br>• Platelet derived growth factor (PDGF)<br>• Fibroblast growth factor (FGF) |
| | Inhibitors | • Cip1 protein— p21<br>• JNK4a protein— p16<br>(p53: Induces p21, delays cell cycle progression) |
| | Ubiquitin dependent proteases | Cyclins are inactivated by protein degradation during anaphase |

## 22. Tests to assess renal tubular function.

- Renal tubules of nephron are involved in reabsorption of:
  - Potassium, phosphates, glucose, amino acids and bicarbonates (proximal tubules)
  - Sodium, chloride, calcium and water and secretion of hydrogen and ammonium ions (distal tubules)
- Thus, tests for renal tubular function is based on assessing these functions of PCT and DCT.

Indications (not performed routinely and useful in evaluation of)

- Acute renal failure due to acute tubular necrosis
- Diabetes insipidius (polyuria)
- Renal tubular acidosis
- Other tubular disorders such as Fanconi syndrome, renal glycosuria, amino acidurias, familial hypophosphatemic rickets (vitamin D resistant rickets).

## Tests of Proximal Tubular Function

a. Serum potassium
   - Hypokalemia suggests impaired proximal tubular function.

b. Serum phosphate
   - Hypophosphatemia results from isolated tubular defect of phosphate reabsorption.

c. Renal glycosuria.

d. Amino aciduria (increased amounts of amino acids in urine)
   i. Renal aminoacidurias
      - Due to impairment of specific transport systems for specific amino acids (cystinuria, Hartnup disease, glycinuria and dibasic aminoaciduria)
      - By generalized renal tubular damage (nonspecific or generalized amino aciduria)

   ii. Overflow amino aciduria (exceeded renal threshold for amino acids)
      - Accumulation of one of the specific amino acids due to specific metabolic defect (phenylketonuria).

e. Tubular proteinuria
   i. B2 microglobulin, a low molecular weight protein is completely filtered by the glomeruli and reabsorbed from the proximal renal tubules
   ii. Urinary excretion of B2 microglobulin is a sensitive indicator of proximal tubular damage.

f. Proximal tubular bicarbonate reabsorption [Proximal renal tubular acidosis (type 2 RTA)]
   i. Isolated proximal tubular acidosis
      - Decreased plasma pH, decreased plasma bicarbonate, hypokalemia and hyperchloremia.

   ii. Fanconi syndrome
      - Glucosuria, phosphaturia, aminoaciduria and uric aciduria.

Revised Scheme 2 & 3

## Tests of Distal Tubular Function

a. Urine-specific gravity
   - Reflects concentration of dissolved total solids and specific gravity is linearly related to osmolality
   - It usually reflects changes in concentration of sodium chloride or urine volume, provided marked glycosuria or proteinuria are excluded.

| *Normal* | *Increased* | *Decreased* | *Fixed specific gravity (1.010)* |
|---|---|---|---|
| 1.016–1.022 | Diabetes mellitus and adrenal insufficiency | Diabetes insipidus | Chronic renal damage due to excretion of urine that is isoosmotic with plasma (because of impaired concentration and dilution of glomerular filtrate by damaged tubules) |

b. Osmolality measurements in plasma and urine

| | *Plasma osmolality* | *Urine osmolality* | *Plasma urine osmolality ratio* |
|---|---|---|---|
| Normal | 280–300 mOsm/kg water | 400–850 mOsm/kg water | >1.3 |
| Diabetes insipidus [due to impaired concentrating ability of distal tubules and collecting ducts either because of renal defect (nephrogenic diabetes insipidus) or impaired secretion of ADH due to pituitary or hypothalamic disease (central diabetes insipidus)] | — | Decreased | ≤1.0 |

c. Water deprivation test
   - Used to confirm diagnosis of diabetes insipidus, as well as cause for polyuria
   - Patient is asked to stop taking any fluid for 8 hours (patient should be under constant supervision during this period for danger of dehydration).

| | *Urine* | *Urine osmolality* | *Plasma osmolality* | *Urine-plasma osmolality ratio* |
|---|---|---|---|---|
| Normal person | Concentrated | >700 mOsm/kg | Does not exceed 295 mmol/kg | ≥2.0 |
| Diabetes insipidus | Not concentrated | <300 mOsm/kg | Exceeds 295 mmol/kg | < 1.0 (between 0.2 and 0.7) |

d. ADH stimulation test after water deprivation
   - Used to distinguish central diabetes insipidus from nephrogenic diabetes insipidus.

| | *Urine* | *Urine osmolality* | *Plasma osmolality* |
|---|---|---|---|
| Central diabetes insipidus (due impaired secretion of ADH) | Increased concentration | >700 mOsm/kg | — |
| Nephrogenic diabetes insipidus (impaired renal tubular function) | — | Not increased | Not decreased |

e. Urine acidification test (acid load test)
   - Used to confirm Type I distal renal tubular acidosis
   - Patient is given ammonium chloride orally in gelatin capsules (0.1 g/kg body weight) and urine samples are collected for next 8 hours at hourly intervals.

| | *Urinary pH* |
|---|---|
| Normal person | At least one specimen will have a pH <5.3 |
| Distal renal tubular acidosis | Rarely falls below 6.0 in random specimen and never falls below 5.3 |

# MBBS PHASE I EXAMINATION

## DECEMBER 2017

## (Revised Scheme 2 & 3)

### LONG ESSAYS

**1. Describe the reactions of glycolysis indicating the enzymes. Add a note on net yield of ATP under aerobic and anaerobic conditions.**

Refer Question No. 4 June 2014 (RS2).

**2. What are the sources, functions, deficiency manifestations and daily recommended allowance of thiamine?**

Refer Question No. 8 June 2005 (RS2).

### SHORT ESSAYS

**3. Describe the fate and formation of glycine. List four compounds formed from glycine.**

Refer Question No. 1 December 2005 (RS2).

**4. What are isoenzymes? Explain the clinical significance giving two examples.**

Refer Question No. 1 December 2007 (RS2).

**5. What are nitrogen producing substances in the body? Explain how they are excreted from the body.**

| Nitrogen producing substances in the body | Excretion of nitrogen from body |
|---|---|
| • Amino acids → Ammonia (urea cycle) → Urea (90%)<br>– Cysteine<br>– Serine<br>– Threonine<br>– Glutamine (purine and pyrimidine ring)<br>– Aspartate<br>– Alanine<br>– Aspartic acid<br>– Valine<br>– Leucine<br>– Isoleucine<br>– Arginine (nitrous oxide) | • Amino acids release nitrogen in form of ammonia which is detoxified by urea cycle<br>**For urea cycle**<br>Refer Question No. 1 December 2011 (RS2). |
| • Amino acids → Creatine → Creatinine<br>– Glycine<br>– Arginine | • Creatine phosphate is spontaneously converted into creatinine and excreted in urine |
| • Purines → Uric acid | • Uric acid is metabolic end product of purine metabolism which is excreted |
| • Pyramidines → Ammonia | • Ammonia is detoxified by urea cycle |

**Significance**

- An healthy adult is said to be in nitrogen balance or nitrogenous equilibrium when amount of intake of N in food (mainly as dietary proteins) is balanced by an excretion of an equal amount of N in urine (in form of urea mainly, uric acid, creatinine and creatine) and in feces (mainly as unabsorbed N).

### 6. Describe the fluid mosaic model of membrane structure.

Refer Question No. 4 December 2009 (RS2).

### 7. Name the ring structure present in cholesterol. Write the key regulatory step in the synthesis of cholesterol. Name four compounds derived from cholesterol.

**For regulation of cholesterol synthesis**

Refer Question No. 1 June 2016 (RS2).

**For compounds derived from cholesterol**

Refer Question No. 3 June 2009 (RS2).

### 8. Define point mutation. Explain the effects of point mutation.

Refer Question No. 11 June 2005 (RS2).

### 9. Briefly explain the lac operon concept.

Refer Question No. 10 December 2013 (RS2).

### 10. Discuss the features of genetic code.

Refer Question No. 2 June 2011 (RS2).

### 11. Discuss the regulation of water by rennin-angiotensin system.

Refer Question No. 9 December 2011 (RS2).

### 12. What is Wilson's disease? State the cause and treatment policy.

- Wilson's disease (hepatolenticular degeneration) is a rare genetic disorder of copper metabolism where copper is accumulated abnormal amounts in liver and lenticular nucleus of brain hepatolenticular degeneration.

| *Cause* | *Pathophysiology* | *Inheritance* |
|---|---|---|
| • Mutation in gene coding for copper binding P type ATPase in liver | • Defect in intestinal excretion of copper through bile → increased copper content in hepatocytes → inhibition of incorporation of copper to apoceruloplasmin → ceruloplasmin level in blood is decreased → accumulation of copper in liver and subsequently in other tissues of body (basal ganglia, cerebral cortex, cornea, lens, kidney) | • Autosomal recessive |

| *Clinical features* | *Biochemical findings* | *Treatment* |
|---|---|---|
| • Hepatitis or cirrhosis of liver<br>• Neurologic features are tremor, dysarthria, involuntary movements and dementia<br>• Copper deposits as green or golden pigmented ring at limbus of cornea (Kayser-Fleischer ring)<br>• Amino aciduria and glycosuria (Fanconi-like syndrome) | • Decreased serum copper<br>• Decreased ceruloplasmin (<20 mg/dL)<br>• Increased serum copper excretion in urine<br>• Marked accumulation of copper in liver biopsy specimens | • Diet low in copper<br>• Administration of D-penicillamine, a copper chelating agent |

## SHORT ANSWERS

### 13. Detoxification.

Refer Question No. 7 December 2005 (RS2).

### 14. Chemiosmotic hypothesis.

Refer Question No. 1 June 2010 (RS2).

### 15. Von Gierke's disease.

Refer Question No. 4 December 2006 (RS2).

### 16. Multienzyme complex.

Refer Question No. 1 June 2006 (RS2).

### 17. Rapoport Luebering cycle.

Refer Question No. 7 June 2010 (RS2).

### 18. Hypoalbuminemia.

Refer Question No. 8 December 2012 (RS2).

### 19. What are DNA probes? Mention the types DNA probes.

- A probe is defined as a single stranded piece of DNA (oligonucleotide), labeled (either with radioisotope 32P or with nonradioactive label), the nucleotide sequence of which is complementary to the target DNA.

| *Types* | *Features* | *Size* | *Labelling* |
|---|---|---|---|
| a. Oligonucleotide probes | Chemically synthesized | 15–50 nucleotides | End labeled |
| b. DNA probes | Cloned DNA or PCR products | 0.1–100 kb | End labeled or internally labeled during in vitro replication |
| c. cRNA (complementary RNA) probes or riboprobes | Single stranded molecules | 1–2 kb | Internally labeled during in vitro replication of cloned DNA |

**DNA probe**

- DNA probe or gene probe is a segment of DNA that is tagged with a label (i.e. isotope)
- They are synthesized using DNA polymerase.

*Types*

a. Radioactive labeled
   - Consists of 32P labeled nucleotide
   - Identified with photographic plate
b. Flourescent labeled
   - Identified when they emit light

Preparation of DNA probes (by random primer method)

- In double stranded DNA containing the sequence that is to act as the probe is denatured and an oligonucleotide sample containing all possible sequences of six nucleotides is added
- In the presence of Klenow fragment and four deoxyribonucleotides, one of the four deoxyribonucleotides is labeled
- Bound oligonucleotides act as primers for DNA synthesis

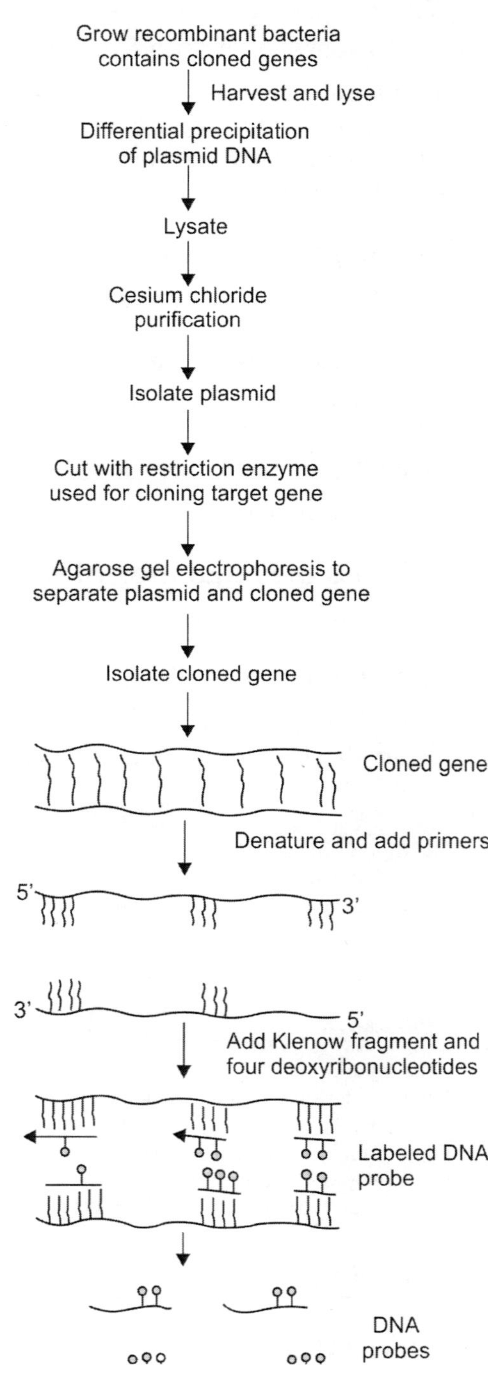


**Fig. 1:** Preparation of labeled probes

- Synthesized DNA is labeled and can be used as a probe to detect the presence of a complementary DNA sequence in a source DNA sample.

*Applications*

- In southern blot and northern blot to identify DNA and RNA fragments respectively
- In DNA fingerprinting
- In diagnosis of infectious and genetic disorders
- For determining specific target sequence in a DNA by hybridization
- Chromosome specific DNA probes tagged with fluorescent dye are used in fluorescent in situ hybridization.

## 20. Describe how plasma proteins are separated in the clinical laboratory.

Refer Question No. 18 December 2015 (RS2).

## 21. Discuss the nutritional role of milk and dairy products.

- Milk and daily products comprises milk, milk powder, yogurt (curd), butter milk, butter and cheese.

### Nutritive Value

| *Rich source of* | *Deficient in* |
|---|---|
| Calcium, phosphorus, riboflavin, high quality protein (Casein) and vitamin D | Iron, copper and vitamin C |

### Nutritional Role

| | |
|---|---|
| Proteins | • Chief protein of milk is casein which occurs in combination with calcium as calcium caseinogenate<br>• Other proteins are lactalbumin and lactoglobulin<br>• Milk proteins contain all the essential amino acids<br>• Animal milks contain nearly three times as much protein as human milk<br>• Human milk proteins contain greater amounts of tryptophan and sulfur-containing amino acids (especially cystein) |
| Lipids | • Fat content of milk varies from 3.4% in human milk to 8.8% in buffalo milk<br>• Human milk contains a higher percentage of linoleic acid and oleic acid<br>• Milk fat is a good source of retinal and vitamin D |
| Carbohydrate | • Carbohydrate in all milks is lactose or milk sugar which is found nowhere else in nature<br>• It is less sweet than cane sugar and is readily fermented by lactic acid bacilli<br>• Human milk contains more sugar than animal milk |
| Minerals | • Milk contains almost all known minerals needed by the body such as calcium, phosphorus, sodium, potassium, magnesium, cobalt, copper, iodine, etc.<br>• Milk is particularly rich in calcium; it is however a poor source of iron |
| Vitamins | • Milk is a good source of all vitamins except vitamin C |

### Significance

- Milk and milk products are the best and most complete of all foods
- It is a fine blend of all the nutrients necessary for growth and development of the young ones as it provides calcium, phosphorus and vitamin D for bone growth and high quality proteins for body growth.

## 22. Discuss the role of carbonic anhydrase in the acid-base regulation.

- Carbonic anhydrase is an metalloenzyme containing zinc.

### Location

- RBCs and renal tubular cells.

## Reaction

- Catalyses the formation of carbonic acid ($H_2CO_3$) from $CO_2$ and $H_2O$ which dissociates into hydrogen and bicarbonate ions.
  Carbonic Anhydrase

$$CO_2 + H_2O \longrightarrow H_2CO_3 \longrightarrow H^+ + HCO_3^+$$

## Role in Acid-Base Regulation

In regal tubules, carbonic anhydrase helps in regulation of acid-base balance as follows:

| | *Excretion of* | *Resorption of* |
|---|---|---|
| Acidosis | $H^+$ | $HCO_3$- |
| Alkalosis | $HCO_3$- | $H^+$ |

# SAMPLE PAPERS

# MBBS PHASE I EXAMINATION

## SAMPLE PAPER-1

### LONG ESSAYS

**1. Write about DNA replication and repair.**

**For Replication**

Refer Question No. 2 Oct. 2010 (RS2).

**DNA Repair**

- DNA proofreading is not 100% accurate hence errors in DNA replication are common which are repaired by DNA repair mechanisms.

*Types*

a. Base excision repair
- A type of DNA repair mechanism

Role
- Removal of non-DNA bases like uracil, hypoxanthine and xathine formed in DNA due to depuriation of cytosine, adenine and guanine respectively
- This depuriation may occur spontaneously or on exposure to radiation or chemicals

Enzymes involved
- DNA glycosylases, AP endonucleases, helicases, phosphodiesterase, DNA polymerase and DNA ligases

Mechanism
- Defective DNA is acted upon by specific N-glycosylase resulting in removal of non-DNA base
- This is followed by cutting of deoxyribose phosphate backbone near defect and removal of basic sugar by apurinic endonucleases
- Gap thus created is filled by action of repair DNA polymerase which inserts appropriate base and DNA ligase which seals phosphodiester bond

Significance
- Spontaneous depurination is very common phenomenon occurring at rate of 10,000 per cell per day therefore base excision repair mechanism is very important process preventing mutation in DNA structure

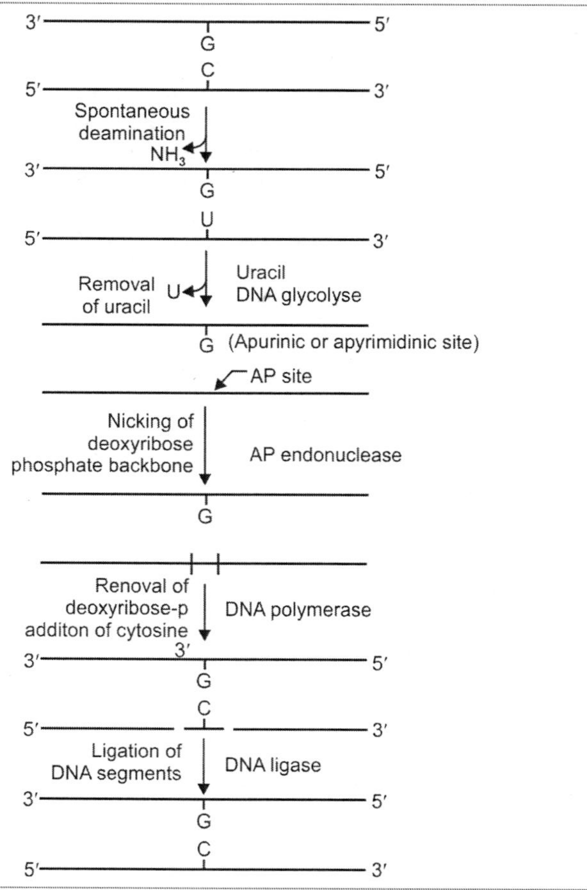

b. Nucleotide excision repair

Role
- Repairs defects like modification of certain bases, strand breaks, cross linkages (covalent bonding between adjacent thymine bases and adjacent thymine-cytosine bases) caused due to ultraviolet light, ionizing radiation and other environmental factors

Enzymes involved
- Exicision nucleases, DNA polymerase and DNA ligase

Mechanism
- After detection of defect in DNA sequence, damaged part is exposed by unwinding of DNA
- DNA on either side of damaged DNA is cut by enzyme excision nuclease which is later degraded
- Gap thus created is filled by regular DNA by enzyme DNA polymerase using undamaged strand as template and DNA ligase seals phosphodiester bond

Significance
- Defect in nucleotide excision repair mechanism results in rare autosomal recessive condition called Xeroderma pigmentosa

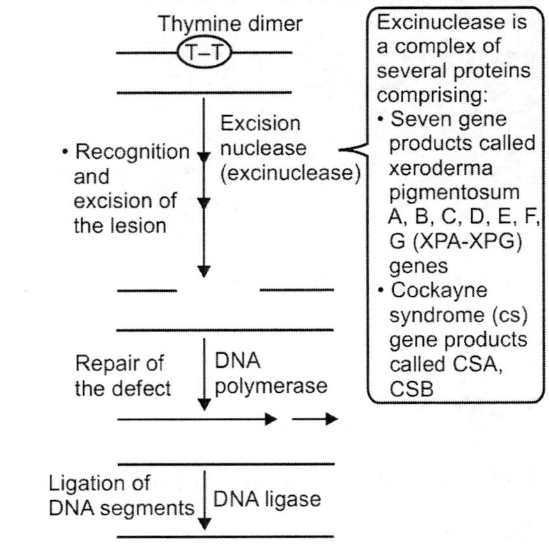


c. Mismatch repair

Role
- Repairs distortions caused by mismatching of bases
- For example, it corrects incorporation of cytosine instead of thymine opposite adenine

Enzymes involved
- Mismatched repair protein complex, DNA polymerase and DNA ligase

Mechanism
- Newly synthesized DNA strand is non-methylated which allows its identification by mismatch repair protein complexes
- Defectively synthesized DNA strand is cut of adjacent to methylated GC sequence by enzyme GC endonuclease which is then degraded
- Damaged DNA strand is now replaced by newly synthesized DNA

Significance
- Defect in mismatch repair is linked to etiology of hereditary non-polyposis colon cancer

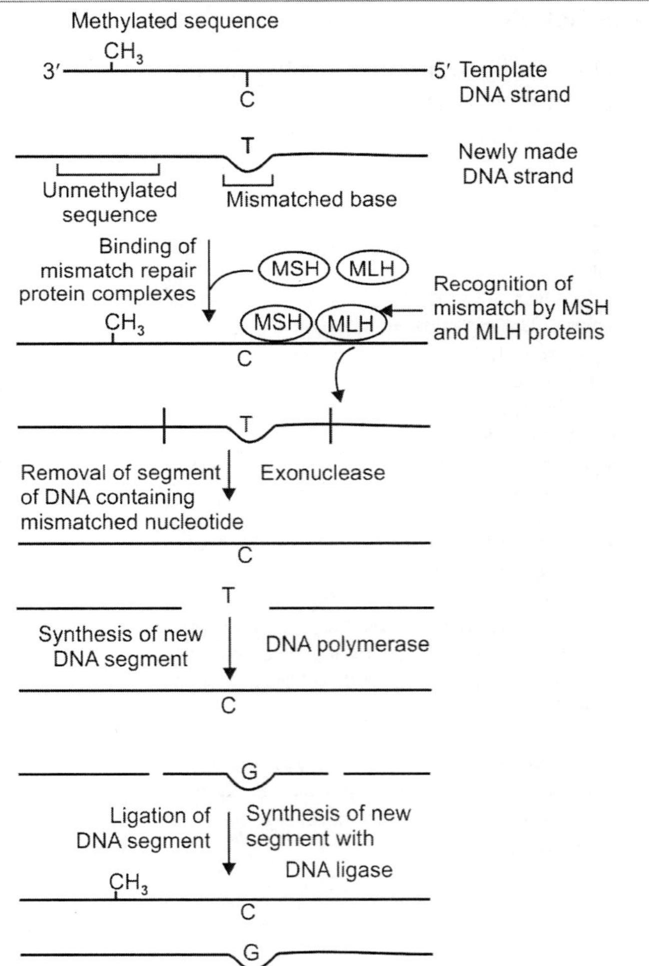

| | |
|---|---|
| d. Double stranded break repair<br>Role<br>– Repairs double stranded breaks caused by ionizing radiations, oxidative stress and chemicals<br>Enzymes involved<br>– Ku protein with helicase activity, DNA dependent protein kinase, exoncuclease and ligase<br>Mechanism<br>– Ku protein binds to both ends of DNA double stranded DNA segments and then recruits DNA dependent protein kinase which approximates 2 separate strands<br>– Ku protein then unwinds two ends of DNA and causes formation of base pairing between approximated DNA ends<br>– Extra nucleotides are removed by exonucleases and gap is filled by ligase<br>Significance<br>– Double strand breaks results in genetic recombination leading to translocation, broken chromosomes and finally cell death | Binding of $K_u$<br>$K_u$<br>Detection of lesion by $K_u$<br>Binding of DNA pk<br>DNA protein kinase (DNA–pK)<br>Approximation of DNA ends<br>Dissociation of DNA–pK<br>Unwinding<br>Unwinding by helicase activity of $K_u$<br>Base pairing<br>Removal of extra nucleotides<br>Nuclease<br>Filling of gap ligation<br>Ligase |
| e. Direct repair<br>Role<br>– Repairs DNA damage involving formation of alkylated base, pyramidine dimmers and modified bases<br>Enzymes involved<br>– Methyltransferases<br>Mechanism<br>– Alkylating agents cause modification of bases usually formation of O-methylguanine which preferentially base pairs with thyamine instead of usual cytosine<br>– Methyltransferases removes methyl group and becoming permanently inactivated<br>Significance<br>– If such substitutions not repaired results in base substitution mutations | |

## 2. Describe the regulation of enzyme activity.

- In a living biological system, there are various factors regulating the activity of a particular enzyme.

### Modes of Enzyme Regulation

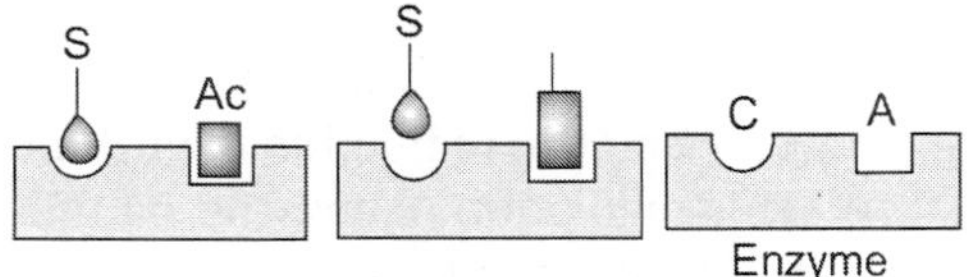


C = Catalyst site; A = Allosteric site; S = Substrate
I = Inhibitor; Ac = Activator

**Fig. 1:** Mechanism of regulation of enzyme activity

a. Allosteric regulation
   - It is a mixed kind of regulation where the activator or inhibitor binds to the enzyme at a special site on a different region known as allosteric site
   - Such enzymes are known as allosteric enzymes.

   Mechanism
   - The allosteric effector when binds to activator site, it increases the enzyme activity and is known as allosteric activator whereas if it binds to inhibitor site, it decreases the enzyme activity and is known as allosteric inhibitor
   - Binding of the inhibitor is reduced in presence of the excess substrate and substrate bound at the active site. Thus allosteric inhibition is effective when the substrate concentration is low, which is important metabolically.

   Features
   - Does not follow the normal Michaelis-Menten hyperbolic kinetics but gives a sigmoid kinetics

- Allosteric inhibitor doesn't bear similarly to the substrate
- Inhibition is partially reversible in presence of excess substrate
- Km value is increased and $V_{max}$ is reduced.

Example:

| *Enzyme* | *Allosteric inhibitor* | *Allosteric activator* |
|---|---|---|
| Phosphofructokinase (Glycoslysis) | ATP | AMP, ADP |
| Isocitrate dehydrogenase (TCA cycle) | ATP | ADP, NAD+ |
| Acetyl CoA carboxylase (Fatty acid synthesis) | Palmitate | Isocitrate |

- Feedback inhibition is a kind of allosteric inhibition where the end product itself allosterically inhibit an enzyme in the pathway to regulate the synthesis of the end product.

Example:
- HMG CoA is the rate limiting enzyme of the cholesterol biosynthesis pathway which is allosterically inhibited by the cholesterol.

b. Irreversible covalent activation of latent enzymes
- Some enzymes are secreted in an inactive form known as proenzymes or zymogens which are activated by irreversible covalent activation by breakdown of one or more peptide bonds
- These once activated cannot be reconverted to proenzymes form.

Example:

| Zymogen | Active enzyme |
|---|---|
| Pesinogen | Pepsin |
| Trypsinogen | Trypsin |
| Plasminogen | Plasmin |

c. Reversible covalent activation
- Some enzymes can be activated and inactivated reversibly as per the requirement by addition or removal of a phosphate or adenylate group
- This mechanism is under influenced of hormone and is mediated through cyclic AMP
- These reactions are catalyzed by cAMP dependent protein kinase and phosphatase.

Example:
- Phosphorylated form of the enzyme muscle phosphorylase is active and it can be rendered inactive by removal of the phosphate group.

d. Compartmentation of metabolic pathways
- Generally the catabolic and anabolic pathways for a particular molecule operate at different subcellular levels
- The pathways are operated by regulating the transport of the common intermediates across the cell organelles depending on the need of the body.

Example:
- Fatty acid oxidation takes place in the mitochondria whereas the enzymes for its synthesis are present in the cytosol.

e. Control of enzyme synthesis
- Most of the enzymes have a very short half life and are present in very low concentration in the body especially the rate limiting enzymes
- This helps in regulation of enzyme activity
- This regulation of enzyme synthesis is done by gene by means of induction (increased synthesis) or repression (decreased synthesis).

Types of enzyme (based on body concentration)
- Constitutive enzymes: Present in a fairly constant concentration all the time
- Adaptive enzymes: Whose concentration is raised or lowered as per the body requirement

Example:
- Insulin induces synthesis of enzymes involved in glucose catabolism like glycogen synthase, glucokinase, etc.
- Glucose represses the enzyme pyruvate carboxylase, a key enzyme in gluconeogenesis pathway.

f. Enzyme degradation
- Enzymes are degraded after their requirement is over
- This is especially rapid in case of the key regulatory enzymes that have short half life.

g. Isoenzymes
   – Multiple forms of a same enzyme also helps in regulation of the enzyme activity by virtue of their tissue specificity and their different Km and $V_{max}$ values for a same reaction.

## Significance

- Regulation of enzyme action is very essential for body integrity as uncontrolled enzyme action can lead to auto-digestion of bodily organs.

## SHORT ESSAYS

### 3. Metabolism of fructose.

- Fructose is an important dietary sugar, largely derived from the intestinal hydrolysis of sucrose, fruits and honey.

## Fructose Metabolism

*Catabolism of Fructose*

| | *Fructokinase pathway* | *Hexokinase pathway* |
|---|---|---|
| Tissue site | Liver | Muscles and adipose tissue |
| Intracellular site | Cytosol | Cytosol |
| Substrate | Fructose | Fructose |
| Products | Glyceraldehyde 3-phosphate<br>Dihydroxyacetone phosphate | Fructose 6-phosphate |
| Steps | Fructose<br>↓ Fructokinase (ATP, $Mg^{++}$ → ADP)<br>Essential fructosuria<br>Fructose–1–phosphate<br>↓ Aldolase B<br>Heriditary fructose intolerance<br>Glyceraldehyde + Dihydroxy acetone phosphate<br>Glyceraldehyde ↓ Triose kinase (ATP, $Mg^{++}$ → ADP)<br>Glyceraldehyde 3–phosphate ↔ Dihydroxy acetone phosphate<br>↓ Aldolase A/Aldolase B<br>Fructose 1,6–bisphosphate<br>↓ Fructose 1,6–bishosphatase ($H_2O$ → Pi)<br>Fructose 6–phosphate<br>↕ Phosphohexose isomerase<br>Glucose 6–phosphate<br>↓ Glucose 6–phosphatase ($H_2O$ → Pi)<br>Glucose | Fructose<br>↓ Hexokinase (ATP, $Mg^{++}$ → ADP)<br>Fructose 6–phosphate<br>↓<br>Pyruvate |
| Significance | Products formed from this pathway are either used for gluconeogenesis or glycolysis | Fructose 6-phosphate is metabolized similar to glucose 6-phosphate via glycolytic pathway to yield pyruvate |

## Fructose Biosynthesis

*Polyol Pathway*

| *Tissue site* | *Substrate* | *Product* |
|---|---|---|
| Seminal vesicles | Glucose | Fructose |

*Steps*

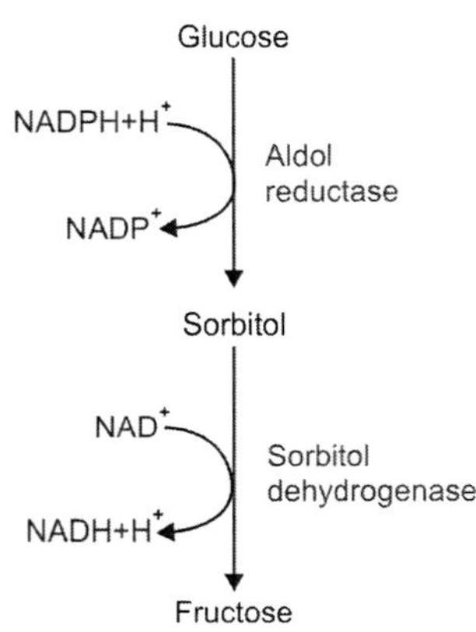


**Fig. 2:** Steps of fructose biosynthesis

*Significance*

- Under normal conditions, polyol pathway provides a means for formation of fructose from glucose which is secreted in seminal fluid as energy source for sperms
- In diabetes mellitus, sorbitol may accumulate causing complications like cataract.

## Fructose Intolerance

Inability to metabolise fructose

| | *Hereditary fructose intolerance* | *Essential fructosuria* |
|---|---|---|
| Deficient enzyme | Aldolase B | Fructokinase |
| Inheritance | Autosomal recessive | Autosomal recessive |
| Clinical features | • Seen in children<br>• Failure to thrive, hypoglycemia, liver failure<br>• Accumulation of fructose 1-phosphate allosterically inhibits liver glycogen phosphorylase to reduce glycogenolysis leading to phosphoglycemia | Benign and harmless |
| Diagnosis | • Urine—positive Seliwanoff's test paper<br>• chromatography<br>• Liver biopsy—decreased aldolase B | Urine—fructosuria |

## 4. Synthesis of triacylglycerol in adipose tissue.

- Triacylglycerol synthesis or lipogenesis is the synthesis of triacylglycerol through acylation of glycerol.

## Pathways

| | *Dihydroxyacetone phosphate pathway* | *Glycerol pathway* | *2-Monoacylglycerol pathway* |
|---|---|---|---|
| Tissue site | Adipose tissue and liver | Liver | Small intestine |
| Subcellular site | Cytosol and microsomes | Cytosol and microsomes | Cytosol and microsomes |
| Source of substrate | • Hydrolysis of triacylglycerol present in chylomicrons and VLDL<br>• De novo synthesis of fatty acids (in adipose tissue) from acetyl CoA that is derived from glucose. | • Fatty acyl CoA from de novo synthesis of fatty acids from acetyl CoA derived from glucose.<br>• Glycerol from adipose tissue lipolysis or breakdown of triacyl glycerol present in chylomicrons and VLDL (which is phosporylated to form glycerol 3-phosphate by enzyme, glycerol kinase) | • 2-monoacylglycerol derived from hydrolysis of dietary triacylglycerol by action of pancreatic lipase<br>• Fatty acid is activated to form acyl CoA using ATP by acyl CoA<br>• Synthetase |

**Steps**

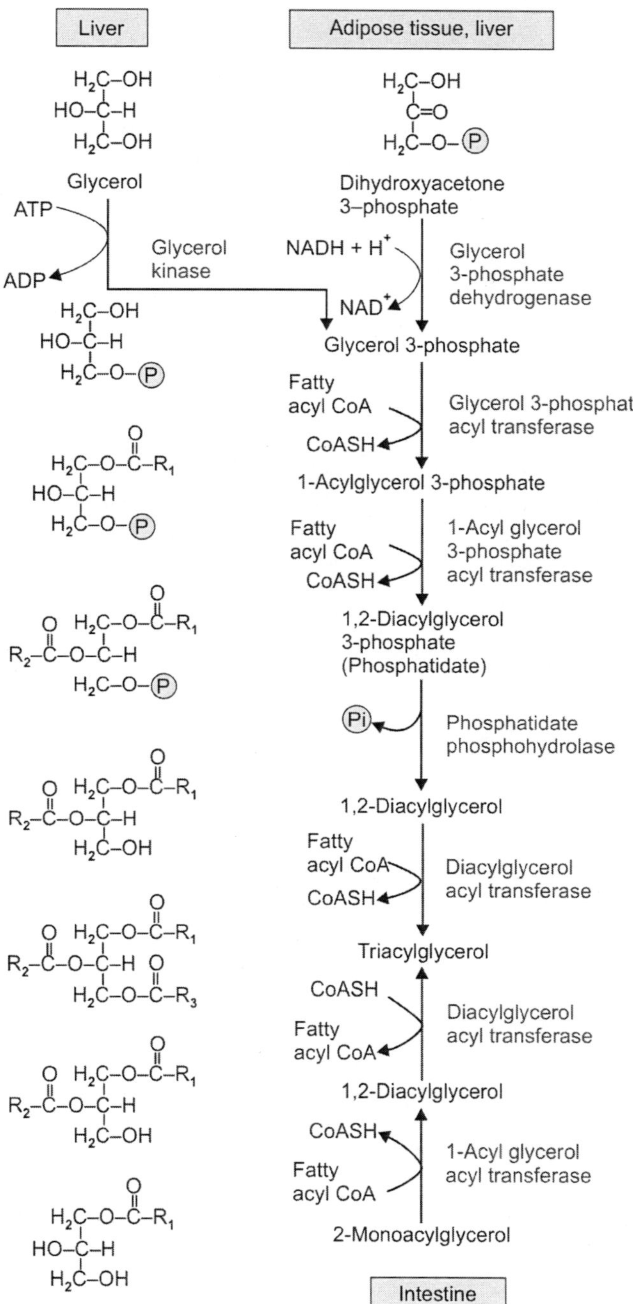


**Fig. 3:** Pathways of lipogenesis

*Regulation*

- High carbohydrate diet stimulates lipogenesis by increased availability of dihydroacetone phosphate (intermediate of glycolysis)
- Stimulation of HMP shunt and de novo synthesis of fatty acids also contribute to enhanced lipogenesis
- Insulin also stimulates glycolysis, pentose phosphate pathway and synthesis of fatty acids thus causing increased lipogenesis.

## Significance

- Lipogenesis is very important in storage of excess carbohydrate in form of fat in adipose tissue for later date use in starvation.

## 5. Jaundice.

- Jaundice is yellowish discoloration of sclera, skin and mucosa due to increased deposition of bilirubin
- Clinical jaundice becomes evident when bilirubin level exceeds 2 mg/dL.

## Classification (Etiological)

a. Hemolytic (prehepatic) jaundice.
b. Hepatocellular jaundice.
c. Obstructive (posthepatic) jaundice.

## Features

| *Features* | *Hemolytic* | *Hepatocellular* | *Obstructive* |
|---|---|---|---|
| Causes | Excessive RBC breakdown<br>i. Liver failure<br>ii. Renal disorder<br>iii. Hypersplenism<br>iv. Burns<br>v. Infections (malaria)<br>vi. Hemoglobinopathies (Hbs)<br>vii. Drugs inducing hemolysis<br>viii. Autoimmune diseases | Infective or toxic damage to liver<br>i. Infective hepatitis<br>ii. Alcoholic hepatitis<br>iii. Cirrhosis of liver<br>iv. Toxic chemicals | Obstruction to bile outflow<br>i. Gall stones<br>ii. Cancer of biliary system or pancreas |
| Location of pathology | Prehepatic | Hepatic | Posthepatic |
| Biochemical investigations | | | |
| a. Blood | Anemia, reticulocytosis and abnormal RBCs | Normal | Normal |
| i. Van der Bergh test | Indirect positive | Biphasic | Direct positive |
| ii. Total serum bilirubin | Elevated | Elevated | Elevated |
| iii. (Direct) conjugated | Normal | Elevated<br>(due to inability to completely excrete conjugated bilirubin) | Elevated<br>(due to obstruction to outflow of conjugated bilirubin through bile) |
| iv. (Indirect) unconjugated | Elevated<br>(due to excessive destruction of RBCs resulting in increased production of bilirubin which hepatocytes are unable to conjugate) | Elevated<br>(due to inefficient conjugation of bilirubin by injured hepatocytes) | Normal |
| v. Serum Alkaline phosphatase | Normal (5–13 KAo units/dL) | Slightly elevated initially (due to released from damaged hepatocytes) but marked elevation later (due to blockage of bile canaliculi by swollen hepatocytes preventing its excretion in bile) | Markedly elevated (due to complete obstruction of bile ducts) |
| vi. Plasma proteins | Normal serum protein levels and normal A/G ratio | Reduction of albumin level (due to less synthesis by damaged liver cells) and elevated globulin (in response to infection) and A/G ratio decreased | Usually normal albumin level but reduced in late stages, normal globulin level and A/G ratio normal |
| vii. Thymol turbidity | Nil | Markedly increased<br>(due to increased g globulin levels) | Usually slight |
| b. Urine | Normal | Deep yellow | Deep yellow |

| Features | Hemolytic | Hepatocellular | Obstructive |
|---|---|---|---|
| i. Urobilinogen | Increased (due to increased formation of stercobilinogen | Decreased (due to decreased stercobilinogen levels) | Absent (due to complete obstruction of bile outflow) |
| ii. Conjugated bilirubin | Absent | Present | Present |
| c. Stool | Dark brown | Pale | Clay colored |
| i. Stercobilinogen | Markedly increased (due to increased quantity of conjugated bilirubin reaching intestine) | Reduced (due to reduced conjugated bilirubin excreted through bile) | Absent (as conjugated bilurubin does not reach intestine) |
| ii. Fat | Normal | 40–50% increase (due to inadequate emulsification and absorption) | 40–50% increase (due to inadequate emulsification and absorption) |
| d. Liver function tests | Normal (because liver cells are normal) | Impaired (due to hepatic damage) | Normal or mildly impaired |

## 6. Discuss the interpretation of oral glucose tolerance test.

- Glucose tolerance is the capacity of body to store and metabolise glucose
- GTT is usually employed to asses ability of the body to tolerate the load of glucose administered.

### Types

| Oral GTT | Intravenous GTT | Stress induced GTT |
|---|---|---|
| • Standard GTT<br>• Routinely done by giving glucose orally<br>• Indicated for diagnosis of diabetes mellitus and to differentiate various types of glycosuria and hypoglycemia | • Indicated in impaired intestinal glucose absorption (gastrectomy or intestinal disease) or inability to administer glucose orally<br>• 20% of 25 g glucose solution is administered intravenously with rest of procedure same as for oral GTT | • Rarely done<br>• Indicated to detect latent or chemical diabetes. |

### Oral Glucose Tolerance Test

*Indications*

- Diagnosis of diabetes mellitus
- Differential diagnosis of glycosurias
- Diagnosis of gestational diabetes mellitus
- Assessment of prognosis during the follow up of treatment of diabetes mellitus.

*Patient Preparation*

- Patient should be normally active.
- Overnight fasting (12 hour after overnight meal)
- Carbohydrate rich diet (300 g/day) for 3 days
- Avoidance of drugs that affect blood glucose (diuretics and glucocorticoids).

*Procedure*

- On test day, morning fasting sample of blood and urine are taken
- Solution of 75 g glucose (1-1.5 g/kg body wt) in 250 mL of water is given to drink slowly to avoid vomiting
- Blood and urine samples are collected at ½ hour intervals for 2–3 hours
- Glucose content of blood is determined by glucose oxidase method and urine is checked for presence of glucose by Benedict's reagent
- A graph is plotted with blood glucose values on Y axis and time on X axis
- Curve thus obtained is called "Glucose tolerance curve".

*Interpretation*

| ***Glucose level*** | ***Fasting*** | ***Peak (30–120 min)*** | ***2 hours*** | ***Urine*** | |
|---|---|---|---|---|---|
| Normal | 60–90 mg% | <160 mg% | <140 mg% | Absent | 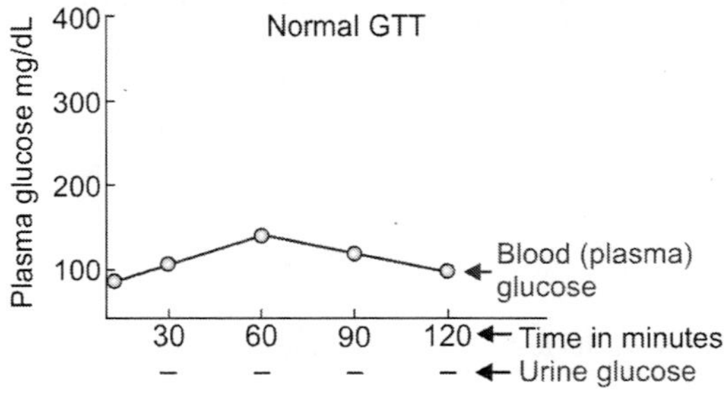 Normal GTT |
| Diabetes mellitus | >126 mg% | >200 mg% | >200 mg% | Present in some samples | 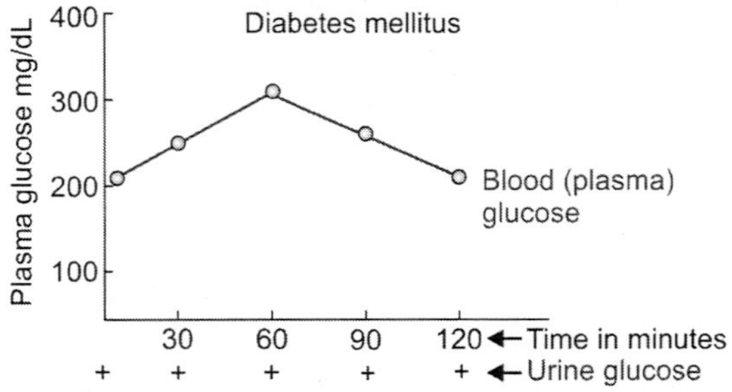 Diabetes mellitus |
| Impaired glucose tolerance | <126 mg% | <199 mg% | 140–199 mg% | May be present or absent | 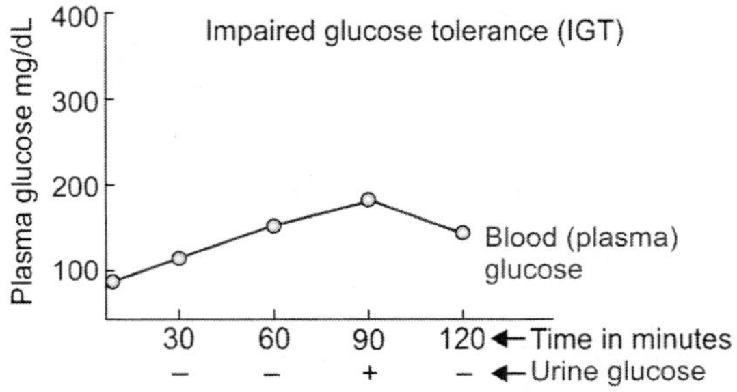 Impaired glucose tolerance (IGT) |
| Alimentary glycosuria | <110 mg% | >160 mg% | <140 mg% | Present in some samples | 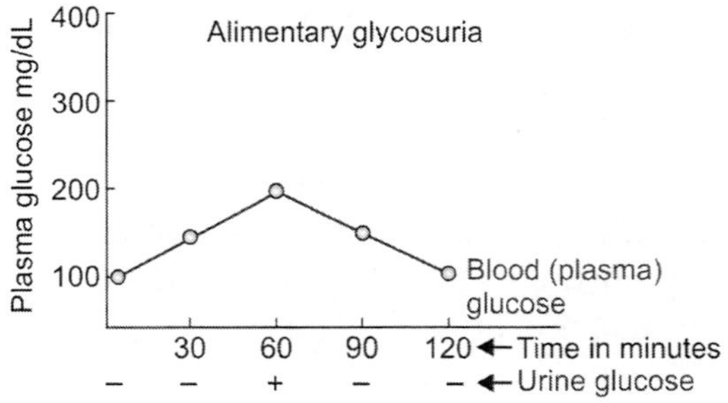 Alimentary glycosuria |
| Renal glycosuria | <110 mg% | <160 mg% | <140 mg% | Present in all specimen | 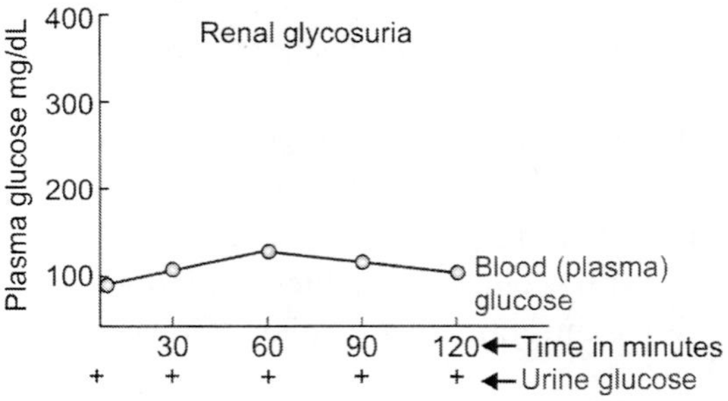 Renal glycosuria |

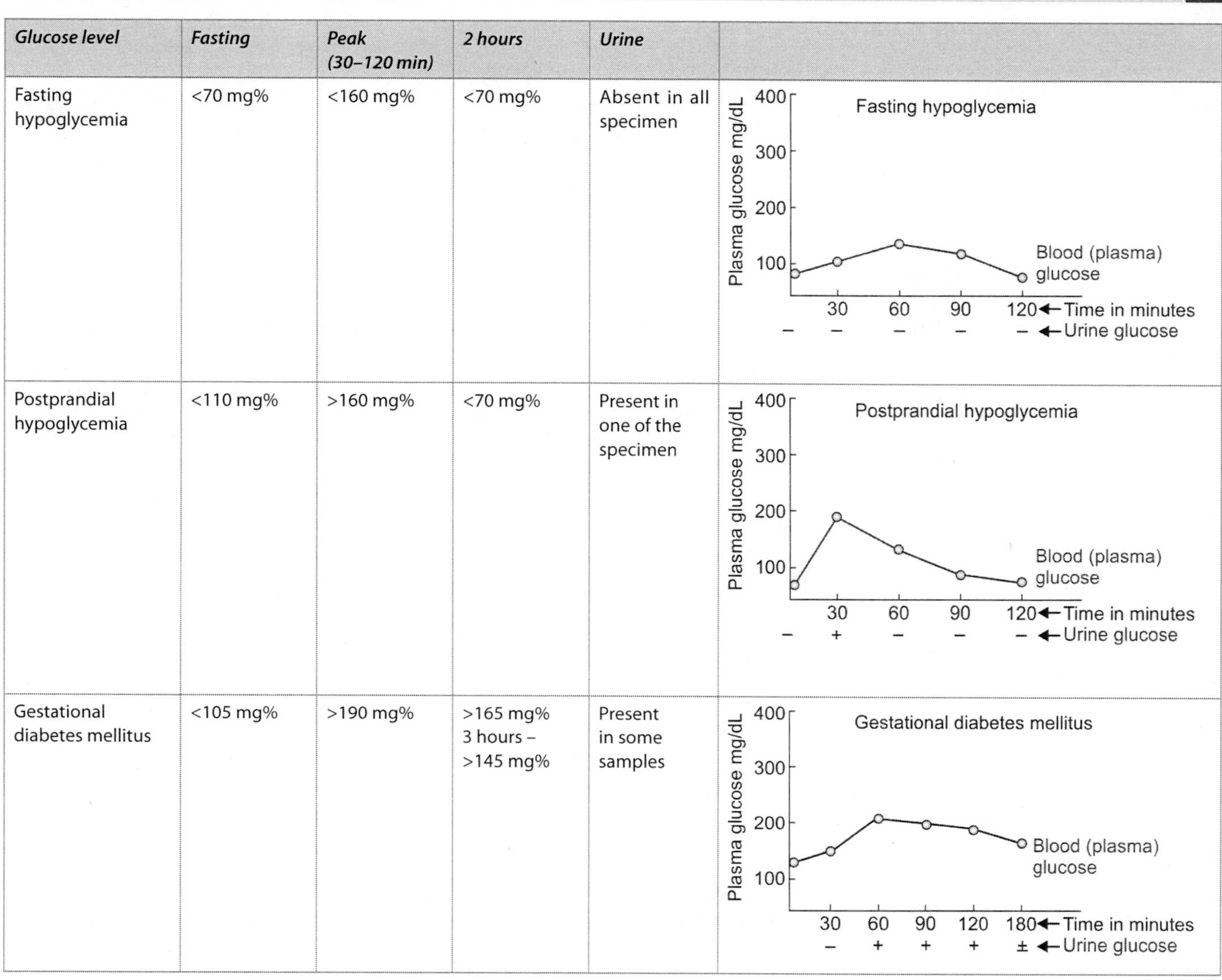

| *Glucose level* | *Fasting* | *Peak (30–120 min)* | *2 hours* | *Urine* | |
|---|---|---|---|---|---|
| Fasting hypoglycemia | <70 mg% | <160 mg% | <70 mg% | Absent in all specimen | |
| Postprandial hypoglycemia | <110 mg% | >160 mg% | <70 mg% | Present in one of the specimen | |
| Gestational diabetes mellitus | <105 mg% | >190 mg% | >165 mg% 3 hours – >145 mg% | Present in some samples | |



WHO recommendation for range of blood sugar level in GTT

| | **Normal** | **Diabetes** |
|---|---|---|
| Fasting | <100 mg/dL | >140 mg/dL |
| 1 hour (Peak) | <160 mg/dL | — |
| 2 hour | <140 mg/dL | >200 mg/dL |

*Significance*

- GTT helps to diagnose glucose intolerance, impending diabetes mellitus, renal glycosuria and other endocrinopathies.

## 7. Regulation of water balance.

- Water balance includes balance between sources of water and losses of water.

| *Sources of water* | *Water losses* |
|---|---|
| • Drinking of water (average 1500 mL)<br>• Water contained in diet (700 mL)<br>• Water derived from food oxidation (400 mL) | • Through urine (average 1600 mL)<br>• Through feces (100 mL)<br>• Through expired air (400 mL)<br>• Through perspiration (500 mL) |

### Regulation of Water Balance

| | *Regulation of water intake (by thirst mechanism)* | *Regulation of renal excretion of water (by vasopressin release)* |
|---|---|---|
| Stimulus | • Increased ECF osmolality (caused by increase in plasma $Na^+$) | • Increased plasma osmolality (caused by increase in plasma $Na^+$, urea and glucose) → stimulation of osmoreceptors in hypothalamus → release of vasopressin<br>• Hypovolemia → through angiotensin II and baroreceptors in carotid sinus → release of vasopressin<br>• Stress, hypoglycemia, drugs |
| Mechanism | • Stimulation of osmoreceptors in anterolateral hypothalamus by increase in plasma osmolality | Vasopressin binds to V2 receptors on cells of collecting ducts<br>⇓<br>Activation of adenyl cyclase<br>⇓<br>Increased levels of cyclic AMP<br>⇓<br>Insertion of water channels into luminal membrane<br>⇓<br>Increased permeability of renal collecting ducts to water |
| Effect | • Increased water intake | • Increased reabsorption of water by renal tubules |

## 8. Iron toxicity.

- Presence of excess iron in body is termed siderosis
- Excess iron is present in form of hemosiderin, a iron pigment which seen as golden brown granules in spleen and liver.

### Types

| | *Hemosiderosis (inborn error of iron metabolism)* | *Hemochromatosis* |
|---|---|---|
| Definition | • Accumulation of hemosiderin in liver and other reticuloendothelial system with no significant tissue destruction | Occurs when tissue iron content exceeds 10-12 times normal<br>• Characterized by extensive deposition of hemosiderin with much tissue destruction |
| Causes | a. Primary hemosiderosis (hereditary cemochromatosis)<br>– Autosomal recessive condition due to abnormal gene (HFE1) located on chromosome 6<br>b. Secondary hemosiderosis or hemochromatosis<br>– Excess iron intake (due to cooking in iron vessels, prolonged self medication with iron)<br>– Increased hemolysis<br>– Repeated blood transfusion (as in hemophilia, aplastic anemia)—most common cause | |
| Clinical features | • Benign condition<br>• Usually diagnosed on Prussian blue staining of liver or spleen | • Characterized by a triad of bronze pigmentation of skin, cirrhosis and diabetes mellitus |
| Treatment | • Repeated phlebotomy every week till serum iron and ferritin level reach normal levels<br>• Desferrioxamine, a chelating agent forms ferroxamine with iron which is excreted in urine | |

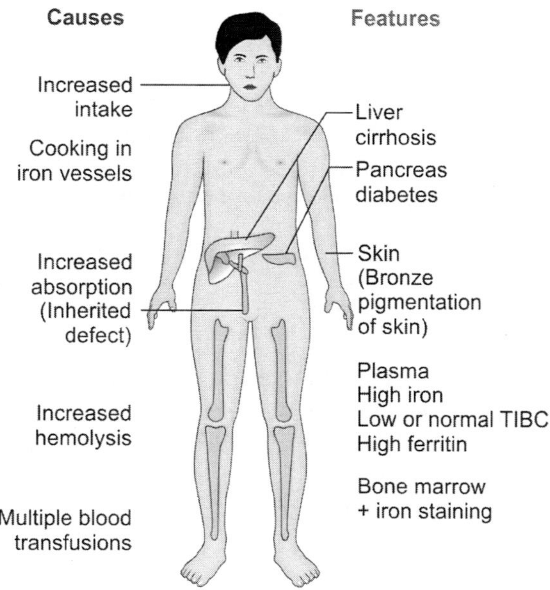


**Fig. 4:** Iron toxicity

## 9. Transamination and deamination.

- Transamination and deamination are processes of amino acid metabolism and major sources of ammonia production.

**For Transamination**

Refer Question No. 2 Oct. 2006 (RS2).

**Deamination**

- Deamination is removal or liberation of amino group ($NH^3$) from amino acids for urea synthesis and converting amino acids into keto acids.

### Types

| | *Oxidative deamination* | *Non-oxidative deamination* |
|---|---|---|
| Definition | • Liberation of free ammonia from amino group coupled with oxidation<br>Tissue site<br>• Liver (glutamate dehydrogenase) and kidney<br>Intracellular site<br>• Mitochondria | • Liberation of free ammonia without undergoing oxidation |
| Examples | a. Glutamate dehydroganse (major and final reaction removing amino group of all amino acids)<br>Glutamate + NAD(P) → $\alpha$ ketoglutarate + $NH_3$ + NAD(P)H + $H^+$<br>b. L – amino acid oxidase (all amino acids except hydroxyl amino acids and dicarboxylic amino acids)<br>L – amino acid + FMN → $\alpha$ keto acid + $NH_3$ + $FMNH_2$<br>c. D – amino acid oxidase (Glycine and bacterial amino acids)<br>D – amino acid + FAD → $\alpha$ keto acid + $NH_3$ + $FADH_2$ | a. Serine dehydratase<br>Serine → Pyruvate + $NH_3$<br>b. Threonine dehydratase<br>Threonine → $\alpha$ ketobutyrate + $NH_3$<br>c. Cysteine desulfhydrase<br>Cysteine → Pyruvate + $NH_3$ + $H_2S$<br>d. Histidase<br>Histadine → Urocanate + $NH_3$ |
| Significance | • Oxidative deamination provides $NH_3$ for urea synthesis and $\alpha$ keto acids for various reactions including energy generation (TCA cycle) | • Non-oxidative deamination reactions are involved in amino acid metabolism besides production of ammonia |

## 10. Write the components and principle of colorimeter.

- Colorimeter is instrument used for measurement of color of the solution which is proportional to the concentration of the solute or compound
- Instrument is operative in visible range (400–800 nm)

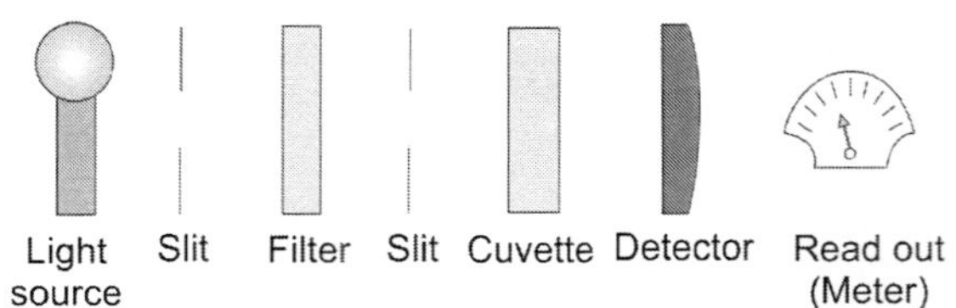


**Fig. 5:** Components of colorimeter

## Parts (Components)

- Light source (tungsten lamp)
- Entrance slit (allowing light to pass through)
- Filter (different filters are used for absorption of color at particular wavelength)
  - Filters will absorb light of unwanted wavelength and allow only monochromatic light to pass through which will have maximum absorbance when passed through a particular colored solution and the color of filter should be complementary to the color of the solution
- Exit slit (allowing light to pass through sample in the cuvette)
- Sample/Cuvette holder
- Detector (photocell)
- Display (galvanometer or digital).

## Principle (Beer-Lambart's Law)

- Colorimeter works on principle of Beer-Lambart's law which explains relation of amount of light absorbed or transmitted by a colored solution
- According to Beer's law, intensity of color is directly proportional to concentration of colored particles in solution
- According to Lambart's law, amount of light absorbed by a colored solution depends on length of column or depth of liquid through which light passes
- Thus to summarize, Beer-Lambart's law states, that amount of light absorbed a colored solution depends upon concentration of absorbing molecules in solution and thickness of medium.

## Application

- To determine analytes in biological fluids such as determination of plasma glucose, urine protein and protein in CSF.

## 11. Glucose transporters.

- Glucose transporters are a family of membrane proteins found in human cells besides most mammalian cells.

| *Structure* | *Mechanism* |
|---|---|
| • Glucose transporters are integral membrane proteins containing 12 membrane spanning helices. Their amino and carboxyl terminals are exposed on the cytoplasmic side of plasma membrane. | • Whenever a glucose molecule binds to one of its binding site by a weak hydrogen bond opening the binded site to imbibe the glucose molecule. Then there occurs a conformational change in the protein, transporting and releasing glucose to the other side of the membrane<br>• Thus the transporter behaves like a gated pore and the process is called ping-pong mechanism |

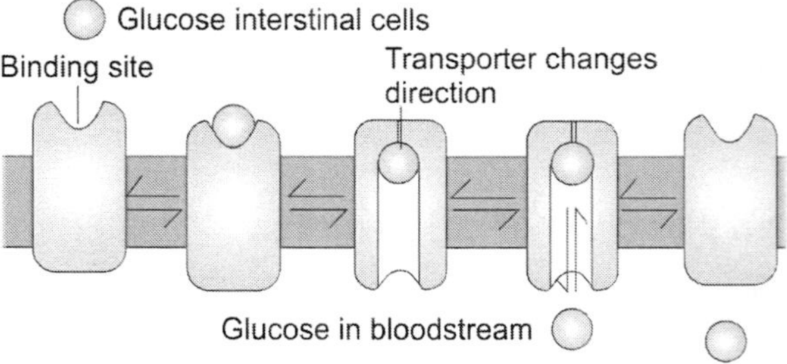


**Fig. 6:** Glucose transporters

## Types

- Three classes based on their pattern of tissue expression, substrate specificity, transport kinetics and regulated expression in different physiological conditions.

| | *Transporter* | *Location* | *Properties* |
|---|---|---|---|
| Class I | GluT1 | RBC, brain, kidney, colon, retina, placenta | Glucose uptake in most of the cells, levels in cell membrane increased by reduced glucose level and vice versa |
| | GluT2 | Serosal surface of intestinal cells, liver, β cells of pancreas | Low affinity (high Km value for glucose), glucose uptake in liver, glucose sensor in β cells, highly specific for D-glucose |
| | GluT3 | Neurons, brain | High affinity, glucose transport in brain |
| | GluT4 | Striated muscles (Skeletal and heart), adipose tissue | Insulin mediated glucose uptake |
| Class II | GluT5 | Small intestine, testis, sperms, kidney | Fructose transporter, poor ability to transport glucose |
| | GluT7 | Liver, endoplasmic reticulum | Glucose from endoplasmic reticulum to cytoplasm |
| | GluT9 | | |
| | GluT11 | | |
| Class III | GluT6 | | |
| | GluT8 | | |
| | GluT10 | | |
| | GluT12 | | |

## Function

- Glucose transporters are uniport, facilitated diffusion system transporting glucose into the cytoplasm of the cell.

## 12. Biotin.

- Biotin is a water soluble B-complex vitamin
- It is also called as anti egg white injury factor because raw egg white contains the protein avidin, which binds biotin causing its deficiency.

| *Chemistry* | *Sources* | *RDA* |
|---|---|---|
| Imidazole derivative containing sulfur | • Eggs, liver, kidney and yeast, pulses, nuts, vegetables (rich sources)<br>• Cereals and dairy products (poor sources)<br>• Synthesis by microbial flora of intestine | 0.3 mg/day—adults |

## Functions

### *Coenzymes*

- Biocytin
- Biotin is a prosthetic group of carboxylase enzyme serving as carrier of $CO_2$.

### *Functions*

Carboxylation reactions
- Reactions where $CO_2$ is donated to an acceptor or substrate.

Mechanism
- In the first step, a molecule of $CO_2$ is captured by the biotin present in the enzyme to become carboxybiotin enzyme in which carboxyl group is covalently attached to a nitrogen of the biotin molecule

- ATP provides energy for this reaction
- Now the activated carboxyl group is transferred to the substrate and a free biotinyl enzyme is regenerated.

Examples

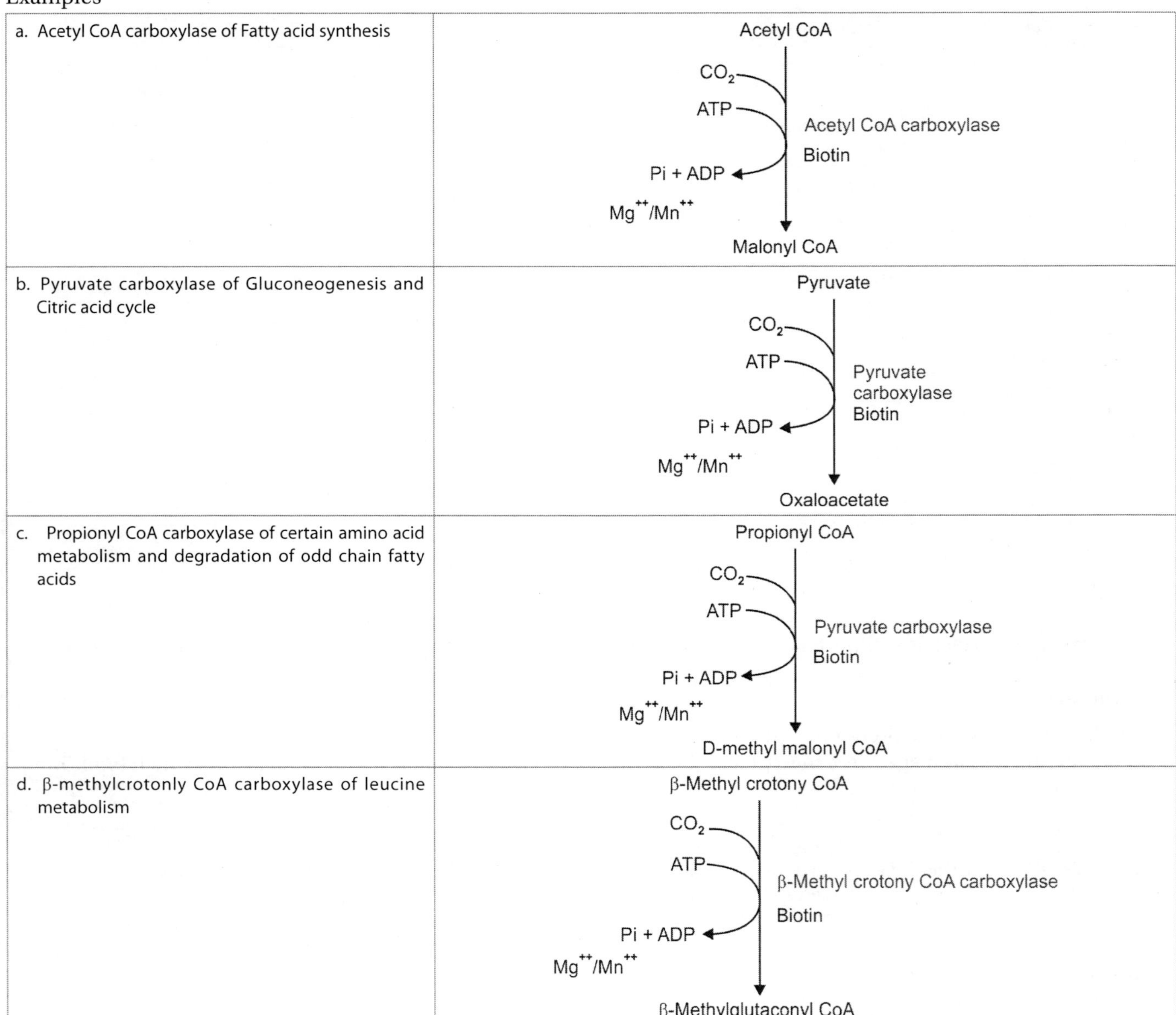

| | |
|---|---|
| a. Acetyl CoA carboxylase of Fatty acid synthesis | Acetyl CoA<br>$CO_2$<br>ATP<br>Acetyl CoA carboxylase<br>Biotin<br>Pi + ADP<br>$Mg^{++}/Mn^{++}$<br>Malonyl CoA |
| b. Pyruvate carboxylase of Gluconeogenesis and Citric acid cycle | Pyruvate<br>$CO_2$<br>ATP<br>Pyruvate carboxylase<br>Biotin<br>Pi + ADP<br>$Mg^{++}/Mn^{++}$<br>Oxaloacetate |
| c. Propionyl CoA carboxylase of certain amino acid metabolism and degradation of odd chain fatty acids | Propionyl CoA<br>$CO_2$<br>ATP<br>Pyruvate carboxylase<br>Biotin<br>Pi + ADP<br>$Mg^{++}/Mn^{++}$<br>D-methyl malonyl CoA |
| d. β-methylcrotonly CoA carboxylase of leucine metabolism | β-Methyl crotony CoA<br>$CO_2$<br>ATP<br>β-Methyl crotony CoA carboxylase<br>Biotin<br>Pi + ADP<br>$Mg^{++}/Mn^{++}$<br>β-Methylglutaconyl CoA |

*Significance*

- Biotin is essential for carboxylation reactions
- However, not all carboxylation reaction require biotin and some important carboxylation reactions independent of biotin are formation of carbamoyl phosphate in urea cycle, incorporation of $CO_2$ in purine synthesis.

## SHORT ANSWERS

### 13. Name any two tests of assessment of gastric function and define the basal acid out.

- Gastric function tests are based on estimation of hydrochloric acid output.

#### Gastric Function Test

a. Pentagastrin stimulation test
   - Consists of estimating acid output every 15 minutes for an hour following administration of pentagastrin (5 mg/kg) and comparing it with basal acid output.

b. Augmented histamine test meal
   - Consists of estimating acid output every 15 minutes for an hour following administration of histamine (0.04 mg/kg subcutaneously) and comparing it with basal acid output.

c. Fractional test meal (not done nowdays)
   - Consists of aspiration of gastric juice every 15 minutes for 2 hours following administration of test meal (black coffee) and analysis of gastric juice for free and total acidity.

d. Alcohol test meal
   - Consists of aspiration of gastric juice every 15 minutes for 1½ hours following administration of 100 mL of 7% alcohol and analysis of gastric juice for free and total acidity.

e. Insulin meal test (Hollander's test)
   - Assess completeness of vagotomy by observing acid output in response to induced hypoglycemia by insulin (0.1 unit/kg)
   - No increase in acid output indicates successful vagotomy.

*Interpretations*

a. Basal acid output (BAO)
   - Basal acid output refers to acid output under basal conditions
   - Obtained by single sample from empty stomach collected with any stimulation

b. Maximal acid output (MAO)
   - Maximal acid output refers to acid output following stimulation
   - Obtained by sum of all four 15 minutes samples

c. Peak acid output (PAO)
   - Peak acid output refers to maximum acid output following stimulation
   - Obtained by sum of first two 15 minutes samples and multiplied by 2.

*Normal Values*

| *(In mm mol/h)* | *Men* | | *Women* | |
|---|---|---|---|---|
| | *Lower limit* | *Upper limit* | *Lower limit* | *Upper limit* |
| Basal acid output | — | 10 | — | 3.5 |
| Maximal acid output | 7 | 45 | 5 | 30 |
| Peak acid output | 12 | 60 | 8 | 40 |

*Significance*

- Increased BAO levels are indicative of hyperacidity as in Zollinger-Ellision syndrome
- Chronic duodenal ulcer shows significant elevation of BAO, MAO, PAO.

### 14. Reverse transcriptase.

- Reverse transcriptase is the enzyme responsible for reverse transcription, i.e. producing a single stranded DNA from a RNA acting as a template
- Also called as RNA dependent DNA polymerase.

## Significance

a. Retroviruses
   - Number of viruses called as retroviruses contain RNA as genome instead of DNA and such viruses synthezise DNA (to be incorporated in host DNA) with help of reverse transcriptase
   - Example: Human immunodeficiency virus (HIV causing AIDS).

b. Genetic recombination through transposition
   - Transposition refers to jumping of mobile DNA sequences (also called transposable elements or transposons) from one place in the genome to another place in the genome
   - One of the mechanisms of transposition involves transposable elements jumping through the formation of:
     - RNA intermediates which are later used as template for formation of DNA using reverse transcriptase
     - Transposition contributes to genetic variability of the genome in humans

c. Molecular biotechnology
   - Reverse transcriptase derived from RNA tumor viruses is used to synthesize complementary DNA (cDNA) copies of mRNA templates
   - cDNA is used for cloning or reverse transcription-polymerase chain reaction.

### 15. Invert sugar.

## Invert Sugar

- Sucrose is dextrorotatory in nature (+66.5)
- Hydrolysis of sucrose produces a molecule of glucose (+52.5) and a molecule of fructose (–92)
- Therefore products change the direction of rotation from dextrorotation to leavorotation or plane of rotation is inverted
- This process is known as invertion
- Therefore equimolecular mixture of glucose and fructose formed on hydrolysis of sucrose is called invert sugar.

*Significance*

- Invert sugar is sweeter than sucrose
- Honey contains invert sugar.

### 16. What is isoelectric pH? What is the application of isoelectric pH?

- Isoelectric pH of a protein is that pH where the number of anions and cations present on the protein molecules are equal and the net charge is zero.

| *Properties of protein (at isoelectric pH)* | *Application of isoelectric pH* |
|---|---|
| • Do not migrate in an electrical field<br>• Minimum solubility, buffering capacity and viscosity<br>• Maximum precibility | • Isoelectric pH is used in separation of proteins by electrophoresis |

### 17. Hyperhomocysteinemia.

- Hyperhomocysteinemia is a medial disorder characterized by an abnormally large level of homocysteine in blood. Normal plasma level of homocysteine is between 5-16 mmol/L.

## Causes

- Genetic defects in enzymes involved in homocysteine metabolism (most commonly cystathionine beta-synthase deficiency)
- Nutritional deficiencies in vitamin cofactors like B complex vitamins and folate in particular
- Several therapeutic drugs (methotrexate, theophylline, cyclosporine and most anticonvulsants)
- Chronic disease states (liver and renal disease, hypothyroidism and malignancies).

## Mechanism (Based on Deficient Enzyme)

| *Methionine synthase* | *Methylenetetrahydrofolate reductase* | *Cystathionine beta-synthase* |
|---|---|---|
| • Inadequate supply of vitamin $B_{12}$ leads to failure of conversion of homocysteine to methionine and the net result is an increase in homocysteine | • Involved in formation of 5-methyl tetrahydrofolate which is essential for conversion of homocysteine to methionine<br>• Thus its deficiency leads to increased levels of homocysteine | • Converts homocysteine to cysteine<br>• Thus, its deficiency leads to increased levels of homocysteine |

## Clinical Features

- Skeletal problems like osteoporosis, Charlie Chaplin gait
- Ocular problems like ectopia lentis, myopia and glaucoma
- Mental retardation/developmental delay
- Thrombotic complications due to increased platelet adhesiveness by activation of Hageman's factor.

## Treatment

- Supplementation of vitamins B complex and folate
- Diet low in methionine and high in cystine.

# 18. Glycosuria.

- Glycosuria is condition where glucose is excreted in urine which is detectable by Benedict's qualitative test.

## Causes (Types)

| *Physiological* | *Pathological* | |
|---|---|---|
| | Hyperglycemic glycosuria (increase in amount of glucose entering tubules/min) | Renal glycosuria (decrease in renal threshold of glucose) |
| • Pregnancy | • Alimentary glycosuria<br>• Emotional or nervous glycosuria<br>• Glycosuria due to endocrine disorders (diabetes mellitus, thyrotoxicosis, acromegaly)<br>• Experimental hyperglycemic glycosuria | • Hereditary<br>• Acquired<br>• Diseases of renal tubules<br>• Heavy metal poisoning<br>• Lowering of renal threshold<br>• Experimental renal glycosuria |

## Mechanism

- Quantity of glucose in glomerular filtrate is increases when more glucose is filtered through glomerular membrane due to decreased renal threshold (renal glycosuria) or increased glucose in blood (hyperglycemic glucosuria) and this increased glucose cannot be reabsorbed resulting in excretion of excess glucose in urine
- Renal threshold of glucose is 180 mg/dL, above which glucose appears in urine.

# 19. Golgi complex.

- Golgi complex is a subcellular organelle located near nucleus
- Also called golgi apparatus
- Present in all cells except RBCs

| *Structure* | *Function* |
|---|---|
| • Consists of 4 or more flattened membranous sacs lined cisternae | • Intracellular sorting of proteins and packaging and secretion of proteins<br>• Post transcription modification of proteins (addition of carbohydrates, lipids or sulfate moieties)<br>• Membrane synthesis for subcellular organelles |

# 20. What is restriction fragment length polymorphism? Give one clinical application of same.

- Restriction fragment polymorphism is the slight differences in the individual DNA structure in form of slight variation in base sequence usually once in every hundred base pairs which do not affect the phenotype and is present in more than 1% of total population.

## Clinical Application

- It is useful for diagnosis of molecular diseases like sickle cell anemia
- In forensic medicine, it serves as DNA finger prints which help in identification.

## 21. What is the significance of brown adipose tissue?

- Brown adipose tissue is relatively less in distribution but very active metabolically.

| *Location (in humans)* | *Features* | *Significance* |
|---|---|---|
| • Newborns and in adults at thoracic region (between the scapulas) | • Posses high proportion of mitochondria and cytochromes<br>• In mitochondria of brown adipose tissue, the oxidation and phosphorylation are not coupled | • Brown adipose tissue produces more heat and less ATP<br>• It is responsible for diet induced thermogenesis |

## 22. What are the major differences between hexokinase and glucokinase?

| | *Hexokinase* | *Glucokinase* |
|---|---|---|
| Specificity | Nonspecific; can phosphorylate any of the hexoses | Specific; can phosphorylate glucose only |
| Stability | More stable | Physiologically more labile |
| Present in | Almost all tissues | Only in adult liver |
| Presence in fetus | Fetal liver | No |
| Inhibition by glucose-6-P | Allosteric inhibition | Not inhibited |
| Km | Low = 0.1 mm | High = 10 mm |
| Affinity for glucose | High | Low |
| Influence of diabetes or starvation | No | Depressed |
| Effect of feeding glucose | No change | Increased (stimulated by glucose) |
| Inhibitors | Glucocorticoids and GH | Glucocorticoids and GH |
| Effect of insulin | No effect | Stimulated |
| Isoenzymes | Known in liver | No known isoenzymes |
| Function | Make glucose available to tissues for oxidation at lower blood glucose level | Clear glucose from blood after meals and at blood levels greater than 100 mg/dL |

## 23. Lactose intolerance.

- Lactose intolerance is a disorder of lactose digestion due to inherited or acquired deficiency of enzyme lactase
- Most common disorder of carbohydrate digestion.

### Causes

- Primary severe lactase deficiency—inherited deficiency of lactase; seen mainly in newborn
- Primary low lactase deficiency—inherited deficiency of lactase; seen mainly in adults
- Secondary low lactase deficiency—acquired deficiency of lactase caused by intestinal diseases such as celiac sprue and gastroenteritis; seen in both children and adults.

### Clinical Features

- Diarrhea results from osmotic effect of lactose in the large intestine
- Flatulence (gas accumulation) results from fermentation of lactose by intestinal bacteria to form hydrogen, methane and carbon dioxide gases which gives rise to distention and abdominal cramps.

### Treatment

- Avoiding the intake of milk (lactose) and replacing milk with glucose water in newborns
- Use of live lactobacilli
- Use of yoghurt or curd.

## 24. Carbonic anhydrase.

- Carbonic anhydrase is an metalloenzyme containing zinc.

## Location

- RBCs and renal tubular cells.

## Reaction

Catalyses the formation of $H_2CO_3$ from $CO_2$ and $H_2O$.

$$CO_2 + H_2O \xrightarrow{\text{Carbonic Anhydrase}} H_2CO_3 \longrightarrow H^+ + HCO_3^+$$

## Functions (Significance)

- In RBCs, it helps to transport $CO_2$ and in kidneys, it helps in reabsorption of $HCO^{3+}$
- It is involved in regulation of Acid Base balance by regulating CO2 transport and $HCO^{3+}$ levels.

## 25. Name the lung surfactant. Mention its composition.

- Lung surfactant is also known as dipalmityl lecithin (DPL).

| *Composition* | *Source* | *Role in lungs* |
|---|---|---|
| • Lipoprotein composed of lecithin, amphipathic phospholipids<br>• Contains palmitic acid at both carbon 1 and 2 of glycerol | • Type II (Granular pneumocytes) of lungs | • It lowers the surface tension in lung alveoli thus prevent its collapse following expiration |

## Clinical Significance

- Deficiency of surfactant in premature fetuses causes lungs to collapse leading to respiratory distress syndrome (hyaline membrane disease).

## 26. What is the clinical importance of glycosides?

- Glycoside is a product formed from reaction of hemiacetal or hemiketal hydroxyl group of a carbohydrate with a hydroxyl group of another carbohydrate or a non-carbohydrate.

## Clinical Significance

- Glycosides are of various important uses in medicine:

| *Type of glycoside* | *Example* | *Use* |
|---|---|---|
| Alcoholic glycoside | Salicin (salicylic acid) | Analgesic, antipyretic and anti-inflammatory effect |
| Anthroquinone glycoside | Anthraquinone | Laxative effect |
| Coumarin glycoside | Apterin (coumarin) | Dilatation of coronary arteries and calcium channel blocker |
| Flavonoid glycoside | Hesperidin, naringin, rutin, quercitrin | Antioxidant effect, decrease capillary fragility |
| Phenolic glycoside | Arbutin | Urinary antiseptic effect |
| Saponins | Liquorice | Expectorant effect |
| Cardiac glycosides | Digitialis | Used in congestive cardiac failure and arrhythmias |

## 27. Write part played by ribosomes in proteins biosynthesis.

- Ribosomes are complexes of ribosomal proteins and rRNA.

| *Structures* | *Functions* |
|---|---|
| • Eukaryotic ribosomes are larger in size with a sedimentation coefficient of 80S<br>• They are made of 2 subunits; a larger 60S subunit and a smaller 40S subunit | • Ribosomes take part in translation of mRNA into a polypeptide<br>• They take part in form of polysome of polyribosome on an mRNA fibre<br>• A ribosome is constituted on the mRNA itself by the sequential bindings of its subunits over the first or 5' codon of the mRNA<br>• Each ribosome then moves in 5'–3' direction along the mRNA |

## Role in Protein Biosynthesis

- Each ribosome possesses a peptidyl or P site and an aminoacyl or A site for binding a peptidyl-RNA and an aminoacyl tRNA respectively
- As the ribosome moves over successive codons of mRNA its A site lies over a particular codon each step
- An amino acyl - tRNA bearing complementary anticodon base occupies a site while P site is occupied by the peptidyl-tRNA formed at earlier step
- Then ribosomal peptidyl transferase, transfers the peptidyl group from peptidyl-tRNA to amino acid of amino acyl-tRNA forming a peptide bond
- Thus the earlier aminoacyl tRNA is converted to peptidyl tRNA
- The deaclylated tRNA at P-site continues at the same site
- As the ribosomes moves (translocated) in 5'-3' direction the new peptidyl tRNA at A site automatically comes at P site vacating A site for a new aminoacyl tRNA to occupy
- The deaclylated tRNA is ejected from ribosomes
- This process is repeated till there is a nonsense codon at the A site
- With the 5'-3' ribosomal movement over successive codon, peptide bonds are formed between amino acids coding for respective codon on mRNA from N-terminal to C-terminal of peptide chain
- Each polysome simultaneously continues translating as many peptide chains as the number ribosomes in it at the instant
- Peptide chain gets progressively elongated as the respective ribosome approaches 3' end of genetic code.

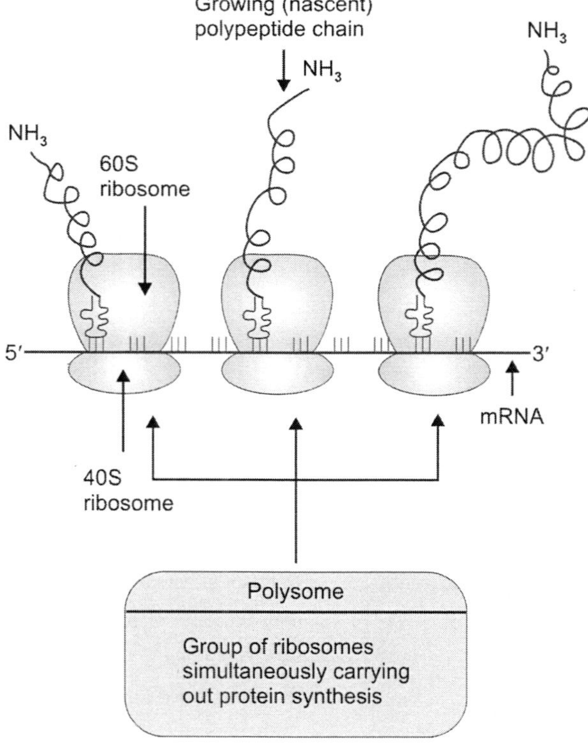


**Fig. 7:** Role of ribosomes in protein biosynthesis

## Significance

- Ribosomes are protein synthesizing machinery of the cell
- Interaction of ribosomes with rRNA, tRNA and mRNA is required for the synthesis of polypetide chain.

## 28. Tests for urobilinogen.

- Urobilinogen in urine is tested by Ehrlich test.

### Ehrlich Test

*Procedure*

- To 10 mL of urine, 1 mL of Ehrlich's reagent (para dimethyl amino benzaldehyde in HCl) is added.

*Observation*

- Development of red color indicates presence of urobilinogen.

*Significance*

- Urobilinogen is excreated in cases of fever, liver diseases and hemolysis.

# SAMPLE PAPERS

# MBBS PHASE I EXAMINATION

## SAMPLE PAPER-2

### LONG ESSAYS

**1. Define enzymes. Explain the mechanism of enzyme action. Add a note on inhibition of enzymes.**

- Enzymes are important group of biomolecules synthesized by living cells which are biocatalyst, protein in nature, colloidal and thermolabial and specific in their action.

#### Mechanism of Enzyme Action

- For breaking down a substance into lower energy compounds, it has to be placed at a higher energy level (activation energy) where spontaneous degradation takes place
- Enzymes catalyze chemical reactions by reducing this activation energy thus facilitating reaction to proceed at lower temperature and at a faster rate.

#### Michaelis–Menton Theory—1913 (Enzyme-Substrate Formation)

- According to this widely accepted theory, prime requisite for enzyme action is combination of substrate with enzyme at active site of enzyme to form enzyme-substrate complex which dissociates to form products and enzymes
- Enzyme once dissociated from complex is free to combine with another molecule of substrate and form product in a similar way
- Mechanism of enzyme substrate formation can be explained by:

| | *Mechanism* | *Remarks* |
|---|---|---|
| i. Fischer's template theory or Lock and Key model | • According to this theory, enzyme has a rigid conformation and three dimensional structure of active site of enzyme is complementary to substrate, i.e. a substrate fits into enzyme like a key in a lock | • Disadvantages<br>• This theory fails to explain flexibility seen in some enzyme and effect of allosteric modulators |
| ii. Koshland's theory or induced fit model | • According to this theory, conformational changes occur at active site of enzyme following its combination with substrate<br>• Active site is not pre shaped and rigid and there is stereospecific binding between enzyme and substrate leading to secondary binding and then conformational charges<br>• These conformational changes are such that there is precise orientation of catalytic groups and appropriate amino acids of enzyme are repositioned to bring about catalysis | • Advantages<br>• This theory explains mechanism of enzyme denaturation, saturation kinetics, competitive inhibition and allosteric modulations |
| iii. Substrate strain theory | • According to this theory, active site of enzyme is rigid and to fit into this rigid active site substrate is strained by attraction of ionic groups on substrate to opposite groups on the enzyme<br>• Straining of substrate leads to formation of products | |

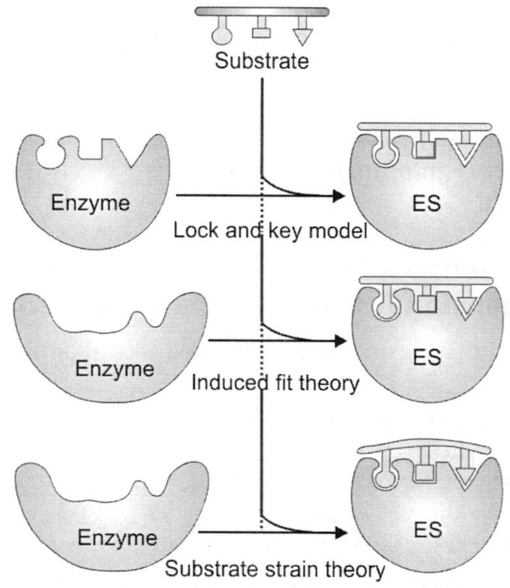


**Fig. 1:** Theories of enzyme substrate complex formation

- Thus, it can be said that a combination of induced fit model and substrate strain is responsible for enzyme action.

*Clinical Significance*

- Studies about mechanism of enzyme action lead to a rational approach to therapy and drug design
- High resolution structural information obtained by X-ray crystallography combined with mechanistic information facilitates drug designing to inhibit the specific enzymes
- Enzyme specificity or catalytic efficiency can be modified using recombinant DNA technology and site directed mutagenesis which facilitates designing and introduction of enzymes of specific desired properties into humans.

## Inhibition of Enzymes

- Enzymes are proteins and can be inactivated by chemical substance known as inhibitor by a process called enzyme inhibition
- An enzyme inhibitor is a substance that binds with enzyme and brings about a decrease in catalytic activity of enzymes.

*Types*

- Reversible inhibition
  - Competitive inhibition
  - Non-competitive inhibition
  - Un-competitive inhibition
- Irreversible inhibition
- Allosteric inhibition

a. **For Reversible inhibition**
   Refer Question No. 3 June 2007 (RS2).
b. **Irreversible inhibition**
   - Here inhibitors bind covalantly with enzyme and irreversibly inactivate them
   - It is similar to reversible non-competitive inhibition in all aspect including kinetics except that inhibition is irreversible

Example:
- Many organophosphorus compounds irreversibly inhibit the enzyme acetylcholine esterase resulting in paralysis and ending fatally.
- British anti-Lewisite (BAL) is used as an antidote in heavy metal poisoning because it irreversibly binds the heavy metal ions and thus reducing their poisonous effects.

c. **For Allosteric inhibition (allosteric regulation)**
Refer Question No. 2 Sample Paper 1.

## 2. How will you differentiate a native protein from a denatured protein? Explain the bonds at different levels of three dimensional structure of a native protein.

- Denaturation is disorganization of native structure of protein with concomitant loss of biological activity.

### Differentiating Native Protein from Denatured Protein

| *Points of difference* | *Native protein* | *Denatured protein* |
|---|---|---|
| Structure | Consists of primary, secondary, tertiary and quaternary structure (native helical structure) | Consists of only primary structure |
| Bonds present | Peptide bonds, hydrogen bonds, disulfide bonds, hydrophic bonds, ionic bonds, van der Waals forces | Only peptide bonds |
| Biological activity | Retained | Lost |
| Solubility | Soluble | Insoluble |
| Viscosity | Low | High |
| Surface tension | High | Low |
| Ionisable and sulfhydral groups of proteins | Low (as used up for hydrogen and disulfide bonds) | High |
| Crystallization | Possible | Not possible |
| Reaction to heat, acid and detergents | Denatured | No effect |

### Bonds Contributing to Native Protein Structure

- Protein has a complex structure formed by amino acids maintained by some bonds which confer proteins the stability and shape that renders them functional.

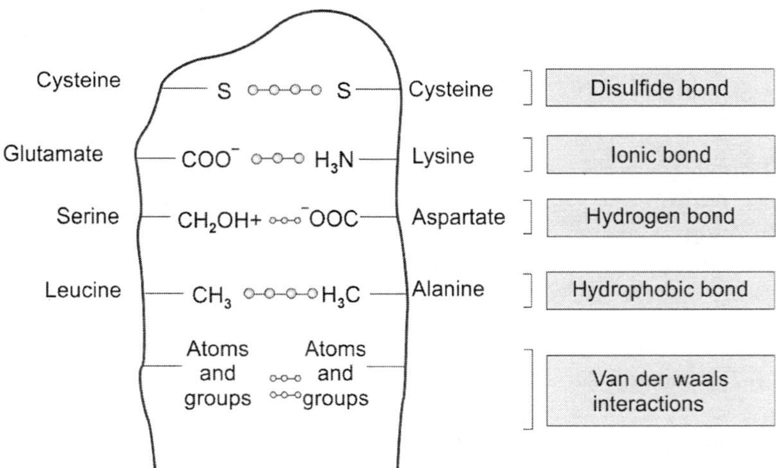


**Fig. 2:** Bonds contributing to protein structure

| Bonds | Definition | Protein structure involved in | Features |
|---|---|---|---|
| a. Peptide bond | • Covalent bond formed by sharing of electrons between C and N molecules of amino acids | • Primary | • Partial double bond, rigid and planar |
| b. Hydrogen bond | • Formed by sharing of an hydrogen between two electrons donors | • Secondary and tertiary | • Hydrogen donating groups are –NH, –OH, $-NH_2$<br>• Hydrogen accepting groups are COO-, C=0 and S-S |
| c. Electrostatic bonds (ionic bonds) | • Attractive forces between two opposite charges, or repulsive between two like charges | • Secondary and tertiary | • Formed between basic amino acids like lysine, argenine or histidine and acidic amino acids |
| d. Hydrophobic bonds | • Formed by interaction between nonpolar hydrophobic side chains of amino acids like alanine, phenylalanine by eliminating water molecules | • Tertiary | • Holds lipophilic side together, i.e. during folding of protein molecule, the hydrophobic groups prefer to be in the interior |
| e. Disulfide bond | • Covalent bond formed between two sulfide groups | • Tertiary | |
| f. Vander Wall's forces | • Attractive forces between all atoms depending upon distance between atoms $1/r^6$ (where r = radius) | • Tertiary and quaternary | • Although very weak, collectively contribute maximum towards the stability of protein structure |

## SHORT ESSAYS

### 3. Metabolism of galactose.

- Galactose is an important dietary sugar obtained from lactose especially in infants and children
- Glycogen metabolism involves three different process.

a. Galactose: Glucose interconversion
Tissue site
- Liver, mammary gland

Substrate
- Galactose

Product
- Glucose-1-phosphate: Undergoes glycolysis to produce energy
- UDP glucose: Used for glycogenesis

Significance
- Also used for synthesis of galactose in liver and mammary glands

Steps

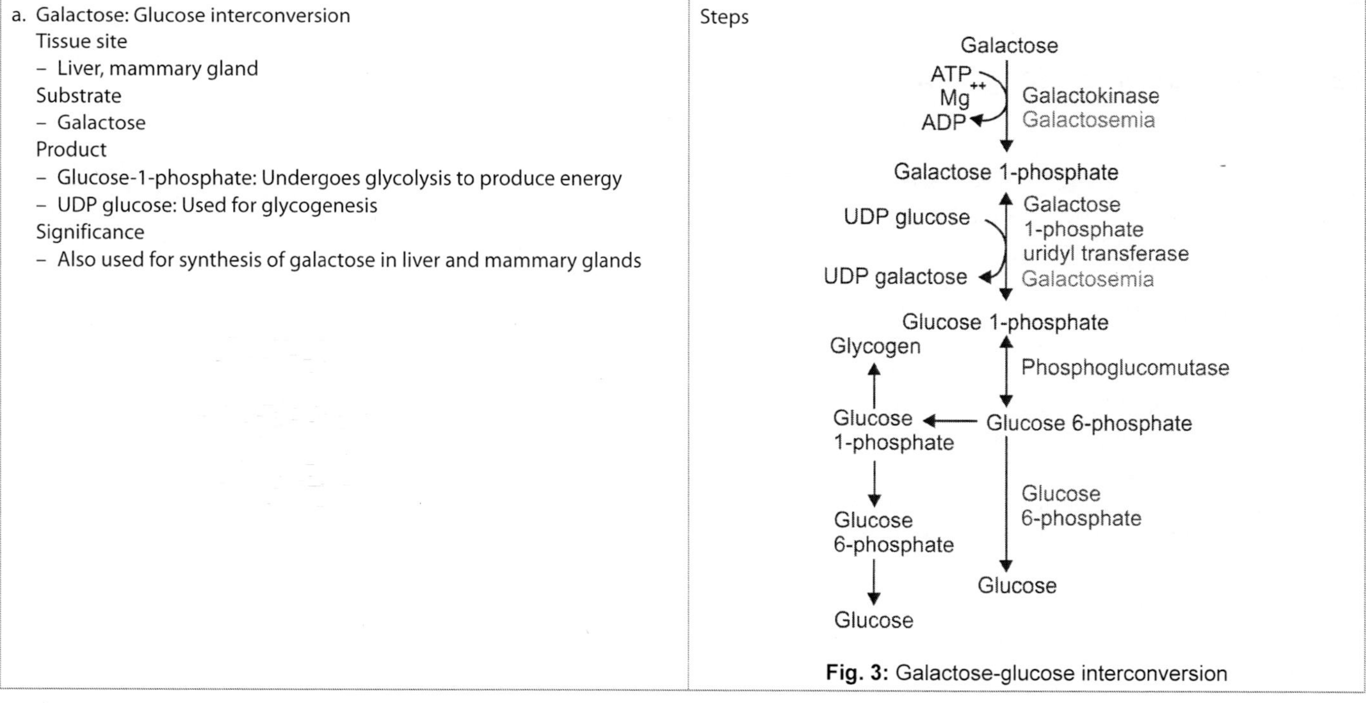


**Fig. 3:** Galactose-glucose interconversion

| | |
|---|---|
| b. Synthesis of glycolipids and glycoproteins<br>Tissue site<br>– Liver, brain and other tissues<br>Subcellular site<br>– Microsomes and Golgi membranes (location of enzyme galactosyl transferase)<br>Significance<br>– UDP galactose formed in the metabolism acts as donor of galactose for synthesis of heteroglycans, glycolipids and glycoproteins | |
| c. Lactose biosynthesis<br>Tissue site<br>– Mammary glands cells | Glucose<br>ATP, $Mg^{++}$ → ADP — Hexokinase<br>Glucose-6-phosphate<br>↕ Phosphoglucomutase<br>Glucose-1-phosphate<br>UTP → PPi — UDP glucose pyrophosphorylase<br>UDP-glucose<br>↕ UDP-hexose epimerase<br>UDP-galactose<br>Glucose → UDP — Lactose Synthase<br>Lactose<br>**Fig. 4:** Lactose biosynthesis |

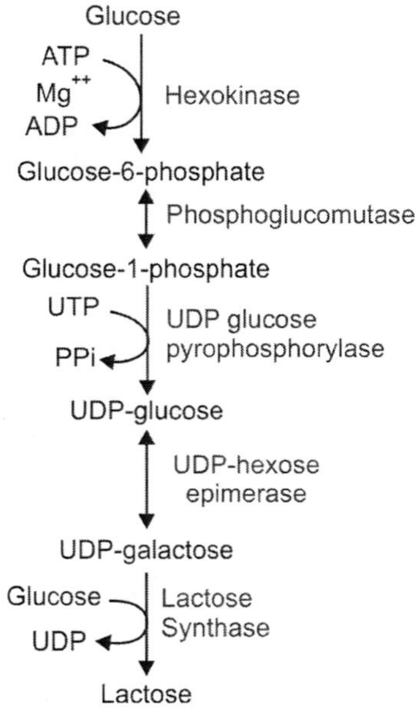

## 4. Microsomal chain elongation of fatty acids.

- Elongation of fatty acids is addition of acetyl fragments to existing fatty acids.

| *Tissue site* | *Subcellular site* | *Substrate* | *Product* |
|---|---|---|---|
| All tissues except brain | Microsomes (smooth ER)<br>- Major site | Acyl CoA (16-C) + Malonyl CoA (Source of 2 carbon units) | Acyl CoA (18-C) |

### Steps (Palmitate to Stearate)

a. Condensation of acyl CoA (C-16 palmitoyl CoA) with malonyl CoA with release of $CO_2$
b. Reduction of acyl CoA group
c. Dehydration of hydroxy acyl CoA
d. Saturation of 2, 3 unsaturated acyl group to form elongated fatty acyl CoA (C-18 stearyl CoA fatty acid)

- This cycle of steps may be repeated a number of times, elongating the acyl chain further by two carbon atom in each cycle.

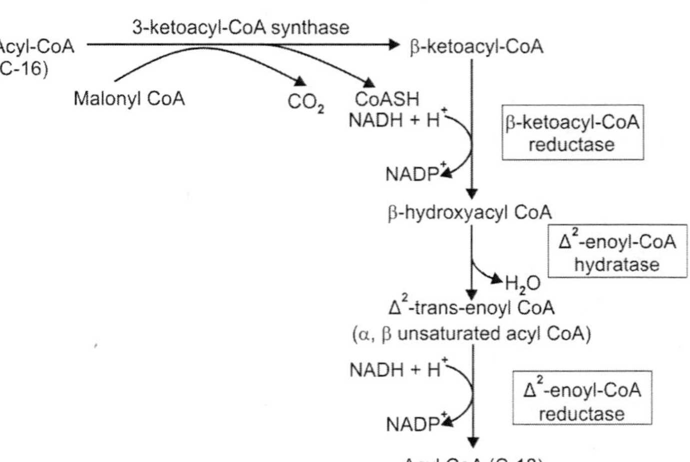


**Fig. 5:** Steps of conversion of palmitate to stearate

## Function

- Microsomal elongation of fatty acid is responsible for synthesis of stearic acid and arachidonic acids from palmitic acid formed in cytosol.

## Significance

- Microsomal elongase system is similar to fatty acids synthase in action but only differences is that the enzymes of elongase system exists as separate integral membrane protein not as multienzyme complex.
- Brain tissue contains a different type of microsomal elongase system
- Other minor pathway of fatty acid elongation is mitochondrial pathway which uses acetyl CoA as source of 2 carbon units.

## 5. Pyruvate oxidation.

- Pyruvate oxidation is 2nd stage in complete oxidation of glucose where in pyruvate formed at end of aerobic glycolysis is further oxidized to Acetyl CoA to be metabolized by TCA cycle.

| *Tissue site* | *Subcellular site* | *Substrate* | *Product* |
|---|---|---|---|
| All tissues | Mitochondria | Pyruvate (end product of aerobic glycolysis) | Acetyl CoA |

**Steps**

a. Mitochondrial entry of pyruvate
   - Pyruvate from cytosol is transported into mitochondria along with $H^+$ (Pyruvate - $H^+$ symport) using inward proton gradient across the membrane

b. Oxidation of pyruvate
   - Enzyme (Pyruvate dehydrogenase complex).

| *Enzymes* | *Co-enzyme* | *Reaction* |
|---|---|---|
| E1 - Pyruvate dehydrogenase | TPP | Oxidative decarboxylation of pyruvate |
| E2 - Dihydrolipoyl transacetylase | Lipoic acid<br>Coenzyme A | Transfer of acetyl group to CoA<br>Reduction of lipoic acid |
| E3 - Dihydrolipoyl dehydrogenase | FAD<br>$NAD^+$ | Oxidation of lipoic acid<br>Reduction of NAD |

**Steps**

i. Pyruvate is decarboxylated to a hydroxymethyl derivative of the thiazole ring of enzyme bound TPP

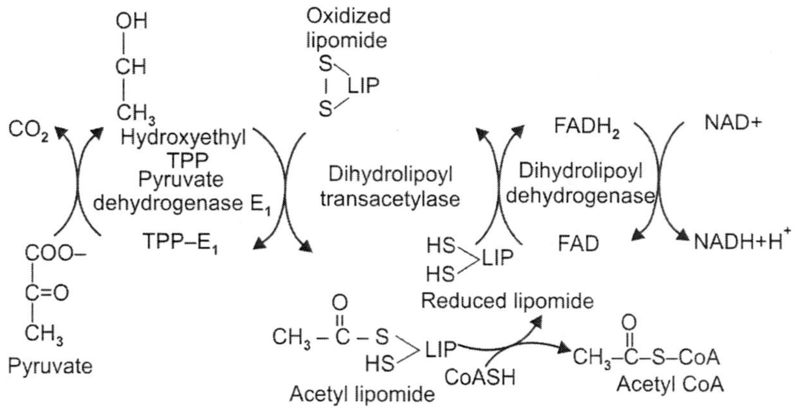

**Fig. 6:** Pyruvate oxidation—pyruvate dehyrogenase complex

Sample Paper-2

ii. Which in turn, reacts with oxidized lipoamide to form 'acetyl lipoamide'
iii. In the presence of dihydrolipoyl transacetylase, acetyl lipoamide reacts with CoA. SH to form 'acetyl CoA' and reduced lipoamide
iv. The latter is reoxidized by a flavoprotein in the presence of dihydrolipoyl dehydrogenase
v. Finally, the reduced flavoprotein is oxidized by $NAD^+$, which in turn transfers the reducing equivalents to the respiratory chain.

*Energetics*

| *Reducing equivalent* | *Mechanism of energy production* | *No. of ATPs* |
|---|---|---|
| $NAD+H^+$ | Oxidative phosphorylation | 2.5 ATPs |

– Thus total ATPs per glucose molecule = 5 ATPs.

*Regulation*

| *Enzyme* | *Regulation* | *Stimulators* | *Inhibitors* |
|---|---|---|---|
| Pyruvate dehydrogenase complex | Covalent modification<br>(Dephosphorylated form—Active<br>Phosphorylated form—Inactive<br>Catalyzed by pyruvate dehydrogenase kinase) | Insulin | Rise in ATP/ADP ratio<br>Rise in $NADH/NAD^+$ ratio<br>Rise in Acetyl CoA/CoA-SH ratio<br>Cyclic AMP levels |
| | Inhibition | | Arsenite, mercuric ions |

## 6. Chromatography.

- Chromatography is a simple technique for the separation of a mixture into its individual components.

### Principle

- Chromatography is carried in 2 media or phases, i.e. a stationary phase and a mobile phase
- Mixture to be separated is dissolved in the smallest possible volume of solvent or buffer and is applied on stationary phase
- As soon as the solution is soaked into the absorbent stationary phase, it is followed by a solvent or buffer.

### Types

| | |
|---|---|
| a. Adsorption chromatography<br>• Stationary phase<br>– Solid stationary medium<br>• Mobile phase<br>– Solvent | • Based on difference in adsorption at surface of a solid stationary medium<br>• Adsorbents are packed into columns and mixture of protein is applied in a solvent on the top<br>• Components get adsorbed with different affinity<br>• Fractions slowly move down; most weakly held move fastest followed by others according to the order of tightness |

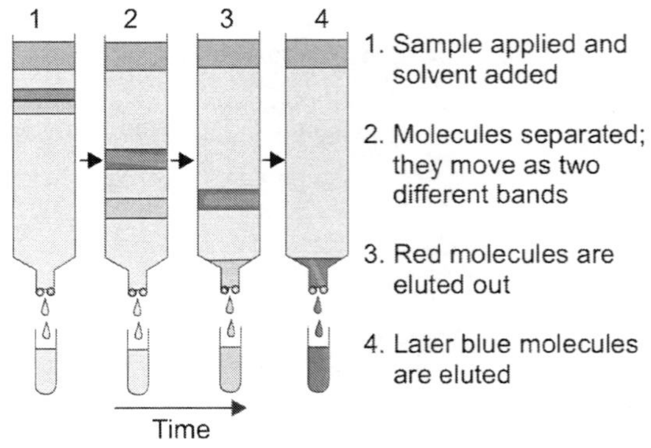

1 2 3 4
1. Sample applied and solvent added
2. Molecules separated; they move as two different bands
3. Red molecules are eluted out
4. Later blue molecules are eluted
Time

**Fig. 7:** Adsorption chromatography

<table>
<tr><td>
b. Partition chromatography<br>
• Stationary phase<br>
– Solid or liquid<br>
• Mobile phase<br>
– Liquid or gaseous<br>
Example<br>
1. Paper chromatography and thin layer chromatography—Used for separation of amino acids and peptides<br>
2. Gas-liquid chromatography—used for separation of lipids
</td><td>
• Components of the mixture to be separated are partitioned between the two phases depending on their partition coefficient of the particular substance<br>
• In Gas-liquid chromatography—stationary liquid phase is supported by inert material in a long narrow column and mixture to be separated is made volatile at one end and vapors are swept over column by an inert courier gas<br>
• Better separation can be achieved by 2 dimensional chromatography, i.e. separation in one direction first and then in direction perpendicular to it:<br>
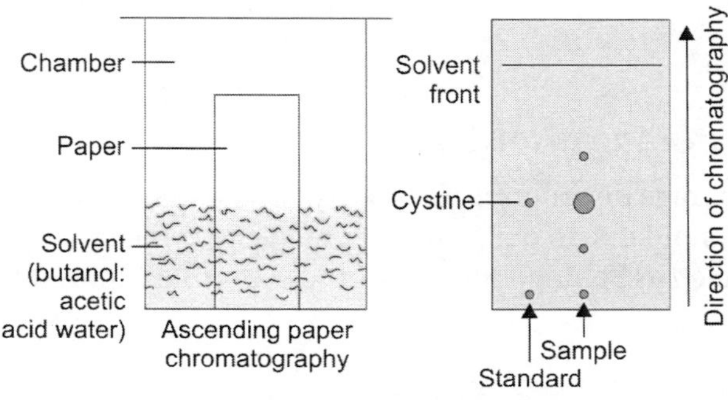
<br>
Fig. 8: Paper chromatography
</td></tr>
<tr><td>
c. Ion exchange chromatography
</td><td>
• Based on electrostatic attraction between charged biological molecules to oppositely charged groups on the ion exchange resin which are cross-linked polymers containing ionic groups<br>
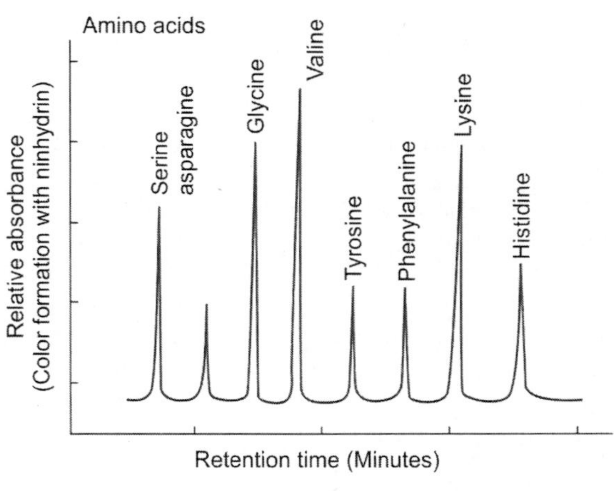
<br>
Fig. 9: Ion exchange chromatography of amino acids
</td></tr>
<tr><td>
d. Gel filtration chromatography (molecular sieving)
</td><td>
• Hydrophilic cross linked gels are used for separation of molecule based on their size<br>
• Used for separation of protein molecules, purification of proteins and molecular weight determinants
</td></tr>
<tr><td>
e. Affinity chromatography
</td><td>
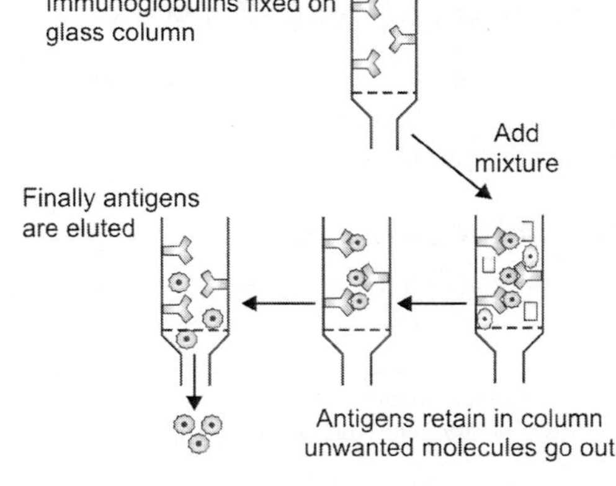
<br>
Fig. 10: Affinity chromatography
</td></tr>
</table>

| | |
|---|---|
| | • Based on the high affinity of specific protein for specific chemical groups<br>• Specific chemical group first covalently attached to the inert matrix, the mixture of proteins are then passed through column and unbound proteins are removed<br>• Particulars proteins retained in column is then eluted<br>• Used for purification of antigens, antibodies or enzymes |
| f. High performance liquid chromatography (HPLC)<br>• Stationary phase<br>– Solid<br>• Mobile phase<br>– Liquid | • Mobile liquid phase passes through the column under high pressure<br>• Separation achieved with better resolution and high speed<br>• Used for all types of compounds |

## 7. Lipid storage disorders.

- Lipid storage disorders are a group of lysosomal storage diseases resulting from failure of breakdown of a particular sphingolipid due to deficiency of a single enzyme
- Also called as Sphingolipidosis as these complex lipids (Sphingolipids) accumulate in the brain and nervous system.

### Features

| *Disease* | *Deficient enzyme* | *LIPID accumulating* | • Features |
|---|---|---|---|
| a. Gaucher's disease | β - glucosidase | Glucocerebroside | • 3 types—adult, infantile, juvenile<br>• Hepatospenomegaly, erosion of bone, moderate anemia, brownish yellow pigmentation of skin, elevated levels of acid phosphatase<br>• CNS involvement is late |
| b. Niemann-Pick disease | Sphingomyelinase | Sphingomyelin | • Profound CNS damage, mental retardation, hepatosplenomegaly, yellowish coloration of skin, cherry red spot in macula<br>• Death by age of 2 years |
| c. Krabbe's leukodystrophy | β-galactosidase | Galactocerebroside | • Severe mental retardation, total absence of myelin in CNS, severe gliosis and globoid bodies in white matter |
| d. Metachromatic leukodystrophy | Sulfatide sulfatase | Sulfogalacta cerebroside (Accumulates in most tissues) | • Neurological deficit, difficulty in speech and finally optic atrophy<br>• Demyelination in late infantile form<br>• Psychological deficit and progressive dementia in adult form |
| e. Fabry's disease | α-galactosidase | Ceramide trihexoside (Accumulates in kidney) | • Progressive renal failure and death by 5 years<br>• Burning and tingling of hands and feet which increase in hot weather, purplish papules on body |
| f. Tay Sach's disease | Hexosaminidase A | Ganglioside ($GM_2$) | • Mental retardation, cherry red spot in macula, progressive deterioration and recurrent infection |
| g. Generalized gangliosidoses | β-galactosidase | Ganglioside ($GM_2$) | • Mental retardation, hepatomegaly, skeletal deformities, foam cells in bone marrow and cherry rod spot in retina |
| h. Lactosyl ceramidoses | β-galactosidase | Lactosyl ceramide | • Affects mainly the CNS and reticuloendothelial system |
| i. Sandhoff's disease | Hexosaminidase A and B | Globoside | • Neurological deficit, mental retardation |

### Common Features of Lipid Storage Diseases

- Usually only one type of sphingolipid accumulates
- Rate of lipid synthesis is normal and only degradation is affected
- Extent of enzyme deficiency is same in all tissues.

## 8. Write about aminoaciduria.

- Amino aciduria is the increased excretion of the amino acid than normal.

| *Causes* | *Types* |
|---|---|
| • Metabolic disorders like defect in either synthesis or breakdown of amino acids or in body's ability to get the amino acid into cells<br>• Chronic liver disease<br>• Renal disorders | a. Overflow aminoaciduria<br>– Defect in metabolic pathway of the amino acid<br>b. Renal aminoaciduria<br>– Defect in renal tubular reabsorption of the amino acid |

## Varieties

| Disorder | Deficiency of | Clinical features | Substance in blood | Substance in urine | Treatment |
|---|---|---|---|---|---|
| a. Phenylketouria (type 1) | Phenylalanine hydroxylase | Mental retardation, hypertonia, seizure | Phenylalanine | Phenylpyruvate | Diet deficient in phenylalanine |
| b. Hypertyrosinemia (type 1) | Fumaryl aceto acetate hydrolase | Mental retardation, hepatorenal damage | Tyrosine, methionine | Tyrosine, PHPPA | Diet deficient in phenylalanine and tyrosine |
| c. Alkaptonuria | Homogentisic acid oxidase | Arthiritis, | Homogentisic acid | Homogentisic acid | Nil |
| d. Homocystinuria (type 1) | Cystathionine beta synthase | Mental retardation, ectopia lentis | Homocysteine, methionine | Homocysteine | Cysteine, methionine |
| e. Homocystinuria (type 2) | Methyl transferase | Mental retardation | Homocysteine | Homocysteine | Folate |
| f. Homocystinuria (type 3) | Methylene THFA | Mental retardation | Homocysteine | Homocysteine | Folate |
| g. Histidinemia | Histidase | Mild mental retardation, speech defect | Histidine, alanine | Imidazole, pyruvic acid | Restrict histidine |
| h. Maple syrup urine disease | Branched chain keto acid decarboxylase | Mental retardation, maple syrup odor | Valine, leucine, isoleucine, keto acids | Valine, leucine, isoleucine, keto acids | Restrict valine, leucine, isoleucine |
| i. Methyl malonic aciduria | Methyl malonyl CoA mutase | Mental retardation, ketosis, hypotonia | Methyl malonic acid | Methyl malonic acid, ketone bodies | Vitamin $B_{12}$ |
| j. Cystathioninuria | Cystathionase | Benign | Cystathionine | Cystathionine | Not required |
| k. Hyperprolinemia | Proline oxidase | Benign | Proline | Proline, hydroxyl proline | -- |
| l. Citrullinemia | Argininosuccinate synthetase | Mental retardation, vomiting, seizures | Ammonia, citrulline | Citrulline | Low protein and high argenine |
| m. Argininemia | Arginase | Spastic diplegia | Arginine, ammonia | Arginine, ornithine | Low protein diet |
| n. Hyperornithinemia | Ornithine decarboxylase | Vomiting, lethargy | Ornithine, ammonia | Ornithine | Low protein diet |
| o. OTC deficiency | Ornithine transcarbamolyase | Lethargy, convulsion | Ammonia | Orotic acid, uracil, glutamine | Low protein diet |
| p. CPS I deficiency | Carbomoyl phosphate synthetase I | Vomiting, lethargy | Ammonia, glutamine | Glutamine | Low protein diet |
| q. Arginino succinic aciduria | Arginino succinate lyase | Vomiting, trichorrhexis nodosa | Arginino succcinate, citrulline | Arginino succcinate, citrulline | Arginine, protein |

## Laboratory Tests

i. Aminoaciduria can be demonstrated in the laboratory by microscopic examination of the urine for amino acid crystals which are very specific for a particular amino acid
 Tyrosine: Turf of fine needles
 Leucine: Yellowish spherical crystals with radial and circular striations
 Cystine: Hexogonal crystals

ii. Ninhydrin can also detect the aminoacid in urine by formation of color complexes called Ruhemann's purple.

iii. Urine chromatography.

## Significance

- Amino acidurias are important clinically as most of them manifest in form of mental retardation and if diagnosed immediately after birth and treatment started, then mental retardation can be prevented
- Even a delay of one week in diagnosis reduces IQ of the child appreciably.

## 9. Sodium-potassium pump.

- Sodium-potassium ($Na^+$-$K^+$) pump is most common transport mechanism found in all parts of body
- Also called $Na^+$-$K^+$ ATPase pump as it uses membrane bound ATPase as a carrier molecule
- Transports sodium out of cell along simultaneous transport of potassium inside cell.

### Location

- Cell membrane of all cells.

| *Structure* | *Mechanism* |
|---|---|
| • Carrier protein, i.e. ATPase is composed of 6 subunits, i.e. 3 $\alpha$ ($\alpha_1$, $\alpha_2$ and $\alpha_3$) and 3 $\beta$ ($\beta_1$, $\beta_2$ and $\beta_3$), all extending through membrane of most cells, however they have specialized function in certain tissues<br>• $\alpha$ subunit transports $Na^+$ and $K^+$ besides which it has:<br>– ATPase enzymatic activity, i.e. ability to convert ATP to ADP thus releasing energy<br>– Binding sites on its intracellular face for $3Na^+$ and 1 ATP molecule and on extracellular face for 2 $K^+$<br>• Function of $\beta$ subunit is unclear | Step 1<br>• Binding of 3 $Na^+$ and ATP to carrier protein inside cell transfers high energy phosphate group from ATP to aspartic acid residue of $\alpha$ subunit of ATPase which causes configuration of protein resulting in transport of 3 $Na^+$ from inside of cell to outside<br>Step 2<br>• When 2 $K^+$ bind to carrier protein on outside of cell, aspartic acid-phosphate bond is hydrolyzed causing second change in configuration of protein resulting in transport of 2 $K^+$ from outside of cell to inside |

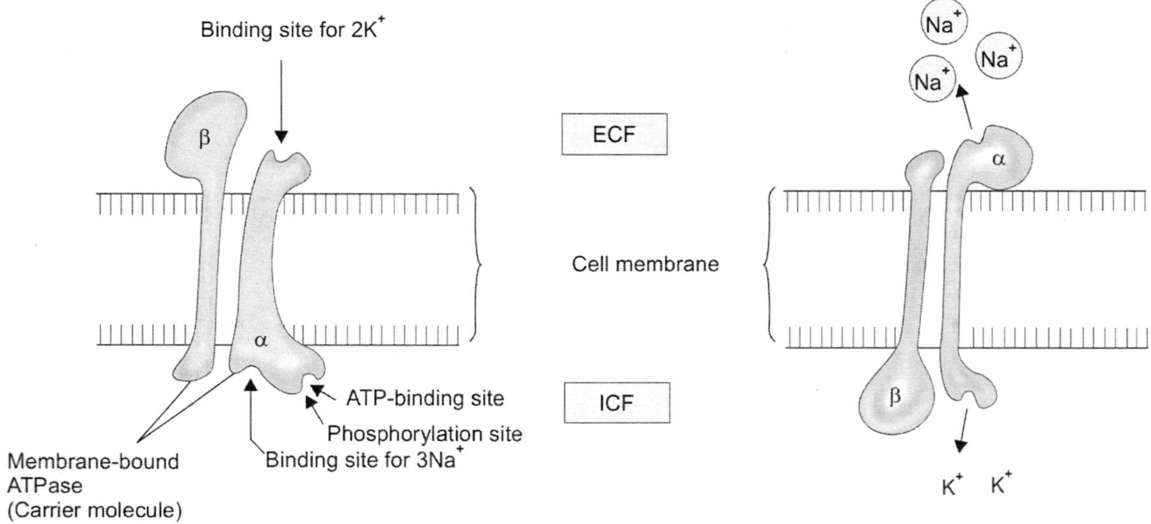


**Fig. 11:** Sodium-potassium pump

| *Inhibitors* | *Stimulators* | *Function (Significance)* |
|---|---|---|
| • Low concentration of either $Na^+$, $K^+$ or ATP<br>• Low temperature<br>• Hypoxia<br>• Metabolic poisons like DNP which prevents ATP synthesis | • Thyroid hormones<br>• Insulin<br>• Aldosterone<br>• G-actin | • Responsible for maintaining the high $K^+$ and low $Na^+$ concentration in cell<br>• Accounts for a large part of the basal metabolism because active transport of $Na^+$ and $K^+$ is one of major energy consuming processes in body<br>• Regulates normal cell volume and pressure<br>• Responsible for development of resting membrane potential |

## 10. Congenital hyperbilirubenemias.

- Congenital hyperbilirubenemias is due to elevation in serum bilirubin level due to inherited defect in the abnormal uptake by liver, conjugation or excretion of bilirubin
- May be conjugated or unconjugated.

## Types

| Disease | Inheritance | Defect in | Features |
|---|---|---|---|
| a. Gilbert's disease | Autosomal dominant | Bilirubin uptake | Patient is asympatomatic except jaundice (bilirubin level up to 3 mg/dL) |
| b. Crigler-Najjar syndrome | Autosomal recessive | Bilirubin conjugation | i. Type 1 (congenital nonhemolytic jaundice)<br>Due to severe deficiency of UDP glucoronyl transferase<br>Jaundice appear in 24 hours of life and results are fatal due kernicterus when bilirubin exceeds 20 mg/dL<br>ii. Type 2 (only 2nd stage of conjugation deficient)<br>Benign disease because serum bilirubin level does not cross 20mg/dL |
| c. Dubin-Johnson's syndrome | Autosomal recessive | Bilirubin excretion | Conjugated bilirubin gets deposited in liver causing blackish discoloration (Black liver Jaundice) |
| d. Rotor syndrome | Autosomal recessive | Bilirubin excretion | No deposition of pigment in liver |

## 11. Describe in detail the de novo synthesis of fatty acids. Add a note on short- and long-term mechanism that regulate lipogenesis.

**For De Novo Synthesis of Fatty Acid**

Refer Question No. 6 Dec. 2013 (RS2).

### Regulation (by Controlling the Activities of the Lipogenetic Enzymes)

i. Short-term or acute control involving allosteric or metabolic regulation and covalent modification of enzymes
ii. Long-term control involving changes in amounts of the enzyme brought about by changes in the rates of synthesis and degradation.

| Short-term regulation | Long-term regulation |
|---|---|
| i. Availability of substrate<br>– Fatty acid synthesis occurs when carbohydrate is abundant and level of fatty acids is low<br>– Availability of citrate in the cytoplasm is the most important short-term regulatory mechanism<br>ii. Acetyl CoA carboxylase<br>– Key enzyme of lipogenesis and earliest unique point for exertion of short-term mechanism<br>– Exists as an inactive protomer or an active polymer<br>– Its activation is promoted by citrate, guanine nucleotides, CoA whereas palmitoyl CoA and malonyl CoA inhibit the enzyme by depolymerization<br>– Also covalently modified, i.e. phosphorylation inactivates acetyl CoA carboxylase<br>iii. Hormonal influences<br>– Glucagon, epinephrine and norepinephrine inactivates acetyl CoA carboxylase by cAMP dependent phosphorylation whereas insulin activates the enzyme by dephosphorylating it. Insulin also promotes lipogenesis by stimulating glucose uptake and its conversion to pyruvate and acetyl CoA | i. Dietary regulation<br>– Consumption of high carbohydrate or fat free diet increases the synthesis of acetyl CoA carboxylase and fatty acid synthase promoting lipogenesis whereas fasting or fat-free diet decreases lipogenesis by reducing the synthesis of these two enzymes<br>ii. Stimulation of acetyl CoA carboxylase, fatty acid synthase, ATP-citrate lyase by insulin |

## 12. Riboflavin.

Riboflavin or vitamin $B_2$ is a water-soluble vitamin.

| Sources | Recommended dietary allowance |
|---|---|
| Rich sources<br>• Milk, meat, eggs, liver, and kidney<br>Moderate sources<br>• Cereals, fruits, green leafy vegetables, fish and yeast | Men: 1.5 mg/day<br>Women: 1.2 mg/day<br>Pregnancy and lactation: 1.5 mg/day |

## Biochemical Functions

*Coenzymes Forms*

a. Flavin mononucleotide (FMN)
b. Flavin adenine dinucleotide (FAD).

*Functions*

a. Energy production
   - FMN and FAD are integral of enzymes called flavoproteins
   - They (mostly FAD and to a lesser extent FMN) participate in many redox reactions responsible for energy production
   - FMN or FAD undergo identical reversible reactions accepting two hydrogen atoms forming FMNH2 or FADH2.

   Example:

| *FAD containing* | *FMN containing* |
|---|---|
| *Protein metabolism* | |
| i. D-amino acid oxidase<br>D-amino acid → $\alpha$-keto acid + $NH_3$<br>ii. Glycine oxidase<br>Glycine → Glyoxylate + $NH_3$ | i. L-amino acid oxidase<br>L-amino acid → $\alpha$-keto acid + $NH_3$ |
| *Carbohydrate metabolism* | |
| i. Pyruvate dehydrogenase complex<br>Pyruvate → Acetyl CoA<br>ii. $\alpha$-ketoglutarate dehydrogenase complex<br>$\alpha$-ketoglutarate → Succinyl CoA<br>iii. Succinate dehydrogenase<br>Succinate → Fumarate | |
| *Lipid metabolism* | |
| i. Acyl CoA dehydrogenase<br>Acyl CoA → $\alpha$, $\beta$ unsaturated acyl CoA<br>ii. Glycerol 3-phosphate dehydrogenase<br>Glycerol 3 phosphate → Dihydroacetone phosphate | |
| *Purine metabolism* | |
| i. Xanthine oxidase<br>Xanthine → Uric acid | |

b. Ectodermal tissue integrity
   - It helps in proper maintenance and health of ectodermal tissues like skin and oral mucosa.

## Deficiency

| *Causes* | *Features* | *Biochemical findings* |
|---|---|---|
| • Inadequate intake<br>• Poor absorption (celiac disease)<br>• Chronic alcoholism | • Mouth soreness, chelosis, angular stomatitis, glossitis<br>• Seborrheic dermatitis, weakness<br>• Corneal vascularization and anemia | • Glutathione reductase activity in RBCs ↓<br>• Riboflavin levels in plasma, RBCs and urine ↓ |

## SHORT ANSWERS

### 13. Formation of glutamine and its importance.

- Glutamine is a non-essential amino acid
- Glutamine is non-toxic and is important tool to dispose ammonia from brain.

| *Formation* | *Functions (importance)* |
|---|---|
| • From ammonia as follows<br>Glutamate + $NH_3$ + ATP<br>↓ Glutamine synthase<br>Glutamine + ADP + Pi | • Transport of ammonia from brain to liver<br>• Ammonia excretion in kidney and hence renal acid base balance<br>• Amino sugar synthesis<br>• NAD biosynthesis from desamido NAD derived from tryptophan<br>• Purine nucleotide biosynthesis by contributing N-3 and N-9 nitrogen atom<br>• Pyrimidine nucleotide biosynthesis by contributing N-3 nitrogen atom<br>• Phenylacetyl glutamine formation (detoxification by conjugation) |

## 14. Methyl folate trap.

- Methyl folate trap is defect in conversion of methyl $FH_4$ to $FH_4$ resulting in trapping of methyl $FH_4$
- Also called methyl group trap or folate trap
- It is called trap because, on one hand, concentration of methyl $FH_4$ continues to rise but, on other hand, due to it being prevented from releasing methyl groups, a 'metabolic dead-end situation' develops, which leads to the inevitable blockage of methylation cycle.

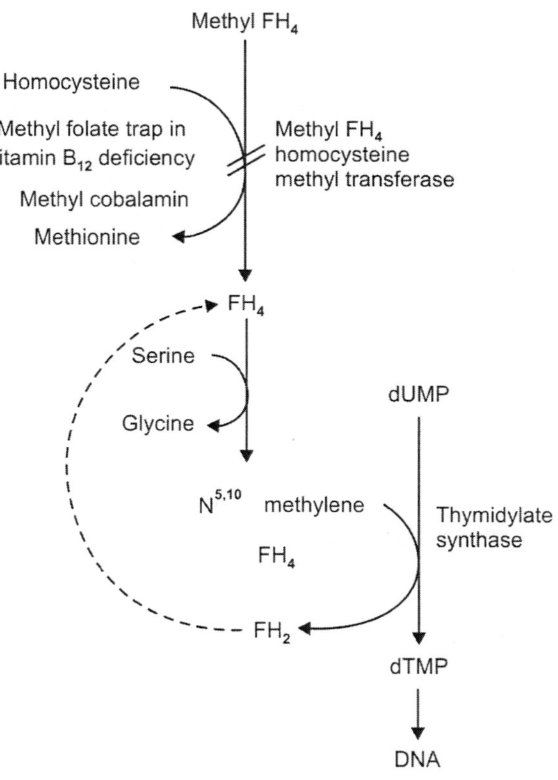


**Fig. 12:** Methyl folate trap

### Cause

- Due to deficiency of vitamin $B_{12}$.

### Effects

- Trapping of methyl $FH_4$ results in non-availability of $FH_4$ derivatives for one carbon metabolism, purine nucleotide and thymidylate synthesis.

## 15. What is hyponatremia? What are its causes?

- Sodium is very important electrolyte playing major role in regulation of plasma volume, acid base balance and also acts as co-transporter.

Normal sodium level
- 130–145 mEq/L.

## Hyponatremia

- Hyponatremia is abnormally low serum sodium concentration lower than 130 mEq/L.

## Causes

| *Hypovolemic hyponatremia (due to sodium and water loss)—characterized by dehydration* | *Euvolemic hyponatremia (due to excess of water intake or SIADH)—characterized by normal sodium* | *Hypervolemic hyponatremia (due to excess of water and sodium retention)—Characterized by oedema* |
|---|---|---|
| a. Extra renal causes<br>– Vomiting<br>– Diarrhea<br>– Gastrointestinal fistula<br>b. Renal causes<br>– Addison's disease<br>– Salt losing nephropathy | a. Due to SIADH<br>– Idiopathic<br>– CNS disorders (meningitis, stroke, tumor)<br>– Pulmonary diseases (tuberculosis, bronchopulmonary carcinoma)<br>– Drugs (chlorpropamide, barbiturates)<br>b. Due to increased water intake<br>– Psychogenic polydipsia<br>– Iatrogenic fluid overload | • Congestive cardiac failure<br>• Cirrhosis of liver<br>• Nephrotic syndrome<br>• End stage chronic renal failure<br>• Acute tubular necrosis |

## Clinical Features

| *Hyponatremia due to excess of water and sodium* | *Hyponatremia due to loss of sodium and water* |
|---|---|
| • Edema, ascites, rales, S3 gallop or raised JVP | • Dehydration, decreased skin turgor, dry mucosa, hypotension and tachycardia |

## Treatment

- Treatment of underlying cause
- Correction of sodium loss for dehydration
- Fluid restriction and diuretics for edema.

## 16. Enumerate the consequences of obesity.

- Obesity is defined as an excess of adipose tissue that imparts health risk, a body of 20% excess over ideal weight for age, sex and height is considered health risk
- It is commonly defined as a body mass index of 30 $kg/m^2$ or higher.

## Health Hazards of Obesity

- Obesity is a risk factor for:
  - Hypertension
  - Diabetes
  - Gallbladder disease
  - Coronary heart disease
  - Certain types of cancers
    - Hormonally related
    - Large bowel cancers
- Obesity predisposes to:
  - Varicose veins
  - Abdominal hernia
  - Osteoarthritis of the knees, hip and lumbar spine
  - Flat feet
- Obesity causes psychological stress especially during adolescence

- Obese persons are at increased risk from surgery
- Obesity may lower fertility.

## 17. Physiological jaundice.

- Physiological jaundice of newborn is mild form of jaundice occurring in newborns on 2nd or 3rd day of life
- Also called neonatal jaundice
- Serum bilirubin rises steadily for a week followed by gradual decline and clinical jaundice manifest when serum bilirubin level >5 mg/dL (but rarely exceeds 12 mg/dL).

| *Pathogenesis* | *Treatment* |
|---|---|
| • Increased serum biliurubin level after birth due to excessive destruction of RBCs<br>• Immaturity of hepatic conjugating enzyme system to metabolize and excrete increased amount of bilirubin | a. Phototherapy<br>– Exposure of newborns with jaundice to white light<br>Role<br>– White light causes structural and configurational photoisomerization of bilirubin to form lumirubin which has shorter life and is water soluble thus is easier to excrete<br>b. Phenobarbitone<br>– Increases glucuronyl transferase levels by enzyme induction |

## 18. Expand ATP. What is its free energy of hydrolysis?

- ATP is an abbreviation of adenosine triphosphate
- It consists of adenosine, ribose sugar and triphosphate moiety
- It is a unique and most important high energy molecule in body.

### Significance

- ATP serves as energy currency of cell.

### Free energy of Hydrolysis

- Free energy of a compound is portion of total energy in a system that is available to do work
- Standard free energy ($\Delta G^o$) is free energy available when reactant or product are at a concentration of 1mol/L at 37°C and pH of 7.0
- Also called chemical potential.

*Free Energy of ATP Hydrolysis*

- Free energy of ATP hydrolysis is 7.3 Kcal/mol
- ATP + $H_2O \rightarrow$ ADP + Pi ($DG^o$ = 7.3 Kcal/mol)
- High energy of ATP is due to relief of change repulsion of adjacent negatively charged oxygen atoms and to stabilization of reaction products.

*Significance*

- Free energy of ATP is used as reference for dividing high energy compounds into high energy phosphates ($DG^o$ > ATP) and low energy phosphates ($\Delta G^o$ < ATP).

## 19. What is second messenger? Give an example.

- Second messengars are group of substances which are produced on interaction of hormone with its receptors on cell membrane.

## Examples

| *Second messenger* | *Hormones* |
|---|---|
| • Cyclic AMP (cAMP) | Glucagon, catecholamine, ACTH, FSH, LH, TSH, ADH, PTH, calcitonin |
| • Phosphotidyl inositol and diacyl glycerol | TRH, GnRH, gastrin, CCK, catecholamines, ADH |
| • Calcium | Acetylcholine |
| • Cyclic GMP (cGMP) | ANP, EDRF |
| • Tyrosine kinase | Insulin, prolactin, GH, oxytocin |

## 20. Peroxisomes.

- Peroxisomes or microbodies are single membrane cellular organelles present in most of eukaryotic cells.

| *Features* | *Functions* |
|---|---|
| • Spherical or oval in shape with 0.3–1.5 µm<br>• Contain enzymes like catalase, peroxidase, uric acid oxidase<br>• Prominent in leukocytes and platelets | • Oxidation of amino acids and long chain fatty acids (C-26 to C-28)<br>• Hydrogen peroxide metabolism into water and oxygen by catalase<br>• Biosynthesis of bile acids, glycolipids and plasmalogens |

## 21. Mention the normal types of hemoglobin.

- Hemoglobin is a conjugated protein consisting of heme and globin
- Heme is an iron protoporphyrin IX complex and globin is a protein consisting of 4 polypeptide chains.

### Normal Types of Hemoglobin

| *Types* | *Polypeptide chains* | *Percentange of total Hb* | *Remarks* |
|---|---|---|---|
| a. Adult hemoglobins | | | |
| – $HbA_1$ | $2\alpha$ and $2\beta$ | 90–95% | Low affinity for oxygen than HbF |
| – $HbA_2$ | $2\alpha$ and $2\ \delta$ | 1–2% | Minor form of Hb |
| – $HbA_{1c}$ (glycosylated Hb) | $2\alpha$ and $2\beta$ | 4–6% | • Glucose derived product of normal adult hemoglobin<br>• Formed by enzymatic addition of glucose to hemoglobin which is irreversible, i.e. one glycosylated hemoglobin is formed it remains in the RBC till its life span<br>Importance<br>• Estimation of glycosylated hemoglobin level in blood in indicator of mean glucose level over previous 10–12 weeks<br>• It is more of a prognostic marker for diabetic patient, i.e. it is used to monitor the blood glucose level of a diabetic patient once every 3 months<br>• Usually glycosylated hemoglobin level should be below 7% and an elevated glycosylated hemoglobin level is indicator of poor control of diabetes mellitus |
| b. Fetal hemoglobin | | | |
| – HbF | $2\alpha$ and $2\gamma$ | 1–2% | • More affinity to oxygen than HbA and less affinity to 2DPG due to lack of $\beta$ chains<br>• Disappears after birth |
| c. Embryonic hemoglobin | | | |
| – Hemoglobin Gover I | $2\varsigma$ and $2\varepsilon$ | – | Minor form of Hb during embryonic development |
| – Hemoglobin Gover II | $2\alpha$ and $2\varepsilon$ | – | Major form of Hb during embryonic development |

## 22. Glycosidic linkage.

- Glycosidic linkages are bonds formed between hemiacetal or hemiketal hydroxyl group of a carbohydrate with hydroxyl or amino group of another carbohydrate or a noncarbohydrate.

| Types | Naming of glycosidic bonds | Examples |
|---|---|---|
| a. O- lycosidic bonds<br>– Glycosidic linkages between two hydroxyl groups<br>b. N-glycosidic bonds<br>– Glycosidic linkages between hydroxyl and amino groups | • Glycosidic bonds are named according to status of anomeric carbon ($\alpha$ or $\beta$) and carbon atom number involved in bond<br>• Glycosidic bond is read from right to left | • Lactose has $\beta$(1-4) glycosidic bond, i.e. bond between $C_1$ of $\beta$-galactose and $C_4$ of glucose<br>• Maltose has $\alpha$(1-4) glycosidic bond, i.e. bond between $C_1$ and $C_4$ of $\alpha$ glucose molecules |

## Significance

- Carbohydrates combine with other carbohydrates or proteins via glycosidic bonds forming di, oligo or polysaccharides or glycoproteins.

## 23. Homocysteine.

- Homocysteine is an intermediate in synthesis of cysteine from methionine.

| Formation | Fate | Normal level |
|---|---|---|
| • From S-adenosyl homocysteine (SAH) by removing adenosyl group | • Can be converted to methionine by addition of a methyl group<br>• Forms cystathionine on condensation with serine in presence of cystathionine $\beta$ synthase | • <15 µmol/L |

## Clinical Significance

- Elevated homocysteine levels are implicated in coronary heart disease by producing reactive free radicals on reaction with collagen and interfering with collagen cross links
- It also increases tendency for atherosclerosis by promoting aggregation of LDL particles.

## 24. What are ribozymes? Mention one use of ribozymes.

- Ribozymes (RNA enzymes) are ribonucleic acids functioning as biological catalysts
- Thus they are non-protein enzymes.

## Functions (Uses)

a. RNA metabolism (splicing)
   – Catalyzing cleavage and synthesis of phosphodiester bond of other RNAs

b. Protein biosynthesis
   – Peptide bond formation during protein synthesis.

## 25. How is histamine formed? What is the role of histamine?

- Histamine is a vasoactive aminwwe formed from histadine.

| Formation | Sources |
|---|---|
| • Histamine is formed by decarboxylation of histadine in presence of enzyme histadine decarboxylase | • Platelets, mast cells, basophils, stomach and brain |

## Role (Functions)

| Tissue | Receptor | Effect |
|---|---|---|
| • Blood vessels | $H_1$ | Pulmonary venous dilatation<br>Superficial temporal artery dilatation (migraine)<br>Dilatation of large veins, smaller venules and capillaries |
| • Cardiovascular system | $H_1$ | Hypotension<br>Increased capillary permeability |
| • Heart | $H_1$ | Chronotropic and ionotropic effect on heart<br>Increased coronary blood flow |

| *Tissue* | *Receptor* | *Effect* |
|---|---|---|
| • Smooth muscles | $H_1$ | Contraction of bronchial muscles (bronchospasm) |
| • Stomach | $H_2$ | Stimulation of gastric acid secretion |
| • Central nervous system | $H_3$ | Increased sensitivity of excitatory responses |

## Significance

- Unwanted effects of serotonin can be minimized by administration of antihistaminic drugs.

## 26. Name the ketone bodies and the tests to detect them.

- Ketone bodies metabolic products of fatty acid oxidation produced due to excessive breakdown of fatty acids.

## Examples

- Acetone
- Acetoacetate
- β-hydroxybutyrate.

## Tests to Detect Ketone Bodies

a. Rothera's test:
   - Most common test to detect ketone bodies in urine

   Principle:
   - Acetone and acetoacetic acid react with sodium nitropruside in presence of alkali to produce purple color

   Procedure:
   - Few mL of ammonia is added to a mixture of 5 mL of saturated urine (with ammonium sulfate) in 3 drops of freshly prepared sodium nitropresside along sides of test tube

   Observation:
   - A violet ring is formed at junction of two fluids if urine contains ketone bodies

   Interpretation (based on intensity of color formed)
   - No change in color Negative
   - Pinkish ring +
   - Red ring ++
   - Deep purple ring +++

b. Gerhardt's test (for acetoacetic acid)
   - Addition of 10% ferric chloride to urine turns it red port in color if ketone bodies are present in urine.

## 27. Phosphate synthetases carbamoyl.

- Carbamoyl phosphate synthetases two sets of enzymes.

## Features

| *Features* | *Carbamoyl phosphate synthetase I (CPS I)* | *Carbamoyl phosphate synthetase II (CPS II)* |
|---|---|---|
| • Involved in | Urea cycle | Pyramidine synthesis |
| • Presence in eukaryotes | Absent | Present |
| • Subcellular location | Mitochondria | Cytosol |
| • Substrates (catalyzes condensation of) | $CO_2 + NH_4$ | $CO_2$ + glutamate |
| • Activators | N-acetylglutamate (allosterically) | PRPP and ATP |
| • Inhibitors | – | UDP, UTP, CDP or CTP |
| • Significance | Rate limiting enzyme | Regulatory enzyme (in animals) |
| • Deficiency | Hyperammonemia type I | – |

## 28. Cyclic adenosine monophasphate.

- Cyclic adenosine monophosphate (AMP) is an adenosine nucleotide.

| *Composition (structure)* | *Metabolism* | *Function* |
|---|---|---|
| • Adenine, ribose and a phosphate | Synthesis<br>• From ATP by membrane bound enzyme adenylate cyclase<br>Degradation<br>• Hydrolysis into 5′ AMP by phosphodiesterase | Acts as second messenger for polypeptide hormones (Group IA)<br>• Adrenocorticotropic hormone (ACTH)<br>• Follicle-stmulating hormone (FSH) and luteinizing hormone (LH)<br>• Thyroid-stimulating hormone (TSH)<br>• Human chorionic gonadotropin (hCG)<br>• Antidiuretic hormone (ADH)<br>• Glucagon<br>• Parathyroid hormone<br>• Calcitonin<br>• Catecholamines<br>Mechanism of action<br>• Activation of protein kinase A which in turn catalyzes phosphorylation of target proteins bringing about desired effect |

# ANNEXURE

## RATE LIMITING ENZYMES

| *Pathway* | *Enzyme* |
|---|---|
| Glycolysis | Phosphofructokinase |
| Gluconeogenesis | Fructose-1,6-bisphosphatase |
| TCA cycle | Isocitrate dehydrogenase |
| Glycogenesis | Glycogen synthase |
| Glycogenolysis | Glycogen phosphorylase |
| HMP shunt | Glucose-6-phosphate dehydrogenase |
| Heme synthesis | ALA synthase |
| De novo pyrimidine synthesis | Carbamoyl phosphate synthetase II |
| De novo purine synthesis | Glutamine PRPP amidotransferase |
| Denovo synthesis of fatty acids | Acetyl CoA carboxylase |
| Fatty acid oxidation | Carnitine acyltransferase I |
| Cholesterol biosynthesis | HMG CoA Reductase |
| Ketogenesis | HMG-CoA synthase |
| Bile acid synthesis | 7-α hydroxylase |
| Urea cycle | Carbamoyl phosphate synthase I |
| Catecholamine synthesis | Tyrosine hydroxylase |
| Melatonin synthesis | Serotonin N-acetylase |

## SUBCELLULAR SITES OF REACTIONS

| *Cytosol* | *Mitochondria* | *Both* |
|---|---|---|
| Glycolysis<br>Glycogen metabolism<br>Hexose monophosphate (HMP) shunt<br>Cholestrol synthesis<br>Protein synthesis<br>Steroid synthesis<br>Amino acid metabolism | β oxidation of fatty acids<br>Oxidative phosphorylation and electron transport chain<br>Ketogenesis and ketolysis<br>Krebs cycle (TCA cycle)<br>Oxidative deamination | Urea cycle<br>Heme synthesis<br>Gluconeogenesis<br>Fatty acid synthesis |

## ENERGETICS

| *Metabolic pathway* | *Energetics* |
|---|---|
| Glycolysis (Aerobic) | 7 ATPs (per glucose molecule) |
| Glycolysis (Anaerobic) | 2 ATPs (per glucose molecule) |
| TCA cycle | 20 ATPs (per glucose molecule) |

*Contd...*

*Contd...*

| *Metabolic pathway* | *Energetics* |
|---|---|
| Glycogenesis | –2 ATPs (to incorporate one glucose molecule) |
| Gluconeogenesis | –6 ATPs (for every glucose molecule) |
| Fatty acid oxidation | 106 ATPs (per palmitic acid molecule) |
| Fatty acid synthesis | –42 ATPs (for synthesis of palmitic acid) |

## VITAMINS

| *Deficiency disorder* | *Vitamin* | *Coenzyme* | *Function* |
|---|---|---|---|
| Xerophthalmia (night blindness) | Vitamin A | – | Night vision<br>Color vision<br>Reproductive function<br>Growth and differentiation |
| Rickets and osteomalacia | Vitamin D | – | Calcium homeostasis<br>Bone mineralization |
| Bleeding disorders | Vitamin K | – | Coagulation |
| – | Vitamin E | – | Antioxidant |
| Scurvy | Vitamin C | Ascorbic acid<br>Dehydroascobic acid | Iron absorption<br>Coenzyme for enzymes |
| Beri beri | Vitamin $B_1$ (thiamine) | TPP (thiamine pyrophosphate) | Cofactor for dehydrogenase enzymes |
| – | Vitamin $B_2$ (riboflavin) | FMN (Flavin mononucleotide) and FAD (flavin adenine dinucleotide) | Electron carriers |
| Pellagra | Vitamin $B_3$ (niacin) | NAD (nicotinamide adenine dinucleotide) and NADP (nicotinamide adenine dinucleotide phosphate) | Reducing equivalents |
| – | Vitamin $B_6$ (pyridoxine) | PLP (pyridoxal phosphate) | Transamination |
| Megaloblastic anemia | Vitamin $B_{12}$ (cyanocobalamin) | Methylcobalamin and deoxyadenosylcobalamin | Essential for folate metabolism |
| – | Biotin | Biocytin | Carboxylation |
| Megaloblastic anemia | Folic acid | FH4 (tetrahydrofolate) | One carbon reactions |
| – | Pantothenic acid | Coenzyme A | Acyl group carrier |

| | *Essential* | *Semiessential* | *Nonessential* |
|---|---|---|---|
| Amino acid | Methionine<br>Threonine<br>Valine<br>Isoleucine<br>Leucine<br>Phenylalanine<br>Lysine | Histidine<br>Arginine | Others |
| Fatty acids | Linoleic acid<br>Linolenic acid | Arachidonic acid | -- |

| *Ketogenic* | *Both ketogenic and glucogenic* | *Glucogenic* |
|---|---|---|
| Leucine | Phenylalanine<br>Isoleucine<br>Tyrosine<br>Tryptophan<br>Lysine | Others |

## INBORN ERRORS OF METABOLISM

| *Metabolic pathways* | *Deficient enzyme or defective system* |
|---|---|
| *Amino acid metabolism* | |
| Phenylketonuria (PKU) | Phenylalanine hydroxylase |
| Malignant PKU | Biopterin cofactor |
| Type 1 tyrosinemia | Fumarylacetoacetate hydrolase |
| Type 2 tyrosinemia | Tyrosine aminotransferase |
| Alkaptonuria | Homogentisic acid oxidase |
| Albinism | Tyrosinase |
| Homocystinuria and hyperhomocysteinemia | Cystathionine-β-synthase or methylenetetrahydrofolate reductase or various deficiencies in formation of the methylcobalamin form of vitamin $B_{12}$ |
| Maple syrup urine disease | Branched-chain ketoacid dehydrogenase complex |
| *Organic acid metabolism* | |
| Propionic acidemia | Propionyl-CoA carboxylase |
| Multiple carboxylase deficiency | Pyruvate carboxylase and 3-methylcrotonyl-CoA carboxylase |
| Methylmalonic acidemia | Methylmalonyl-CoA mutase;<br>Defects in the enzyme systems involved in vitamin $B_{12}$ metabolism |
| *Fatty acid metabolism* | |
| Hyperlipidemia and hypercholesterolemia | Regulation or utilization of lipoproteins |
| Fatty acid oxidation disorders | Very long chain acyl-CoA dehydrogenase; long chain hydroxyacyl-CoA dehydrogenase; dehydrogenase; medium chain acyl-CoA dehydrogenase; short chain acyl-CoA dehydrogenase; short chain hydroxyacyl-CoA dehydrogenase |
| *Glycogen storage diseases* | |
| Type 0 | Glycogen synthase |
| Type I (Von Gierke's disease) | Glucose-6-phosphatase |
| Type II (Pompe's disease) | Acid maltase |
| Type III (Forbe's/Cori's disease) | Debranching enzyme |
| Type IV (Anderson's disease) | Branching enzyme |
| Type VI (Her's disease) | Liver glycogen phosphorylase |
| Type VII (Tarui's disease) | Muscle and erythrocyte phosphofructokinase 1 |
| Type VIII and IX | Phosphoylase kinase |
| *Carbohydrate metabolism* | |
| Galactosemia | Galactose-1-phosphate uridyltransferase |
| Lactose Intolerance | Intestinal lactase |
| Fructose Intolerance | Aldolase B |
| Fructosuria | Fructokinase |
| *Purine and pyrimidine metabolism* | |
| Lesch-Nyhan syndrome | Hypoxanthine phosphoribosyl-transferase |
| Orotic aciduria | Orotate phosphoribosyltrasnferase and OMP decarboxylase |
| *Lysosomal storage disorders* | |
| Gaucher disease | Cerebrosidase |
| Niemann-Pick disease | Sphingomyelinase |
| Refsum's disease | Branched-chain fatty acid buildup |
| Tay-Sachs disease | Beta-hexosaminidase A |
| Fabry disease | α-galactosidase |

*Contd...*

*Contd...*

| *Metabolic pathways* | *Deficient enzyme or defective system* |
|---|---|
| Hurler syndrome, Hunter syndrome | α-iduronidase (Hurler syndrome); iduronate sultatase (Hunter syndrome) iduronate sulfatase (Hunter syndrome) |
| *Urea cycle* | |
| Hyperammonemia type 1 | Carbamoyl phosphate synthetase I |
| Hyperammonemia type 2 | Ornithine transcarbamylase |
| Citrullinemia | Argininosuccinate synthase |
| Argininosuccinic aciduria | Argininosuccinate lyase |
| Hyperargininemia | Arginase |
| *Heme metabolism* | |
| Acute intermittent porphyria | Hydroxymethylbilane synthase (uroporphyrinogen I synthase or PBG deaminase) |
| Porphyria Cutanea Tarda | Uroporphyrinogen decarboxylase |
| Protoporphyria | Ferrochelatase |
| Erythropoietic porphyria | Uroporphyrinogen cosynthase |
| Hereditary coproporphyria | Coproporphyrinogen oxidase |
| Variegate porphyria | Protoporphyrinogen oxidase |
| *Bilirubin metabolism* | |
| Criggler-Najjar syndrome | UDP-glucuronyltransferase |
| Gilbert's disease | Reduced activity of UDP-glucuronyltransferase |



## REFERENCE RANGE

| | *Normal level* |
|---|---|
| Aspartate aminotransferase (AST/SGOT) | 8–20 IU/L |
| Alanine aminotransferase (ALT/SGPT) | 10–35 IU/L |
| Acid phosphatase (ACP) | 2.5–12 IU/L |
| Alkaline phosphatase (ALP) | 40–125 IU/L |
| Amylase | 50–120 IU/L |
| Sodium | 135–145 mEq/L |
| Potassium | 3.5–5 mEq/L |
| Chlorides | 96–106 mEq/L |
| Bicarbonates | 20–26 mEq/L |
| Calcium | 9–11 mg/dL |
| Phosphorus | 3–4.5 mg/dL |
| Proteins | 6–8 g/dL |
| Albumin | 3–5 mg/L |
| Globulin | 2.5–3 mg/L |
| Glucose (fasting) | 70–110 mg/dL |
| Urea | 20–40 mg/dL |
| Creatinine | 0.7–1.4 mg/dL |
| Uric acid | 3–7 mg/dL |
| Cholesterol | 150–200 mg/dL |
| Bilirubin | 0.2–1 mg/dL |
| Direct/conjugated bilirubin | 0.1–0.4 mg/dL |
| Indirect/unconjugated bilirubin | 0.2–0.7 mg/dL |
| Hemoglobin | 13–16 g/dL |

# INDEX


**A**

Acetyl CoA 270
  fate 270
  sources 270
Acid-base balance, renal regulation of 191
Adenosine triphosphate (ATP) 365
  formation, sites of 67
Albinism 162
Albumin 206
Albumin/globulin ratio 207
Aldolase B deficiency 332
Alkalosis 312
Alkaptonuria 161
Allosteric enzymes 184
Alpha-fetoprotein (AFP) 208
Amino acid
  classify 247
  essential 138
  limiting 100
  nutritional classification of 154
Aminoaciduria 358
Anaplerosis 92
Anion gap 15
Anomerism 256
Anticancer agents 244
Anticoagulants 100
Anti-egg white injury factor 341
Antioxidant 94
  vitamins 94
Antiport 181
Apolipoproteins 127
Arachidonic acid 267
Atherosclerosis 300

**B**

Bacterial DNA polymerases 34
Balanced diet 279
Basal metabolic rate (BMR) 45
Base pairing rule 226
Bence-Jones protein 33
Beri-beri 14
Bicarbonate
  buffer 191
  reclamation 192
Bile salts 274
Bilirubin
  conjugation 71
  metabolism 71
Biochemical defect 373
  in albinism 373
  in alkaptonuria 373
  in Criggler-Najjar syndrome 129
  in drug induced hemolytic anemia 129
  in galactosemia 373
  in Gauchers's disease 373
  in Gilbert's disease 373
  in hereditary fructose intolerance 373
  in homocystinuria 373
  in hyperargininemia 373
  in lactose intolerance 373
  in maple syrup urine disease 373
  in methyl malonyl aciduria 373
  in Niemann-Pick disease 373
  in phenylketonuria 373
  in Refsum's disease 373
Biologically active peptides 46
Biotin 341
Biotransformation 27
Biphosphoglycerate pathway 151
Blood
  buffers 190
  sugar, regulation of 131
Brown adipose tissue 346

**C**

Calcitriol 73, 123
Calcium 121
  homeostasis 122
  regulations, parathyroid hormone in 123
Carbamoyl phosphate synthatases 368
Carbohydrate
  digestion
    and absorption of 271
    enzyme in 272
  function of 105
Carbomoyl phosphate synthetase deficiency 180
Carbon and nitrogen atoms
  of purine ring, sources of 214
  of pyrimidine ring, sources of 203
Carbon metabolism 286
Carbonic anhydrase 346
  in acid-base regulation 325
Carboxyhemoglobin 99
Carboxylation reactions 342
Carcinogenesis 142
Carnitine cycle 103
Carnitine in beta-oxidation, role of 103
Catabolism heme 71
Catecholamines 309
Cell
  cycle 318
  diagram of 205
  membrane 138
    functions 138
    transport across 290
Cellular buffers, extra 191
Chargaff's rule 226
Chemiosmotic theory 144
Chloride shift 95
Cholesterol 300
  catabolic products of 124
  functions 300
  substances formed 300
  transport, reverse 280
Chondroitin sulphate 285
Chromatography 356
Chylomicrons 10
Citric acid cycle 90
  amphibolic role of 91
Clearance tests 29
Cobalamin 285
Codon 173
  chain
    initiating 173
    terminating 173
  degeneracy of 173
Coenzymes 242
Colorimeter 339
Competitive inhibition 64
Concentration dilution test 176
Copper 317
Cori's cycle 120
CPK isoenzymes 83
Creatinine clearance test 30
Crigler-Najjar syndrome 361
Cyclic amp 369
Cyclic nucleotides 49
Cysteine 7
Cystinuria 108
Cytochrome 188
  in detoxification reaction 114
  oxidase, inhibitors of 69

**D**

Deamination 339
Decarboxylation reactions 41
De novo synthesis of purine 214
Deoxyribonucleic acid 147
  functions 147
  probes 324
  replication 147
  structure 146
  technology, recombinant 93
Detoxification 27
  by conjugation 28
  of alcohol 129
  of ammonia 178
Diabetes mellitus 106
Dietary
  antioxidants 94
  fiber 264
Digestion of lipids, enzyme in 283
Disaccharides, digestion and absorption of 210
DNA repair mechanism, base excision 327
Dubin-Johnson disease 361

**E**

Eicosanoids 267
Electron transport chain 66
Electrophoresis 295
Embden-Mayerhof pathway 248
Endocytosis 290
Endonuclease and restriction endonuclease, difference between 287
Endopeptidases 127
Endoplasmic reticulum 155
Energy compounds, high 223
Enzyme
  absolute specificity of 194
  action
    factors affecting 213
    mechanism of 350
  activity, regulation of 329
  classify 212
  clinical importance of 236
  diagnostic importance of 173
  inhibition 64
  irreversible inhibition of 351
  mechanism of 350
  specificities 194
Enzyme-therapeutic uses 12
Epimerism 256
Erythropoietic porphyria, congenital 278

**F**

Facilitated diffusion 292
Fatty acid
  beta oxidation of 102
  essential 308
  microsomal chain elongation of 354
  synthase complex 38
Fatty liver 52
Ferritin 79
FIGLU 255
  excretion test 224
Fluid
  and electrolyte, hormonal regulation of 185
  mosaic model 137
Fluoride 317
Fluorosis 99
Folic acid 305
Free radicals 18
Fructose
  intolerance 332
  metabolism 331

**G**

GABA 255
Galactosemia 311
Gastric function test 343
Gene
  expression, regulation of 240
  therapy 85
Genetic code 173
Gilberts syndrome 258
Glucagon 83
Glucokinase 346
Gluconeogenesis 117 120
Glucose
  6 phosphate dehydrogenase deficiency 86
  absorption 273
  alanine cycle 120
  tolerance
    curve 336
    test 335
  transporters 340
Glutamine 362
Glutathione 208
Glycine 22
Glycogen storage disorders 50
Glycogenesis 58
Glycogenolysis 59
Glycolysis 248
Glycosaminoglycans 284
Glycosides 347
Glycosidic linkage 366
Glycosuria 345
Glyscolysis, regulation 250
Golgi complex 345
Gout 63
Growth factors 32

**H**

Hartnup's disease 197
Hemoglobin 229
Hemoglobinopathies 231
HDL cholesterol 10
Heme proteins 110
Hemochromatosis 338
Hemoglobin
  abnormal types 231
  buffering agent 296
  normal types 366
Hemolytic jaundice 334
Hemosiderosis 338
Henderson-Hasselbach equation 252
Hepatocellular jaundice 334
Hexokinase and glucokinase, difference between 346
Hexose monophosphate shunt 234
Hippuric acid test 113
Histamine 367
HMG CoA 297
Homocysteine 367
Homocystinuria 108, 275
Hormones regulating water balance 281
Hyaluranic acid 285
Hydrochloric acid in protein digestion 261
Hydrolysis, free energy of 365
Hydroxy amino acids 247
Hyperbilirubinemia,
  congenital 360
  unconjugated 110
Hyperhomocysteinemia 344
Hyperuricemia 63
Hypervitaminosis A 135
Hypoalbuminemia 207
Hypocalcemia 124
Hypokalemia 165
Hyponatremia 363
Hypothyroidism 304

**I**

Immunoelectrophoresis 99
Immunoglobulin 167
  A (IgA) 168
  G (IgG) 168
  M (IgM) 168
Insulin 6
Intracellular insulin receptor 49
Invert sugar 344
Iodine 174
  metabolism 87
Ionophores 209
Iron 76
  toxicity 338
Isoelectric pH 344
Isoenzymes 82

**J**

Jaundice 334

**K**

Ketogenesis 170
Ketolysis 171
Ketone bodies 170
  test for 368
Ketosis 171
$K_m$ value 164
Kwashiorkor 152

**L**

Lac operon concept 240
Lactose intolerance 346
Lagging strand, replication of 149
LDH isoenzymes 83
LDL cholesterol 10
Lecithin 136
Lesch-Nyhan syndrome 15
Lipid
  classify 201
  compound 201
  digestion and absorption of 283
  functions of 202
  peroxidation 86
  storage disorders 358
Lipogenesis, regulation 361
Lipoproteins 10
Lipotropic factors 53
Liver function
  enzyme assays for 114
  tests 110
Lyases 212
Lysosomes 166

**M**

Magnesium 317
Malate-aspartate shuttle 225
Maple syrup urine disease 126
Marasmus 152
  and kwashiorkor, difference between 152
Melanin synthesis 159

Melatonin 198
Menke's disease 199
Messenger RNA (mRNA) 218
Metabolic acidosis 79, 96
Metabolic alkalosis and respiratory alkalosis, difference between 312
Metabolism 158
 of galactose 353
Methanol poisoning, ethanol in 48
Methemoglobin 302
Methemoglobinemia 302
Methionine 231
Methyl folate trap 363
Michaelis-Menten constant 164
Milk and dairy products, nutritional role of 325
Missense mutation 17
Mitochondria 195
Mitochondrial shuttle systems 224
Monoclonal antibodies 256
Mucopolysaccharides 284
Multienzyme complex 36
Muscle phosphorylase deficiency 51
Mutagens 317
Mutarotation 56
Mutations 16
Myocardial infarction 261
 enzyme profile in 260

**N**

Native protein and denatured protein, difference between 352
Negative acute phase reactants 154
Niacin 220
Niemann-Pick disease 155
Nitrogen
 balance 17
  positive 18
 producing substances 322
Non-competitive inhibition 64
Non-enzymatic antioxidants 94
Non-protein nitrogenous substances 81
Nucleotide 62
 biologically important 20
 excision repair? 328
Nutritional deficiency anemias 35

**O**

Obesity, consequences 364
Obstructive jaundice 244, 334
Okazaki fragments 318
Oncogenes 163
Organelles 205
Orotic aciduria 16
Oxidative and substrate level phosphorylation, difference between 259
Oxidative phosphorylation 144
 uncouplers of 145
Oxygen species, reactive 115

**P**

P:O ratio 69
Pantothenic acid 275
Passive transport 291
Pellagra 221
Pepsinogen 261
Peptide bond 353
Peroxisomes 366
Phenylalanine 158
Phenylketonuria (PKU) 160
Phosphate buffer 191
Phospholipids 136
Phosphorus 221
Physiological jaundice 365
Plasma proteins 266
 separation of 295
Plasmids 75
Point mutation 17
Polyamines 293
Polymerase chain reaction 43
Polyunsaturated fatty acids 308
Porphyria 276
 acute intermittent 277
Post-transcriptional modifications of messenger RNA 139
Post-translational modification 225
Potassium 207
Proenzymes 141
Prostaglandins 268
Prostate specific antigen (PSA) 208
Protein
 acute phase 154
 alpha-helical structure of 182
 beta-pleated structure of 182
 biological value of 315
 biosynthesis 1
  inhibitors of 5
 classify 217
 complementary 316
 complete 142
 denaturation of 156
 digestion and absorption of 261
 energy malnutrition 152
 of blood, transport 126
 primary structure of 181
 quaternary structure of 183
 secondary structure of 182
 structural organization of 181
 structure, bonds contributing to 352
 tertiary structure of 183
Proteolytic enzymes 261
Protooncogenes 163
Provitamins 318
PUFA 255
Purine
 catabolism 62
 salvage pathways of 31
Pyridoxine 40
Pyrimidines, degradation of 97
Pyruvate
 dehydrogenase complex 36
 fate of 355
 oxidation 355

**R**

Radio isotopes 245
Radioactive isotopes 165
Radioactivity 246
Rancidity 98
Rapoport-Luebering cycle 151
Reference range 89, 374
 of albumin 374
 of ALT 374
 of amylase 374
 of AST 374
 of bicarbonates 374
 of calcium 374
 of cholesterol 374
 of creatinine 374
 of fasting blood glucose 374
 of phosphorus 374
 of potassium 374
 of sodium 374
 of total proteins 374
 of urea 374
Refsum's disease 98
Renal
 clearance 29
 distal tubular function tests 320
 function tests 175
 glycosuria 157, 188
 threshold for glucose 167
 tubular function tests 319
Respiratory
 acidosis 79, 265
 alkalosis 289
 quotient 157
 regulation of acid-base balance 193
Restriction endonucleases 287
Restriction fragment length polymorphism 345
Riboflavin 361
Ribonucleic acid (RNA) 218
 polymerase 313
 synthesis 53
  inhibitors of 56
Ribosomal ribonucleic acid (rRNA) 220
Ribosomes in proteins biosynthesis 347
Ribozymes 367
Rickets 74
RNA and DNA, difference between 34

**S**

S-adenosyl methionine 233
SAM 255
Second messenger 365
Secondary active transport 290
Selenium 153
Semiconservative mechanism of replication 147
Serotonin 197
Serum
 alkaline phosphatase 83
 amylase 155
Sickle cell
 anemia 87
 hemoglobin 87
Silent mutation 17
Sodium 207
Sodium-potassium pump 360
Southern blot techniques 258

Specific dynamic action (SDA) 199
Sphingomyelin 136
Standard urea clearance test 194
Starch and glycogen, difference between 289
Starvation 253
Steatorrhea 196
Steroid hormones 95
Subcellular organelles 206
Substrate level phosphorylation 259
Surfactant 347
Symport 181
Synthesis of
  ammonia 140
  bile acids 273
  cholesterol 297
  creatine 23
  glycogen 58
  heme 109
  purine 214
  pyrimidine 203
  triacylglycerol 332
  urea 178
  uric acid 62

**T**

TCA cycle 90
Thalassemia 227
Thiamine 13
Thyroid
  function tests 186
  stimulating hormone (TSH) 143
Trace elements 316
Transamination reactions 41
Transcriptase, reverse 343
Transcription 53
Transmethylation reactions 150
Transport RNA (tRNA) 219
Transport, active 290
Tryptophan
  derivatives 197
  metabolism 300
Tumor markers 69
Tyrosine metabolism 158
Tyrosinemia 162

**U**

UDP-glucuronic acid 280
Uniport 181
Unsaturated fatty acid 308
Urea acycle 180
  disorders 180
Urea cycle 178
Uremia 180
Urine, abnormal components of 245
Urobilinogen, test for 349
Uronic acid pathway 127

**V**

Vander Bergh's reaction 111
Vitamin
  A 133
  $B_1$ 13
  $B_{12}$ 285
  $B_2$ 361
  $B_3$ 220
  $B_5$ 275
  $B_6$ 40
  $B_7$ 341
  C 25
  D 73
  E 46
  K 200
von Gierke's disease 51

**W**

Wald's visual cycle 134
Water balance, regulation of 338
Water by rennin-angiotensin system, regulation of 185
Wilson's disease 323
Wobble hypothesis 226

**X**

Xenobiotics 166
Xeroderma pigmentosa 211
  causes of 211

**Z**

Zinc 43
Zymogens 141